Step Up to Wellness

A STAGE-BASED APPROACH

Jan Galen Bishop

Steven G. Aldana
Brigham Young University

Allyn and Bacon
Boston   London   Toronto   Sydney   Tokyo   Singapore

Publisher: Joseph Burns
Vice President and Editor-in-Chief: Paul Smith
Sr. Developmental Editor: Mary Kriener
Editorial Assistant: Sara Sherlock
Marketing Manager: Richard Muhr
Composition and Prepress Buyer: Linda Cox
Manufacturing Buyer: Megan Cochran
Cover Administrator: Linda Knowles
Photo Director: Susan Duane
Principal Photographer: Anthony Neste
Production Service: Marret Kauffner
Electronic Composition: Omegatype Typography, Inc.

PHOTO CREDITS

All photos by Anthony Neste except the following:
Richard Hutchings/Photo Researchers: p. 12; Will Hart: pp. 31, 41, 201, 283, 285, 323; Anne Marie Weber/The Stock Market: p. 72; Aaron Haupt/Photo Researchers: p. 106; Anthony Blake/Tony Stone Images: p. 160; Robert Harbison: pp. 170, 237, 241, 280, 349; Mark Lewis/Tony Stone Images: p. 183; Educational Media Center Tufts University: pp. 221, 225; Will & Deni McIntyre/Photo Researchers: p. 238; A. Glauberman/Science Source/Photo Researchers: p. 321; Laurence Monnenet/Tony Stone Images: p. 333.

Copyright © 1999 by Allyn & Bacon
A Viacom Company
160 Gould Street
Needham Heights, MA 02494

Internet: www.abacon.com

Library of Congress Cataloging-in-Publication Data

Bishop, Jan Galen.
    Step up to wellness : a stage-based approach / Jan Galen Bishop, Steven G. Aldana.
      p.   cm.
    Includes bibliographical references and index.
    ISBN 0-205-27970-8 (pbk.)
    1. Health--Miscellanea.   2. Health promotion--Popular works.   3. Health behavior--Popular works.
    4. Conduct of life--Health aspects--Popular works.
    5. Self-care, Health--Popular works.   I. Aldana, Steven G., 1962- . II. Title.
RA776.5.B54   1998
613--dc21   98-33568
                                    CIP

Printed in the United States of America
10 9 8 7 6 5 4 3 2 1   VHP   03 02 01 00 99

*To wellness that is born
of good friends and family
and to my husband Rich
and son Noah.*
JGB

*To my wonderful wife, my children,
and a kind God in heaven,
to whom I owe everything.*
SGA

CONTENTS
in Brief

CONTENTS

vii

CHAPTER 3

Cardiorespiratory Endurance 46

CHAPTER 4

Flexibility 70

CHAPTER 5

Muscular Strength and Endurance   102

CHAPTER 6

Striving for Wellness with Proper Nutrition   149

CHAPTER 7

Understanding Body Composition   179

CHAPTER 13

Preventing Sexually Transmitted Diseases 292

CHAPTER 14

Understanding and Avoiding Substance Abuse 313

CHAPTER 15

Living Well in Today's World 347

APPENDICES

FEATURE BOXES

PREFACE

A pioneer in the personal wellness field, *Step Up to Wellness: A Stage-Based Approach* was written with the understanding that accurate wellness information is truly useful only when it is incorporated into an individual's lifestyle. As with most successful wellness texts, this one contains the most current health and fitness research, but it goes a giant step further by integrating wellness knowledge with the most effective behavior change strategies.

Although considerable wellness knowledge has been discovered by the scientific community, comparable amounts of scientific information on human behavior have also been recognized. Yet very little of the most up-to-date science of human behavior change has been made available. The synthesis of the best behavior change strategies and accurate wellness knowledge is what makes this textbook unique.

For many years, it has been generally believed that increasing a person's knowledge about a specific wellness topic will cause that individual to eventually change behaviors. This is true for a few people—those who know how to change their behaviors and are ready and willing to do so. But for everyone else this knowledge only provides the "what" and "why," not the "how" to change. Traditionally, wellness courses have been designed to communicate that "what" and "why" of wellness and have assumed that everyone is ready to make changes. Now we know that few individuals are currently ready to make changes. The failure of the "everyone is ready to make change" approach has been the catalyst that has caused many of the world's best behavioral psychologists to find more effective ways to help all individuals adopt good behaviors.

THE STAGES OF CHANGE MODEL

Over a decade ago, Drs. James Prochaska, Carlo DiClemente, and their colleagues began studying how people change. They learned that change is a multistep process in which success is best attained when intervention strategies match a person's stage of readiness to change. Their work has become what is now known as the Transtheoretical Model of Behavior Change, more commonly referred to as the Stages of Change Model.

The Transtheoretical Model is considered transtheoretical because it implements concepts and processes across a variety of behavior change models and combines them with the idea that behavior change occurs in stages. It suggests that individuals attempting to change a health behavior move through a series of five stages of change: precontemplation (not intending to make changes), contemplation (considering change), preparation (making small changes), action (actively engaging in behavior change), and maintenance (sustaining change over time). People progress through these stages at varying rates, often moving back and forth through the stages before ultimately obtaining the stage of maintenance. In the model, people use different cognitive and behavioral processes of change as they move from one stage to another. Successful change depends on doing the right thing (processes) at the right time (stages). According to this theory, tailoring interventions to match a person's readiness or stage of change is essential. For example, when dealing with people who are not yet contemplating becoming physically active, encouraging a discussion of the benefits of exercise may be more effective and realistic than encouraging them to move directly into an exercise program. The theory has been the subject of hundreds of scientific studies and now dominates the field of behavior change. It continues to expand its influence into all disciplines that include human behavior.

We believe that the key to achieving wellness lies in the individual's ability to make lifestyle change. We have integrated the Stages of Change Model into our text because it provides you with the best opportunity to make successful change. The "everyone is ready to make change" approach to behavior change is therefore replaced with stage-based programming that tailors behavior change to an individual's stage of readiness to change.

BEHAVIOR CHANGE FEATURES

In *Step Up to Wellness* we have integrated the Stages of Change Model into each chapter. You have the opportunity to assess your own stage of readiness on a number of wellness topics and then employ stage-based behavior change strategies. Instructors no longer have to treat all their students the same way. Five different sets of lab materials are provided in virtually every chapter so that you and the instructor can tailor the change process. With this approach, different strategies and activities can be used by different people.

You begin the change process by using the short staging questionnaire at the beginning of the chapter to determine your stage of readiness. After reading the chapter you are asked to complete the behavior change lab that corresponds to your stage of readiness. Embedded in the chapter is a feature called Barrier Busters. Barriers are the reasons people give for failing to start or failing to succeed in adopting a healthier lifestyle habit. For example, typical exercise barriers include not having enough time, not being good at sports, and being too tired. Fortunately there are many ways to overcome these barriers. The Barrier Busters section gives hints and suggestions for overcoming most of the barriers you will encounter.

CONTENT, ASSESSMENT LABS, AND ACTIVITIES

Step Up to Wellness brings together both fitness and health topics as they relate to personal wellness. Compelling arguments are provided for a number of important topics. The first chapter of the text is an introduction to the concept of wellness, followed by a detailed description of key components of the Stages of Change Model and other behavior change strategies and processes. Chapter 2 is an introduction and overview of physical fitness concepts and exercise principles. The new physical activity guidelines are described, compared, and contrasted with previously established guidelines for exercise. You will learn how physical activity and exercise are related to health promotion (disease risk reduction) and quality of life.

The next series of chapters elaborates on each of the health-related components of physical fitness introduced in Chapter 2: flexibilty, cardiorespiratory endurance, muscular strength and endurance, and body composition. Fitness chapters 3–5 include a definition of the particular fitness component ("what"), a detailed description of the physiological and psychological benefits of developing this component ("why"), assessments for identifying your present level of fitness and readiness to change ("Where Am I?"), guidelines for developing this component of fitness ("how"), and finally stage-based behavior change exercises aimed at helping you progress toward a lifestyle of regular physical activity (how to change).

Chapter 6 picks up the final health-related component of fitness—body composition. This chapter is devoted to the discussion of the risks associated with excessive body fat. Various body-fat assessments are available to self-assess your level of body fat. To help you achieve and maintain proper body weight, the weight control chapter (7) discusses the most current scientific information on weight control and guides you through the appropriate activities and labs according to your stage of readiness to change your body weight.

The second half of the book shifts from a fitness-wellness orientation to one of health-wellness. The nutrition chapter (8) appropriately bridges these segments as it plays an integral role in both physical fitness development and the prevention of diseases such as atherosclerosis and cancer. The essential nutrients, their roles, and recommended consumption are described, along with awareness and behavior change activities. In addition, information on how to read a food label is included so that you can become a more savvy consumer. Chapters 9 and 10 shift toward health promotion through disease risk reduction, as they discuss cardiovascular disease and cancer prevention. You are encouraged to understand how these diseases manifest themselves and how to actively prevent their occurrence. Assessments and behavior change activities are provided.

Chapter 11 focuses on stress management, a growing area of concern. Stress is presented as a multifaceted subject and one for which there are both cognitive and physical stress-reduction strategies. Activities provoke student thought concerning good and bad stress and encourage you to experiment with different stress-management techniques.

Healthy relationships (Chapter 12) are a key part of a wellness approach. A topic often overlooked, this chapter focuses on stage-based strategies for building good relationships. These relationships often serve as the foundation for future behavior change, as changes are more easily made when you have the support of friends, family members, and coworkers. Relationships certainly play a role in the next two topics—sexually transmitted diseases (Chapter 13) and substance abuse (Chapter 14). These chapters illustrate the hazards of poor health habits and the benefits of staying disease and substance free. The focus in both cases is on prevention behaviors. The substance abuse chapter is unique in that it not only provides labs for changing abusive habits, it also provides labs for getting involved in helping others stop or never start the abuse of a substance. Each chapter uses the most up-to-date literature to support recommendations for change and each provides clearly written stage-based exercises designed to help you adopt healthy lifestyles. The final chapter of the text (15) presents the concept of personal wellness as it relates to world wellness. This summary chapter helps you view your thinking and actions from a global perspective and demonstrates that real happiness is largely determined by how we relate to the world around us.

Throughout, you are encouraged not only to learn about topics like heart disease and exercise but also to internalize and personalize the information. Student activities are provided for just this purpose. Many of the chapters contain assessments that you can use to evaluate your current levels of health risk. Some of these assessments include nutrition analyses, body fat calculations, and fitness measures. Each of the assessments in the text has been found to be both a reliable and a valid measure of health risk. Once you have completed these, you can determine how you compare to other college age students by using the normative data found in tables throughout the book.

PEDAGOGICAL FEATURES

In addition to the behavior change exercises, this textbook has a number of features to assist both instructor and student.

- Chapters start with clearly stated behavioral objectives. The objectives have two purposes. First they serve to familiarize you with the intent and content of the chapter. Second, after reading the chapter, you can return to these objectives and use them to self-test your understanding and retention of the material.

- Key terms are listed at the start of each chapter and defined in the Glossary at the back of the book. The key term list may be used as a guideline for study along with the Objectives. These same words appear in bold type within the chapter so that their in-text definitions may be located quickly.

- A series of four boxes found at various points within the chapters is used to reinforce concepts, expand upon topic discussion, and assist with the behavior-change process:

  1. General wellness boxes highlight topics of special interest.

  2. Cognitive Corners provide a more critical examination of some topics.

  3. Activity boxes provide you with an opportunity to apply some of the concepts introduced within the text.

  4. Barrier Busters serve as a potential intervention to negative thoughts that can interfere with positive behavior change.

- Chapter summaries revisit the most important concepts presented within each chapter.

INSTRUCTOR SUPPLEMENTS

We offer the following comprehensive set of ancillary material for the instructor to assist with classroom preparation:

Instructor's Manual: The Instructor's Manual contains lecture outlines for each of the chapters, additional student activities and assessment tools, and a printed copy of the examination questions that comprise the computerized test bank. In addition, the Instructor's Manual also contains a special feature called Behavior Boosts, which consist of stage-based intervention activities for each of the wellness topics. Instructors can use these to supplement the book's already strong behavior change theme.

Computerized Test Bank: A computerized version of the test questions that appear in print in the Instructor's Manual. Using this software, instructors can quickly select and organize questions to create tests, study questions, or homework assignments. A combination of multiple choice, short answer, and essay questions is provided.

Nutrition Software: A computer-based nutrition assessment and analysis program is available. Students can work with this software to identify the strengths and weaknesses of their diets.

Overhead Transparencies: A set of color overhead transparencies depicting key wellness concepts is furnished to assist instructors in their dynamic presentation of the material.

Web Site: A number of additional photographs and explanations of flexibility and muscular strength and endurance are available on the Web. Students can visit the site at www.abacon.com to further individualize their exercise routines.

ACKNOWLEDGMENTS

We would like to thank the following reviewers for their valuable suggestions: Cathy Kennedy, Colorado State

University; Ray Reinertsen, University of Wisconsin—Superior; Frank Powell, Furman University; Susan Rossi, University of Rhode Island/Cancer Prevention Research Center; and Kathy Koser, California State University—Fullerton.

This project has benefited from the expertise of two publishing companies, Gorsuch Scarisbrick Publishers (GSP) and Allyn & Bacon. We would like to thank our GSP publisher Gay Pauley and acquisitions editor Colette Kelly for seeing potential in us as writers and starting us on the vision of a unique wellness text. Thanks also to our GSP developmental editor Katie Bradford for putting in countless hours of foundational work on the text. Thanks also to Dr. Susan Rossi, who did an in-depth review of our stages of change material, making sure that our application was a proper extension of the research. At Allyn & Bacon we are indebted to Mary Kriener for picking up our project midstream and helping us turn a manuscript in six colors of ink into a high-quality text. We would like to acknowledge the expertise of Susan Duane, who coordinated the photographs; Jim Walczyk, who made it happen on site; and photographer Anthony Neste (and assistant Chris Edwards), who expertly captured the exercises on film. We would also like to thank our models, whose pictures so wonderfully bring the information alive: Joanna Hollenback, Becky Rhodes, Charles Burchett, Jennifer Fair, Tee Ezell, Clint Hill, Pearl Ocampo, Darin Dixon, James Braswell, and Jim Walczyk. We'd like to extend our gratitude to Marret Kauffner, whose job was to shepherd our manuscript through production but who did far more than that as she coordinated two long-distance authors and kept track of a dizzying number of details. Finally, our very special thank-you belongs to our friends and family, and most especially our spouses Richard Bishop and Diana Aldana for their five years of armchair editing, patience, and loving support.

JGB
SGA

CHAPTER 1

Discovering the Wellness Lifestyle

Terms

- Quality of life
- Dysfunctional living
- Health
- Self-responsibility
- Wellness
- Precontemplators
- Contemplators
- Preparers
- Action takers
- Maintainers
- Supports
- Barriers

Objectives

1. Define and contrast *health* and *wellness*.

2. Define quality of life as it affects your future and how it can be affected by a wellness lifestyle.

3. Describe the illness-to-wellness continuum.

4. Explain why each of the five dimensions of wellness is important for you.

5. Identify ways in which lifestyle is related to each dimension of wellness and give examples from your personal life.

6. List and explain the four factors responsible for all causes of death.

7. Identify the different aspects of the physical dimension of wellness.

8. Describe the five stages of the behavior change model.

9. Explain how you can increase the quality of your life by changing some of your unhealthy behaviors.

Eat Healthy Foods

Exercise Often

Die Anyway

These greeting card–style words poke fun at all of us who struggle to "do the right thing" and remind us of our certain mortality. What *difference* does it make if we do things such as eat right, exercise, manage our stress, protect our skin from the sun, and work to achieve relationships with others? The answer is in *how* we want to live our lives—in the quality of life, and perhaps the length of life we want to have. There is now evidence that people who practice certain healthy behaviors increase their likelihood of living longer and with less disease. People who exercise regularly, for example, will on the average live longer than those who don't. There are no guarantees—you can be jogging and be hit by a car—but why not take control of the things you can, practice prevention, limit your risk of premature death, and live the best quality of life possible?

A healthy lifestyle encompasses many different areas, much like a college program that includes courses from a variety of disciplines. Your academic goal is not only to pass all your courses with good grades, but also to acquire the work and study habits that will enable you to do well in a career. Similarly, the overall goal of a wellness program is to adopt an array of habits that will enable you to optimize your health throughout your life.

If you decide to strive for a wellness lifestyle, you will probably have to make changes. Change can be difficult, and it requires commitment and resources. Readiness to change is influenced by many factors including personality, living and work environments, and family support. Thus, not everyone is ready to make the same change at the same time and in the same way. In the past, programs such as smoking cessation courses assumed that everyone enrolled was equally ready for change, and this assumption helped contribute to a low rate of success. New materials and programs, including this text, try to match change strategies with an individual's needs. It is important to recognize that you can be in a different stage of readiness than someone else, *and* that you can be more ready to make one lifestyle change than another. Becoming aware of this can help you choose the best change strategies.

As we will discuss later, there are five stages of readiness for making a lifestyle change (see pages 12–17). They range from not wanting to change at all to wanting to maintain a good habit. It is common to be in different stages with different wellness behaviors. For example, a person can be thinking about eating a better diet, not interested at all in modifying drinking habits, and already exercising regularly.

Here are four examples of people who could be starting this course. Notice the differences in readiness to change within each person—everything from no interest in change, to thinking of change, to maintaining some good wellness habits.

A. I've been thinking maybe I should change some of the things I do. I've heard that exercise will give me more energy and I could certainly use some energy with this course load. And I have put on that "freshman 15" everyone talks about. . . . But while other freshmen are stressing out, I feel okay. I am good about saying "no" to things that will over-commit me, and my roommate and I are getting along well. I've heard that I shouldn't suntan so much, but I look so much more attractive with a tan that I'm not going to worry about that until I'm out of college.

B. It took me a while to adjust to college and get organized, but for the past eight months I've been eating right, getting regular exercise, and managing my stress. I had to make changes like getting a new roommate and joining a health club, but it is paying off in how I feel now. Yeah, sure, I smoke cigarettes and a little marijuana, but so do a lot of other people and I'm not concerned about the consequences right now.

C. I really enjoy partying and for once I don't have to worry about what my parents would say—besides I'm not an alcoholic or anything. Plus if I'm going to have sex, I always use a condom—at least I think I do. I don't always remember the sex when I've been drinking. I quit using drugs though, I was afraid of where that was leading me. I've been drug free for six months. My best friend really stuck by me while I was quitting, and I've started doing a lot better in my classes.

D. I'm watching what I eat but find it hard not to eat a bunch of junk food at the parties or grab a fast-food meal before rushing off to class. I also stopped drinking, but I'm getting teased a lot by friends about being a "goody two shoes." The same is true about my decision to abstain from sexual activity. I'm trying to keep up my new habits, but I'm afraid temptation and peer pressure will get to me. My friends say I should get more exercise, but I don't have time and I get embarrassed because I have two left feet and am still overweight.

This text gives you an opportunity to determine where *you* are with regard to your readiness to change your behaviors. Before we discuss the five stages of behavior change, let's take a look at what it means to be "well."

WHAT IS WELLNESS?

The concept of wellness has evolved from a holistic point of view that sees the human body as a complex mixture of physical, emotional, social, mental, and spiritual factors, all of which are dependent on each other

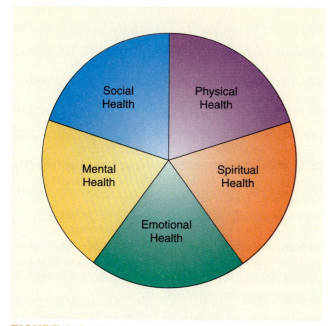

FIGURE 1.1   The dimensions of wellness.

and interact to create a sense of who we are and what we can become (see Figure 1.1). When one of the factors is neglected or overemphasized, the other aspects of a person's life may suffer. For example, individuals with great social lives may not be taking the time to exercise, study, or eat right. The concept of wellness places an equal amount of importance on each of these different factors and encourages the continuous balancing of them.

To get an accurate understanding of what wellness is, we need to view life from behind a wide-angle lens. Such a view shows that life is a web of interdependent influences and associations shared with other family members, friends, neighbors, and total strangers. If we widen our perspective even further, we see that the earth contains a finite amount of resources to be used and enjoyed by all, and that our personal choices influence and affect our families, our community, society, the world, and perhaps the universe. Wellness can be described with a few simple words: fulfillment, contentment, happiness, and self-esteem. One of the best descriptors of wellness is **quality of life.**

Wellness Means Striving for Quality Living

The wellness way of life focuses on expanding not only the length of your life, but even more important, the quality of your life. A high quality of life means feeling good about yourself and being able to do most of the things you want to do despite any limitations you may have. In contrast, a low quality of life might involve being dependent on others for basic needs, having a poor self-concept, being too ill to effectively communicate or take part in a relationship, or being unable to do the things you want to do.

A poor quality of life is also known as **dysfunctional living,** or the inability to perform activities required for daily living, such as bathing, dressing, and eating. Difficulty in performing these tasks ultimately leads to dependence upon medical, family, and community services. In 1995 the average life span was 75.8 years, including 63.7 years of healthy (quality) living and 12.1 years of dysfunctional living.[1] Today, the average life span is slightly higher, but the ratio of healthy to dysfunctional years hasn't changed much since 1995.

We all have limitations with which we may have to live, but by which we do not have to be controlled. Our limitations may be physical, emotional, spiritual, mental, or social in nature. Positive lifestyle choices help us overcome our limitations. For example, Veronica is a quadraplegic who draws pictures with a pencil in her mouth. She could have chosen to be totally dependent on others, but instead she is an artist, earning money and communicating with those around her, thus improving her quality of life. Computer technology has offered many other people with physical limitations a way to communicate and be connected to others, as well as to earn a living. Even though she is somewhat dependent on others, Veronica has taken control of her life and finds happiness through her accomplishments.

Much evidence suggests that adoption of wellness lifestyles not only can reduce the number of dysfunctional years but also can increase one's life span.[2] For example, the average person who quits smoking lives longer and enjoys better health than someone who doesn't. The same holds true for persons who become physically active. Although we do not have total control over our health or length of life, we can take action to limit our risk of premature death or unnecessary injury.

The aim of a wellness program is to help you find ways to increase the quality of your life—to live your life to its fullest. As the next section discusses, the way to reach a high quality of life and improved health is to proactively adopt wellness behaviors.

Wellness Means Being Proactive

Most of us are content with the way we are living as long as we feel good. This is usually true even when we engage in poor health behaviors. For example, people who are unfit, eat a diet high in fat and cholesterol, and smoke may be very content with their level of health if they feel free of symptoms and disease, or if they ignore the symptoms that are creeping up on them slowly. Fortunately for us, medical services provided in the United States are among the best in the world, but medicine can't always cure. We're finding out that prevention and early intervention are more successful strategies than leaning on medicine as a cure-all. Good lifestyle habits and regular checkups put prevention on the front line and allow medicine to play an effective second line of defense.

The evolution of the term **health** into a *wellness* concept reflects this new thinking. At one time health was

Now Is the Time for Wellness

In the course of this century, average life span in the United States has increased from 47 years in 1900 to 75.5 in 1993. However, over the past 10 years there have been relatively small increases in the average life span.

It is possible to break the past century into historical periods that represent the major causes for the increases in life span.

Age of Environment (1900–1936).   This period was characterized by a continual improvement in life expectancy. City health departments, federal health campaigns, insulin, other medical discoveries, and public health measures such as the pasteurization of milk all helped extend life by reducing illness and disease.

Age of Medicine (1937–1949).   The discovery of bacteria-killing drugs radically changed the way medicine was practiced. Antibiotics like penicillin did much to cure some diseases. The average life span increased to 65 years, and lifestyle and heredity became the leading factors in premature death.

Age of Lifestyle (1950–1989).   Approximately 75 percent of all premature deaths were preventable by 1989. It was clear that by changing the way they live their lives, people could live longer. For example, controlling blood pressure and cholesterol levels, wearing seatbelts, stopping tobacco use, and awareness of safety all characterized this period. Sophisticated medical procedures such as transplants and open heart surgery also emerged during this period, but they have had little effect on the extension of life.

Age of Wellness (1990–   ).   Though we currently enjoy all of the medical breakthroughs developed in the past, the average life span has increased little in the past decade. Any additional increase in life span will likely result from continued lifestyle changes and new discoveries about the human body. The Age of Wellness combines lifestyle change with an emphasis on improving quality of life. When the physical, mental, social, emotional, and spiritual dimensions of life are balanced, quality of life increases. High quality of life is the goal of wellness.

Adapted from Vickery, D.M. *Life plan for your health.* Reading, MA: Addison-Wesley, 1978; and *Health United States 1994,* U.S. Department of Health and Human Services, DHHS Publication No. (PHS) 95-1232, Hyattsville, MD, May 1995.

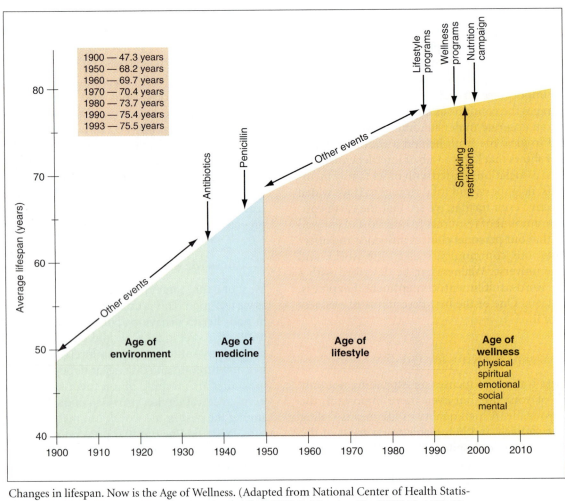

Changes in lifespan. Now is the Age of Wellness. (Adapted from National Center of Health Statistics. *Health United States, 1994 and prevention profile.* DHHS Publication No. (PHS)90–1232. Hyattsville, MD: U.S. Department of Health and Human Services, 1995.)

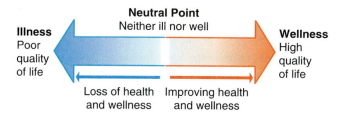

FIGURE 1.2 The illness-to-wellness continuum.

defined as "the absence of disease." But one can be free of disease and still not enjoy a full, wholesome, satisfying life. Recognizing this, the World Health Organization broadened its definition of health to be "a state of complete physical, mental, and social well-being and not merely the absence of disease or infirmity."

Wellness begins with this broader definition of health but carries it a step further, placing the responsibility of our health back into our own hands. Thus, **wellness** is being engaged in attitudes and behaviors that enhance quality of life and maximize personal potential. Wellness does not assume that you live free of disease or disability or some other limitation. It does assume a proactive stance.

The illness-to-wellness continuum in Figure 1.2 shows death and debilitating illness on one end and complete wellness on the other. Everyone falls on the continuum somewhere, and most people are likely to be found in the middle, which is characterized by the absence of any major symptoms or illness. Quality of life is not as high as it could be, but generally, little pain or physical suffering is being experienced. Individuals in this middle section sometimes ask, "I feel fine, so why should I change my life?" Others might ask, "I've lived like this for years. Why should I do anything differently?"

The role of most conventional medicine is to move the sick and dying back toward the center of the illness-to-wellness continuum, where symptoms and pain are gone. The wellness way of life, on the other hand, encourages individuals not only to be free from as much illness and pain as possible but also to move away from the center to the wellness, or far right, end of the continuum. In order to move to the right, you must be able to take conscious control of the way you live. A proactive stance for achieving wellness means participating in regular physical activity, controlling stress, developing proper nutrition habits, practicing cancer and cardiovascular disease prevention, managing body weight, avoiding harmful substances and infectious diseases, enjoying healthy relationships, encouraging spiritual development, and caring for the environment. These aspects of a well life are discussed in more detail in the chapters that follow.

UNDERSTANDING THE COMPONENTS OF WELLNESS

A person concerned with wellness tries to balance the spiritual, physical, emotional, social, and mental dimen-

sions of his or her life. Each dimension is connected to every other dimension in many ways.

Learning to manage the dimensions of life, and taking responsibility for decisions that affect you, describe a wellness lifestyle. Consistent wellness lifestyle habits are what maintain your quality of life when sudden trials or problems come upon you. A wellness life is not about being perfect in every dimension, but rather juggling the several dimensions in such a way as to maximize quality of life and happiness.

The Balloon Theory

Many people picture their lives as a juggling act—a college student today may have to juggle academic pressures, club or athletic commitments, job demands, family responsibilities, and social obligations. Jugglers, however, have only two choices: catch the ball or drop it. Life is not so definitive: it is more fluid, contains many gray areas, and is very interconnected. Failing one test, for example, does not mean you have dropped the academic ball altogether.

The Balloon Theory is a metaphor in which each balloon is a summation of the factors that influence one aspect of wellness. The balloons float up or drop down according to the conditions of your life. The Balloon Theory as developed below is a perspective-keeper (see Figure 1.3), one that is useful when you feel divided and

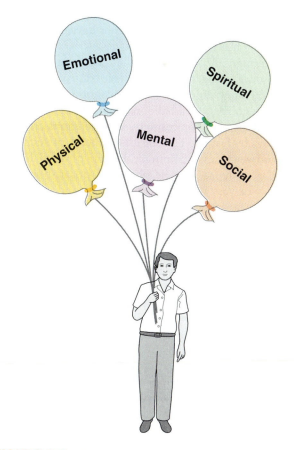

FIGURE 1.3 The Balloon Theory.

need to take a good look at your overall status, get your bearings, and go on. It is also a way to help you visualize the wellness concept central to the theme of this book.

Imagine that you are standing on the ground holding on to five balloons. Each balloon represents a part of you—the emotional, mental, social, spiritual, and physical parts of you. Your five balloons can inflate or deflate with helium, depending on what is happening in your life. Most of the time, the balloons have some helium in them and you are pulled upward. Your social life balloon may pull hard when you have a good on-going relationship with someone, a supportive family, or a good network of friends. A big date may have your social balloon tugging you to the stratosphere, while breaking up with someone could temporarily pop it, sending you back to earth. Your mental health balloon may be inflated by a compliment from a professor, while a problem with financial aid could weaken your emotional balloon. A good night's sleep and some well-rounded meals can fill the physical balloon, while all-nighters, too many drinks, or a night with a crying baby can definitely send you lower.

Because all of the balloons are connected, any upward or downward motion of one balloon will create a pulling effect on the others. If, for example, you abuse the physical health balloon (through sleep deprivation, poor diet, chronic injury, or drugs, for example) you will also be affected mentally, emotionally, socially, and spiritually. Similarly, prolonged or intense mental and emotional stress can result in physical ailments such as headaches or stomach upset. The reverse is also true. People with good social relationships have, on the average, longer, healthier lives.

Although all the balloons that encompass your life are loosely tied together, you do have control in that you can deliberately choose to deflate a balloon. Occasionally it may be good to let a balloon deflate while you attend to something else. For example, some religions celebrate holy days by fasting. The spiritual benefits of such rites may outweigh any temporary loss in physical health. Sexual abstinence may be physically unsatisfying, but also may be very rewarding emotionally and spiritually. Caring for a sick child, parent, or sibling, or helping a friend in crisis may detract from your ability to progress academically, but fulfilling this social role as a good friend or family member may be more important during critical times. If you are inspired on a project and you work intensely at it, your diet, sleep, and social life will no doubt suffer, but the accomplishment may have powerful mental and emotional rewards. These swings are okay as long as they do not come one right after another and no one balloon is neglected for a prolonged period. If you lead a fairly balanced life and consciously decide when to alter the balance, you will have the reserve needed to handle surprises and emergencies, and the energy to take advantage of opportunities. In new situations such as entering college or starting a new job, everything can look important and it takes a little time to

sort out priorities and find a balance. Problems occur most often when an imbalance lasts too long or the sacrifice is too large.

Learning to manage your balloons (your life) and taking responsibility for decisions that affect you describes a "wellness lifestyle." Consistent wellness lifestyle habits fill the balloons even when a sudden disturbance occurs. For example, spiritually sound individuals can pull on their faith when faced with a traumatic experience. This helps them stay emotionally and mentally stable—the spiritual balloon lifts the other two, preventing a total loss of self. There may be times when all of your balloons are deflating. Sometimes this is the result of poor personal choices. Substance abuse, for example, can plummet you into disaster. In these cases, seeking help from friends, clergy, or physicians or other health care professionals may be necessary to get your balloons back in the air. You will weather lows better if you have built a good wellness network around you.

Every rare now and then, you will find that everything in your life is going "just right." All the balloons are filled to their maximum, and it feels good. Take a deep, satisfying, relaxing breath and admire the world around you. You are feeling very "well" indeed! These moments are to be savored. However, if you consider anything short of this a failure, then most of your life will be judged as such. Life is full of change and living a well life is not about having all the balloons filled all the time. Living a well life means keeping a positive attitude as you manage your balloons and successfully handle the changes that come your way.

Physical Dimension

In recent years, participation in regular physical activity has become a notable part of our society. Ordinary people from all walks of life walk, jog, bicycle, and play organized sports. Although it seems that more people are exercising today than ever before, over 60 percent of adults fail to exercise regularly.[3] The number of people who do not exercise is more than twice as high as the number of individuals who smoke, have high blood cholesterol, or have high blood pressure. Because so many people are not exercising, health experts believe that large improvements in national health could be realized if the sedentary portion of the population were to adopt physically active lifestyles.[4]

The physical fitness component of wellness includes several different areas:

- Cardiorespiratory endurance
- Joint flexibility
- Muscular strength and endurance
- Body composition

Each of these fitness components has a distinct effect on physical health and well-being. Some of these effects include increased endurance, less fatigue, decreased risk of certain cancers and cardiovascular diseases, decreased risk of obesity and subsequent diabetes, decreased chance of osteoporosis, increased immune response, improved sleep, and a host of other physical and emotional benefits.

How much activity is required to reap the health benefits of physical activity? Some people believe a person has to participate in an extensive exercise program to ensure good health. There is still some debate as to exactly how much exercise is required, but most experts believe that moderate intensity activity is sufficient to produce health benefits.[5] The health-related benefits that come from exercise do not depend on speed, agility, balance, coordination, or reaction time, important factors in sports and athletics. Increases in health are seen when the cardiovascular system becomes more efficient, when muscles are able to cope with the demands of everyday living, when blood pressure and cholesterol levels are improved, when stress is relieved, and when other threats to health are eliminated through regular participation in physical activity. Extremely high levels of fitness, like those seen in marathon runners or high-performance athletes, are difficult to achieve and maintain. This level of physical fitness is required for peak performance, but is not a requirement for good health or wellness. In fact, some research indicates that for those persons who are expending extreme amounts of energy in physical activity, health benefits may actually decrease.[6]

A previously sedentary individual may experience substantial health benefits by becoming moderately active, such as walking 1 to 2 miles a day for a total of 7 to 14 miles a week. This same amount of activity could be achieved by walking for approximately 30 minutes, three times a week. Long-term studies of various levels of fitness and causes of death have demonstrated that improved levels of fitness are associated with decreased risk of death due to cardiovascular diseases and cancer.[7] (See Figure 1.4.)

People with poor fitness levels have eight times higher risk of death due to cardiovascular disease and five times higher probability of dying from cancer than do persons who have good or excellent levels of fitness. This is true for both men and women. Overall, persons with low levels of fitness are three times as likely to die of cancer or cardiovascular diseases as are individuals with elevated fitness levels. The health-promoting effects of physical fitness are not confined only to those individuals who have moderate to high levels of fitness. In fact, the greatest benefit is attained when a previously sedentary individual becomes moderately physically active.[8]

When high levels of fitness are accompanied by reductions in cholesterol, blood pressure, smoking, and body fat, even greater decreases in death rates occur. Other aspects of the physical dimension that are covered in this text are managing stress, preventing alcohol and drug abuse, and avoiding sexually transmitted diseases.

Although the use of cigarettes is actually on the decline, the tobacco industry is responsible for 2.5 percent

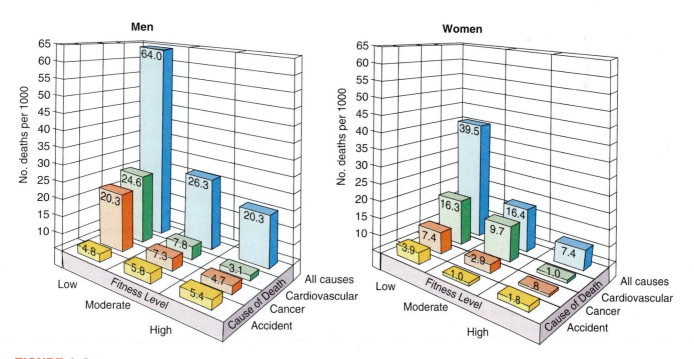

FIGURE 1.4   The relationship between fitness and all-cause mortality. The risk of death increases as fitness levels decrease. (Adapted by permission from S. N. Blair, H. W. Kohl III, R. S. Paffenbarger, Jr., D. G. Clark, K. H. Cooper, and L. W. Gibbons. Physical fitness and all-cause mortality: A prospective study of healthy men and women. *Journal of the American Medical Association* 262(17):2398 (Figure 2), 2399 (Figure 3), 1989. Copyright 1989 by the American Medical Association.)

of the gross national product of the United States.[9] Only recently have political powers been convinced of the detrimental effects of tobacco smoke. An estimated 400,000 people die each year from tobacco smoke. Even people who do not smoke but live or work in smoke-filled environments are at risk of death. The American Cancer Society calculates that environmental tobacco smoke is responsible for 50,000 deaths a year.[10] A wellness lifestyle involves not only abstinence from tobacco products, but also avoidance of environmental tobacco smoke.

Perhaps one of the most socially accepted of the harmful substances, alcohol is clearly the silent factor in the death and misery of many individuals. Over half of all fatal traffic accidents, suicides, murders, cases of child abuse, rapes, drownings, and on-the-job accidents are alcohol related. We often get so concerned about toxic wastes or body fat that we forget about this number one abused drug in America. A wellness lifestyle includes avoidance or moderation in the amount of alcohol one consumes.

Spiritual Dimension

When the spiritual dimension of wellness is discussed, the terminology can be confusing. For example, what does it mean when people say they have developed an inner self? What is happiness? Why are we here? What happens when we die? Spiritual wellness is not as obscure as these questions might suggest. It involves taking a proactive stance in acquiring a higher quality of life. For many, spiritual wellness consists of coming to peace with one's self and discovering a sense of purpose. Sometimes spiritual wellness is accompanied by the realization that all humanity is somehow interrelated and that true happiness involves more than the acquisition of material goods. For each person spiritual wellness is unique, and we do others a disservice when we assume that we all define spiritual well-being the same way. This dimension of wellness might include

- The ability to identify and change personal weakness
- Decreased emphasis on financial security
- Recognition of some unifying force; for some, this force is a divine power
- Humility
- A desire to comfort and help others
- Demonstration of hope and faith
- The desire to show gratitude and generosity
- The ability to admit you are wrong
- The desire to contribute to society
- Willingness to listen to other points of view

For many, religion is a central component of spiritual wellness. The various religions of the world teach many of the same ideals: love others as yourself, be kind

Wellness Lifestyle—Adopted!

Cognitive Corner

In an effort to evaluate the long-term effects of adoption of healthy lifestyles from the physical dimension, an eight-year study of 12,000 members of the Church of Jesus Christ of Latter-Day Saints (Mormons) was conducted.[a] The study participants had followed a healthy lifestyle characterized by abstention from alcohol, tobacco, coffee, and tea. They also consumed diets high in grains, cereals, fruits, and vegetables, with meat being consumed sparingly. Proper amounts of sleep and regular physical activity were an integral part of their daily lives. Amazingly, the men demonstrated an 11-year increase in the average male life span, with women adding an extra six years to the typical U.S. life span. Rates of death due to cancer, cardiovascular diseases, and all causes of death combined were half the U.S. average (see Figure 1.4). These large increases in longevity are some of the lowest death rates ever reported and demonstrate that adoption of wellness lifestyles can have a tremendous impact on both longevity and quality of life.

[a]Enstrom, J. E. Health practices and cancer mortality among active California Mormons. *Journal of the National Cancer Institute* 81: 1807–1814, 1989.

and caring, give of yourself and you will be happy. These ideals all contribute to an individual's overall wellness.

Spiritually healthy people believe in and adhere to an assortment of personal morals and values. This set of personal guidelines acts as a secure anchor when difficult times arise. A sense of spiritual well-being can help us view present events and misfortunes from a long-range perspective and is a necessary component of a high quality of life.

Emotional Dimension

Various medical and other health professionals are researching the relationship between mind and body. Many of their findings are leading to the same conclusion: the human mind may have more ability to exercise control over how our bodies recover from disease and injury than was previously realized. Your emotional state is the sum of the emotions or feelings you are experiencing at any given time. Emotional wellness refers to your ability to handle emotions in a constructive way resulting in a positive emotional state. Happiness is an important aspect of emotional wellness. Happiness that is based on short-term events or dependent on other individuals typically does not last and thus does not contribute to emotional wellness. The old saying that money cannot buy true happiness characterizes the reality that material goods are incapable of providing true enduring happiness and that there is more to happiness than being surrounded by inanimate objects.

Our ability to gain self-confidence, to avoid selfishness, and to like ourselves despite our flaws will ultimately affect whether or not we are truly happy. A positive self-concept or self-image can build confidence and lead us to successful experiences, which in turn further increase our self-esteem. Truly happy people have the ability to love themselves and other people and feel loved in return. Those who are unable to love often live lives of loneliness or despair, and may develop both physical and mental illnesses.

Having a sense of value or feeling loved by others can add to our personal happiness; the ability to make friends or to become a valued family member depends on how we treat others. Anger and hostility not only destroy relationships but decrease the personal value others place in us. Someone who "flies off the handle" or demonstrates unremitting anger is not only demonstrating emotional difficulties but also is destroying personal relationships.

The personality trait of hostility is one of the most powerful predictors of heart attacks.[11] Several detrimental biochemical and physical changes that occur in our bodies when we are angry can ultimately lead to heart disease and even premature death. Anger, hostility, selfishness, hate, fear, and depression can all affect the quality of our relationships with others. People with emotional wellness are able to control their anger and emotions and find other ways to vent their frustrations safely, thereby leaving relationships intact. Learning to express personal feelings outwardly is a sure sign that emotional wellness is being practiced.

One inevitable aspect of life is the occurrence of trials and adversity. No one is immune to "bad days" and hardship, but each of us has the ability to react to these difficulties in an optimistic manner. A cheerful attitude can be a tremendous tool in the reduction of stress and anxiety. Learning to handle stress in a safe and therapeutic manner is essential to attaining emotional wellness and requires an optimistic outlook on life and the hope that tomorrow will bring a better day.

Studies on the mind/body relationship are beginning to demonstrate that the power of positive suggestion and attitude can have a significant effect upon health and well-being. This optimistic attitude, sometimes referred to as "hardiness," is an important part of a wellness lifestyle.

Emotional wellness also includes the ability to laugh and to stimulate laughter in others. Laughter is a healthy, outward expression of emotional balance and happiness, and those who possess the uncanny ability to laugh at themselves have mastered an even more important aspect of emotional well-being. To be able to admit that you messed up or did something that was silly demonstrates to yourself and to others that you acknowledge your imperfect nature and are willing to make improvements. Accepting your limitations and making the best out of a bad situation indicates a balanced emotional state.

Social Dimension

All interactions between ourselves and others are part of the social dimension of wellness. Hugging, holding hands, smiling, singing, owning a pet, writing and receiving letters, and visiting with relatives and friends are all parts of the social dimension of wellness. Throughout the centuries, most of the world's moral and spiritual leaders promoted one surprisingly similar teaching: treat other people the same way you would like to be treated. This belief is not only a religious doctrine, it is a biologically and physically sound health principle.[12] Outside of any spiritual or emotional benefits that might result from such living, there are documented medical and psychological benefits to this type of lifestyle. In short, nice people tend to have a higher quality of life. Niceness has to do with being sensitive to and loving others, treating people with respect, being honest, fair, and trustworthy, and being kind to others.

In his own words, Dr. Bernie Siegel, a clinical professor of surgery at Yale Medical School, describes how the social dimension of wellness can affect quality of life. "If I told my patients to raise their blood levels of immune cells, no one would know how. But if I can teach them to love themselves and others fully, the same thing happens automatically. The truth is: Love heals."[13]

Researchers do not understand how love can improve immune function, but the evidence strongly suggests that it does. Loving others has been shown not only to increase a person's antibodies and white blood cells, but also to decrease susceptibility to colds, increase tolerance to pain, and even extend life.[14]

Much of the social interaction that occurs on a daily basis takes place in a family setting. Although the public's concept of family has evolved over the years, several characteristics of healthy families remain unchanged. A clear sense of value and trust resides in healthy homes, where a spirit of teamwork abides and individual family members are thought of as important, distinctly different persons. Interpersonal relationships are strong, especially between parent and child. In a healthy social environment, these same characteristics carry over into occupational and school settings. Churches and community organizations also provide a vital role in supplying social networks and services that are important in maintaining social wellness.

Mental Dimension

A retired grandmother was asked by her doctor to describe the symptoms and pain she was feeling from an injury she sustained during a recent sports-related accident. Thoroughly impressed at her knowledge of injuries and injury management, the doctor asked her how she knew so much about the human body and the nature of her injury. She replied, "I read about it in a book." The doctor soon discovered that his patient was also fluent in several languages and was currently taking a watercolor painting class at the local community center. This patient demonstrated how mental wellness can positively affect quality of life and the adoption of wellness lifestyles. Knowledge is a powerful tool in preventing disease and avoiding problems. By knowing how to take care of your body you will avoid unnecessary illness and be able to take care of yourself when you do become ill or injured.

The mental dimension of wellness is comprised of the intellectual and creative aspects of our minds. The mind is constantly able to learn, adapt, and change as it processes new experiences and information. This dimension of wellness includes the continued enjoyment of gaining new knowledge and participating in new experiences. We should eagerly approach new challenges and activities with the hope of becoming a better person. Mental wellness also includes viewing difficult situations as challenges and opportunities for growth.

Mental wellness involves an element of curiosity. How does something work? Is there another way to solve a certain problem? The only way to satisfy curiosity is to obtain new knowledge. The ability to think clearly and to assimilate new information is vital to making good decisions and to enjoying all that a high quality of living has to offer. New problems and choices confront us every day and require us to make decisions. Continued learning is the only way to acquire the necessary information needed to make wise choices.

The mental aspect of wellness is also characterized by the desire or ability to be creative. New ideas, thoughts, and creations are the result of imaginative thinking. This stretching of the mind with new information is a healthy way to keep ourselves mentally alert and young in spirit. Continuing education, night school, conferences, and professional seminars provide opportunities to revive forgotten information and to learn and express new ideas.

FACTORS INFLUENCING WELLNESS

According to Murphy,[15] all deaths can be attributed to four major factors: heredity, environment, inadequate health care, and lifestyle. Heredity refers to the genetic endowment that each of us receives from our natural parents. For example, it is possible to inherit a certain combination of muscle fibers that allows you to run exceptionally fast or jump very high. In the same way, a person who inherits the gene mutation for a certain disease has an increased likelihood of getting the disease.

The second factor, environment, refers to everything around us, including weather, pollution, soil, culture, and sunlight. Environmental factors can determine what we eat, whether or not we exercise, what we do with our free time, who our friends are, when and where we work, and what kind of clothes we wear. Many of these influences can have an impact on the quality and quantity (duration) of our lives. Examples of dangerous environments include living in a high crime area, breathing and drinking polluted air and water, and living in areas of severe weather, contaminated soils, or radon exposure. Although you cannot control all of the factors in your environment, you can control some of them. For example, you can eat and live in a smoke-free environment, wash your vegetables to eliminate pesticide residue, surround yourself with positive people, and wear sunscreen to the beach. You will be presented with more ideas in the following chapters.

Inadequate or nonexistent medical service is another contributor to illness and premature death. Although we live in a society with modern medical care that can enhance and extend life, some people have limited access to this care because they do not have health insurance, or they live in remote areas where medical services are limited. Even if services are available, some people do not seek medical help in a timely manner or choose not to follow their physician's recommendations.

In battle, a good tactic is to know and understand the enemy. Some of the greatest enemies to wellness are those lifestyles that can lead to a reduced quality of living. As we have indicated, some illnesses and deaths are related to just one factor, but usually all four factors contribute to the problem. (See Table 1.1.) Notice that lifestyle contributes a minimum of 23 percent and as much as 70 percent to these causes of death. This means that through lifestyle choices, you can control a lot of your risk of premature death.

An important key to a wellness lifestyle is the idea of **self-responsibility.** All of us have a great deal of influence in determining who we are and what kind of life we want to live. Through self-responsibility the adoption of behaviors can lead to improved health and heightened life satisfaction. Thus, a wellness lifestyle is composed of a consistent pattern of healthy choices, including making choices that minimize risks. For example, people who walk to their cars at night with keys and pepper spray in hand are much more likely to avoid an attack or to survive an attack if it occurs than those who stand fumbling for their keys in the dark. Motorcyclists who wear helmets are more likely to survive an accident.

By understanding the factors that can lead to illness and premature death, you will be better able to identify unhealthy behaviors and make changes that will prevent problems.

TABLE 1.1 ■ Estimated Contribution of Four Factors to the Ten Leading Causes of Death Before Age 75

Causes of Death	FACTORS AND PERCENT CONTRIBUTION			
	Lifestyle (%)	Environment (%)	Biology/Heredity (%)	Inadequate Health Care (%)
Heart disease	54	9	25	12
Cancer	37	24	29	10
Motor vehicle accidents	69	18	1	12
Other accidents	51	31	4	13
Stroke	50	22	21	7
Homicide	63	35	2	0
Suicide	60	35	2	3
Cirrhosis	70	9	18	3
Influenza/pneumonia	23	20	39	18
Diabetes	34	0	60	6
All 10 causes together	51.2	20.3	20.1	8.4

Source: Terborg, J. R. Health promotion at the worksite: A research challenge for personnel and human resource management, in K. H. Rowland and G. R. Ferris, eds., *Research in personnel and human resource management,* Vol. 4. Greenwich, CT: JAI Press, 1986, pp. 225–267. Reprinted by permission.

REACHING WELLNESS THROUGH LIFESTYLE CHANGE

We all have the capacity to achieve health and quality living through changing behaviors. If we choose to make behavior changes, we will see improvements in the various dimensions of wellness and may even to some degree prevent future illness. But to move successfully in the direction of wellness, we need to replace high-risk behaviors with healthier ones. One purpose of this book is to provide you with knowledge and tools to change high-risk behaviors.

To adopt new behaviors, we must first know how to distinguish between positive and negative behaviors. This text provides assessments to make you aware of the aspects of your life that may need changing as well as those that are currently leading toward wellness. Then, based on your stage of readiness, the text will identify behavior change strategies and techniques that you can use to progress toward wellness.

Awareness

Wellness doesn't just happen. We need knowledge and effort to modify and replace detrimental lifestyle habits with healthy behaviors. To be aware is to know what high risks are and how to identify them. How much fat can I consume every day and still enjoy my food, but not put myself at risk for certain diseases? How much body fat is too much? How will my life be different if I exercise regularly? Just how high does a person's blood cholesterol level have to be before he or she has increased risk of cardiovascular disease? These questions will be addressed throughout this book, particularly in the discussion of assessing behavior change.

Assessment

It is often difficult to determine whether we need to improve in the various dimensions of wellness. For example, in the physical dimension of wellness, you will need to have your blood cholesterol level measured to determine if it is normal or high. We will cover measurement of blood pressure, dietary habits, percentage of body fat, personal fitness, stress, muscle strength and endurance, flexibility, and use of harmful substances in this text. Because so many aspects of wellness are difficult to measure, health risk appraisals exist to assist in evaluating levels of self-reported risk. One such appraisal is Lab 1.1 at the end of this chapter. It is a paper-and-pencil survey of the various fitness and wellness aspects of your life. After completing this survey, and after you collect information about the various physical parameters of risk, you will assess your level of risk and compile a list of positive and negative behaviors to provide an overall picture of the good and bad aspects of your current lifestyle. The assessment phase of behavior change involves doing a complete evaluation of the different health risks and determining which behaviors can be left as they are and which need to be changed.

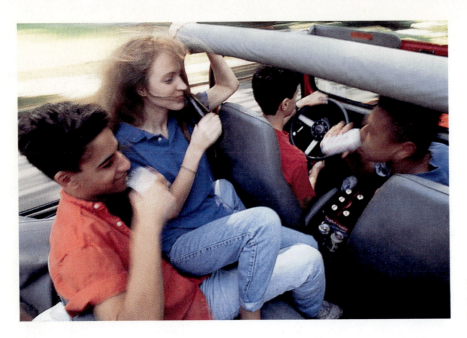

The first step in changing behaviors that can threaten personal wellness is to recognize them as potential risks.

STAGES OF CHANGE

Drs. James Prochaska and Carlo DiClemente and colleagues pioneered what has now become known as the Transtheoretical Model of Change and revolutionized what we know about how people change.[16] This has also been referred to as the Stages of Change Model. It's not uncommon for health professionals to expect lifelong smokers to go from a two-pack-a-day smoking habit to being nonsmokers. Overweight individuals are expected to lose weight and keep it off—for life. Even dietitians would like everyone to stop eating high-fat food and consume five servings of fruits or vegetables every day. The difficulty of making large-scale behavior change is reflected in the low success rates of most behavior change programs. Only 5 percent of dieters are able to reach and maintain an optimal body weight after two years. Many Americans continue to smoke despite ample opportunities to participate in smoking cessation programs, and few adults eat enough fruits or vegetables.

Frustrated by the lack of success of most behavior change programs, Dr. Prochaska and his colleagues began studying how people change and developed categories to describe people who are in different stages of readiness to change. The five stages of change include precontemplation, contemplation, preparation, action, and maintenance.

Precontemplators are people who are *not thinking* about changing their behavior. In contrast, **contemplators** are people who are *seriously thinking* about changing their behavior but have not done so. Those who are **preparers** have *made the decision* to change their behavior but have not taken consistent action to change it. Preparers intend to make changes in the immediate future (30 days), but often have an ill-formed plan about how they will go about it. If they have tried to change their behavior at all, preparers practice the new behavior at a level below the desired level. **Action takers** have actually made changes and consistently adhere to the new behavior although they have been doing so for *less than six months*. At this stage, individuals have achieved the desired level for the behavior they are changing. **Maintainers** are strongly committed to their changed behavior: they have adhered to the behavior and have maintained the desired level for *more than six months*. Unlike the action taker, the maintainer's risk for relapse to previous behavior is relatively low.[17]

Now that you have some basic definitions to work with, let's take a look at how these five stages relate to a health area such as nutrition. A precontemplator eats a high-fat diet and is unlikely to change his diet because he is not seriously thinking about changing it. When it comes to eating a proper diet, most people are precontemplators. In contrast, a person who is seriously considering cutting down on fat within the next few months is considered a contemplator. A preparer is a person who is ready to change her diet but is not taking action or is not doing so consistently. If she tries to avoid high-fat foods, she doesn't consistently reduce her overall intake of fat to reach the desired fat level in her diet. An action taker is one who has reduced his fat intake to the recommended level within the prior six months, and a maintainer is one who has reduced fat intake to the desired level and adhered to a low-fat diet for more than six months. These five stages can be applied to all aspects of wellness. For example, Figure 1.5 shows how a person can move through each of the stages with regard to exercising, starting with the precontemplation stage and ending with the maintenance stage.

It is possible to be in different stages for different health behaviors. For example, a young man might be able to reach and maintain ideal body weight and not smoke. He would be in the maintenance stage for these two behaviors. However, his blood pressure may be ele-

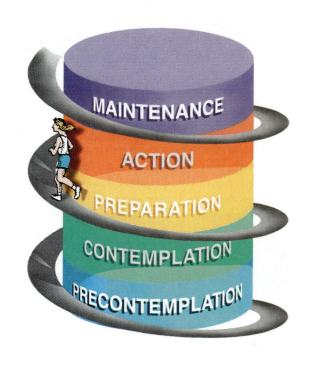

FIGURE 1.5 Stages of Change.

vated and he may suffer from excessive work stress. According to his current behavior and intentions, he might be in the precontemplation stage for controlling his blood pressure and in the action stage for reducing stress. The ultimate objective of the stages of change model is to assist individuals in attaining the maintenance stage for all healthy behaviors. Occasionally, people complete a self-assessment and conclude that nothing about their lives needs to be modified. However, they can almost inevitably find some small aspect of their lives that needs modification if they will only look a little more closely at their lifestyle.

Remember that the key to successful behavior change is not the short-term attainment of the maintenance stage. Real lifestyle change and wellness is attained when we gradually progress from one stage to the next, ultimately reaching and maintaining the new behavior. Movement is vital to reach the maintenance stage. What strategies people use to move between the stages vary depending on the stage they are in. To help you be more successful in adopting new behaviors and attaining wellness, the following sections offer general strategies to assist you in moving from stage to stage.

Most behavior change strategies have varying degrees of effectiveness depending on the stage in which they are used. These behavior change strategies are also called *processes of change*. One of these processes involves gaining awareness of problem behaviors and learning about good behaviors. Learning how our behavior affects those around us is also an important process. Our behavior affects others and the behavior of others can have an impact on us; therefore, the example of others or a role model can encourage good behaviors.

Characteristics of the Five Stages of Change

Precontemplators

- Have no intention of changing
- Often get defensive at suggestions that they change
- Resist efforts to change
- Firmly believe that the cons against making the change outweigh the benefits or pros of making the change (pros < cons)

Contemplators

- Are generally indecisive about changing
- Lack commitment to make change
- Think about making change, but don't want to change
- Find that all arguments against making a change are equally balanced with the benefits of making a change (pros = cons)
- Believe that temptation is too great to overcome

Preparers

- Want to change but don't know how
- Believe that reasons for change outweigh reasons to not change (pros > cons)
- Lack confidence in ability to maintain the new behavior
- Still experience strong temptations to do the old behavior

Action Takers

- Have made changes in behavior in last six months
- Have a plan of action
- Have goals, but goals may be unrealistic
- Are committed to new behavior
- Believe that benefits of change outweigh arguments against change (pros > cons)
- Experience the greatest risk of relapse
- Can get discouraged
- Find that confidence slowly increases

Maintainers

- Have sustained action for six months or more
- Recognize and enjoy benefits of change
- Are less likely to relapse
- Have adopted the new behavior as a lifestyle change
- Experience confidence in the new behavior that continues to get stronger
- Find that temptations are fewer and less enticing

Journal writing helps us to reevaluate ourselves in a critical manner. Our values, beliefs, and self-image are clarified and challenged when we use journal writing as a process of change. A contract is a binding agreement we can make to achieve an outcome. Use of contracts is helpful in getting an individual to commit to make a change. Most often a contract will have some stated goal or outcome. The purpose of the goal is to encourage additional effort to change. In addition to these processes of change, rewards, incentives, and social support are equally effective. As you read the remainder of this chapter, you will see how each stage of readiness to change uses these and other processes.

How to Move from Precontemplation to Contemplation

Precontemplators are the most resistant to change. Their reasons not to change still outweigh any benefits that might result from adopting a new behavior. To become a contemplator, it is important to get a clear understanding of the benefits associated with adopting a new behavior. For example, the benefits of adopting a physically active lifestyle include reduced risk of cardiovascular disease, increased fitness, decreased body fat, improved self-concept, and others. This book will explain the benefits of a wellness lifestyle so that precontemplators will perhaps consider thinking about adopting wellness lifestyles. Even if precontemplators are aware of the benefits of change, barriers against making change appear to be too difficult to overcome and supports appear too few.

Supports and Barriers

When we get reinforcement for our actions, we feel good about what we've done and we are more likely to continue the behavior. Without some sort of reward, most behaviors will simply stop. When we plan to make changes, those facets of our lives that support our decision to change are important segments of successful behavior change. **Supports** can come in the form of monetary rewards, special attention paid to us, improved self-esteem, improved health, better grades, more social approval, and even improved quality of life. One important way for precontemplators to overcome the barriers to change is to list those supports that will assist and encourage successful change. The list can act as a reminder of what will happen once the good behavior has been adopted.

In contrast, **barriers** keep us from succeeding in our efforts to change our poor behaviors. They are the main reasons why we don't succeed or fail to start. For example, if getting a balanced diet was my new goal, some barriers to this new behavior might be: I work at a bakery, my friends have very poor diets, my family always eats unhealthy foods, I can't resist chocolate-covered doughnuts.

By listing several supports and barriers, we gradually move toward becoming a contemplator. Each chapter of this text after this one contains a list of Barrier Busters, or suggestions and ideas that you can use to overcome the many different barriers and make permanent lifestyle changes.

Pressing Forward: Contemplation to Preparation

Contemplators are considering change. They are not only thinking about their current behavior, but they are seriously considering making a change. Increased health awareness, peer pressure, personal desires to improve, and readiness for change may all motivate the contemplator to make a commitment to change

Goals

Goals are visions or ideas toward which we direct our aspirations, efforts, and motivations. With goals, you have a better chance of making changes. To make changes, you need to take a good look at what you are presently doing, identify problem areas, and set goals. College-age students who have set wellness-related goals as part of a behavior change project often list the following goals:

Lose weight

Get regular physical activity

Sleep seven to eight hours every night

Stop smoking or using smokeless tobacco

Eat a balanced diet every day

Control anger and stress

Maintain ideal body weight

Eat a balanced breakfast every day

Reduce intake of dietary fat

Increase muscular strength

One notable aspect of these goals is that they do not include several different behaviors as part of one grand goal. Too often our intentions are so grandiose that we try to change everything at once, and in the end we fail at altering the poor behavior. Every goal needs to be broken down into secondary goals that can be individually reached as we gradually move toward our ultimate objective. For example, the goal to become more physically fit is great, but it can be broken down into smaller, more specific, more easily attainable, short-term goals such as: I will walk for three miles every time I walk; I will play basketball at least three times each week; each time I work out by lifting weights, I will take a partner with me to keep me going.

As people reach each secondary goal, their primary goal of acquiring increased fitness will eventually be reached. Too often, people fail because they never specified their secondary goals. Keep your goals simple and confined to one behavior. You will inevitably fail if your goal reads something like this: I want to increase my quality of life by increasing personal fitness, reducing body fat, getting proper nutrition, and managing my time so as to help me get better grades. Keep it simple and start with priority goals.

A good technique to help you decide which goal to work toward is to imagine how your life will be different if you successfully alter a specific behavior. Will the spiritual, physical, emotional, mental, or social aspects of your life be different? In what ways will your new behavior change your current life? Choose a goal that will best meet your expectations and enable you to improve your life.

With a goal in mind, you need to recognize and address the behaviors associated with the poor behavior. Smoking is typically associated with certain situations: social gatherings, parties, studying, even eating. Smoking may also be associated with specific friends or colleagues; stress and smoking often occur together. Every behavior we possess is associated with other environmental and daily occurrences. We often eat at certain times of the day or eat specific foods when they are presented to us. Observe the various characteristics of your behaviors and pay special attention to how they reinforce your lifestyle.

Moving from Preparation to Action

To make this move, you will need a plan. A plan of attack consists of the strategies you will use to modify your behavior. It is here where knowledge of your supports and barriers is very important. Each barrier needs to be confronted and planned for accordingly. By addressing each barrier, the ultimate outcome of the behavior change is more likely to be successful.

You have probably seen that your behaviors are connected or chained to other events and choices. A plan of attack is a guide to breaking the chains that connect behaviors. Excessive weight gain is likely the result of overeating and lack of exercise. A weight-loss program consisting only of dietary intervention and no regular physical activity is doomed to failure. Exercise can break the link between weight gain and inactivity. There are specific strategies you can use with each behavior, and, when used correctly, you can successfully adopt new lifestyles. Each chapter of this text deals with a different wellness topic and contains specific guidelines and strategies to help you modify your behaviors.

People in the action stage are at the greatest risk of relapse. Dealing with relapse is critical. The average person who permanently quits smoking tried to do so at least three times in seven years before having success. Relapse is a common occurrence in behavior change. Problems arise when we fail to get back on our plan of action and slowly gravitate back to the old behavior. Relapse can be overcome by recommitting ourselves to the new behavior and planning ahead for the time when relapse may occur so that when we do slip, we can regroup and take precautions to be more careful next time. Setbacks are common but we can gain strength by learning from our mistakes.

Perhaps your methods are not working. Successful behavior change will require flexibility and the willingness to change your plan of action to accommodate the unforeseen and unexpected. Take time to reevaluate your methods, successes, and failures and make changes to your strategies. Remember that if a strategy is not working, do not be afraid to try something else. Be patient and don't let anything deter you from reaching your goal.

Measuring Your Progress

To measure progress, you must have a starting point. By using the various assessment tools in this text you will be able to measure and chart your progress. Each assessment is described in detail on the designated lab provided at the back of each chapter. The norms provided with these tests should give you a general idea of how well you scored. It is important to compare your earlier scores with more current ones. Tangible evidence of improvement can be a strong motivator. You may discover that you are doing well in one dimension of wellness, but not so well in another. Follow a program that lets you maintain your strengths and improve your weaknesses.

Evaluating Your Progress and Goals

After you have been making a concerted effort for four to eight weeks, take an objective look at your plan to see whether you are accomplishing what you intended. Look at your goals and the results of your assessments. Be critical of your progress toward each specific goal. If the results of your program don't indicate achievement toward your goals, pause and try changing the goals or the program.

Sometimes goals change. For example, teenagers often base their goals on a desire to have an "incredible body," while adults place more emphasis on weight control and overall physical health. As they approach retirement, people tend to shift their goals again, this time toward sociability and maintaining physical independence. Keep your goals up-to-date and adjust your program whenever your goals change.

Sometimes a plan of attack is working, but it is not reflected in the goals. Take, for example, a person whose goal is to lose weight. After eight weeks of physical activity, she is discouraged because she has gained weight. On closer examination, however, she discovers that she has lost inches and has a lower percentage of body fat; she actually lost fat and gained muscle. Since muscle weighs more than fat, she gained weight. The program worked, but her goal did not reflect her improvement.

Making the Move from Action to Maintenance

Successful lifestyle change happens when you are able to maintain a new behavior for the rest of your life. The maintenance stage is dynamic because it requires constant adjustment and relapse prevention. The initial period of the maintenance stage is typically full of enthusiasm and determination. Personal commitment to make permanent change is high, motivation is high, new behaviors are very appealing, but, with the passage of time, most of the reasons to change slowly diminish and fade from our minds and our determination weakens.

Finding Motivation

There are two forms of motivation: intrinsic and extrinsic. Intrinsic motivation comes from inside you. For example, if you exercise because you want to look and feel better, then you are intrinsically motivated. Extrinsic motivation comes from outside you. It may be in the form of a television commercial selling soda and exercise, a girlfriend offering you a lobster dinner if you exercise for three months, or a friend calling up to see whether you would like to exercise together.

When you personally believe in something, you will be more motivated to do it than if someone else is telling you to do it. Therefore, to motivate yourself to exercise, you want to find a form of exercise that you enjoy, one you can do in a location and at a time convenient for you. If you are aware of these intrinsically motivating factors, you will be more likely to stick with exercising.

You may be one of those rare and wonderful people who has the internal desire and discipline to maintain a behavior change all your life. But if you are like most of us and need a push to keep motivated, here are a few sources of extrinsic motivation you can tap:

1. **Writing in a journal** at least three times per week forces you to think about your efforts or lack of efforts in making changes. Writing causes you to reflect upon successes and failures and helps you to stay focused on the task at hand. Most behavior goals can be quantified in some manner; thus, record keeping is a useful way to evaluate your progress. Records might include pounds of body weight lost or percent of body fat decreased. Good records can be kept on those behaviors that are measurable. For example, reducing the amount of stress in a person's life is important, but measuring stress is not easy. As the behavior change process goes on, regular measurement of the behavior should be taken and recorded. These measurements can then be graphed to show how the behavior has changed over time. Graphical representations of successful change can help to keep you motivated and focused.

2. **Role models** can be effective tools in helping make positive changes. Identify someone who possesses the behavior you want to attain, and ask that person how he or she did it, including any advice or suggestions that might help you make changes. Role models give us an example to follow and can be helpful in providing encouragement and support.

3. **Rewards and incentives** can help us stay focused. The cost of smoking two packs of cigarettes a day adds up to approximately $120 a month, or $1,440 annually. The money saved by not smoking could be used as a reward for quitting. New clothes, entertainment, or even travel could be purchased with the savings. Rewards should consist of healthy, wellness-promoting gifts. Candy, alcohol, or other less healthy foods do not make the best rewards. As goals are met, incentives can be used to provide encouragement and reinforcement for further success.

4. The **inclusion of others** in your plan of attack can increase your commitment and determination to continue. If friends, roommates, or family know that you are determined to lose weight, they may be more willing to assist you in your efforts. By informing others, we become obligated to change our behavior and they in turn will make efforts to assist us by not placing us in difficult or tempting situations. One particularly effective tool is the use of a buddy or partner. In adopting a new exercise schedule, you may feel more inclined to exercise when you remember that your partner is expecting you to show up and is probably standing around waiting for you.

Before You Begin

A wellness lifestyle requires adopting new behaviors in all dimensions of our lives. Use of the Stages of Change Model applies to each of our behaviors. To help you succeed at adopting a wellness lifestyle, each chapter in this text includes laboratory exercises. Some of them will help you assess your current behavior, but the majority of the labs will give you clear, concise methods on how to progress to the next stage of change. You might already have adopted and maintained some of the wellness lifestyles discussed in this text. In that case, you can congratulate yourself and move directly to the labs on maintenance, which will help you continue with your healthy behavior. Those who are precontemplators, contemplators, in preparation, or in the action stage can go to the labs that best describe their current stage of readiness to change. *Remember, the important thing is to make progress from one stage to the next.*

Behavior change comes down to whether or not a person really wants to change. You have to want to make changes or it just will not happen. Motivation is the key to making real changes. Unfortunately motivation fluctuates from day to day and is affected by all aspects of our lives. Two of the most powerful motivators are pain or coming close to death.

Patients with heart disease not only experience great pain, but many come close to dying because of their condition. The majority of cases of heart disease are lifestyle-related and can be avoided by living wellness-oriented lives. For these patients, however, the damage is already done and most will undergo difficult and expensive surgery if they want treatment for the disease. After surgery, these patients are required to participate in rehabilitation where they learn about wellness lifestyles, including proper nutrition, stress reduction, regular physical activity, and other health-promoting and disease-preventing lifestyles. Rehabilitation is intense and often difficult, but these patients are usually very motivated to change their old lifestyle. The memory of almost dying is often enough to make most patients want to do something about their behaviors.

For these persons, daily exercise is required, only low-fat foods are to be eaten, smoking cessation is mandated, and stress-reduction techniques are encouraged. One patient was overheard saying, "How many weeks do I have to continue exercising before I can quit?" The adoption of a wellness lifestyle is not intended to last eight weeks or even a year. It must become an integral part of the rest of our lives. Movement from one stage to the next may not occur during a semester; it usually takes more than sixteen weeks to become a maintainer. So be patient and see whether your pros have increased and your cons decreased.

Throughout the rest of this book, various activities will help you determine your own level of readiness. The labs are designed to accommodate individual differences in stages of readiness. For each chapter, determine your current stage of change and complete the appropriate laboratory exercises.

SUMMARY

A wellness lifestyle can improve your life and its quality. Of the many factors that determine how long we live, lifestyle is the most important, affecting each of the five dimensions of wellness. Because lifestyle is such an important part of wellness, strategies have been developed to help you modify your lifestyle by replacing your negative behaviors with positive ones. The Stages of Change Model can help you progress through behavior change, leading to the maintenance of positive behaviors. Through stages of change, everyone can achieve wellness.

SUGGESTED READING

Pelletier, K. R. *Sound mind, sound body: A new model for lifelong health.* New York: Simon & Schuster, 1994.

Prochaska, J. O., J. C. Norcross, and C. C. DiClemente. *Changing for good: The revolutionary program that explains the six stages of change and teaches you how to free yourself from bad habits.* New York: William Morrow, 1994.

Name _____   **Section**   **Date** _____

Health and Wellness Inventory

Instructions

Please circle the appropriate answer to each question and total your points as indicated at the end of the questionnaire. Circle 5 if always true, 4 if frequently true, 3 if occasionally true, 2 if seldom true, and 1 if never true.

1.	I am able to identify the situations and factors that overstress me.	5 4 3 2 1
2.	I eat only when I am hungry.	5 4 3 2 1
3.	I don't take tranquilizers or other drugs to relax.	5 4 3 2 1
4.	I support efforts in my community to reduce environmental pollution.	5 4 3 2 1
5.	I avoid buying foods with preservatives and artificial coloring.	5 4 3 2 1
6.	I rarely have problems concentrating on what I'm doing because of worrying about other things.	5 4 3 2 1
7.	My employer (school) takes measures to ensure that my work (study) place is safe.	5 4 3 2 1
8.	I use medications carefully and only when necessary.	5 4 3 2 1
9.	I am able to identify certain bodily responses and illnesses as my reactions to stress.	5 4 3 2 1
10.	I question the use of diagnostic x-rays.	5 4 3 2 1
11.	I try to alter personal living habits that are risk factors for heart disease, cancer, and other lifestyle diseases.	5 4 3 2 1
12.	I avoid taking sleeping pills to help me sleep.	5 4 3 2 1
13.	I try not to eat foods with refined sugar or corn sugar ingredients.	5 4 3 2 1
14.	I accomplish goals I set for myself.	5 4 3 2 1
15.	I stretch or bend for several minutes each day to keep my body flexible.	5 4 3 2 1
16.	I support immunization of all children for common childhood diseases.	5 4 3 2 1
17.	I try to prevent friends from driving after they drink alcohol.	5 4 3 2 1
18.	I minimize extra salt intake.	5 4 3 2 1
19.	I don't mind when other people and situations make me wait or lose time.	5 4 3 2 1
20.	I walk four or fewer flights of stairs rather than take the elevator.	5 4 3 2 1
21.	I eat fresh fruits and vegetables.	5 4 3 2 1
22.	I use dental floss at least once a day.	5 4 3 2 1
23.	I read product labels on foods to determine their ingredients.	5 4 3 2 1
24.	I try to maintain normal body weight.	5 4 3 2 1
25.	I record my feelings and thoughts in a journal or diary.	5 4 3 2 1

Source: Edlin, G., and E. Golanty. *Health and wellness,* 4th ed., pp. 17–19. © 1992. Sudbury, MA: Jones and Bartlett Publishers. www.jbpub.com. Reprinted with permission.

26. I have no difficulty falling asleep.   5 4 3 2 1

27. I engage in some form of vigorous physical activity at least three times a week.   5 4 3 2 1

28. I take time each day to quiet my mind and relax.   5 4 3 2 1

29. I am willing to make and sustain close friendships and intimate relationships.   5 4 3 2 1

30. I obtain an adequate daily supply of vitamins from food or vitamin supplements.   5 4 3 2 1

31. I rarely have tension or migraine headaches, or pain in the neck or shoulders.   5 4 3 2 1

32. I wear a safety belt when driving.   5 4 3 2 1

33. I am aware of the emotional and situational factors that lead me to overeat.   5 4 3 2 1

34. I avoid driving my car after drinking any alcohol.   5 4 3 2 1

35. I am aware of the side effects of the medicines I take.   5 4 3 2 1

36. I am able to accept feelings of sadness, depression, and anxiety, knowing that they are almost always transient.   5 4 3 2 1

37. I would seek additional professional opinions if my doctor recommended surgery for me.   5 4 3 2 1

38. I feel that nonsmokers should not have to breathe the smoke from cigarettes in public places.   5 4 3 2 1

39. I feel that pregnant women who smoke harm their babies.   5 4 3 2 1

40. I feel that I get enough sleep.   5 4 3 2 1

41. I ask my doctor why a certain medication is being prescribed and inquire about alternatives.   5 4 3 2 1

42. I am aware of the calories expended in my activities.   5 4 3 2 1

43. I am willing to give priority to my own needs for time and psychological space by saying no to others' requests of me. 5 4 3 2 1

44. I walk instead of drive whenever feasible.   5 4 3 2 1

45. I eat a breakfast that contains about one-third of my daily need for calories, proteins, and vitamins.   5 4 3 2 1

46. I prohibit smoking in my home.   5 4 3 2 1

47. I remember and think about my dreams.   5 4 3 2 1

48. I have routine yearly checkups rather than seeking medical attention only when I have symptoms or feel that some (potential) condition needs checking. 5 4 3 2 1

49. I endeavor to make my home accident free.   5 4 3 2 1

50. I ask my doctor to explain the diagnosis of my problem until I understand it.   5 4 3 2 1

51. I try to include fiber or roughage (whole grains, fresh fruits and vegetables, or bran) in my daily diet.   5 4 3 2 1

52. I can deal with my emotional problems without alcohol or other mood-altering drugs.   5 4 3 2 1

53. I am satisfied with my work at school and on the job.   5 4 3 2 1

54. I require children riding in my car to be in infant seats or shoulder harnesses.   5 4 3 2 1

55. I try to associate with people who have a positive attitude about life.   5 4 3 2 1

56. I try not to eat snacks of candy, pastries, or other "junk" foods.   5 4 3 2 1

57. I avoid people who are "down" all the time and bring down those around them.   5 4 3 2 1

58. I am aware of the calorie and fat content of the foods I eat.   5 4 3 2 1

59. I brush my teeth after meals.   5 4 3 2 1

60. (for women only) I routinely examine my breasts.   5 4 3 2 1
    (for men only) I routinely check for signs of testicular cancer.

How to Score

Each of the questions above relates to a specific category of wellness. Next to the question number on the next page enter the numbers you've circled and total your score for each category. Then determine your degree of wellness for each category, using the wellness status key.

Emotional Health	Body care	FITNESS Environmental Health	Stress	Nutrition	Medical self-responsibility
6 _____	15 _____	4 _____	1 _____	2 _____	8 _____
12 _____	20 _____	7 _____	3 _____	5 _____	10 _____
25 _____	22 _____	17 _____	9 _____	13 _____	11 _____
26 _____	24 _____	32 _____	14 _____	18 _____	16 _____
36 _____	27 _____	34 _____	19 _____	21 _____	35 _____
40 _____	33 _____	38 _____	28 _____	23 _____	37 _____
47 _____	42 _____	39 _____	29 _____	30 _____	41 _____
52 _____	44 _____	46 _____	31 _____	45 _____	48 _____
55 _____	58 _____	49 _____	43 _____	51 _____	59 _____
57 _____	59 _____	54 _____	53 _____	56 _____	60 _____
total _____	total _____	total _____	total _____	total _____	total _____

Wellness Status

To assess your status in each of the six categories, compare your total score in each to the following key:

0–34 Need improvement; 35–44 Good; 45–50 Excellent

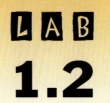

Healthy Lifestyles Evaluation

After completing Lab 1.1, answer the following questions:

1. Using the results of Lab 1.1, list your strongest and weakest dimensions of wellness.

    Strongest   *Weakest*

2. List the wellness behaviors you have that need to be modified.

3. Why are these behaviors part of your lifestyle?

4. If you were to decide to alter any one of these behaviors, what benefits would you expect to receive?

5. What barriers might prevent you from changing this behavior?

6. List any supports you might receive if you were to try to modify a poor health behavior.

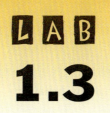

L A B

1.3

Behavior Change Contract

1. I desire to change the following behavior: _____
   _____
   _____

   My long-term goal is _____
   _____
   _____

2. How often and where does this behavior occur? _____
   _____
   _____
   _____

3. How will my life be different if I successfully change this behavior?
   a. _____
   b. _____
   c. _____

4. What might happen if I fail to change this behavior?
   a. _____
   b. _____
   c. _____

5. I will change my behavior by attaining these short-term, measurable goals:
   a. _____
   b. _____
   c. _____

6. Here are a few of the supports and barriers I might encounter as I strive to alter my behavior:

   Supports   *Barriers*

   _____   _____
   _____   _____
   _____   _____
   _____   _____
   _____   _____
   _____   _____

7. Details of the plan of attack I will use to change this behavior:

_____

_____

_____

_____

_____

_____

_____

_____

8. My long-range goal will be attained by the following date: _____

9. I, _____, agree to try my best to attain this goal.

Signature: _____

Date: _____

Witness signature: _____

CHAPTER 2

The Fitness-Wellness Connection

Terms

- Physical activity
- Exercise
- Physical fitness
- Health-related components of physical fitness
- Skill-related components of physical fitness
- Cardiorespiratory endurance
- Body composition
- Flexibility
- Muscular endurance
- Muscular strength
- Endorphins
- Homeostasis
- Anaerobic
- Aerobic
- Warm-up
- Workout
- FIT
- Cross training
- Threshold of training
- Fitness target zone
- Cool-down
- Developmental stretch
- Principle of individuality
- Principle of overload
- Principle of overuse
- Principle of progression
- Principle of specificity
- Principle of reversibility

Objectives

1. Discuss the benefits of physical activity on each of the five wellness dimensions.

2. Explain how an expanded knowledge base in physical fitness and exercise has changed our perception of what types of activity are important to health and wellness.

3. Name and define the five health-related components of physical fitness.

4. Explain the importance of both health-related and skill-related components of physical fitness.

5. Organize and list by bodily system the physical benefits of exercise.

6. Define physical activity, exercise, and physical fitness.

7. Use the components and principles of physical activity to design a physical activity session using an activity of your choice.

ACTIVEWEAR AND ACTIVE LIFESTYLES

They used to be called sneakers. Now they are basketball shoes, tennis shoes, running shoes, court shoes, aerobic shoes, and a new version of the all-around sneaker: cross trainers. Americans are in love with their athletic shoes. They use them as back-to-school shoes, to-and-from-work commuter's shoes, get-around-campus shoes, sport shoes, stable supportive shoes for the elderly, nurse's and surgeon's work shoes, and occasionally even wedding shoes! We even have special shoes for walking. What is this American love affair with athletic shoes about? It is a symbol of how times have changed. Athletic shoes, T-shirts, sweatsuits, and stretch pants demonstrate a move toward comfortable casualwear—a desire for freedom of movement and a relaxed lifestyle.

Now the irony: even though at some point during the day American adults are dressed in activewear, more than 60 percent do not achieve the recommended amount of regular physical activity. In fact, 25 percent are not active at all.[1] One-quarter of us have our athletic shoes propped up on a footstool! And twice as many more of us are taking much too long to wear them out.

As it has become more and more evident that physical activity is linked to good health, getting the American public to exercise has moved up the public health priority list. Physical inactivity is now considered to be as important a risk factor for CHD disease as smoking, high blood cholesterol, and high blood pressure. It is clear that we cannot afford to sit still. According to the Surgeon General,[2] inactivity is presently more common among: (1) women than men, (2) African American and Hispanic adults than whites, (3) older than younger adults, (4) less affluent than more affluent people, and (5) more educated than less educated adults.

The good news is that there has been a trend of increasing physical activity among Americans starting in the 1960s and extending into the 1980s. More recently, however, this trend seems to have plateaued.[3] We also know that social support from family and friends is positively related to physical activity and that the amount and nature of exercise once thought to be needed for health benefits has changed.

Until the 1960s, exercise was primarily thought of as calisthenics, military training, and sports play. In 1968, Dr. Kenneth Cooper introduced the idea of aerobic exercise and revolutionized people's thinking about exercise and health. He took the adjective *aerobic,* meaning "with oxygen," added an "s," and created the noun *aerobics.* His popular book bearing that title, and his subsequent books, explain to people how they can achieve the many health benefits of aerobic activity, which Cooper defines as any sustained rhythmic large-muscle activity. Men and women took to the streets, jogging for their health. The first activity boom was off and "running."

In the 1970s, tennis and racquetball became the "boom" sports, and by the late 1970s Jackie Sorenson had introduced aerobic dance—the boom activity of the 1980s. During the 1970s, university professors began to specialize in exercise research. Much of the early physiological research focused on performance measures—how to go farther, faster, and so on—but a second focus emerged in the 1980s, one that combined fitness and health. The medical community began to shift its emphasis from "fix" to "prevent," and health and fitness professionals started teaming up to share their wealth of combined knowledge with the public. Charles Corbin and Ruth Lindsey designed the first college course and textbook[4] for those not majoring in physical education, emphasizing exercise concepts and principles and personal involvement in fitness assessment and exercise programming. (This approach is very different from traditional courses in which an instructor teaches a specific sport or series of sports.) What they started as a "Fit for Life" movement has on many college campuses grown into a wellness movement. At many universities today, physical education and health faculties have joined together to offer courses that teach both physical fitness and health in a wellness context.

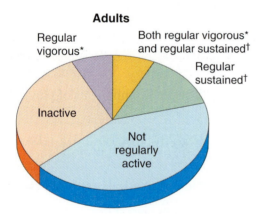

Adults

Regular vigorous*

Both regular vigorous* and regular sustained†

Regular sustained†

Inactive

Not regularly active

*Regular vigorous—20 minutes 3 times per week of vigorous intensity
†Regular sustained—30 minutes 5 times per week of any intensity

FIGURE 2.1 Regular physical activity by adults. (Adapted by permission from S. N. Blair, H. W. Kohl III, R. S. Paffenbarger, Jr., D. G. Clark, K. H. Cooper, and L. W. Gibbons. Physical fitness and all-cause mortality: A prospective study of healthy men and women. *Journal of the American Medical Association* 262(17): 2395–2401, 1989. Copyright 1989 by the American Medical Association.)

PHYSICAL ACTIVITY, EXERCISE, AND PHYSICAL FITNESS

The three terms *physical activity, exercise,* and *physical fitness* are closely related but not synonymous. **Physical activity** is the broadest term and it can be defined as "any bodily movement produced by skeletal muscles that results in energy expenditure."[5] This means that physical activity includes everything you do during the day, including brushing your teeth, walking, and blinking. It also includes any exercise you perform. **Exercise** is generally thought of as a planned event, a structured workout that will make you more physically fit. **Physical fitness** describes what you become, a set of attributes you obtain, attributes that allow you to perform physical activities. For example, physically fit persons are strong, flexible, and energetic. People who are physically fit can participate in more physical activities with less fatigue.

HEALTH-RELATED FITNESS VERSUS SKILL-RELATED FITNESS

In response to a growing concern among professionals that fitness training and tests were concentrating too much on skill and not enough on health, the American Alliance of Health, Physical Education, Recreation and Dance (AAHPERD) charged a committee with the job of reevaluating the tests. In 1980, AAHPERD published a booklet describing two categories of physical fitness—one called "health-related components of physical fitness," the other, "skill-related components"—and a new set of tests for the health-related components of fitness.[6] Prior to this, fitness tests consisted largely of skill items such as the softball throw and the shuttle run. In addition, only those individuals who scored in the top 15 percent received awards, which meant that most of the recognition went to athletes. In 1980, the emphasis shifted from athleticism toward monitoring improvement in and giving recognition for healthy levels of fitness. This was great news for those who had struggled and failed on skill-related tests and who could see no relevancy between their lives and sport-specific skills. Health-related tests such as the one-mile run, sit-and-reach flexibility, and sit-ups were introduced. At the same time, team sport curriculums were modified to include lifetime activities such as tennis, golf, and archery. Today schools and communities offer activities as diverse as ropes courses, orienteering, and cross-country skiing. For people who don't enjoy team sports, these are welcome changes and opportunities.

How is exercising for health different from training for competition? To fine-tune your performance for competition, you must train long hours at high intensities. You may also have to place your body in mechanically difficult positions. For example, volleyball players and weight lifters drop into deep knee bends, placing stress on their knee ligaments; gymnasts hyperextend their backs, putting extra pressure on their vertebral discs; and pitchers put their elbows at risk when they throw curve balls. The motivation for intense practices and high-level performances comes from a deep-seated drive to excel and a desire to win recognition and awards.

Many positive outcomes are associated with competition, and health is one of them. However, a higher risk of musculoskeletal injury is also associated with high-intensity training. (Injuries and burnout may also occur when coaches and parents expect too much too soon from their athletes and children.) Surprisingly, not all highly trained competitors are physically fit. For example, some excellent golfers and baseball players are over-fat and lack good cardiorespiratory endurance. And marathoners usually sacrifice upper-body strength for a highly trained cardiorespiratory system. Furthermore, elite athletes have to focus so much of their lives on training that the physical dimension of wellness often overshadows the social, mental, emotional, and sometimes spiritual dimensions. Therefore, being highly skilled or extremely well developed in one aspect of fitness does not ensure overall health or wellness.

If you are exercising for health rather than performance, you can train at a more moderate intensity, one that provides physiological and psychological benefits and limits the risk of injury. You need not "exercise until you drop" or "kill yourself to get fit." Lifetime fitness is built on activities that are enjoyable and, when done correctly, free from pain.

There are five **health-related components of physical fitness:** cardiorespiratory endurance, body composition, flexibility, muscular endurance, and muscular strength. Any improvement in these five areas will improve your health. (Sometimes muscular strength and endurance are considered one component, making the total number of health-related components four.)

There are also six **skill-related components of fitness:** coordination, agility, balance, reaction time, power, and speed. Sometimes kinesthetic awareness (knowing where your body is in space—for example, a diver knowing when to open from a tuck) is considered a seventh component. Many of us enjoy playing sports and want to play well. To be skillful, we need to be coordinated, agile, and quick; but to be *healthy*, we don't need such attributes. Too many people have shunned exercise because they think they must be great athletes. *Not true!* With even basic sport skills, you can have fun joining recreational activities such as volleyball, picnic softball, or pick-up football games. You can stay fit through playing sports, but there are many other ways, too, as you will see.

Let's focus on the five health-related components of fitness, because they have the most influence on your wellness. To develop specific sports skills, seek out qualified instructors and coaches, and/or consult some sport drill and technique books.

HEALTH-RELATED FITNESS: THE FIVE COMPONENTS

Cardiorespiratory Endurance

Cardiorespiratory endurance is the ability to perform large-muscle movements over a sustained period of time. In other words, it is the ability of the circulatory (heart, blood, blood vessels) and respiratory systems (lungs, diaphragm, and so on) to deliver fuel, especially oxygen, to the muscles during continuous exercise. Fit individuals have a heart-lung capacity that allows them to persist in physical activity for relatively long periods of time without undue fatigue. The terms *cardiovascular endurance* and *cardiorespiratory endurance* are often used interchangeably. We will use the latter in this text because it reflects the important relationship between the respiratory and circulatory systems. Cardiorespiratory endurance is also commonly referred to as cardiorespiratory fitness.

Cardiorespiratory endurance can be achieved through sustained large muscle movements such as brisk walking, jogging, and swimming (see Chapter 3). Some of the health benefits associated with cardiorespiratory endurance include a stronger heart, improved circulation to the heart, increased oxygen transportation by the blood, a lower risk of coronary heart disease (CHD), a better chance of surviving a heart attack, a decreased level of blood fat (cholesterol), an increased level of high-density lipoproteins (HDL), a lowered resting heart rate, lower blood pressure, and a better chance of living a longer, healthier life.

Body Composition

Body composition refers to the relative amounts of lean body mass and fat in your body. Lean body mass includes bones, muscles, and connective tissue. Fat includes subcutaneous fat (the fat deposits stored between the muscles and the skin) and intramuscular fat (the fat stored within the muscles). The percentage of fat you have can be measured in several ways, including the skinfold technique and underwater weighing (hydrostatic weighing) (see Chapter 7). A certain amount of fat is essential for health, but too high or too low a percentage of fat is unhealthy.

Body composition can be improved by decreasing the amount of fat or increasing the amount of lean body mass, or both. A sound diet keeps off excess fat and exercise can burn off fat and put on muscle (lean body mass). Increasing muscle mass has the added benefit of increasing your resting metabolic rate, which means your body is burning more calories while at rest. This can help you maintain a healthy weight after a weight-loss diet.

The benefits of maintaining a healthy percentage of body fat include reducing your CHD risk, building an attractive physique, increasing your self-concept, and improving your body's capacity to work. To picture an increased work capacity, imagine climbing six flights of stairs while carrying a thirty-pound sack. Now imagine the difference if you weren't toting that sack. The less excess fat you have, the more energy you have available. Next, think what would happen if you added a little muscle power (lean body mass)—how much more you would be able to accomplish without getting tired! Climbing the same six flights with stronger legs would seem so much easier, you might even be tempted to run up them.

Flexibility

Flexibility is the ability to move a joint through its full range of motion. Loss of function occurs when a joint is too loose or too tight. When muscles and connective tissue tighten and shorten, the range of motion in the joint is restricted. Simple tasks such as turning around in a car seat to check traffic or picking something up off the floor can become difficult. Too loose a joint can result in slippage, injury, and possible dislocation. Strengthening muscles around a loose joint can help stabilize it.

You can work on flexibility by stretching during the warm-up and cool-down or by performing a specific flexibility program. (If you have been diagnosed with "loose" joints as a result of injury or heredity, you should not stretch them.) Health benefits associated with good flexibility include freedom of movement, greater movement efficiency, less risk of muscle or joint injury, and decreased risk of lower back pain.

Muscular Endurance

Muscular endurance is the ability of a muscle, or group of muscles, to (1) apply a submaximal (less than all-out) force repeatedly, or (2) sustain a muscular contraction for a period of time. Leg lifts are an example of a repeatedly applied submaximal force. Holding the leg in a raised position for 10 seconds is an example of a sustained contraction. You can improve muscular endurance by performing a relatively high number of repetitions of a movement against light to moderate resistance or by increasing the amount of time you hold a position. The benefits of improving muscular endurance include less fatigue during regular activity, an increased ability to do work, and a reduced risk of injury.

Muscular Strength

Muscular strength is the ability of a muscle, or group of muscles, to exert force against a resistance. The number of pounds you can lift one time is a measure of maximal muscular strength. You can improve your muscular strength by lifting relatively heavy weights for a low number of repetitions. Weight training is one of the best ways to increase strength. While weight machines, bars, and plates are needed for moderate to heavy resistance, you can obtain light to moderate resistance by using exercise bands, wrist and ankle weights, weighted balls, or water resistance (for example, deep-water running or water aerobics).

The health benefits related to muscular strength include an increased ability to do work, particularly physically challenging work, and a decreased risk of injury, particularly to the back.

HOW MUCH PHYSICAL ACTIVITY IS ENOUGH?

Two major philosophical shifts have occurred concerning fitness and exercise in the past 15 to 20 years. The first, as described earlier, was a movement away from strictly skill-based programs toward programs that included activities and tests promoting health-related physical fitness. The second shift, a more recent one, concerns the debate over how much physical activity is enough.

In 1978 and again in 1990, the American College of Sports Medicine (ACSM) published a set of guidelines on the recommended quantity and quality of exercise for healthy adults. The 1990 guidelines, especially regarding cardiorespiratory fitness, became the gold standard for physical fitness. The recommendations encouraged people to perform 20 to 60 minutes of moderate- to high-intensity endurance exercise three to five times a week. People were also urged to perform a minimum of one set of eight to twelve repetitions of eight to ten exercises involving the major muscle groups twice a week to develop and maintain muscular strength and endurance[7] (see Chapters 3 and 4). These recommendations were based on research that studied how exercise training regimens affected physical performance measures. For example, researchers tested how many times a week, and at what intensities, someone had to run to increase aerobic capacity (the ability to use oxygen to fuel muscle contractions). Experts assumed that health benefits accompanied this type of training but these benefits were not specifically studied in the beginning.

More recently, when researchers looked at how much exercise was needed to acquire health benefits (as opposed to performance measures), they were surprised to discover that performing a lower intensity activity than previously recommended would still yield substantial health benefits and that even small increases in activity at low levels of intensity make a significant difference in the health of sedentary people.

Figure 2.2 demonstrates this relationship between physical activity and health. Health benefits rise quickly as inactive or low-active persons increase their activity to a moderate level. Additional health benefits are attained by those who become highly active, but notice that the increase in benefits is modest in comparison. The good news, then, is that moderate-level activities like a brisk 30-minute walk, a round of golf (pulling or carrying your clubs), or three 10-minute sessions of serious housecleaning can garner the majority of health benefits. Since these kinds of activities are easier to adopt and

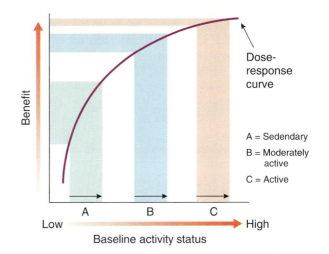

FIGURE 2.2 This graph represents relationship between physical activity (dose) and health benefits (response). Sedentary people who increase their physical activity receive the greatest increases in health benefits. Active people already enjoy many of the health benefits and consequently experience the smallest gains. (Adapted from R. R. Pate et al. Physical activity and public health: A recommendation from the Centers for Disease Control and Prevention and the American College of Sports Medicine. *Journal of the American Medical Association* 273(5):402–407, 1995.)

maintain than high-intensity exercise,[8] it is hoped that this new information will encourage more people to add physical activity to their lifestyle.

Experts brought together by the Centers for Disease Control and Prevention (CDC) and the American College of Sports Medicine reviewed the available body of research and in 1995 published a set of physical activity guidelines. These guidelines are meant to complement existing guidelines, not replace them. Their recommendation on the quantity of physical activity needed for disease prevention and health promotion is that every U.S. adult accumulate 30 minutes or more of moderately intense physical activity on most, preferably all, days of the week.[9] Moderately intense is described as roughly the equivalent of brisk walking (3 to 4 miles per hour for most adults).

The *amount* of activity you do is more important than *what* activity you do. Table 2.1 gives examples of moderate amounts of activity. If 30 minutes of sustained activity does not fit your schedule, you can accumulate your 30 minutes in short time periods, such as three 10-minute activities. For your 30 minutes you might walk to lunch the long way, throw around a Frisbee or ball, or drop off that book you've been meaning to return to the library. Libraries, by the way, are one of the best places for walking multiple flights of stairs. These types of activities take more time, but not a whole lot more time, which makes them manageable even in a busy schedule.

Physical activity can be categorized by the number of calories burned per unit of time. Studies have shown

TABLE 2.1 ■ Examples of Moderate Amounts of Activity	
• Washing and waxing a car for 45–60 minutes	Less Vigorous, More Time
• Washing windows or floors for 45–60 minutes	
• Playing volleyball for 45 minutes	
• Playing touch football for 30–45 minutes	
• Gardening for 30–45 minutes	
• Wheeling self in wheelchair for 30–40 minutes	
• Walking 1¾ miles in 35 minutes (20 min/mile)	
• Basketball (shooting baskets) for 30 minutes	
• Bicycling 5 miles in 30 minutes	
• Dancing fast (social) for 30 minutes	
• Pushing a stroller 1½ miles in 30 minutes	
• Raking leaves for 30 minutes	
• Walking 2 miles in 30 minutes (15 min/mile)	
• Water aerobics for 30 minutes	
• Swimming laps for 20 minutes	
• Wheelchair basketball for 20 minutes	
• Basketball (playing a game) for 15–20 minutes	
• Bicycling 4 miles in 15 minutes	
• Jumping rope for 15 minutes	
• Running 1½ miles in 15 minutes (10 min/mile)	
• Shoveling snow for 15 minutes	More Vigorous, Less Time
• Stairwalking for 15 minutes	

U.S. Department of Health and Human Services, *Physical activity and health: A report of the Surgeon General.* Centers for Disease Control and Prevention, National Center for Chronic Disease Prevention and Health Promotion. Atlanta: The President's Council on Physical Fitness and Sports, 1996.

that burning as little as 500 to 1,000 calories a week through exercise reduces the premature death rate, but experts recommend expending a minimum of 1.35 calories per pound of body weight per day to ensure the health benefits related to physical activity. For most people, this represents about 1,000 to 2,000 calories a week, or 150 to 300 calories per day. Table 2.2 (pages 32 and 33) lists activities according to how many calories they burn per minute per pound of body weight. Multiply the number of pounds you weigh by calories listed by the number of minutes you engage in the activity. Do not feel limited to 150 to 300 calories; this is the amount needed to achieve the majority of health benefits; more activity (not excessive activity) will build greater fitness and further increase your health benefits.

THE BENEFITS OF PHYSICAL ACTIVITY AND EXERCISE

Thirty minutes of daily physical activity is the foundation of fitness and the minimum requirement for wellness. For many college students a brisk walk around campus meets this requirement and fits a busy schedule. If, however, you desire a more active lifestyle, you will need a higher level of fitness, one that is achieved through vigorous cardiorespiratory activity and moderately challenging strength and muscular endurance exercises. This kind of program will give you the energy and stamina for activities such as competing in an intramural league, bicycle touring, doing step aerobics, and lifeguarding at a pool. People who wish to be more highly conditioned and compete at a higher level reach an even higher level of physical fitness. High-intensity activities and competitive sports offer little additional advantage in terms of health benefits; in fact, musculoskeletal injuries are more common. They do, however, offer excitement, challenge, and fulfillment. Some people thrive on pushing themselves to the limit and some enjoy the intensity of high-level competition. There is something for everyone within the scope of fitness—and health benefits are part of the package at every level.

Social, Emotional, Spiritual, and Mental Benefits

Exercise is something that most people enjoy doing with others. You can transform a lonely day into a pleasant one just by inviting a friend to go for a walk. Many corporations and hotels have established walking trails for their employees and customers. Parks, community pools, hiking trails, and dance classes are wonderful places to meet active, energetic people who share your interests.

Exercise lifts your spirits. Aerobic exercises in particular (walking, swimming, rowing) may help ease depression and reduce stress.[10,11] If you are exercising outdoors, the bright sunlight is good for your mental outlook. Studies show that people who spend time in bright light are less apt to be depressed.[12] Sunlight is 1,200 times brighter than normal indoor light, so if your job or studies keep you indoors most of the time, an outdoor event may be the spirit booster you need.

Aerobic exercise is also believed to increase the number of endorphins circulating in your bloodstream. **Endorphins** are natural painkillers thought to

1. Calculate the minimum number of calories you need to burn through exercise to ensure exercise-related health benefits.

   Examples

   110-lb person × 1.35 = 150 calories

   222-lb person × 1.35 = 300 calories

   148-lb person × 1.35 = 200 calories

   _____ × 1.35 = _____ calories
   your body weight

2. Identify one or more physical activities you like to do and find the number of calories per pound per minute that activity burns by looking at Table 2.2.

Activity	**cal/lb/min**
_____	_____
_____	_____
_____	_____

   Example

   Moderate-intensity bicycling = 0.049 cal/lb/min

3. Calculate the number of calories you will burn per minute doing your activity of choice by multiplying your weight in pounds by the number of cal/lb/min.

   Example

   110 lb × 0.049 cal/lb/min (bicycling) = 5.39 cal/min

   _____ × _____ = _____ cal/min
   your wt   cal/lb/min/ for
              activity of choice

4. Calculate the number of minutes you will need to perform your activity by dividing the number of calories you calculated in Step 1 by the calories per minute you calculated in Step 2.

   Example

   150 calories ÷ 5.39 cal/min = 28 minutes

   _____ calories ÷ _____ cal/min = _____ minutes

   _____ calories ÷ _____ cal/min = _____ minutes

be responsible for the euphoric feeling many people feel after exercising. This good feeling is often referred to as the "runner's high," but it is not limited to runners or to running; any aerobic activity can produce it. It may take you six to eight weeks of doing regular exercise before you experience this "high." Unfortunately, many people stop their program before then. Those who have exercised enough to experience this feeling of well-being often continue exercising because of it. So, you might begin exercising to "look good" but your motivation to keep exercising may also become to "feel good." For some individuals, spiritual insights are

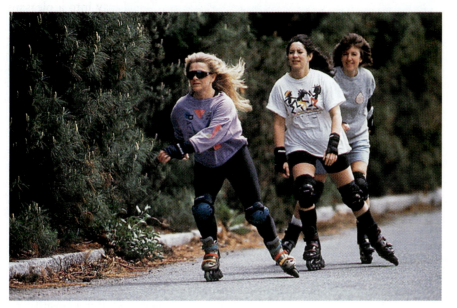

Whether exercising alone or with friends, the realized benefits are numerous.

TABLE 2.2 ■ Summary of Sports and Activities

This table classifies sports and activities as high (H), moderate (M), or low (L) in terms of their ability to develop each of the five components of physical fitness. The skill level needed to obtain fitness benefits is noted: Low (L) means little or no skill is required to obtain fitness benefits; moderate (M) means average skill is needed to obtain fitness benefits; and high (H) means much skill is required to obtain fitness benefits. The fitness prerequisite—conditioning needs of a beginner—is also noted: Low (L) means no fitness prerequisite is required; moderate (M) means some preconditioning is required; and high (H) means substantial fitness is required. The last two columns list the calorie cost of each activity when performed moderately and vigorously.

Components
CRE: cardiorespiratory endurance
BC: body composition
MS: muscular strength
ME: muscular endurance
F: flexibility

Sports and Activities	COMPONENTS					Skill Level	Fitness Prerequisite	APPROXIMATE CALORIE COST (CAL/LB/MIN)	
	CRE	BC	MS[a]	ME[a]	F[a]			Moderate	Vigorous
Aerobic dance	H	H	M	H	H	L	L	0.046	0.062
Backpacking	H	H	M	H	M	L	M	0.032	0.078
Badminton, skilled, singles	H	H	M	M	M	M	M	—	0.071
Ballet (floor combinations)	M	M	M	H	H	M	L	—	0.058
Ballroom dancing	M	M	L	M	L	M	L	0.034	0.049
Baseball (pitcher and catcher)	M	M	M	H	M	H	M	0.039	—
Basketball, half court	H	H	M	H	M	M	M	0.045	0.071
Bicycling	H	H	M	H	M	M	L	0.049	0.071
Bowling	L	L	L	L	L	L	L	—	—
Calisthenic circuit training	H	H	M	H	M	L	L	—	0.060
Canoeing and kayaking (flat water)	M	M	M	H	M	M	M	0.045	
Cheerleading	M	M	M	M	M	M	L	0.033	0.049
Cross-country skiing	H	H	M	H	M	M	M	0.049	0.104
Fencing	M	M	M	H	H	M	L	0.032	0.078
Field hockey	H	H	M	H	M	M	M	0.052	0.078
Folk and square dancing	M	M	L	M	L	L	L	0.039	0.049
Football, touch	M	M	M	M	M	M	M	0.049	0.078
Frisbee, ultimate	H	H	M	H	M	M	M	0.049	0.078
Golf (riding cart)	L	L	L	L	M	L	L	—	—
Handball, skilled, singles	H	H	M	H	M	M	M	—	0.078
Hiking	H	H	M	H	L	L	M	0.051	0.073
Hockey, ice and roller	H	H	M	H	M	M	M	0.052	0.078

Source: Adapted from *Your guide to getting fit,* by Ivan Kusinitz and Morton Fine, Table 7.1. Copyright © 1991 by Mayfield Publishing Company. Reprinted by permission of the publisher.
[a]Ratings are for the muscle groups involved.

gained through challenging physical activity. A healthy body also frees you to concentrate on mental and spiritual events.

In addition to lowering stress, physical activity may help clear your mind. People who exercise will tell you that they feel refreshed and ready to tackle problems after a workout. Solutions or creative ideas may even come to you while you are physically active.

Being toned and fit usually helps you to feel better about yourself—you are doing something positive to

TABLE 2.2 ■ **Summary of Sports and Activities** (*continued*)

Sports and Activities	CRE	BC	MS[a]	ME[a]	F[a]	Skill Level	Fitness Prerequisite	APPROXIMATE CALORIE COST (CAL/LB/MIN) Moderate	Vigorous
Horseback riding	M	M	M	M	L	M	M	0.052	0.065
Interval circuit training	H	H	H	H	M	L	L	—	0.062
Jogging and running	H	H	M	H	L	L	L	0.060	0.104
Judo	M	M	H	H	M	M	L	0.049	0.090
Karate	H	H	M	H	H	L	M	0.049	0.090
Lacrosse	H	H	M	H	M	H	M	0.052	0.078
Modern dance (moving combinations)	M	M	M	H	H	L	L	—	0.058
Orienteering	H	H	M	H	L	L	M	0.049	0.078
Outdoor fitness trails	H	H	M	H	M	L	L	—	0.060
Popular dancing	M	M	L	M	M	M	L	—	0.049
Racquetball, skilled, singles	H	H	M	M	M	M	M	0.049	0.078
Rock climbing	M	M	H	H	H	H	M	0.033	0.033
Rope skipping	H	H	M	H	L	M	M	0.071	0.095
Rowing	H	H	H	H	H	L	L	0.032	0.097
Rugby	H	H	M	H	M	M	M	0.052	0.097
Sailing	L	L	L	M	L	M	L	—	—
Skating, ice and roller	M	M	M	H	M	H	M	0.049	0.065
Skiing, alpine	M	M	H	H	M	H	M	0.039	0.078
Soccer	H	H	M	H	M	M	M	0.052	0.097
Squash, skilled, singles	H	H	M	M	M	M	M	0.049	0.078
Stretching	L	L	L	L	H	L	L	—	—
Surfing (including swimming)	M	M	M	M	M	H	M	—	0.078
Swimming	H	H	M	H	M	M	L	0.032	0.088
Synchronized swimming	M	M	M	H	H	H	M	0.032	0.052
Table tennis	M	M	L	M	M	M	L	—	0.045
Tennis, skilled, singles	H	H	M	M	M	M	M	—	0.071
Volleyball	M	M	L	M	M	M	M	—	0.065
Walking	H	H	L	M	L	L	L	0.029	0.048
Water polo	H	H	M	H	M	H	M	—	0.078
Water skiing	M	M	M	H	M	H	M	0.039	0.055
Weight training	L	M	H	H	H	L	L	—	—
Wrestling	H	H	H	H	H	H	H	0.065	0.094
Yoga	L	L	L	M	H	H	L	—	—

take care of yourself and you like the way you look. Having a good self-image gives you more confidence.

Our bodies were designed to be active, and as the technological revolution continues to make our physical life easier and our stress higher, we need an outlet. Physiologically, our bodies respond the same way when facing a menacing tiger or confronting the challenge of a difficult examination. In both cases, fear results in a pounding pulse, sweaty palms, an adrenaline rush, blood surging to our muscles: a general gearing up for "fight or flight." Although we might want to, we seldom run screaming from a test or deadline; instead, we typically bottle up our anxiety. If your body continually suppresses all this sense of "readiness for action," you eventually retaliate with things

Benefits of Physical Activity

Skeletal System

Increases bone density and strength.

Helps prevent osteoporosis (brittle bones).

Helps maintain good bone alignment, which is especially important to the spine.

Cardiovascular System

Decreases blood pressure.

Decreases blood cholesterol. Increases HDL.

Decreases risk of cardiovascular disease.

Decreases resting heart rate (workload on the heart).

Increases cardiac muscle strength.

Increases the number of capillaries.

Increases systemic and coronary circulation.

Increases blood/oxygen exchange to muscles.

Increases aerobic capacity.

Increases stroke volume (the amount of blood the heart ejects in one beat).

Increases the functional capacity of asthmatics.

Respiratory System

Increases lung capacity.

Increases blood/oxygen exchange in the lungs.

Increases waste removal efficiency (CO_2).

Muscular System

Increases muscular efficiency and coordination (neuromuscular benefit).

Increases strength and/or endurance.

Increases muscle size (to a greater extent in men than women).

Increases the ability of the muscle to use oxygen.

Increases fiber length.

Reproductive System

May enhance sexual pleasure due to increased muscular flexibility, endurance, and control.

May result in healthier babies, and fewer complications during birth.

May result in a speedier recovery after giving birth.

Nervous System

In combination with the muscular system, increases muscular efficiency and coordination.

Increases motor skill.

Other

Increases regular digestion and excretion.

Improves sleep quality.

Psychological Benefits

Improves self-image, self-concept.

Decreases stress.

May decrease depression and anxiety.

Increases endorphins, sense of well-being.

May provide a means for increasing socialization.

---

like ulcers or headaches. A good way to rid yourself of anxiety and stress is literally to take flight—by running, cycling, swimming, or doing whatever physical activity feels good to you. (Less vigorous activities like gardening and walking the dog can also ease tension.) Some people would rather fight, by joining a boxing club, taking part in combat aerobics, doing battle on the basketball court, or conquering a mountain. The key is to provide your body a physiological release.

Physical Benefits

The human body is made up of a set of intricately engineered and fantastically coordinated systems. Each of these systems is in some way influenced and benefited by exercise. The many benefits of physical activity and exercise on the cardiovascular, respiratory, skeletal, and muscular systems are summarized in the box above, but are not addressed here because they have already been mentioned in the discussion on health-related fitness and will be elaborated on in detail in Chapters 3 through 6. Instead, let us mention some of the benefits to other body systems. Exercise enhances the nervous system's ability to coordinate its signals, and as a result improves muscular efficiency and coordination. Exercise benefits the reproductive system in several ways. There is some evidence that more-fit mothers have healthier babies, experience fewer complications during birth, and have speedier recoveries after giving birth. Exercise may also enhance sexual pleasure because it increases muscular flexibility, endurance, and control. It is also believed to increase regular digestion and excretion.

Regular physical activity has some very important influences on the five modifiable risk factors for coronary heart failure. A sedentary lifestyle is obviously eliminated. High blood cholesterol and hypertension are lowered as the cardiorespiratory system is improved. Body fat decreases and obesity can in time be eliminated. Finally, exercise can help people quit smoking by acting as a substitute activity, one that helps keep one's mind off smoking and eating. Some people tend to eat more when they quit smoking. Exercise can help burn some of these unwanted calories and help prevent calorie consumption by offering an activity that is usually not associated with food.

One final physical benefit of exercise—the better shape you are in, the more likely you are to survive an accident or trauma and the more able you are to fight illness and disease. It makes sense that healthy lungs, heart, bones, and muscles are an asset during illness or injury. It takes a lot more to knock down a well-fortified wall than it does to fell a poorly maintained one.

Exercise and Asthma

Asthma is a disease in which the muscles surrounding the airways constrict, causing shortness of breath, wheezing, and coughing. Allergies, infections, emotion, and exercise can trigger an attack. When exercise is the trigger, the condition is called exercise-induced asthma (EIA). The labored breathing caused by bronchial constriction may discourage people with asthma from exercising. But research has shown that for most asthmatics, aerobic exercise improves their cardiorespiratory system, which in turn raises the exertion level at which symptoms begin to occur. Therefore, people with controlled asthma can and should exercise. If you have asthma, consult with your physician before beginning an exercise program. If you experience EIA, try to recognize early symptoms and then lower your intensity or take a break. If you use a bronchodialator medication, keep it with you and use it at the first sign of wheezing. Long, gradual warm-ups and cool-downs may ease symptoms. Drink plenty of fluids and be particularly careful on days in which environmental conditions are more likely to trigger an attack, such as hot or cold, high-pollen-count, or smog-alert days. Set an appropriate exercise intensity in consultation with your physician and instructor and then work to gradually increase your symptom-free exercise time.

Exercise and Diabetes

Diabetes mellitus is a metabolic disease in which the pancreas fails to produce sufficient insulin (Type I) or the body is unable to use the insulin it does produce (Type II). Insulin's role is to regulate the amount of sugar (glucose) in the blood. Regular moderate exercise helps persons with diabetes maintain normal blood glucose levels and in some cases may reduce the need for insulin. Many diabetics are overweight and have an elevated risk for heart disease; exercise helps control body fat and lowers heart disease risk. If you have diabetes and are beginning or changing your exercise program, discuss it with your physician so that it can be part of an integrated health plan. Some exercise guidelines include the following:

- Avoid exercising on an empty stomach. Exercise one to two hours after a meal and eat something like crackers and juice about half an hour before exercising. Carry a rapid-acting carbohydrate snack in order to prevent low blood sugar incidence.
- Know when and where to take insulin shots. Shots prior to exercise in a major muscle may result in faster circulation and absorption than desired.

- Wear good socks and keep your feet dry. See a doctor immediately if you experience foot problems.
- Try to exercise at the same time of day (avoid peak insulin times).
- Wear a medical alert tag and tell friends (instructors) you are diabetic.

THE METABOLIC SYSTEMS: TURNING FOOD INTO ENERGY

Because nutrition and exercise are intricately intertwined, it is helpful to understand how foods are used to produce energy for movement. The metabolic systems, often referred to as the body's energy systems, convert the food you eat into chemical energy. Muscle cells then convert this chemical energy into mechanical energy to produce movement. Different energy systems metabolize different nutrients. In order to get the most out of your body you need to combine the right foods with the right exercises. Being able to match exercises and foods with energy systems will help you know how to lose fat and how to gain muscle. For example, to maximize fat loss you need low-fat foods and exercises that use a fat-burning energy system. Energy systems can be trained and improved just like muscles and the result is more efficient movement and improved performance.

The food you eat is digested and chemically processed to produce adenosine triphosphate (ATP), a high-energy phosphate molecule that, when split, releases energy for your body's cells. Muscle cells use ATP to fuel the contraction process. Movement is possible as long as ATP is available. ("Rigor mortis" occurs when ATP is not available!) There are two types of metabolic systems that produce ATP: aerobic and anaerobic.

The intensity and duration of activity you are engaged in determine how much energy each system produces. It is important to note that no activity is run purely by one system or the other. When an activity is referred to as "aerobic," that means the energy for movement is predominantly, but not exclusively, supplied through aerobic metabolism. When you perform exercises that emphasize aerobic metabolism, you get a different kind of conditioning than when you emphasize anaerobic metabolism. Familiarity with each of the metabolic systems can help you select activities to reach your fitness goals.

Anaerobic Metabolism

Anaerobic means "without oxygen." During short, intense bursts of activity, such as running up a flight of stairs, the body cannot meet the muscles' demand for oxygen. For this situation, the body is equipped with two energy-producing systems that do not depend on oxygen: the phosphagen and lactic acid systems. These anaerobic systems are rapid sources of ATP for short periods of time. In a sense, the cells are making energy while they hold their breath.

Phosphagen System

The most rapid anaerobic system is called the phosphagen system. This form of stored energy is used to get you going at the beginning of exercise, especially if you start quickly. It also allows you to leap out of your seat when someone yells "Free concert tickets!" Small amounts of high-energy phosphagens are stored directly in the muscle cell. As ATP is broken down, the high-energy phosphagens build it back up. The muscle can store only enough high-energy phosphagens to produce ATP for one to six seconds of activity. Training this system is only important if you want to compete in sports such as weight lifting or sprinting. The lactic acid and aerobic systems are much more important to lifetime fitness. As the phosphagen system is depleted, the lactic acid system (also known as anaerobic glycolysis) takes over as the main energy producer.

Lactic Acid System

The lactic acid system produces ATP by breaking down carbohydrate (glucose) without oxygen. Along with energy, lactic acid and heat are produced. If the anaerobic activity is intense enough, the lactic acid builds up and makes the muscle feel heavy and "burn." The buildup of lactic acid is associated with muscle exhaustion.

When you stop exercising or drop to a lower intensity, the concentration of lactic acid decreases. The excess heat is dissipated through sweat. You breathe hard after an anaerobic bout of exercise because your body requires oxygen to clear up the lactic acid and to return the cardiorespiratory system to homeostasis.

Activities that depend on anaerobic metabolism for energy are usually short, intense, and powerful. Predominantly anaerobic activities last for less than a minute. Sprints and strength-training exercises are examples of anaerobic exercises. Many exercises are partly anaerobic and partly aerobic. Anaerobic glycolysis also plays a major role in intense activities that last for one to three minutes. People like Bonnie Blair, an Olympic gold medalist in speed skating, who can perform well in a middle-distance event, must be in both excellent anaerobic and aerobic shape.

A number of exercise benefits are associated with anaerobic training. The most important are muscular strength and endurance and cardiorespiratory fitness. The latter is achieved using interval training, which involves a series of short intense bouts of exercise, such as sprints. Only short breaks are allowed between bouts. Since anaerobic training increases tolerance to lactic acid, someone in good anaerobic condition can sustain high-intensity activity for longer than someone who is not.

Aerobic Metabolism

The aerobic system produces energy more slowly than the anaerobic systems, but it is capable of producing more energy per unit of food. **Aerobic** means "with oxygen." The aerobic system breaks down carbohydrate (aerobic glycolysis) and fat (fatty acid oxidation) in the presence of oxygen to produce ATP (energy), carbon dioxide, water, and heat. Carbon dioxide is transported by the blood to the lungs, where it is exhaled from the body. Heat and water are released primarily through sweat.

It is easiest for the body to metabolize carbohydrate, so that is the primary source of fuel for the aerobic system. When the body is convinced that it will have to meet an elevated energy demand for a long period of time, it will conserve carbohydrate and use fat. It takes more energy to burn fat than carbohydrate, but fat is a much richer source of energy. The burning of fat is called fatty acid oxidation, also called beta oxidation.

Fatty acid oxidation must be coaxed into operation. To benefit from this process you need to exercise for at least 20 minutes. If your goal is to burn fat, you would benefit more from exercising for a longer time at a moderate intensity than for a short time at a high intensity. High-intensity activities primarily burn carbohydrate whereas low-to-moderate-intensity activities burn both fat and carbohydrate. Low-intensity activities tend to burn a higher percentage of fat but also fewer calories per minute than moderate-intensity activities. As a result you must sustain a low-intensity activity for a longer period of time than a moderate one in order to burn the same amount of fat. For example, you would have to walk longer than jog to get the same fat-burning benefit.

Fat and carbohydrate are both being burned at rest and during exercise, but the percentages of each and the overall consumption of each vary with the intensity of activity. While longer-duration activity is more apt to result in fat burning, any activity that burns calories will help prevent storage of fat. If you burn more calories than you take in, you will encourage fat loss and discourage fat storage.

Aerobic exercises are continuous, rhythmic activities using large-muscle groups. Swimming, cycling, brisk walking, cross-country skiing, and "fast" dancing are all aerobic activities. The many health benefits associated with aerobic conditioning are discussed in more detail in the chapter on cardiorespiratory fitness. Cardiorespiratory endurance, weight management, and muscle endurance are some benefits of aerobic training.

Aerobic fitness cannot guarantee you a long, healthy life (you could be hit by a bus tomorrow), but it does increase your odds of longevity and allows you to function more efficiently and independently throughout your life. The physical dimension is only one part of the wellness equation. If you want to change your lifestyle, developing and sticking to a physical activity program is one of the best things you can do. Physical health is a strong foundation for overall well-being. And as you have learned, the health benefits of physical activity can be attained through simple, regular physical activity.

GETTING OFF TO A GOOD START

Medical Clearance

It is important to make sure "all systems are go" before you start a new activity or launch into an exercise program. If you have any special conditions or health concerns, discuss them with your doctor first. Before you embark on a vigorous exercise plan, have a thorough medical examination with a stress test performed by a physician if you are a male over 40, a female over 50 years of age, or have a chronic disease or risk factors for chronic disease.

Dress for Success: What to Wear

The type of clothing and corresponding equipment will vary a great deal depending on the activities you select. For example, the difference between gardening, weight-lifting, golf, bowling, and cycling gloves is considerable!

Physical Activity Readiness
Questionnaire - PAR-Q
(revised 1994)

PAR - Q & YOU

Regular physical activity is fun and healthy, and increasingly more people are starting to become more active every day. Being more active is very safe for most people. However, some people should check with their doctor before they start becoming much more physically active.

If you are planning to become much more physically active than you are now, start by answering the seven questions in the box below. If you are between the ages of 15 and 69, the PAR-Q will tell you if you should check with your doctor before you start. If you are over 69 years of age, and you are not used to being very active, check with your doctor.

Common sense is your best guide when you answer these questions. Please read the questions carefully and answer each one honestly: check YES or NO.

YES	NO	
☐	☐	1. Has your doctor ever said that you have a heart condition <u>and</u> that you should only do physical activity recommended by a doctor?
☐	☐	2. Do you feel pain in your chest when you do physical activity?
☐	☐	3. In the past month, have you had chest pain when you were not doing physical activity?
☐	☐	4. Do you lose your balance because of dizziness or do you ever lose consciousness?
☐	☐	5. Do you have a bone or joint problem that could be made worse by a change in your physical activity?
☐	☐	6. I your doctor currently prescribing drugs (for example, water pills) for you blood pressure or heart condition?
☐	☐	7. Do you know of <u>any other reason</u> why you should not do physical activity?

If you answered

YES to one or more questions

Talk with your doctor by phone or in person BEFORE you start becoming much more physically active or BEFORE you have a fitness appraisal. Tell your doctor about the PAR-Q and which questions you answered YES.

- You may be able to do any activity you want — as long as you start slowly and build up gradually. Or, you may need to restrict your activities to those which are safe for you. Talk with your doctor about the kinds of activities you wish to participate in and follow his/her advice.
- Find out which community programs are safe and helpful for you.

NO to all questions

If you answered NO honestly to <u>all</u> PAR-Q questions, you can be reasonably sure that you can:
- start becoming much more physically active—begin slowly and build up gradually. This is the safest and easiest way to go.
- take part in a fitness appraisal — this is an excellent way to determine your basic fitness so that you can plan the best way for you to live actively.

DELAY BECOMING MUCH MORE ACTIVE:
- if you are not feeling well because of a temporary illness such as a cold or a fever — wait until you feel better; or
- if you are or may be pregnant — talk to your doctor before you start becoming more active.

Please note: If your health changes so that you then answer YES to any of the above questions, tell your fitness or health professional. Ask whether you should change your physical activity plan.

FIGURE 2.3 Physical activity readiness questionnaire (PAR-Q). Before increasing your activity, take a minute to answer these questions and follow up as recommended. (Reprinted by permission from the 1994 revised version of the Physical Activity Readiness Questionnaire (PAR-Q and YOU). The PAR-Q and YOU is a copyrighted, pre-exercise screen owned by the Canadian Society for Exercise Physiology.)

BARRIER Busters

I don't have time.

- Use the 7 minutes of commercial time between TV programs.
- Get friends or family involved so that it is also social time.
- Build activity into your daily routine.
- Make time; this may require a shift in priorities.

I'm too tired.

- Pick a time of day when you won't be exhausted or interrupted.
- Stick with the program long enough to feel the energy boost.
- Put on some energizing music while you put on your exercise clothes.
- Rethink your lifestyle—why are you tired?
- If you are getting sick, take the day off, guilt-free.

I don't like sports.

- There are many activities that are not sport-related.
- One of the new sports like inline skating may appeal to you.
- Be active not to acquire sport skills but for health-related reasons.

I've gotten this far without exercise.

- Is the quality of your life what you want?
- The effects of aging can be delayed by being active now.
- Are there any activities you'd like to be doing but aren't in good enough shape to do?

I don't see any reason to exercise since I never get hurt and feel fine.

- Prevent injuries, especially low-back pain, before they occur.
- Maintain full joint movement as function may be lost as you get older.

I've exercised before with no results.

- Did you follow the fitness concepts presented here?
- Were you involved in a quality program?
- Did you stay with it long enough to get results?
- Make sure your technique and exercises are correct.

Exercise hurts.

- See a physician and find out whether there is any way to control the pain and any activities that would be recommended for your condition.
- Make sure you are using proper techniques.
- Substitute exercises or activities that don't hurt for those that do.
- Perform a good warm-up and cool-down to minimize exercise-related soreness.

I hate getting sweaty.

- Swim.
- Do lower-level activity interspersed throughout the day.

Seek out an expert for activity-specific needs. Here are a few guidelines:

1. Wear nonrestrictive clothing that allows heat and moisture to escape. Nylon does not breathe; cotton, Lycra, and Spandex do.
2. Wear supportive undergarments, such as a sports bra or an athletic supporter.
3. Wear layers of clothing so that you can peel off layers as you get hot and add layers as you get cold.
4. Wear comfortable and supportive shoes.

The technology behind shoe design in the 1990s is remarkable; if you can afford a quality shoe made for a specific activity, you will be getting the best design and support. If you cannot afford a closet full of shoes, a good cross-training shoe is usually the way to go. With cross-training shoes, you can play volleyball one day and cycle the next, wearing the same footwear. These shoes are designed to be effective for a number of sports activities. Quality cross-training shoes provide good lateral stability, shock absorption, and arch support. They are excellent for walking and for court games like volleyball, tennis, and racquetball. They do not, however, supply enough shock absorption or have a flared enough heel for jogging. Nor do they have enough forefoot shock absorption for aerobic dance. Buying shoes designed especially for these activities is your best bet.

Goal Setting

Goal setting is an integral part of getting yourself started on the way to physical fitness. An individual's goals determine the exercise program. As you proceed through this book, setting goals will help keep you headed in the right direction. The following steps will be helpful to you.

Steps to Goal Writing

1. In general terms, decide what it is you want to do.
   Example: I want to lose weight.
2. Assess where you are right now.
   Example: I will measure, or have a professional measure, my percentage body fat.
3. Make your general goal more specific, using information from your assessment (Step 2).

- Plan enough time after exercising for a hot shower or bath. Early morning or evening usually work best.

I'm embarrassed to exercise in front of people.

- Start with a walking program or something like step aerobics that can be done in your home. When you feel more comfortable you can join a group if you want.
- If you can afford it, go with one-on-one training to boost your confidence or slim down your figure.
- Wear baggy, comfortable clothing.

There is no convenient place to exercise.

- Select activities that can be done in or near your home: walking, jump roping, exercise machine, step aerobics.

There is no safe place to exercise.

- Organize a group of people. For example, work out with coworkers in the lobby after hours.
- Exercise in your home or walk at the mall or join a club.
- Walk or jog around the perimeter of a field where recreational or school teams are practicing.

I don't have a partner or friend who can exercise with me.

- Select activities that can be performed alone.
- Join a club and meet others.
- Ask around; maybe someone will surprise you and join you.

I have too many family obligations.

- Make one of the obligations to exercise together.
- Intersperse activity throughout your day.

I have nothing to wear.

- Wear what's comfortable and serviceable—don't be overly concerned about fashion.
- Make the first step of your activity plan to select or buy some exercise clothes.
- Lay out your exercise clothing the night before.

It's too cold or rainy today. I'll do it (start) tomorrow.

- Plan an alternative indoor activity ahead of time so when the bad weather hits you are ready. For example, mall walk, exercise machine such as a treadmill, house repairs or cleaning, especially things that take you up and down stairs.

I just can't seem to get started.

- Post your starting date in a visible place.
- Get your clothes ready ahead of time.
- Start small and work your way up.
- Find a partner and make a pact.
- Join a program that appeals to you.

Example: I want to move from 30 percent body fat to 24 percent body fat.

4. Decide how you are going to accomplish your goal.
   Example: I will combine three days of walking and three days of low impact aerobics with my present weight-loss diet.

5. Add a time frame:
   Example: I will lower my body fat by 6 percent in the next six weeks. (For a woman weighing 100 to 200 pounds this represents a 6 to 12 pound loss, a 1 to 2 pound per week loss.)

6. Write a very specific goal incorporating all the information from the first five steps.
   Example: I will lose 5 percent body fat in the next six weeks, using thirty minutes of brisk walking on Tuesday, Thursday, and Saturday and attending a low-impact aerobics class on Monday, Wednesday, and Friday. I will combine this with my present 1500-calorie balanced diet.

7. Decide how you will evaluate and monitor your progress.
   Example: I will have my body fat taken again in six weeks.

PLANNING YOUR EXERCISE SESSION

Whether you engage in moderate or vigorous physical activity and whether it is an exercise workout or an activity like building a drama set, you'll want to apply a few fundamental program components and principles of physical activity. For example, a warm-up should precede vigorous or heavy exercise. If you are practicing for an intramural soccer game this would mean having a thorough warm-up before running difficult plays or demanding conditioning drills. If you are building the drama set, warm up your back, arms, and legs by doing light work before you move the heavy pieces.

Components of a Physical Activity Session

The following terms have been applied primarily to exercise but they can apply to any physical activity. Exertion is exertion whether it is formal exercise or an activity you are trying to accomplish. An exercise plan is a more formal attempt to include moderate to vigorous activity in your life. The basic parts of an exercise plan and some principles of exercise are explained here.

Physical exertion should start off easily, get progressively harder, and then taper down again. The most difficult or demanding part of your activity should be in the middle, when you are thoroughly warmed up and not yet fatigued. Then do a good cool-down to give your body a chance to recover and to prevent muscle soreness. Here are some suggestions for each of these components.

Warm-up

The **warm-up** is a series of movements and stretches to prepare your body for activity. Start off slowly and gradually build up to a brisk pace. This gives your body a chance to adjust. If your muscles are tight from sitting in class, working at a desk, bending over machinery, or sitting in a car, they need to be awakened, warmed up, and stretched out. If you like to exercise early in the morning or are physically active at an early morning job, the warm-up is even more important, since your muscles have been inactive all night.

First, you literally need to make your body warm. Easy, active movements, possibly performed to energizing music, start the blood circulating and raise the body's temperature.

Work up to a moderate pace. You want to move vigorously enough to raise your body temperature and increase circulation but not so fast that momentum carries your limbs beyond a comfortable range of motion. Walking, light jogging, easy dance steps, and light arm work are all good body-warming activities.

As muscles warm up, they become more elastic. Warm muscles are also capable of more forceful and rapid movements than cold muscles and are less vulnerable to injury. Starting slowly gives the cardiorespiratory system time to adjust gradually to the increasing oxygen demand of the muscles. Sudden vigorous activity is hard on your body, and the shunting of blood to the muscles may leave you light-headed. Just think how you feel when you sprint to catch a bus or quickly jump out of the way of danger. A good warm-up prevents this jarring feeling. Work with smooth movements—flowing, sustained movements allow your body to comfortably make the transition from being sedentary to being active.

Warm-up activity also signals the release of synovial fluid. This fluid, secreted into the joints, acts as a lubricant. Much like the Tin Man in *The Wizard of Oz*, you need to "oil up your joints." Start out with small movements, and as the joints and muscles respond, work up to larger ones. For example, start a shoulder warm-up by just lifting and rotating your shoulders while your arms hang relaxed at your sides. Next, do a circling motion with your arms, letting your elbows draw the circle. Last, work the circles with straight, but not locked, arms.

The warm-up is also a good time to prepare yourself mentally for exercise. Set aside the worries of the day and focus on the positive aspects of the activity ahead. For some people, physical activity represents a time for quiet contemplation, for others a chance to socialize or turn on loud music and blow off steam.

The second part of the warm-up consists of stretching exercises. Although experts disagree on the importance of stretching before an activity, many people feel more ready for exertion after stretching. Professionals do agree that flexibility is important and that stretching after physical activity will develop flexibility, which in turn improves physical performance and reduces the risk of injury.[13] If the activity you are about to engage in is vigorous, you will probably want to do some prestretching. If the activity is less vigorous, such as walking, stretch beforehand if it feels good to you. Many people enjoy interspersing stretches with warm-up movements. For example, you can walk for a few minutes, stop and stretch a little, walk some more, stretch some more, and perform arm circles while walking. It usually takes 5 to 10 minutes to warm up, although longer warm-ups may be required for highly demanding activity and/or cold days. More detailed information on stretching can be found in Chapter 4.

The Workout

The workout is the main activity you plan to do and for which you have been preparing by warming up. It should be a natural extension of the warm-up. Gradually continue to increase the intensity of the activity until you reach the level at which you wish to work out. An exercise workout might include one or more of the following components: flexibility, muscle strengthening, muscle endurance, or cardiorespiratory endurance. Your personal needs determine the specifics of your own exercise plan. For general health, it is usually recommended that you perform some type of aerobic workout as well as activities that strengthen and stretch the major muscle groups.

If physical fitness is one of your goals, your workout needs to incorporate the elements of an approach called the FIT Principle.

The FIT Principle. A workout can be defined by three variables: **Frequency (F)**, **Intensity (I)**, and **Time (T)** or FIT (see Chapter 3 for a more in-depth discussion). Sometimes "FIT" is expanded to "FITT" to include the Type (T) of activity you select. Performing more than one activity is called **cross training.** Cross training offers people the advantage of variety and of working different muscles in many ways. Participation in a variety of activities also helps keep motivation high.

As you plan a fitness workout, decide how many times a week you want to exercise. This is your exercise frequency. Then, using the goals you've set for yourself,

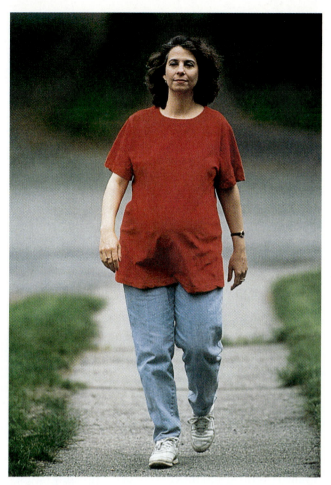

Pregnant women can continue to exercise and derive health benefits from even mild to moderate exercise.

out. However, remember that activities performed below target zone intensities are still worthwhile and can enhance your health if done regularly over a period of years.

Exercise and Pregnancy Exercise is a positive health habit that in most cases can be continued through pregnancy. It is important, however, to recognize the demands it places on a woman's body and to make adjustments accordingly. It is better to start an exercise program before pregnancy, but it is certainly possible to begin with light exercising during pregnancy. Women who have been exercising regularly prior to conception may be able to continue their program for a while as long as they make appropriate adjustments to their intensity and avoid contraindicated exercises. Most hospitals and other organizations offer special exercise programs for pregnant women. As pregnancy advances, many women prefer to take a class specifically designed for pregnant women or continue with a nonweight-bearing activity such as cycling or swimming. If you are pregnant or considering pregnancy, discuss an exercise plan with your physician. The American College of Obstetricians and Gynecologists (ACOG) has published exercise guidelines for healthy pregnant women. For a complete set of guidelines contact ACOG directly. See the resources list at the end of the chapter for their address.

These recommendations are intended for healthy women with normal pregnancies. Discuss pregnancy and exercise with your physician to determine if these guidelines apply to you or if they need to be modified. In some cases, exercise is not recommended, but usually with the right precautions, exercise can enhance your pregnancy and help you regain your shape after giving birth.

determine how hard or how intensely you will need to exercise. Finally, decide how much time you can afford to dedicate for each session. This will be the duration or length of your workout.

A minimum amount and intensity of exercise must be performed before fitness improvement begins. This minimum level of exercise is called the **threshold of training.** To improve your physical fitness, you must exercise above your threshold of training, which for a sedentary person is relatively low. As you become more fit, your threshold of training increases. However, beyond a certain amount of exercise and level of fitness, the benefits diminish and the risk of injury increases.

The optimal intensity range for exercise is called the **fitness target zone.** The lower limit of the zone is the threshold of training; the upper limit is the maximum amount of exercise that is beneficial. The best-known target zone is the one for cardiorespiratory endurance. However, target zones exist for each of the health-related components of fitness. The next three chapters will discuss how to adjust the frequency, intensity, and duration of your exercise so that you get the most out of your work-

Cool-Down

The **cool-down** is the activity that follows the workout; its purpose is to bring the body gradually back down to a resting state. During moderate to vigorous activity, a large portion of the blood (usually 30 to 50 percent but can be as high as 70 percent) circulates to the limbs to supply the big working muscles with oxygen. At the end of a workout, it is important to keep moving so the blood is returned to the heart and lungs to be reoxygenated instead of being pooled in the limbs. If you stop exercising suddenly, you might feel light-headed from the lack of oxygenated blood in the brain. In fact, fainting is your body's way of getting you level so that the blood doesn't have to be pushed against gravity to get back to the heart, reoxygenated, and circulated to the brain. There is no need to feel light-headed or dizzy following a workout; simply keep moving and gradually reduce your activity level. Avoid movements that cause you to drop your head, such as toe touches or squat thrusts, as they may cause light-headedness.

When you move the big muscles of your arms and legs during the cool-down, the muscles contract around

the veins and help push or massage the blood upward. This aids the venous pump, the system of moving blood up through the veins against gravity. Venous blood is pumped up through the veins by the pressure created from the heart's contractions. Between heartbeats (contractions), blood is held in its newly elevated position by one-way valves inside the veins. Muscle contractions added to the heart's contractions help move the blood more quickly, which in turn helps you recover more speedily.

After physical exertion, your body has to clear waste materials, replace stores of energy, and supply a still-elevated metabolic rate. For these reasons you will continue to need extra oxygen, which means you will breathe heavily and your heartbeat will continue to be elevated. As your bodily systems get caught up and reset, your breathing and heart rate will slow down and you will begin to cool off.

The actual movements and technique required for the cool-down are just like the warm-up, only you reverse the process. Start with big, active movements and slowly wind down to smaller, easier movements. Continue the cool-down until your breathing is back to normal and your pulse is less than 120 beats a minute.

Developmental Stretch

The **developmental stretch** is the last segment of an activity session (usually considered part of the cool-down). Its purpose is to relieve muscle tension and develop flexibility. The same stretches and stretch technique used during the warm-up are used for the closing stretch, with one exception: the stretches should be held longer. Although a 10-second hold may improve your flexibility, optimum stretching occurs when you hold for 20 to 60 seconds. One recommended regimen is to hold for 15 seconds, four times in a row. The best time to do this is at the end of the cool-down, since your cardiorespiratory system will have had time to recover but your muscle temperature is still high. Muscles will respond like warm taffy and stretch more easily.

If you are enrolled in an exercise class and have to leave early, step out of class with enough time to cool down. Using the same logic, if you arrive late, take the time to prepare your body for vigorous exercise. Although you may be tempted to jump right in, your body needs a little transition time.

Principles of Physical Activity

As you learn more about how to design an exercise program or as you become more involved in a new physical activity, keep the following general principles in mind. Applications of these principles will be provided in Chapters 3 to 5.

Principle of Individuality

Everyone is unique, including each person's response to exercise. The **principle of individuality** holds that no two people react exactly the same way to exercise. Two men with the ability to lift the same amount of weight can have significantly different muscle circumferences. Two women eating the same diet, attending the same exercise class, and working out at the same intensity will lose inches or pounds in different places at different rates. This means that the only person you can really compare yourself to is yourself. Your rate of progress and the way you progress is unique to you.

Many fitness tests provide norms, averages, or percentiles for you to compare your scores against. These are helpful guidelines, but they are not a "gold standard." Norms simply state what a tested group of people were able to do. For example, the norms for a sit-up test performed by athletes would be considerably higher than the norms for a sit-up test performed by senior citizens. The best fitness test norms are age-adjusted and are based on scores from large populations. The fitness tests included in this book were selected with these criteria in mind. Compare yourself to these norms, but most important, compare yourself to yourself.

Principle of Overload

When the human body is stressed repeatedly over a period of time, it responds by either adapting or breaking down. Good physical activity puts enough stress on the body to cause positive adaptations like muscle strength and movement efficiency. In physical fitness terms, stress is called overload and the concept of overloading (stressing) the body is called the **principle of overload.** Do not be fooled by the word "overload"; in this context it does not mean too much of something; proper overloading means placing a more than normal amount of stress on the body with the intent of safely achieving fitness gains. You can achieve overload in any of the following ways:

- To improve flexibility, the muscle is overloaded by being stretched longer than its normal length.
- To improve strength, overload is achieved by increasing the amount of resistance against which the muscle normally moves.
- To increase muscular endurance, overload is accomplished by repeatedly performing a movement more times than normal or by holding an isometric contraction for a longer period of time.
- To improve cardiorespiratory endurance, overload consists of placing a greater than normal demand on the heart and lungs through sustained aerobic activity.

When you overload, you are temporarily increasing the intensity of an exercise. As your body adapts, you experience a training effect, meaning that your body is adapting and the exercise is becoming easier. To continue to improve your physical fitness, you have to continue to overload. For example, if you can normally do ten push-ups, create an overload to the arm and chest muscles by doing eleven or twelve. When twelve becomes easy, overload again by doing thirteen or fourteen, and so on. When you reach your desired level of fitness you can stop overloading. To maintain your fitness level, continue to perform your new "normal" amount. Doing less than normal will result in deconditioning.

Overuse is a result of violating the principle of overload. When you overdo, you can incur injuries, especially chronic injuries such as shinsplints and tendinitis. Some people actually become addicted to exercise. One sign of addiction is the refusal to exercise fewer than seven days a week despite evidence that this much activity can be harmful. Addiction leads to overtraining. Overtraining, again, can result in chronic injuries and an elevated resting heart rate. Overuse may also be the result of a violation of the principle of individuality. A person trying to keep up with another person may overload too quickly. One hundred push-ups may be an appropriate load for one individual but may be overuse for another.

Principle of Progression

The **principle of progression** is an extension of the principle of overload; it means to overload gradually over a period of time. Too slow an increase will delay or prevent improvement. Too rapid an overload can make you stiff and sore or may even result in injury. Progression can be thought of as a staircase where each stair is a comfortable challenge. The phrase "progressive overload" is often used to describe the application of these principles. In the previous example of adding push-ups, the additional push-ups were the overload and the progression was the gradual addition of push-ups over a period of days or weeks.

Principle of Specificity

Would you ever practice stretching your shoulders so that you could touch your toes or do a set of curl-ups (sit-ups) to tone your legs? Of course not. You would select exercises designed to accomplish your goal. When you make these selections you are using the **principle of specificity,** which states that placing a specific demand on the body results in a specific adaptation.

If you create a demand on the body by doing strength exercises, the body adapts by building stronger muscles. If you create a demand by doing aerobic exercises, the body adapts by improving the cardiorespiratory system. The adaptation is specific to the demand.

Different occupations place different demands on the body. For instance, ice-cream scoopers have one arm that is stronger than the other, pianists have strong fingers, construction workers have well-developed shoulder and arm muscles, and aerobic dance instructors have toned muscles and healthy hearts. If an occupation creates muscle imbalances, like the ice-cream scooper with one stronger arm, a tailored exercise program can usually correct the imbalance.

Principle of Reversibility

Sometimes referred to as detraining or the use-disuse principle, the **principle of reversibility** is defined by the well-known phrase, "use it, or lose it." How fast and how much you lose depends upon a number of factors, including your training regimen, your present fitness level, and the type and length of disuse (bed rest, cast, or normal daily activity but no exercise). Roughly speaking, within two weeks of the time you stop, you will begin to lose cardiorespiratory conditioning. Strength losses tend to take longer. Competitive athletes can lose their edge even more quickly but some of this is due to a loss in skill performance (that is, timing) as opposed to physiological losses.

Once you are in good shape, you must continue to exercise hard enough to sustain it. If you don't, your body adapts to the new lower demands and begins to lose cardiorespiratory fitness, muscle tone, and flexibility. Nobody is protected from "losing it." Even varsity college athletes who stop exercising when they graduate are soon no better off than people who never exercised.[14] The only way to be fit is to keep moving!

Principles at Work

You might not know it, but you are probably an expert at using the principles of physical activity and exercise. For example, have you ever increased the frequency, intensity, or duration of a workout to make it more challenging? (overload and progression) Have you ever asked someone to teach you a better exercise to achieve a goal like a flatter abdomen or thinner thighs? (specificity) Have you ever wondered why your friend is adapting more quickly or more slowly than you are to certain types of exercise? (individuality) Have you ever noticed how you have more energy when you are on an exercise program than when you stop your program? (reversibility) Now you can consciously put these principles to work for you as you create, modify, or maintain your physical activity program. Plan a session using the exercise and nonexercise components of physical activity. Try to identify how each of the principles was incorporated or considered.

MAINTAINING AN EXERCISE PROGRAM

People start exercise programs full of energy and good intentions, but 30 to 70 percent of those who start drop out within six months. If you are a "fitness dropout," don't despair. Perhaps you set your goals too high at first. Review the guidelines and try again. If you have never started exercising consider how much you can benefit from even low-intensity activity. Changing a behavior, in this case adding or modifying your physical activity, is always a challenge. To help you stick with it, here are some suggestions for selecting activities. Choose activities that

- Are enjoyable
- Can be done near home, work, or campus
- Are financially comfortable
- Are supported by family and friends
- Are a natural extension of your daily routine

Assessment

Tracking your progress can be very motivational. Physical fitness can be assessed using expensive equipment in established exercise laboratories or through fairly simple field tests. While the first may be the more accurate, the latter provide good estimates of physical conditioning and are easy to administer. In many cases you can self-administer a test or accomplish it with the help of a friend. A set of assessment labs accompanies each of the fitness chapters that follows.

INJURY PREVENTION AND CARE

If you are in pursuit of health and fitness, there is no reason to beat your body into the ground. Leave the pain and agony to the professionals who are paid handsomely to put their bodies at risk. Some soreness at the beginning of a program is normal, but if you are hurt, exhausted, or run-down after a workout, something is wrong. You might feel temporarily tired, and then actually get a lift of energy from the workout.

When an injury occurs and the cause of injury can be identified, your activity, the equipment you are using, or the environment in which you are active can often be modified to eliminate or minimize the risk of injury. For example, if your shins hurt after a jog, you can (1) work to correct foot-plant technique errors that may be causing the problem, (2) purchase better shock-absorbing shoes, (3) run on more even surfaces, or (4) change to a nonimpact activity like cycling.

Strong and flexible muscles can prevent many injuries. For example, back pain can often be prevented or relieved by adopting a stretching and strengthening program. Good posture and exercise technique are also critical to injury prevention.

People beginning physical activity with a history of orthopedic problems run a slightly higher risk of injury. To reduce this elevated risk, they should start slowly, overload gradually, and avoid exercises that hurt. They should also get medical clearance before beginning a new activity.

Unfortunately, there will always be unforeseeable accidents. When an accident occurs, the best thing to do is to administer prompt, proper first aid. If you exercise at

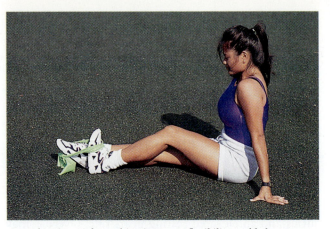

A good regimen of stretching improves flexibility and helps prevent injury. For example, stretching the shin muscles can help prevent shinsplints.

a gym or other facility, make sure they are prepared to handle emergency situations.

Learn how to put prevention in your program. Listed in Appendix C are some of the injuries that can occur during regular physical activity. The common causes, preventive actions, and proper first aid for each injury are given.

SUMMARY

Physical activity is a powerful change agent. By adding formal exercise or by adding moderately intense physical activity to your lifestyle, you can dramatically affect your health. As you work through the next three chapters, you will have an opportunity to assess your level of fitness, determine where you fall on the continuum of behavior change described in Chapter 1, and decide on your next steps.

Skill development is not as directly related to health but being skilled certainly makes sport activities enjoyable. This in turn provides motivation to be active. And physical activity leads to health. Health-related components of physical fitness are central to wellness, and developing skill may enhance activity adherence since people tend to stick to things they are good at and enjoy. The health-related components include cardiorespiratory fitness, muscular strength and endurance, flexibility, and body composition. The skill-related components are agility, balance, coordination, power, speed, and reaction time.

We live in the information age and knowing how and why something works enables you to decide if it is important and relevant to you. Knowing how the body works and how exercise works on the body will help you take responsibility for your own health. You can choose the benefits that are important to you and make sure that the exercises that result in those benefits are included in your activity or exercise program.

Behavior changes are most successful when you have "bought in," when you feel that the change is important for you and/or those around you. For this reason, one of the goals of this and the next three chapters is to supply you with quality information to help you make decisions about physical activity.

There are a lot of "right ways" to get or stay in shape. You can join an exercise class, lift weights, take a walk with your pet, go for a swim, fix the house, or choose the stairs rather than the escalator at the mall. Staying active is the key to physical wellness.

Here are the bottom lines:

1. Any type of activity is better than none. If you apply Nike's "Just Do It" saying to wellness, the "It" doesn't matter as much as the "Do."

2. Substantial health benefits (as much as 80 percent) can be achieved by performing moderately intense activity, as long as you do it for 30 minutes on most days.

3. Greater health benefits and cardiorespiratory endurance are achieved when you perform vigorous activities as compared to moderately intense activities.

SUGGESTED READING

American College of Sports Medicine. *Guidelines for exercise testing and prescription,* 4th ed. Philadelphia: Lea & Febiger, 1991.

American College of Sports Medicine. The recommended quantity and quality of exercise for developing and maintaining cardiorespiratory and muscular fitness in healthy adults. *Medicine and Science in Sports* 22(2):265–274, 1990.

Brunick, T. Choosing the right shoe. *The Physician and Sportsmedicine* 18(7):104, 1990.

Fletcher, G. F., et al. American Heart Association: Statement on exercise. *Circulation* 86:2726, 1992.

International Society of Sport Psychology. *Physical activity and psychological benefits: Position statement* 20:179, 1992.

Paffenbarger, R. S. Jr., R. T. Hyde, A. L. Wing, and C. C. Hsieh. Physical activity, all-cause mortality, and longevity of college alumni. *New England Journal of Medicine* 314:605–613, 1986.

Pate, R. R., et al. Physical activity and public health: A recommendation from the Centers for Disease Control and Prevention and the American College of Sports Medicine. *Journal of the American Medical Association* 273(5):402–407, 1995.

Shephard, R. J. *Aerobic fitness & health.* Champaign, IL: Human Kinetics, 1994.

U.S. Department of Health and Human Services. *Physical activity and health: A report of the Surgeon General.* Centers for Disease Control and Prevention, National Center for Chronic Disease Prevention and Health Promotion. Atlanta: The President's Council on Physical Fitness and Sports, 1996.

U.S. Department of Health and Human Services. *Healthy people 2000: National health promotion and disease prevention objectives.* DHHS Publication No. (PHS) 91-50213. Washington, D.C.: U.S. Government Printing Office, 1990.

Wilmore, J. H., and D. L. Costill. *Training for sport and activity: The physiological basis of the conditioning process,* 3rd ed. Champaign, IL: Human Kinetics, 1993.

RESOURCES

The American College of Obstetricians and Gynecologists
409 12th Street, S.W.
P.O. Box 96920
Washington, D.C. 20090–69200
www.acog.com

CHAPTER 3

Cardiorespiratory Endurance

Terms

- Cardiorespiratory endurance
- Heart rate
- Stroke volume
- Resting heart rate (RHR)
- Cardiac output
- Blood pressure
- Aerobic
- Anaerobic
- VO_2max
- Threshold of aerobic training
- Pulse
- Training heart rate range (THR)
- Target heart rate zone (THR)
- Maximum heart rate (MHR)
- Exercise heart rate (EHR)
- Ratings of perceived exertion (RPE)

Objectives

1. Describe the health benefits associated with cardiorespiratory activity.

2. Explain the physiological impact of physical activity on the cardiorespiratory system.

3. Describe the target zone for aerobic exercise in terms of frequency, intensity, and time.

4. Calculate and monitor a target heart rate zone.

5. Assess your cardiorespiratory endurance and set appropriate goals for improvement or maintenance.

6. Establish an activity plan—either a formal exercise program, or informal physical activities to be built into your daily routine.

7. Describe how to exercise safely in the heat, cold, and high altitude.

Stages of Change

Where Am I?

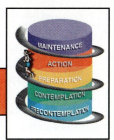

MODERATELY INTENSE ACTIVITY*

Precontemplator _____ I am currently physically inactive, and I do not intend to change in the next six months.

Contemplator _____ I am currently physically inactive, but I am thinking about starting moderately intense physical activity in the next six months.

Preparer _____ I am currently doing moderately intense physical activity, but not regularly.

Action Taker _____ I am currently doing moderately intense physical activity, but I have only begun doing so in the last six months.

Maintainer _____ I am currently doing moderately intense physical activity and have done so for longer than six months.

VIGOROUS EXERCISE

Precontemplator _____ I currently do not exercise, and at this point I do not intend to start.

Contemplator _____ I currently do not exercise, but I am thinking about starting to exercise.

Preparer _____ I currently exercise some, but not regularly.

Action Taker _____ I currently exercise regularly, but I have only begun doing so in the last six months.

Maintainer _____ I currently exercise regularly and have done so for longer than six months.

Source: Adapted from personal communication with Dr. Bess Marcus and from B. H. Marcus, J. S. Rossi, V. C. Selby, R. S. Niaura, & D. B. Abrams, The stages and processes of exercise adoption and maintenance in a worksite sample, *Health Psychology* 11, 386–395, 1992; and B. H. Marcus, B. C. Bock, B. M. Pinto, L. H. Forsyth, M. B. Roberts, & R. M. Traficante, Efficacy of an individualized motivationally-tailored physical activity intervention, *Annals of Behaviorial Medicine,* in press.

*See the definitions of moderately intense activity and vigorous exercise on the next page.

This chapter is about the kind of activities you need to do to improve cardiorespiratory endurance. This level of activity is above the base level of physical activity discussed in Chapter 2. However, because the 30 minutes a day of moderate-intensity activity is so important to your health, and because it is a good preparation for more vigorous activity, behavior change material is provided for both levels of activity. Select the stage of behavioral change that best describes you in terms of moderately intense activity and/or in terms of more vigorous activity. To be considered an action taker or maintainer, you must meet the criteria described in the following definitions:

Moderately Intense Activity. Moderate physical activity or exercise includes activities such as brisk walking, gardening, and heavy housecleaning, with exertion similar to brisk walking. Generally, heavy housecleaning does not include activities such as dusting or washing dishes. For moderate activity to be regular, it must add up to a total of 30 minutes or more a day and be done at least 5 days a week. For example, you could climb stairs for 10 minutes, three times a day.

Vigorous Exercise. Vigorous physical activity or exercise includes activities such as jogging, aerobics, swimming, or biking. For vigorous activity to be regular, it must last at least 20 minutes each time, and be done at least 3 days a week.

How valuable is a shiny red Porsche if the insides are rusted out? Our image of being beautifully fit often stops with outside appearances when, in fact, remembering to take a good look under the hood may lengthen our lives. When you picture a physically fit person, do you see only muscles or do you also picture a strong heart, clean, clear lungs, smooth flexible arteries, and rich blood, free of extra fat? You should; a fit cardiorespiratory system promotes health, increases energy, improves stamina, and defends against coronary heart disease.

WHAT IS CARDIORESPIRATORY ENDURANCE?

Cardiorespiratory endurance is the ability of the cardiovascular and respiratory systems to provide fuel, especially oxygen, to the muscles and the ability of the muscles to use this fuel for sustained physical work. The better your cardiorespiratory endurance, the longer and harder you can be physically active without getting tired.

Aerobic exercise is the preferred type of exercise for increasing cardiorespiratory endurance because it specifically trains the cardiovascular, respiratory, and muscular systems to better consume, transport, and use oxygen. Anaerobic exercise also contributes to cardiorespiratory endurance by improving the delivery of oxygen in the blood, increasing blood flow, and strengthening the heart. Anaerobic exercise does not, however, improve the muscle cells' ability to use the oxygen to produce more energy.

Plus, to benefit from anaerobic training, you must train at very high all-out intensity efforts for short amounts of time alternated with short rest periods. Many people dislike the physical discomfort that accompanies this level of training. It takes high levels of motivation to work out at near maximal exertions—one reason drop-out rates for high-intensity activities are higher than for moderately intense activities.[1] High-intensity training also puts a person at higher risk for musculoskeletal injury, another reason people stop exercising. Nor is high-intensity exercise good for beginners or most older people.

Most people prefer to train their cardiorespiratory system using aerobic exercise. The more moderate intensity and continuous nature of aerobic conditioning tends to be more comfortable and therefore more enjoyable. Aerobic exercise also provides the kind of fitness base that supports daily and recreational activities. Anaerobic training is more performance-oriented and is therefore more important for those training for competitive sports.

In Chapter 2, you learned that moderate-intensity activities can substantially reduce the risk of cardiovascular disease and provide many of the other health benefits associated with physical activity, and that for someone of low fitness, this level of activity may be sufficient to increase fitness. However, if you want to attain a moderate to high level of cardiorespiratory endurance, you must exercise vigorously enough to produce a training effect. We will focus on how to do this in the second portion of this chapter.

THE CARDIORESPIRATORY SYSTEM AT WORK

Let's look at how the cardiorespiratory system works and some of the advantages of training it. The term *cardiorespiratory system* encompasses both the cardiovascular and respiratory systems. The combination of these systems can be thought of as an elaborate grocery delivery and waste removal system. Groceries (oxygen and food) enter via the mouth and nose and travel to the stomach (food) and lungs (oxygen). The food continues down through the digestive system and eventually enters the bloodstream as glucose, vitamins, and minerals. Meanwhile, the oxygen enters the blood at the loading docks (alveolar–capillary interface) in the lungs, is carried (by the red blood cells) down the outbound roadways (the arteries), and is delivered (capillary–tissue interface) to the doorstep of the muscle cells. The cells take in the oxygen (and other nutrients) and unload waste products, such as carbon dioxide, into the blood. The blood travels back to the central plant (the heart) via the inbound roadways (the veins), stopping to dump waste products off at the appropriate sites (liver, kidneys, and lungs).

Heart: The System's Pump

The heart, a four-chambered organ composed of cardiac muscle, is the pump that drives the whole system (Figure 3.1). Its size and rate of contraction determine the volume and speed at which oxygenated blood is delivered to the working muscles. The rate of contraction is called the **heart rate** (HR) and the volume of blood ejected out of the heart with each contraction is called the **stroke volume** (SV). The **resting heart rate** (RHR) is the number of heart contractions needed per minute to supply oxygen to the resting body and establish an aerobic homeostasis. During low-intensity activity the correspondingly low increase in oxygen demand is easily met. When you are more active, such as during exercise, your heart rate, stroke volume, and respiration increase more dramatically to meet the new oxygen demand and reestablish homeostasis at a higher metabolic level. When vigorous physical activity stops, the oxygen demand decreases sharply, and to accommodate, the heart rate drops rapidly for 1 to 2 minutes. After this, the heart rate continues to decline, but at a slower rate, until homeostasis is reestablished at a resting level.

Cardiac output (CO) is the amount of blood pumped out of the heart in 1 minute. Cardiac output is the product of stroke volume, the amount of blood the heart ejects in one beat, and the heart rate (SV × HR = CO). When you exercise, both the stroke volume and the heart rate increase, but the heart rate increases more dramatically, especially with vigorous exercise. When the heart beats very quickly, the stroke volume may actually decrease if the chambers of the heart don't have enough time to fill completely.

Benefits of Exercise

The heart muscle becomes stronger with exercise. Like skeletal muscle, the cardiac (heart) muscle can improve in strength. The left ventricle (the chamber that ejects blood into the body) adapts differently depending on the kind of physical training performed. The walls of the ventricle thicken in response to anaerobic training and the volume of the chamber increases with aerobic training. The increased volume means an increased stroke volume, which means the heart can pump more blood with each beat or the same amount of blood with fewer beats. The average resting stroke volume is 70 to 90 milliliters per beat. During exercise, this can increase to 100 to 120 milliliters per beat. People who train with regular aerobic exercise may have resting stroke volumes equal to exercise stroke volumes of nonfit individuals (100 to 120 milliliters per beat) and exercise volumes up to 150 to 170 milliliters per beat. This improved stroke volume and contractility of the heart result in a decrease of the resting heart rate. The average healthy heart has a resting heart rate of 70 to 80 beats per minute (bpm), but with participation in regular aerobic exercise this can drop 10 to 20 bpm or more. Just a 10-beat decrease would save the heart about 5,256,000 beats over a year and 262,800,000 beats over 50 years.

The resting heart rate is influenced not only by the strength of the heart muscle but also by the efficiency of other parts of the circulatory system. Among aerobically fit individuals (maintainers), it is not uncommon to hear about resting heart rates in the 60s, 50s, and even 40s. Heredity also plays a role in establishing the resting heart rate. Some individuals who may or may not be aerobically fit have inherited a low resting heart rate. Similarly, some highly trained individuals have average (70 to 80 bpm) resting heart rates. Allowing for these individual differences, in general, as you train, your resting heart rate declines.

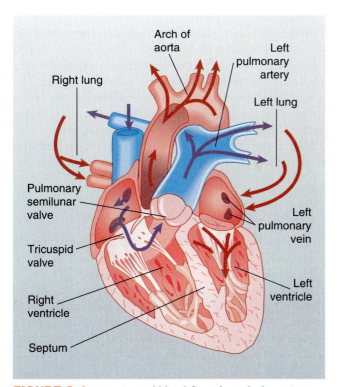

Right lung

Arch of aorta

Left pulmonary artery

Left lung

Pulmonary semilunar valve

Left pulmonary vein

Tricuspid valve

Right ventricle

Left ventricle

Septum

FIGURE 3.1 Oxygenated blood flows from the lungs into the left atrium, to the left ventricle, and out to the body. Deoxygenated blood enters the heart at the right atrium, flows to the right ventricle and then goes to the lungs to be reoxygenated.

Arteries: Pipelines of the System

Large arteries starting near the heart branch off into smaller and smaller arteries. The smallest arteries, called capillaries, deliver oxygen to the cells. The blood in the heart does not supply the heart muscle with oxygen. Instead, heart cells are nourished with oxygen-rich blood through the two coronary arteries—small arteries that branch off the aorta (main artery) near the heart.

Benefits of Exercise

Exercise increases the number of capillaries. More capillaries mean better oxygen and carbon dioxide exchange between the blood and the muscle cells. In addition, if an artery becomes blocked, blood flow can be diverted to other healthy branches. Think how much stress is avoided when there are alternate routes to take when there is a car accident on a main street.

Exercise also increases the number of branches on the coronary arteries. This means that if one pathway becomes blocked, oxygen-rich blood can be rerouted and delivered to the heart muscle. This can prevent or decrease the severity of a heart attack. In the brain, a greater network of arterial capillaries helps prevent a stroke, which is caused by a lack of oxygen to the brain cells.

When you exercise, your **blood pressure,** the pressure created by the blood against the arterial walls, rises because your heart contracts more often and pushes higher volumes of blood through your arteries. Healthy arteries stretch and can handle the extra blood flow without any problem. In other words, blood pressure stays in a healthy range even with the added "stress" of exercise. To appreciate the ability of the arteries, imagine an airport or train station with hallways that can expand at prime time to accommodate extra travelers.

Regular physical activity and a good diet can help prevent arterial diseases, lower your blood pressure, and decrease the levels of fat in the blood. Exercise also increases the amount of HDL (good cholesterol), which helps carry fat out of the bloodstream, preventing it from forming plaque along the arterial walls.

Blood: The System's Carriers

Blood is a complex liquid that performs a number of critical functions, including the transportation of oxygen and carbon dioxide. Microscopically, blood is composed of solids (including red and white blood cells and platelets) and plasma, a liquid containing dissolved substances. Hemoglobin is contained in the red blood cells and is capable of combining with oxygen and carbon dioxide and transporting them through the blood vessels.

Benefits of Exercise

Blood volume increases in response to regular aerobic exercise. Most of the expansion is due to an increase in blood plasma, the liquid portion of the blood. This lowers the viscosity of the blood, allowing it to flow through the blood vessels with less resistance, which in turn results in lower blood pressure. Red blood cells and the hemoglobin content of the red blood cells also increase. This means that the blood has a greater oxygen and carbon dioxide carrying capacity. The ability of the blood to load oxygen also improves, which means it travels to the cells more fully saturated. At the cellular end, muscle cells become more effective at extracting oxygen and other nutrients from the blood in the capillaries. All of this means a more plentiful supply of oxygen for energy production.

High-altitude exercise over a period of time can further increase the number of red blood cells in your blood. At sea level, these extra red blood cells are an advantage as they can help carry even more oxygen to the muscle cells. It is no accident that the Olympic Training Center is located in Colorado Springs, Colorado.

Lungs: The Blood's Oxygen Depot

When you breathe in, you draw oxygen through the trachea and down the bronchial tubes into the lungs. The bronchi branch repeatedly and eventually become small alveolar ducts. At the ends of these ducts are numerous alveoli and alveolar sacs. It is between these alveoli and the tiny arteries and veins that oxygen and carbon dioxide are exchanged.

Benefits of Exercise

Cardiorespiratory endurance exercises strengthen the respiratory muscles and increase the amount of air you can breathe into and out of your lungs (pulmonary ventilation). An average untrained person can ventilate about 120 liters of air per minute. Pulmonary ventilation increases to about 150 liters of air following fitness training, and highly trained athletes can ventilate more than 180 liters per minute.[2] More surface area of the lung also becomes available for the exchange of oxygen and carbon dioxide.

Metabolic Processes: The Power Plants

The **aerobic** and **anaerobic** systems were introduced in Chapter 2. The anaerobic processes take place in the cytoplasm of the muscle cell while the aerobic processes take place inside the mitochondrion, a structure floating in the cytoplasm. The mitochondrion is often referred to as the "powerhouse" of the cell, as it is inside this little "factory" that simple sugars (carbohydrates after digestion) are converted into cellular energy (ATP).

Benefits of Exercise

Aerobic conditioning results in an increase in the number of mitochondria (which increases the potential for

I can't motivate myself to do cardiorespiratory exercise.

- If you picture exercise as something like running for 20 minutes, try instead to picture yourself doing a moderately intense physical activity like those listed on page 30.
- Think about the kinds of things you are motivated to do and see if physical activity can become part of them. For example, if you like to shop, first take several brisk walks around the mall (window shop) and then slow down and browse. Or if you are going to watch a football game, use halftime to go out and run while throwing a ball around with a friend. If spring break finds you on the beach, take a swim, walk along the shore, or play a friendly game of beach volleyball.

I have good intentions but can't seem to stick to an aerobic exercise program.

- Surround yourself with supportive people: workout buddies, family, or an exercise class.
- Select aerobic activities you enjoy.
- Plan vacations that involve or provide the opportunity for aerobic activities.
- Treat yourself to a reward for sticking with your program.

I never seem to have time for cardiorespiratory exercise.

- Try to establish a regular exercise time so that it won't be easily interrupted.
- Select activities that fit most easily into your day. Keep in mind that weekend days may be very different from weekdays and therefore the activities may be different.
- Place home exercise equipment in front of the TV, near the phone, or in another place where you tend to sit and socialize.

I can always find an excuse not to exercise.

- Get your workout clothes and equipment ready ahead of time.
- Acknowledge the importance of physical activity/exercise and give it the priority it deserves.
- Select activities that you enjoy so that you look forward to exercise rather than dread it. It also helps to do the activity with someone with whom you want to spend time.

I'm bored with my cardiorespiratory workout.

- Do your activity in a new place for variety: Take your bike to a new trail or country road, walk a new path or reverse your normal route, swim in a lake during the summer instead of doing laps in a pool.
- Change activities if you are getting bored. Cross training (participating in more than one activity) appeals to a lot of people.
- Train for a competition: There are competitive aerobic events for every age group.
- Volunteer for a walkathon or similar charitable event.

For additional barriers and barrier-busting ideas see the list in Chapter 2.

ATP production) and enzymes responsible for fat utilization. These adaptations make more energy available for physical activity, and in the case of aerobic activity, more fat can be mobilized. Anaerobic conditioning results in greater storage of glycogen and high-energy phosphagens [ATP and creatine phosphate (CP)] inside the muscle cells. The more energy a cell can store and/or produce, the longer an activity can be sustained. Just think of all the ATP mitochondria have to produce for an hour of aerobics or for a marathon run!

Other Benefits of Aerobic Exercise

Physical activity, and aerobic exercise in particular, has a positive influence on social, emotional, and mental well-being. These influences were described in Chapter 2, and will be recurrent themes throughout this book. In brief, then, aerobic exercise helps alleviate some depression, anxiety, and insomnia. It decreases the secretion of hormones triggered by stress and provides an emotional outlet for pent-up anger. It also boosts the number of endorphins circulating in the bloodstream, which act to mask pain and to produce feelings of euphoria—the "runner's high."

HOW TO IMPROVE CARDIORESPIRATORY ENDURANCE

Improving your cardiorespiratory endurance occurs when you do physical activity at a high enough intensity to cause a training effect. The training effect is optimized when you exercise within the aerobic target zone as outlined by the FIT Principle: frequency, intensity, and time.

Frequency

Optimal aerobic training occurs when you exercise three to five times a week. The majority of improvement in aerobic capacity occurs with three days of exercise a week. Some additional improvement occurs with four or five days of training; after that, improvement starts to plateau. Exercising six or seven days a week results in little or no apparent improvement, except in weight loss. If weight loss is a primary goal, frequency can range from three to seven days a week, depending on intensity, duration, and mode of exercise. High-frequency exercisers can reduce risk of injury by cross training using a variety of weight- and nonweight-bearing exercises.

Exercise addicts are people who feel compelled to work out every single day. As a result, they often suffer from overuse injuries such as shinsplints and tendinitis. Some individuals develop such an obsession for exercise that they begin to value it above everything else. Like any addiction, this leads to an unhealthy lifestyle. Physical fitness must always be balanced with other wellness components such as emotional, intellectual, and spiritual health. Exercise three to five times a week and feel good about using the other two to four days to do something else. (If, however, you are using lower-intensity physical activity, daily activity is recommended.)

Intensity

This section contains a number of abbreviated terms.[3] To make your reading easier, here is a quick reference list:

HR = heart rate

RHR = resting heart rate

EHR = exercise heart rate

MHR = maximum heart rate

HRR = heart rate (maximum) reserve

THR = target heart rate zone or training heart rate range

VO_2max = maximum volume of oxygen consumed per minute per kilogram body weight

The more intensely you exercise, the more oxygen your muscles need. Your breathing becomes faster and deeper to bring in more oxygen and your heart beats faster to speed up the delivery of oxygen to your muscles. As exercise becomes more and more intense, the rate and volume of oxygen entering the body continue to increase until finally the body is consuming oxygen as rapidly as it can. This maximum volume of oxygen consumption (measured in liters per minute or milliliters per minute per kilogram body weight) is called **VO_2max.** (This volume may also be called MOU or maximum oxygen uptake.) If exercise intensity is increased any further, the muscles' demand for oxygen cannot be met. You can exercise at these very high intensities above VO_2max for only a short time before exhaustion makes you stop. Age,

heredity, and physical training influence VO_2max. Experts believe that about 80 percent of a person's VO_2max is genetically determined whereas about 20 percent can be determined through training. VO_2max declines slowly with age, but there is evidence that it declines more slowly in people who remain physically active.

Exercising at VO_2max is very strenuous and not a lot of fun for most people. The good news is that aerobic conditioning begins at just 50 percent of VO_2max, an intensity aptly referred to as the **threshold of aerobic training.** The American College of Sports Medicine (ACSM) recommends that the average normal healthy adult exercise aerobically at an intensity between 50 and 85 percent of VO_2max. During exercise it is normal to fluctuate a little in your intensity; knowing what an acceptable range is allows you to exercise without being concerned about maintaining a precise intensity. However, you will want to target the lower, middle, or upper portions of the range, depending on your fitness level.

So how do you know at what percentage of VO_2max you are exercising? To get a direct measure you would have to exercise in a laboratory while scientists measured the amount of oxygen you consumed. Fortunately researchers have found an easier way for us to get a good estimate. Exercise scientists discovered an almost linear relationship between the number of times the heart beats per minute and the volume of oxygen consumed per minute. This means that you can use your heart rate to estimate oxygen consumption. By simply taking your **pulse,** which is the wave of pressure felt in the arteries when the heart beats, you can measure your heart rate and monitor your exercise intensity.

Heart rate information can be used to calculate a range of intensities similar to the 50 to 85 percent VO_2max range. This range is called the **training heart rate range** (THR) or **target heart rate zone.** To achieve aerobic conditioning you must exercise hard enough to keep your heart rate within your THR. To calculate your THR you will need to know your **maximum heart rate** (MHR), which is the fastest rate your heart can beat. The most accurate way to determine your MHR is to exercise to absolute exhaustion while your heart rate is monitored by an EKG (electrocardiograph) machine. Fortunately, there is an easier, faster way—simply subtract your age from 220. Sixty to 90 percent of this MHR represents a good aerobic conditioning range according to ACSM. Another, more individualized formula that uses both age and resting heart rate is called the Karvonen formula (see Table 3.1). Using this formula, ACSM recommends a range of 50 to 85 percent of heart rate reserve (HRR). HRR is the difference between your MHR and your RHR.

Although a training effect occurs throughout each of these ranges, the very high intensities are significant only for competitors. Competitive athletes have to exercise at high intensities to maintain the winning edge, but fitness gains for those interested in achieving health-related cardiorespiratory fitness can be achieved at more moderate intensities.

For health-related fitness, the training heart rate range is generally set in the middle of the cardiorespiratory training ranges previously discussed. Beginners are encouraged to start at the lower values, and more-fit individuals can exercise in the middle to upper parts of the following ranges:

60–80 percent of VO_2max

70–85 percent of MHR

60–80 percent of HRR (Karvonen formula)

To calculate your THR using the Karvonen formula, see Activity 3.1.

Exercise Heart Rate

Your **exercise heart rate** (EHR) is the speed at which your heart is beating during exercise. Your EHR should fall within your THR. If your EHR is higher than your THR, you are exercising too intensely. If it is lower, you aren't exercising hard enough. To find your EHR, either take your pulse while you are exercising or complete your count within 15 seconds of the time you stop. When you stop exercising, your heart rate stays at a level close to your EHR for about 15 seconds, then drops off quickly as your body recovers. During the first 15 seconds you have time to locate your pulse (most people require 2 to 4 seconds) and take a 10-second pulse count. Multiply the number of beats you count in 10 seconds by 6 to determine your pulse in beats per minute. For example,

$$\frac{25 \text{ beats}}{10 \text{ seconds}} \times \frac{\overset{6}{\cancel{60 \text{ seconds}}}}{1 \text{ minute}} = \frac{150 \text{ beats}}{\text{minute}}$$

Exercisers often take a 6-second count, since mentally multiplying by 10 is easy. The problem with this method is that if you miscount your heart rate, you are multiplying your error by 10. When your heart is beating very fast, it is easy to miscount by 1, even 2 beats. A 2-beat miscount becomes an error of 20 beats. If instead you use the 10-second count, a 2-beat miscount represents only a 12-beat error. Almost all fitness experts recommend the 10-second count.

To eliminate the problem of mentally multiplying by 6, convert your THR from beats per minute to beats per 10 seconds by dividing the top and bottom of the range by 6 and rounding off to the nearest whole number.

Taking Your Pulse

When you press gently on an *artery* you can feel the pulsing of the blood as it is pushed through the arteries by the heart. The arteries most commonly used for taking the pulse during exercise are the radial and carotid arteries.

The *radial artery* is located on the inside of your wrist. You can feel it beside your forearm tendons on the thumb side. The *carotid artery* is just to the side (either side) of your voice box (larynx). You can feel it in the valley between your Adam's apple and your neck muscles.

To feel your pulse, use two fingers to press gently but firmly on the artery. Do not use your thumb; it also has a pulse and will cause you to miscount. If you can't feel your pulse, you may be pressing too lightly or too hard. Pressing too hard on an artery squeezes it shut so that you can no longer feel any pulsing. Try different pressures while sitting quietly until you can feel and count your pulse easily. Then practice taking it while you move around the room. If you have a lot of trouble counting your pulse, place your hand over your heart and count beats.

Although most people can use the carotid site without experiencing any problems, a word of caution is in order. Special receptors located in the walls of the carotid artery are responsible for detecting changes in pressure. If you put pressure on these baroreceptors while taking your pulse (or massage them while looking for your pulse), they send a message to the heart to slow down. This slowing heart rate can cause dizziness or faintness in some people. If your heart rate does slow down, your pulse count will not be accurate. Try taking your pulse at both your carotid and your radial sites. If you find the carotid gives you a slower count, use the radial site.

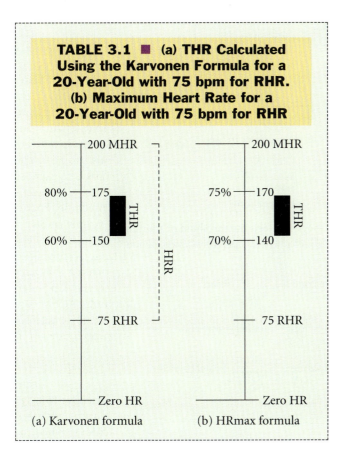

TABLE 3.1 ■ (a) THR Calculated Using the Karvonen Formula for a 20-Year-Old with 75 bpm for RHR. (b) Maximum Heart Rate for a 20-Year-Old with 75 bpm for RHR

(a) Karvonen formula — 200 MHR; 80% → 175; THR; 60% → 150; HRR; 75 RHR; Zero HR

(b) HRmax formula — 200 MHR; 75% → 170; THR; 70% → 140; 75 RHR; Zero HR

1. Find your **resting heart rate (RHR).** Take your pulse for one minute when you have been lying still for 30 minutes or more. First thing in the morning is a good time as long as you haven't been startled awake by the alarm clock. (A note on your clock will remind you to take your pulse.) Take your RHR on three different occasions and find the average.

   Example

80	225 divided by 3 = 75 bpm
75	
70	
225	

   1st time _____

   2nd time _____

   3rd time _____

   total _____ ÷ 3 = [_____]
           RHR

2. Find your **maximum heart rate (MHR)** by subtracting your age from 220.

   Example 220 – 20 years old = 200   220 – _____ = [_____]
                 your age MHR

3. Find your **maximum heart rate reserve (HRR)** by subtracting your RHR from your MHR.

   Example 200 – 75 = 125   _____ – _____ = [_____]
               MHR RHR HRR

4. Multiply your HRR by 0.60 (60%).

   Example 125 × 0.60 = 75   _____ × 0.60 = _____
               HRR

5. To find your threshold of training add your RHR to your answer in Step 4.

   Example 75 + 75 = 150 bpm   _____ + _____ = [_____]
             answer in RHR threshold
             Step 4   of training

6. Multiply your HRR by 0.80 (80%).

   Example 125 × 0.80 = 100   _____ × 0.80 = _____
               HRR

7. Find the upper end of your target zone by adding your RHR to your answer in Step 6.

   Example 100 + 75 = 175 bpm   _____ + _____ = [_____]
             answer in RHR upper end
             Step 6   of target zone

The target heart rate zone in this example is 150–175 bpm, or the range between the threshold of training and the upper end of the target zone. To convert the above range (zone) into beats per 10 seconds, divide the top and bottom of the above range by 6.

   Example 150/6 = 25 bpm   My target heart rate zone is _____ bpm

         175/6 = 29 bpm

The target heart rate zone is now 25–29 beats in 10 seconds. What is your target heart rate zone for beats per 10 seconds?

   _____ ÷ 6 = _____   My target heart rate zone is _____ beats/10 seconds

   _____ ÷ 6 = _____

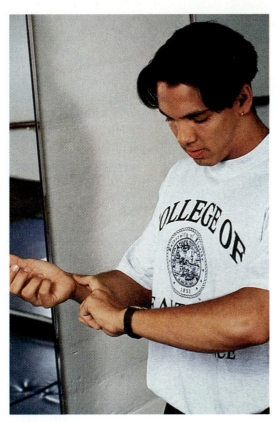

Radial artery.

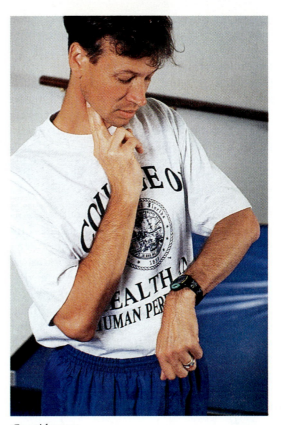

Carotid artery.

When taking your pulse, count complete cardiac cycles. A pulse throb constitutes the end of a cardiac cycle. If the instructor says *go* and you immediately feel a throb, don't count it (or call it zero). If the instructor says *go* and there is a pause and then a beat, go ahead and count it as number one. Continue to count until the instructor stops you.

Ratings of Perceived Exertion Scale and the Talk Test

A Swedish physiologist named Gunnar Borg discovered a relationship between the perception of exercise intensity and heart rate. He developed the **ratings of perceived exertion** (RPE) scale shown in Table 3.2. To use this scale, look at the numbers and word descriptions and select the number that best represents how hard you feel (perceive) you are exercising. Perceived exertion ratings between 12 and 18 produce a training effect. Research evidence indicates that the RPE scale is an effective way for adults to monitor aerobic intensity.

When first using the RPE scale, it is a good idea to make ratings and then check your heart rate. When you know which ratings coincide best with your target heart rate range and are consistently labeling the same heart rate with the same RPE, you can start to phase out taking your pulse and rely more on ratings of perceived exertion. In essence, what you are doing is learning how to listen to your body so you can know how hard you are working.

TABLE 3.2 ■ The Borg RPE Scale	
Score	**Degree of Exertion**
6	No exertion at all
7	Extremely light
8	
9	Very light
10	
11	Light
12	
13	Somewhat hard
14	
15	Hard (heavy)
16	
17	Very hard
18	
19	Extremely hard
20	Maximal exertion

Source: © Gunner Borg, 1970, 1985, 1998. Reprinted by permission.

RPE also works when heart rate is not reliable. If, for example, you are on a medication that affects heart rate, or if you aren't good at taking a pulse count, RPE can be a good method for estimating workout intensity.

Another quick, easy (and less scientific) method for estimating intensity is the talk test. You should be able to talk comfortably while working out. If you can't, your workout intensity is too high. If you can sing comfortably, your intensity is probably too low.

When to Monitor Intensity

Using the pulse check, the RPE scale, or the talk test, you should monitor your level of exertion periodically during your workout. It is a good idea to check your intensity level 5 to 10 minutes into the aerobic workout to make sure you have reached your training intensity. Check again at the peak of the aerobic section to make sure you aren't too high. Check once again toward the end of the aerobic section to see whether you were able to maintain the training intensity to the end. If you check your intensity only at the end and find that you are too high or too low, it is too late to modify your workout. In addition, your finishing heart rate may not be indicative of the intensity of your entire workout.

Time

ACSM describes the optimal duration of a cardiorespiratory workout as 20 to 60 minutes. This range is a guideline for all aerobic activities and is not specific to any one type of exercise. You may wish to limit those activities with higher impact stress, such as running, to shorter periods of time and use activities such as swimming, cycling, or walking for longer workouts. Dr. Cooper, Director of the Institute for Aerobics Research in Dallas, recommends running be limited to 80 to 90 minutes a week at three times a week for 30 minutes or four times a week for 20 minutes. He believes that the additional benefits gained by running more (other than weight loss) do not outweigh the increased risk of bone, joint, and muscle injury.

Performing any kind of aerobic activity for more than 60 minutes brings diminishing returns. In other words, you get less and less additional benefit for your hard work. In fact, after 30 to 40 minutes, the amount of benefit, except calorie expenditure, begins to decrease. If you want to exercise for longer periods of time in order to lose fat, consider some of the low-impact activities or a variety of low- and high-impact activities.

APPLYING THE PRINCIPLES OF PHYSICAL ACTIVITY/EXERCISE TO CARDIORESPIRATORY ENDURANCE

1. Principles of Progression and Overload
   - If your cardiorespiratory endurance is low, start with short bouts of activity of easy intensity then increase the number and/or length of bouts until you have achieved 30 minutes of moderately intense activity or 20 minutes of vigorous activity.
   - Increase intensity only after achieving the appropriate duration.

2. Principle of Individuality
   - Select activities that meet your needs and your schedule.
   - Fat loss through aerobic exercise will occur in different places for different people at different rates. Spot reducing is a myth. Fat comes off all over the body, but it always seems like it comes off the place you want it off the most, last!
   - Resting heart rates will decline at different amounts and at different rates for different individuals.
   - Everyone can improve cardiorespiratory endurance; however, beginners will show more dramatic improvement than advanced participants because beginners have more room for improvement.

3. Principle of Specificity
   - Aerobic activities of sufficient intensity encourage fat mobilization and are less apt to cause musculoskeletal injury than anaerobic activities.
   - Anaerobic activities emphasize carbohydrate metabolism, encourage energy storage, are less comfortable for most people, and have a higher risk of injury than aerobic conditioning.

The FIT Principle and Aerobic Conditioning

Moderate Physical Activity

F = every (most) days

I = moderately intense

T = accumulated 30 minutes

Vigorous Physical Activity (Exercise)

F = 3–5 times per week
    6–7 for weight loss

I = 70–85 percent MHR, 60–90 percent VO$_2$max
    12–18 RPE

T = 20–60 minutes per session

---

4. Principle of Reversibility
   - Health benefits are maintained only as long as you stay active.
   - Almost everyone has a problem with relapses; the important thing is to start again. The more support you have and the more you enjoy the activities, the more likely you will be to stay active. Aim to make physical activity as routine in your life as brushing your teeth.

DESIGNING YOUR CARDIORESPIRATORY PROGRAM

When setting up a program for improving your cardiorespiratory endurance, the following steps can be useful. Use Lab 3.5 to record your program.

1. Assess your present level of cardiorespiratory fitness. You may use one or more of the cardiorespiratory fitness tests provided on pages 64 to 67.

2. Using the assessment information from Step 1 and after contemplating the level of fitness you would like to have, write a general goal.

   Examples

   I would like to be able to walk up two flights of stairs and not be breathless.

3. Select one or more cardiorespiratory activities for your program. Try to select activities that you enjoy and that are feasible in your present situation in terms of fitness level, time commitment, convenience, equipment, facility availability, and financial outlay.

4. Determine the frequency, intensity, and duration to perform your chosen activity or activities. Using this information, write one or more specific goals.

   Example

   I want to be able to walk/run 1 mile in 8 minutes without exceeding my THR.

5. Set a date to begin. Commit to it by planning time in your schedule, by telling a supportive friend, by inviting someone to join you, or by signing up for an activity.

EXERCISE AND THE ENVIRONMENT

As you implement your exercise plan, it is important to take into account the environment in which you will be active. Here are some tips on how to handle some of the environmental conditions you may experience.

Air, Noise, and Water Pollution

- If air quality is an issue where you live, exercise in the early morning or later evening when the air quality is best.
- Avoid high-traffic areas where exhaust will affect your breathing.
- If there is a smog alert or enough of an air quality problem to affect your respiratory system, exercise indoors.
- Select an exercise route that avoids high-noise areas such as construction sites.
- Call the local government to find out which bodies of water are swimmable.

Hot and Sunny Weather

- Dress in lightweight fabrics that breathe (that is, fabrics that allow air and moisture to pass through them).
- Wear light colors to reflect heat.
- Wear a sunblock to prevent sunburn.
- Wear a wet bandanna loosely around your neck.
- If you are on the water, wear sunglasses to cut the glare and filter out harmful UV (ultraviolet) light.
- Start slowly. Add to your exercise program as your tolerance to the heat improves.
- Drink one to two glasses of water to retain fluid (avoid high sugar or caffeinated drinks) before exercising and then drink four to eight ounces of fluid every 10 to 15 minutes during exercise. Drink even more with very intense exercise.

Apparent temperature (what it feels like)

Air temperature (F°)	70°	75°	80°	85°	90°	95°	100°	105°	110°	115°
0%	64°	69°	73°	78°	83°	87°	91°	95°	99°	103°
10%	65°	70°	75°	80°	85°	90°	95°	100°	105°	111°
20%	66°	72°	77°	82°	87°	93°	99°	105°	112°	120°
30%	67°	73°	78°	84°	90°	96°	104°	113°	123°	135°
40%	68°	74°	79°	86°	93°	101°	110°	123°	137°	151°
50%	69°	75°	81°	88°	96°	107°	120°	135°	150°	
60%	70°	76°	82°	90°	100°	114°	132°	149°		
70%	70°	77°	85°	93°	106°	124°	144°			
80%	71°	78°	86°	97°	113°	136°				
90%	71°	79°	88°	102°	122°					
100%	72°	80°	91°	108°						

(Relative humidity — left vertical scale)

Apparent temperature	Heat stress risk with exertion
90° – 105°	Heat cramps and heat exhaustion possible.
105° – 130°	Heat cramps or heat exhaustion likely; heat stroke possible.
130° and above	Heat stroke highly likely with continued exposure.

FIGURE 3.2 Heat and humidity chart. To determine the risk of exercising in the heat, locate the outside air temperature on the top horizontal scale and the relative humidity on the left vertical scale. Where these two values intersect is the *apparent temperature.* For example, on a 90°F day with 70 percent humidity, the apparent temperature is 106°F. Heat cramps or heat exhaustion are likely to occur, and heat stroke is possible during exercise under these conditions. (Adapted from U.S. Department of Commerce, National Oceanic and Atmospheric Administration, Heat index chart, in *Heat wave: A major summer killer.* Washington, D.C.: Government Printing Office, 1992.

- Pay attention to the combined effects of heat and humidity. (See Figure 3.2.) Exercise in an air-conditioned facility when the indices are too high for safe outdoor exercise. Or consider a water activity.

- Take rest breaks in the shade.

- Exercise in the coolest parts of the day: mornings and evenings.

Cold Weather

- Dress in layers. All clothing should allow moisture to escape but keep heat in. As you get warm during exercise, take off enough layers to prevent sweating. Body heat is lost through sweat, and when you stop exercising in the cold, you do not want body heat to be lost. (See Figure 3.3.)

- Wear sunscreen on exposed skin, including your face, neck, and hands.

- Wear sunglasses or goggles to cut snow and ice glare.

- Drink plenty of water. It is less obvious that you are losing fluids since sweat is being controlled.

- Be sure that someone knows where you have gone and when to expect you back. Do not deviate from your plan.

- Take along some food, such as trail mix. Eating warms the body, and if you are lost or tired this will buy you some time.

High Altitude

- Start slowly. Give yourself one to two days to acclimate. For example, ski half-days or hike lower, easier trails for the first couple of days.

- Drink plenty of water. Mountain air tends to be drier, which makes dehydration easier. Avoid caf-

Ambient Temperature (°F*)														
40	35	30	25	20	15	10	5	0	−5	−10	−15	−20	−25	−30
Effective Temperature (°F)														

Wind speed (mph)

Wind speed	40	35	30	25	20	15	10	5	0	−5	−10	−15	−20	−25	−30
Calm	40	35	30	25	20	15	10	5	0	−5	−10	−15	−20	−25	−30
5	37	33	27	21	16	12	6	1	−5	−11	−15	−20	−26	−31	−35
10	28	21	16	9	4	−2	−9	−15	−21	−27	−33	−38	−46	−52	−58
15	22	16	11	1	−5	−11	−18	−25	−36	−40	−45	−51	−58	−65	−70
20	18	12	3	−4	−10	−17	−25	−32	−39	−46	−53	−60	−67	−76	−81
25	16	7	0	−7	−15	−22	−29	−37	−44	−52	−59	−67	−74	−83	−89
30	13	5	−2	−11	−18	−26	−33	−41	−48	−56	−63	−70	−79	−87	−94
35	11	3	−4	−13	−20	−27	−35	−43	−49	−60	−67	−72	−82	−90	−98
40	10	1	−6	−15	−21	−29	−37	−45	−53	−62	−69	−76	−85	−94	−101

Little danger   **Danger**   **Great danger**

*°C = 0.556 (°F −32)
Convective heat loss at wind speeds above 40 mph have little additional effect on body cooling.

FIGURE 3.3 Windchill index. To determine exercise risk in the cold, locate the outside temperature on the top horizontal scale and the wind speed on the left vertical scale. Where the two scales intersect is the effective temperature and a safety rating. (Adapted by permission of Williams & Wilkins from C. W. D. McArdle, F. I. Katch, and V. L. Katch, *Exercise, physiology, energy, nutrition, and human performance*, 3rd ed. Philadelphia: Lea and Febiger, 1991)

feinated beverages, which act as diuretics and can further dehydrate you.

- Beware of alcohol's effect. Alcohol, in excess, will impair coordination and judgment more quickly than at low altitudes. Alcohol may also add to a dehydration problem. A hangover may mask symptoms of altitude sickness such as headache or nausea.

- Avoid sleeping pills. They may cause shallow breathing while you sleep and make it more difficult for you to get enough oxygen.

- Know the symptoms of altitude sickness and listen to your body. Common symptoms are tiredness, headache, nausea, and slight dizziness. If these symptoms don't get better in one to two days, see a health care provider. More severe symptoms include a persistent cough, shortness of breath while resting, noisy breathing, loss of balance, confusion, or vomiting. If you have any of these symptoms see a physician or other health care provider immediately.

SUMMARY

Cardiorespiratory endurance may be the most important health-related component of fitness due to its large impact on coronary heart disease risk factors and other chronic diseases. It provides us with stamina and extra energy for recreational activities. Aerobic training provides stress release and may result in the euphoric "runner's high." Physical activity at a moderate intensity for 30 minutes a day provides substantial disease protection and improves health, while vigorous activity promotes a higher level of fitness and physical performance.

To improve aerobic fitness you must exercise above your aerobic threshold and within your aerobic target zone. The target zone is described by the FIT variables: frequency, intensity, and time. Optimum cardiorespiratory fitness occurs when you exercise three to five times a week, at 60 to 80 percent of heart rate reserve, for 20 to 60 minutes. Beginners should work at the lower end of the target zone, while more fit individuals can work out at intensities near the high end.

SUGGESTED READING

American College of Sports Medicine. The recommended quantity and quality of exercise for developing and maintaining cardiorespiratory and muscular fitness in healthy adults. *Medicine and Science in Sports* 22(2):265–274, 1990.

American Heart Association. *The healthy-heart walking book: The American Heart Association Walking Program.* New York: Macmillan, 1993.

Cooper, K. H. *The aerobics program for total well-being.* New York: M. Evans, 1982.

Dishman, R. K., ed. *Advances in exercise adherence.* Champaign, IL: Human Kinetics, 1994.

Iknoian, T. *Fitness Walking: Technique, motivation, and 60 workouts for walkers (fitness spectrum).* Champaign, IL: Human Kinetics, 1995.

Pate, R. R., et al. Physical activity and public health: A recommendation from the Centers for Disease Control and Prevention and the American College of Sports Medicine. *Journal of the American Medical Association* 273(5):402–407, 1995.

U.S. Department of Health and Human Services. *Physical activity and health: A report of the surgeon general.* Centers for Chronic Disease Control and Prevention, National Center for Chronic Disease Prevention and Health Promotion. Atlanta: The President's Council on Physical Fitness and Sports, 1996.

U.S. Department of Health and Human Services. *Healthy people 2000: National health promotion and disease prevention objectives.* DHHS Publication No. (PHS) 91-50213. Washington, D.C.: U.S. Government Printing Office, 1990.

Wilmore, J. H., and D. L. Costill. *Training for sport and activity: The physiological basis of the conditioning process.* Champaign, IL: Human Kinetics, 1993.

Behavioral Lab 3.1

What Can I Do?

At the beginning of this chapter, you determined your stage of readiness to change with regard to moderately intense physical activity or vigorous cardiorespiratory exercise. Complete the corresponding section of this lab: precontemplator, contemplator, preparer, action taker, or maintainer. Notice that sometimes two statements are offered within an item; one statement applies to moderately intense physical activity, the other to vigorous cardiorespiratory (aerobic) exercise.

Precontemplator

1. Try to identify the main reasons you are against or not motivated to be physically active. *Or* Try to identify the main reasons you are against or not motivated to participate in vigorous cardiorespiratory exercise.

2. Can you think of any reason why physical activity/ vigorous cardiorespiratory (aerobic) exercise would be good for you?

3. Are there times when you *don't* do something because you don't have enough energy or stamina? Start something and then have to stop because you are tired or breathing hard? How much would you like to be able to do these activities? *Or* Are there times when a lack of cardiorespiratory fitness has limited your ability to do something, maybe even stop? Or limited the quality of your performance? How much would you like to change this?

4. In addition to inactivity, do you have any other risk factors for coronary heart disease? How would becoming physically active affect your risk? *Or* If you have taken a cardiorespiratory test, do the scores support a need for change?

5. Do you feel any differently about increasing your physical activity or vigorous exercise after reading the Barrier Busters on pages 38–39 and/or 51? Are there solutions to the problems you listed in item 1 that appeal to you?

6. Do your answers in items 2 to 5 (pros) outweigh your answers in item 1 (cons)?

7. Will you think about adding physical activity or vigorous exercise to your lifestyle? If yes, what activities or type of exercise appeals to you?

Contemplator

1. What moderately intense physical activity/vigorous exercise are you thinking about doing?

2. What changes (benefits) will this action (item 1) bring about that are important to you? Why are they important?

3. Is there something you need to know more about in order to move ahead?

4. What do you need in order to consider making this change? Try to finish this statement:

   Examples

   I would consider changing if . . . .

   I had a partner.

   It wouldn't cost me any money.

   I could easily fit it into my day.

   I knew more about what to do.

   (yours) _____

5. How can you overcome or accomplish the items listed in item 4? Who can help you overcome them?

6. If you were going to become physically active, what are the top three to five activities you would consider doing? *Or* Make a list of three to five cardiorespiratory endurance activities you think you would enjoy doing.

7. Write down your schedule for a typical day. Now brainstorm ideas for how, when, and where you could perform one or more of the activities/exercises you listed in item 6. Identify the ones that fit most easily into your day.

Preparer

1. What do you specifically want to accomplish? (For directions on goal setting see Chapter 2.)

2. What type of activities will accomplish this goal? (For programming ideas see pages 30, 32–33, and 57.)

3. Identify several moderately intense physical activities or vigorous cardiorespiratory endurance activities that you *think* you would enjoy doing on a regular basis.

4. Brainstorm ways that you can experiment with the activities/exercises you selected in item 3 in order to find out which ones you would enjoy doing on a regular basis. (For example, try walking at different time of day or borrow a friend's exercise machine.)

5. Restate your goal from item 1 using the moderately intense physical activity or vigorous cardiorespiratory endurance exercise you selected in item 4. Then break the goal down into small steps.

6. What kinds of things might tempt you to put off starting the activity/exercise plan you outlined in item 5?

7. What strategies can you use to eliminate or neutralize these temptations? (For example, rewards, buddy system)

8. What first step are you prepared to take toward your goal? What makes you believe you can accomplish this first step?

9. If the first step you choose doesn't work for you, what will you do?

10. Complete the following statement:

    I am going to take my first step on _____ .

    date within 30 days

Action Taker

1. What type(s) of moderately intense physical activity are you doing? For how many minutes each day? How many days a week? *Or* What vigorous cardiorespiratory endurance activity(ies) are you doing? How often? At what intensity? For how long?

2. Do you look forward to doing the activities you listed in item 1? If not, can you name an alternative activity to try?

3. Are you keeping track of your progress? If yes, how? (For example, journal, log sheet, fitness tests)

4. What positive rewards you are experiencing from being physically active/exercising?

5. Are you receiving support for your efforts? If yes, what kind? If no, why not? How might you gain support?

6. How confident are you that you will continue?

7. Can you think of anything that might cause you to stop or tempt you to stop?

8. Is there any way to prevent the temptations you listed in item 7? Or to strengthen your resolve against them?

9. How would you get started again if you did stop?

10. Are your physical activity/cardiorespiratory exercise goals clearly and specifically stated? If not, see Chapter 2 on how to write goals.

11. Do you believe that you can reach your goal(s)? Why or why not? If you are not confident you can reach your goal(s), what or who could help boost your confidence?

12. What strategies are you presently using or would you like to use to decrease the temptation to stop your physical activity/exercise and increase your confidence to continue?

Maintainer

1. For how long have you maintained your daily (or near daily) 30 minutes (or more) of moderately intense physical activity? *Or* For how long have you maintained your vigorous cardiorespiratory exercise program?

2. What are the top two reasons that make you want to continue?

3. Have you been tempted to stop? If so, what tempted you?

4. How confident are you that you can resist temptations to stop being physically active/exercising? If your confidence level has changed, can you identify why?

5. How do you convince yourself to continue when you are tempted to stop or skip a day? (What strategies do you use?)

6. Can you prevent temptations from occurring? If so, how?

7. Are you happy with your current fitness level, or do you wish to improve? If you are content, move on to item 8. If you want to improve, state your goal, establish a first step, and identify a day to begin.

8. Are you keeping track of your progress? If yes, how? Does this motivate you to continue?

9. Do you receive support for your efforts? If yes, what kind of support? If no, can you think of ways to develop more support?

10. How have you changed, or how have you changed the environment around you to accommodate a healthier lifestyle through physical activity/exercise?

11. Is there anything else you need (for example, information, time) to promote your continued maintenance?

12. If you listed something in the previous statement, can you think of a way to attain it or can you think of someone who can help you with it?

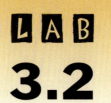

LAB
3.2

One-Mile Rockport Walk Test

This is a maximum-effort test so, although it is a walking test rather than a running test, a person should still precede the test with six to eight weeks of brisk walking.

Equipment

1. Stopwatch or a regular watch that displays seconds; if possible have two available

2. Measured, flat one-mile path, free of traffic lights or other obstacles that could delay a walker

3. Partner (optional)

4. Pencil or pen

Directions

1. Warm up and stretch.

2. Walk one mile as fast as you can, maintaining a steady pace.

3. On completion, record, or have your partner record, your time to the nearest second. This should be done quickly so that you can immediately count your pulse as described in Step 4. If you have two timers (such as a stopwatch and a watch), you can leave the one-mile time on the stopwatch and use the other to count your pulse.

   1-mile walk time: _____

4. Continue walking, but slow down the pace. Count your pulse for 15 seconds and multiply by 4 to obtain your heart rate in beats per minute. Record your results:

   15-second post-mile heart rate: _____ × 4

   = _____ beats per minute

5. Cool down by walking slowly for several minutes and performing some stretches; especially stretch your legs and hips.

6. Turn to the appropriate Rockport Fitness Walking Test charts according to your age and sex. These show the established fitness norms from the American Heart Association. Using your relative fitness level chart, find your time in minutes and your heart rate per minute. Follow these lines until they meet and mark this point on the chart. This point is designed to tell you how fit you are compared to other individuals of your age and sex. For example, if your mark places you in the Level 4 section of the chart, you are in better shape than the average person in your category. The charts are based on weights of 170 pounds for men and 125 pounds for women. If you weigh substantially less, your relative cardiovascular fitness level will be slightly underestimated. Conversely, if you weigh substantially more, your relative cardiovascular fitness level will be slightly overestimated.[a]

   Date: _____   fitness level: _____

Notes: For additional information about the Rockport Fitness Walking Test, see www.rockport.com.

[a]© (1993) The Rockport Company, Inc. All Rights Reserved. Reprinted by permission of The Rockport Company, Inc.

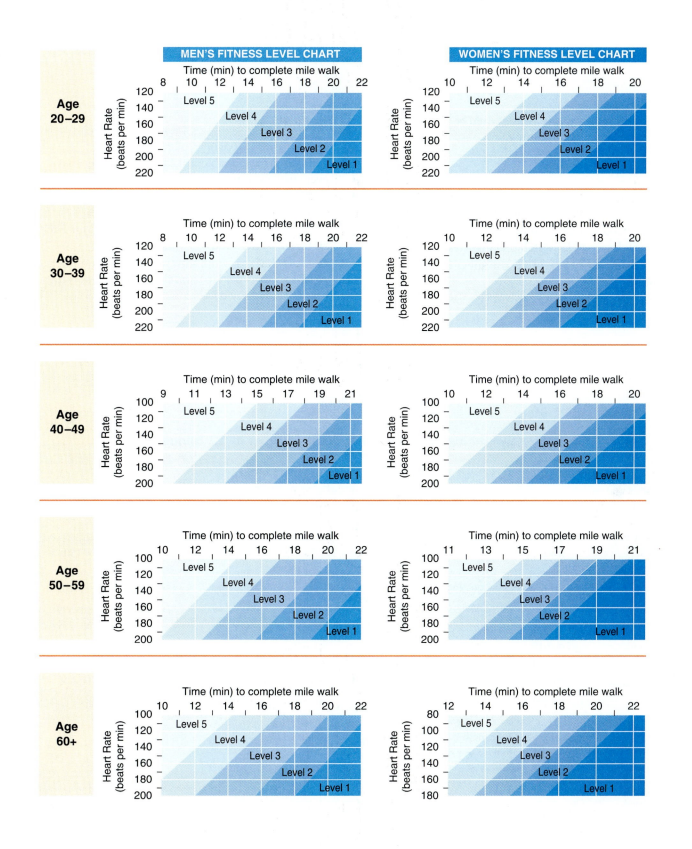

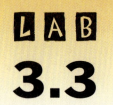

Name _____   **Section**   **Date**

LAB 3.3

12-Minute Swim Test

This is a maximum-effort test and should be preceded by six to eight weeks of conditioning.

Equipment

1. Swimming pool or other body of water with no current, where distance is clearly marked.
2. Partner to count laps and time the swim using a stopwatch or regular watch that displays seconds.
3. Paper and pencil to record the number of laps swum.
4. Calculator (optional) to convert laps swum to yards swum.

Directions

1. Warm up and stretch.
2. Swim as far as possible in 12 minutes using whatever stroke you prefer and resting as necessary. During the swim, have a partner time you, and count and record the number of laps swum.
3. Cool down by swimming at a slower speed for 5 to 10 minutes, followed by some stretching.
4. Convert the laps swum into yards swum (number of laps × yards per lap) and find your fitness rating on the chart provided below.

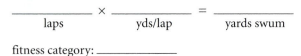

_____ × _____ = _____
   laps   yds/lap   yards swum

fitness category: _____

Fitness Category		AGE (YEARS)					
		13–19	**20–29**	**30–39**	**40–49**	**50–59**	**60 +**
I. Very poor	(men)	< 500[b]	< 400	< 350	< 300	< 250	< 250
	(women)	< 400	< 300	< 250	< 200	< 150	< 150
II. Poor	(men)	500–599	400–499	350–449	300–399	250–349	250–299
	(women)	400–499	300–399	250–349	200–299	150–249	150–199
III. Fair	(men)	600–699	500–599	450–549	400–499	350–449	300–399
	(women)	500–599	400–499	350–449	300–399	250–349	200–299
IV. Good	(men)	700–799	600–699	550–649	500–599	450–549	400–499
	(women)	600–699	500–599	450–549	400–499	350–449	300–399
V. Excellent	(men)	> 800	> 700	> 650	> 600	> 550	> 500
	(women)	> 700	> 600	> 550	> 500	> 450	> 400

12-Minute Swimming Test: Distance (Yards) Swum in 12 Minutes[a]

Source: "Swimming Test" from *The aerobics program for total well-being* by Kenneth H. Cooper, M.D., M.P.H., p. 142. Copyright © 1982 by Kenneth H. Cooper. Used by permission of Bantam Books, a division of Bantam Doubleday Dell Publishing Group, Inc.

[a]The swimming test requires you to swim as far as you can in 12 minutes, using whatever stroke you prefer and resting as necessary, but trying for a maximum effort. The easiest way to take the test is in a pool with known dimensions, and it helps to have another person record the laps and time. Be sure to use a watch with a sweep second hand.

[b]< Means "less than"; > means "more than."

1.5-Mile Timed Run Test

This is a maximum-effort test. It is recommended that you exercise regularly for six to eight weeks prior to taking this test.

Equipment

1. Stopwatch
2. Measured course
3. Pencil or pen

Directions

1. Warm up and stretch.
2. On the start signal, run/walk the 1.5-mile course as quickly as possible. (An even pace throughout the course is recommended.)
3. Record your time at the end of the course:

   _____ minutes
4. Cool down with a slow jog or brisk walk and do some stretches, especially for your legs.
5. Consult the chart to find your fitness rating:

   fitness category: _____

Time in Minutes for 1.5-Mile Run Test						
		AGE (YEARS)				
Fitness Category		**13–19**	**20–29**	**30–39**	**40–49**	**50–59**	**60 +**
I. Very poor	(men)	>15:31[a]	>16:01	>16:31	>17:31	>19:01	>20:01
	(women)	>18:31	>19:01	>19:31	>20:01	>20:31	>21:01
II. Poor	(men)	12:11–15:30	14:01–16:00	14:44–16:30	15:36–17:30	17:01–19:00	19:01–20:00
	(women)	16:55–18:30	18:31–19:00	19:01–19:30	19:31–20:00	20:01–20:30	20:31–21:00
III. Fair	(men)	10:49–12:10	12:01–14:00	12:31–14:45	13:01–15:35	14:31–17:00	16:16–19:00
	(women)	14:31–16:54	15:55–18:30	16:31–19:00	17:31–19:30	19:01–20:00	19:31–20:30
IV. Good	(men)	9:41–10:48	10:46–12:00	11:01–12:30	11:31–13:00	12:31–14:30	14:00–16:15
	(women)	12:30–14:30	13:31–15:54	14:31–16:30	15:56–17:30	16:31–19:00	17:31–19:30
V. Excellent	(men)	8:37–9:40	9:45–10:45	10:00–11:00	10:30–11:30	11:00–12:30	11:15–13:59
	(women)	11:50–12:29	12:30–13:30	13:00–14:30	13:45–15:55	14:30–16:30	16:30–17:30
VI. Superior	(men)	<8:37	<9:45	<10:00	<10:30	<11:00	<11:15
	(women)	<11:50	<12:30	<13:00	<13:45	<14:30	<16:30

Source: "1.5 Mile Tests" from *The aerobics program for total well-being* by Kenneth H. Cooper, M.D., M.P.H., p. 141. Copyright © 1982 by Kenneth H. Cooper. Used by permission of Bantam Books, a division of Bantam Doubleday Dell Publishing Group, Inc.

[a] < Means "less than"; > means "more than."

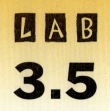

LAB 3.5

Developing Your Cardiorespiratory Endurance Program

1. Set a general goal for your program:

2. Select activities and organize your exercise program:

Activity	Frequency (times per week)	Intensity	Duration	Days of the Week	Time of Day

3. Set specific goals:

4. Set a start date: _____

3.5 *(Continued)*

5. Use the following log to record your progress:

Date	Activity	Intensity	Duration	Comments

CHAPTER 4

Flexibility

Terms

- Flexibility
- Range of motion (ROM)
- Connective tissue
- Tendons
- Ligaments
- Lordosis
- Kyphosis
- Scoliosis, functional
- Scoliosis, structural
- Stretch reflex
- Inverse myotatic reflex
- Reciprocal innervation
- Passive stretch
- Active stretch
- Static stretch
- Ballistic stretch
- PNF stretching

Objectives

1. Establish flexibility as a valuable attribute.

2. Explain at least three ways that flexibility can enhance the quality of your life.

3. Explain the advantages and disadvantages of static, ballistic, and PNF stretching.

4. Identify the factors that influence muscular flexibility.

5. Demonstrate examples of static, ballistic, and PNF stretching, including active and passive static stretching.

6. Using proper technique and alignment, demonstrate a series of flexibility exercises for the major muscle groups of your body.

7. Identify at least three ways that you can prevent low-back pain.

8. Determine personal flexibility needs and establish a flexibility plan that will meet those needs.

Where Am I?

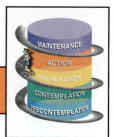

Precontemplator _____ I currently do not do any flexibility exercises and I do not intend to start in the next six months.

Contemplator _____ I currently do not do any flexibility exercises, but I am considering starting within the next six months.

Preparer _____ I currently do some flexibility exercises but do not do them regularly and/or I perform flexibility exercises only for some of the major muscles (joints) of my body.

Action Taker _____ I currently perform flexibility exercises regularly but have been doing so only within the last six months.

Maintainer _____ I currently perform flexibility exercises regularly and I have done so for longer than six months.

The behavior goal for flexibility is to perform flexibility exercises for the major muscles (joints) of the body, five to seven days a week. This would equate to roughly eight to ten stretches covering the calf, thigh (front and back), hips, back, chest, shoulders, arms, and neck. To be an action taker or maintainer you must practice this goal behavior.

If you fall short of this goal but are able to perform some flexibility exercises on a regular basis, you should still give yourself a lot of credit. Being able to sustain even a portion of the goal behavior is a major accomplishment and a real confidence booster. Look at the statements above and select the one that best describes your flexibility stage of change.

Fl-e-e-e-xibility is so easy to take for granted until . . . Ouch!—you stretch too far. How flexible are you? Does seeing people doing the limbo at a wedding look like fun or torture? Would you survive unscathed a sudden split on a patch of ice or a slippery floor? Can you still literally "put your foot in your mouth" like you could when you were a baby? Does it matter? How much flexibility is enough?

No one is quite sure how much flexibility is ideal, but one thing is clear: when muscle tightness interferes with your ability to move, you aren't flexible enough. A good "wellness" guideline is to have enough flexibility to perform daily tasks and enjoy recreational activities comfortably and efficiently, with a minimum risk of injury. Individualizing this guideline is important. For

some people, daily tasks mean being able to walk, bathe, cook, and so on, while for others it includes a physically demanding job or participation in competitive athletics. Similarly, recreational activities range from simple walking to white-water rafting. The types of movements, and the level at which you want to perform them, will determine the degree of flexibility you need. Rock climbing, for example, requires more flexibility than trail hiking, and rock climbing for beginners with relatively closely placed footholds requires less flexibility than an advanced climb with widely spaced footholds.

The best approach is to develop enough flexibility to meet your activity needs. Unfortunately, many people do the opposite; they change or limit their activities to accommodate their present level of flexibility. Are

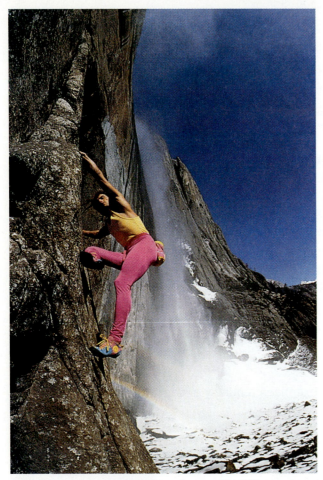

Different activities require different degrees of flexibility.

you guilty of letting that hard-to-reach Frisbee or ball go by because you would have had to stretch just a little too far . . . or do you get out of the car to reach something in the back seat because twisting and reaching from the front seat is too difficult? Or eat the food located in the front of the refrigerator rather than bend and reach to the back shelf? Adjusting your activities to your present level of flexibility can create a downward spiral where the less active you become, the less flexible you become; the less flexible you become, the fewer activities you can do.

Poor flexibility is like wearing a blazer that's too tight in the shoulders or a narrow skirt that limits the length of your stride. Fortunately, you don't have to put up with this unnecessary confinement. Freedom of movement can be preserved or achieved by being physically active and regularly moving your joints through their full range of motion. People of every age can increase their flexibility.[1–3] Starting young, however, has the advantage of slowing down the aging effect and putting you in a position of maintaining flexibility rather than regaining it. The bottom line: it is never too late to start, but sooner is better than later.

WHAT EXACTLY IS FLEXIBILITY?

Flexibility is defined as the **range of motion (ROM)** around a joint or a group of joints. Raising your arm from alongside your body to an overhead position is an example of a full ROM in a single joint (the shoulder joint). The ROM you can achieve when attempting to touch your toes is an example of multi-joint flexibility since this motion requires movement of both the hip and low back joints. Many joints are multidirectional, which means that they have ranges of motion in several directions. Your shoulder joint, for example, allows you to move your arm forward, backward, and sideways. Maintaining flexibility in one direction does not ensure it in another. Because we tend to use our arms more in front of our body, flexibility is more apt to be lost to the back or side. To have optimal shoulder flexibility, you need to maintain full ranges of motion in all directions. Stretching exercises can help offset any muscle tightness that results from daily activities or the lack thereof.

THE ANATOMY OF STRETCHING

Before stretching, it is useful to have an idea which tissues in your body should be stretched, which should not, and how to accomplish the first without accidentally doing the second. An understanding of the muscles, bones, and connective tissues that compose a joint is helpful.

From here on, the word *joint* will refer to a synovial joint. In healthy joints, movement is limited to a normal range of motion by the bony structures and connective tissues that make up the joint. Synovial joints, like those in the arms and legs, allow a lot of movement and are the joints important to flexibility.

Connective tissue binds, supports, and strengthens other tissues of the joint. Its properties range, depending on its function, from flexible and elastic, to stiff, strong, and plastic. Elastic connective tissue, like a rubber band, will return to its original shape when it is not being stretched; plastic connective tissue does not have the same ability to retract after stretching. Both kinds of connective tissue are involved in joints.

The joint capsule, a saclike structure made of tough fibrous connective tissue, surrounds the ends of the bones that make up joints. Synovial fluid in the joint cavity lubricates the cartilage on the ends of the bones, making it possible for them to slide and rotate with less friction. A good warm-up encourages the release of synovial fluid into the joint. Warm-up motions also help synovial fluid become less viscous—a change something like converting soft margarine to oil.

Deep fascia, the connective tissue that surrounds and subdivides muscle tissue, is quite elastic. The outer layer envelops the whole muscle, and inner layers surround individual muscle fibers and fiber bundles. These layers of deep fascia join at the ends of muscle to form **tendons,** connective tissue that links muscle to bone.

Tendons that have been kept in a shortened position, such as the Achilles tendon after wearing high heels, or the patellar tendon after wearing a leg cast, should be carefully stretched to regain their normal length.

While you want your joints to have a full range of motion, you also want them to be snug fitting. **Ligaments** are connective tissue that attach one bone to another. Healthy ligaments hold bones together in their proper positions. If a ligament is too long—the result of an inherited condition, injury, or overstretching—the joint will be looser than it should be; this is known as joint laxity. "Double-jointed" individuals have "relaxed" ligaments that allow more than normal motion in the joint. If joint laxity interferes with function, surgery may be necessary to "tighten" the ligaments and restore normal function.

Because of their more plastic nature, injured (overstretched) ligaments and tendons tend to remain somewhat lengthened, resulting in a condition of joint instability. You may have heard the phrase, "A bad sprain is worse than a break." This is because bones usually heal more easily than ligaments and tendons. If a joint already has some laxity, you shouldn't stretch it. Instead, consider strengthening the muscles around the joint to add stability to the area. To avoid damaging ligaments and tendons during stretching, pay close attention to technique and alignment, and avoid the "bad" stretches identified on pages 86–94.

Assuming that your bone structure is normal and your ligaments and tendons are healthy, most of the flexibility of a joint is determined by the muscles and their fascia. Muscle tissue is elastic—sarcomeres (the contractile units that make up muscle fibers) can be stretched to 150 percent of their resting length[4]—but to achieve good muscle stretch, the muscle fibers need to be relaxed. As the muscle elongates, the deep fascia becomes taut and then stretches. The muscle and muscle fascia will adapt to a stretching program by becoming less resistant to elongation and by increasing their resting length. The net effect is more freedom of movement. When doing stretching exercises, the goal is to stretch the elastic muscle (and deep fascia), to stretch the tendon somewhat, and to avoid stretching ligaments.

FACTORS THAT INFLUENCE FLEXIBILITY

Age

The unchecked erosion of flexibility happens slowly over the years and the tendency is to adjust unconsciously to a more limited range of motion. Is it uncomfortable to sit with your legs extended in front of you? (Many people have to lean back or bend their knees to sit in a bathtub.) Is it difficult to pick up something you've dropped? Does someone have to help you with a zipper or an itch on your back? When flexibility decreases enough, it interferes with our ability to function effectively and live independently. Many of our elderly cannot bend over to put on their shoes, or have trouble getting up out of a chair. Is that your future or will you be one of the growing number of senior citizens playing golf, swimming, dancing, and enjoying their grandchildren?

You might think the ability to increase flexibility is all downhill after you reach school age, but it's not. Flexibility studies on American schoolchildren show that flexibility increases each year between the ages of 6 and 18,[5,6] with girls being more flexible than boys. A Canadian study of 6-, 9-, 12-, and 15-year-olds had similar findings,[7] also noting that the difference in male and female flexibility widened with age. Flexibility in these studies was measured using the sit-and-reach test (see Lab 4.2), a test of low-back, hip, and leg flexibility. Additional studies have found that flexibility increases slow down and stabilize during the late teens and early twenties.[8] After this, flexibility begins to decline.

Physical Activity

Although flexibility seems to decline with age, recent studies indicate that the amount of decline is largely up to the individual. Sedentary individuals are relatively inflexible, while active individuals of all ages tend to maintain or even increase their flexibility. In a shoulder flexibility study,[9] researchers found that flexibility decreased after age 10 but that the decrease was minimal for those who remained active. Connective tissue does lose some of its elasticity and hydration with age, but as more and more senior citizens remain physically active, we are seeing that flexibility is more related to activity level than age.

One day, while doing something that used to be easy, you may discover your body has changed. This wake-up signal to poor flexibility is often, but not always, a sports movement or a pulled muscle from a quick movement. Most likely you will try to blame this new limitation on aging, when the real culprit is probably your activity level. Remember the secret to healthy, flexible joints is to use them—to move and be active!

The activities that we choose affect our flexibility. People who spend most of their time sitting can lose flexibility in their hip joints. Runners who don't stretch often experience a tightening of the leg muscles because their stride uses a limited range of motion. When muscles are totally immobilized they can quickly lose range of motion. For this reason, nurses and physical therapists work with patients who are bedridden by moving the patients' limbs and exercising their muscles. Similarly, people who use wheelchairs need to move their limbs and back through full ranges of motion to prevent stiffness. To test the idea that "use" maintains flexibility, put your dominant hand (the one you write with) overhead and down your back as if you are washing the back of your neck. Reach behind your back and up with the opposite arm. Try to bring your fingertips together without arching your back. This is a measure of shoulder flexibility. Now, switch your arms, nondominant hand up. Are you more

BARRIER Busters

I don't know which stretches would be good for me.

- Consult the exercise list on pages 86–94 of this chapter, a fitness specialist, or an article or book written by a professional.
- Join a class and follow the instructor's routine. Watch a quality video.
- Perform some flexibility tests (see the labs in this chapter).

I don't have enough time to do both cardiorespiratory exercise and stretches.

- Build stretching into your routine. For example, walk ¼ mile, stretch calves, walk ¼ mile, stretch hamstrings, and so on. If you are more active (for example, running, cycling), build them into the warm-up and cool-down. Swim a slower lap, stretch shoulders against the wall, swim another lap, stretch calves against the wall, and so on.
- With very limited time, select the most important stretches and do them.
- Include stretching in your daily routine. While waiting on hold on the telephone, do ankle circles and then ankle flexion holds. After climbing the stairs, take a moment on the top stair to stretch your calves. During a study or work break, bend over in your chair and gently stretch your low back.

Stretching is painful.

- Stretch gently, with proper technique, and after a warm-up. If you still feel pain, see a physician.
- For some people, stretching in warm water is more comfortable. Stretch gently during or after a shower or bath, or exercise in a swimming pool. Diving pools and therapeutic pools are kept warmer than regular pools. Saunas and whirlpools can also effectively warm your body, but avoid any significant exertion since the temperature is so high. (Do not use a sauna or whirlpool if your physician has advised against it.)

I've never been injured and I've never stretched before.

- When you say you have never been injured, are you counting any episodes of low-back pain? Also consider that as you get older your joints tend to stiffen, which can make you more susceptible to injury. Stretching can help prevent some of the stiffening.

I don't play sports.

- Flexibility is as important to daily activity as it is to sports activity. Failure to maintain joint mobility cuts more and

---

flexible with one arm up than the other? Which one? Why? Were you aware of a loss of mobility on one side? If your shoulders are equally flexible (less usual), can you think of a reason why? The flexibility tests in Labs 4.2 and 4.3 will help you identify muscle imbalances and check for healthy ranges of motion. By identifying which of your muscles are kept in a shortened position, you can concentrate on flexibility exercises for them.

Muscle Temperature

Warm muscles stretch more easily than cold ones. Warming up increases blood circulation to the muscles and decreases the viscosity of fluids in the joint capsule and connective tissues. Warming up allows tissues to slide across one another more easily, which promotes flexibility and coordinated muscle movement.

When you perform flexibility tests, it is important to perform successive tests under the same conditions, since test scores taken after a warm-up or workout will be better than those taken when your muscles are cold. Make note of the conditions under which you take the test and try to repeat the conditions in subsequent tests. It is generally recommended that flexibility exercises be done after a body-warming experience. This can be a short, easy aerobic workout like walking or easy jogging, or it can be the result of an external source of warmth, such as a warm bath or sauna.

Gender

Women and girls tend to be more flexible than their male counterparts. The reasons for this are not totally understood; however, flexibility findings between genders may have been influenced to some extent by the nature of activities in which each gender has traditionally participated. For example, more girls and women have traditionally selected flexibility-enhancing activities like dance and gymnastics than men. As men and women (boys and girls) participate in a broader range of activities, future research may find less of a gender difference in flexibility.

Body Composition

There are only two instances in which body composition plays a role in flexibility. One is when there is an abundance of adipose tissue. Too much tissue simply gets in

more into the quality of your life.

I don't have a partner to help me stretch.

- Most stretches do not require a partner. If you need a partner for motivational purposes, join a club to meet people, find someone on the Internet and send motivational messages back and forth, or ask your family and friends to support your efforts. Ask around to see whether anyone is interested in starting a stretching program with you.

I am naturally flexible.

- That's wonderful. Knowing that flexibility is joint-specific, are you naturally flexible in all your joints? And are you equally flexible in both hamstrings? Quadriceps? Other muscles?

I've done it before—with no results.

- First reexamine the program you used. Did it follow the fitness concepts and guidelines presented in this text? Did you stay with the program long enough to get an effect? It can take six to eight weeks to start to see gains. Reexamine the types of stretches you used. Consult your instructor or other professional for advice.

I've gotten this far without it.

- Okay, but is the quality of your life poorer as a result? Can you do all the activities you want to do or does lack of flexibility limit your movements somewhat? As you age, will a lack of flexibility affect you?

I've been trying to do some stretching but I don't have any confidence in my ability to keep it up.

- Try to identify the situations that tempt you to stop or skip your stretching. Then, brainstorm ways to prevent the temptations from occurring or to nullify their effect. You may want to ask a professional for ideas.
- Reward yourself for each small step in the right direction.
- Get an outside opinion about your progress. Maybe you are doing very well but aren't giving yourself enough credit.

I've made a tentative plan of action but haven't been able to get started.

- You are talking a good story but need to move from a verbal commitment to action. Pick just one small thing to do and get started.
- Involve another person in the process of getting you started . . . sometimes all we need is a "kick in the pants."
- Review your schedule and make a decision about when you will start. Post this information in a highly visible location.

the way. The second is a very rare phenomenon in which there is so much muscle bulk that one muscle butts up against another and limits joint movement. It is not true that people who weight train will lose muscle flexibility due to muscle boundness. In fact most muscular individuals have excellent flexibility because they have trained their muscles through a full range of motion.

Disease

Diseases like arthritis can make it uncomfortable or even very painful to move joints. When inflammation is low, exercises are often prescribed in an effort to maintain joint mobility. If you suffer from a joint-affecting disease, you should consult your physician for suggestions. The "freezing up" of joints can be very debilitating and should be prevented whenever possible.

Injury

Injury can severely limit range of motion, but often a good rehabilitation program can help you regain all or a good portion of your flexibility and strength. Sports medicine doctors and physical therapists work very hard with top athletes to help them regain their range of motion. You shouldn't settle for less. When injury or disease causes permanent damage, it is critical to regain as much movement as possible.

BENEFITS OF FLEXIBILITY

Good flexibility allows for more efficient and effective movement. Compare the biomechanically efficient and fluid butterfly stroke of the flexible swimmer with the choppy movement created by a swimmer with less shoulder flexibility. Shoulder rotation is also an important part of throwing a ball. The further back you can lay your arm, the more leverage you will have. Kicking a ball also requires flexibility to follow through properly. A dancer's apparent effortlessness of motion depends on good flexibility too. You certainly don't have to be as flexible as Olympic Gold Medal athletes like diver Greg Louganis or gymnast Shannon Miller to enjoy sports, but you will find that as you increase your flexibility, certain skills and movements will become easier to perform.

Relaxation is another benefit of stretching. It feels good to stretch and bend after sitting for long periods at a desk or in a car. Muscle tension is released and movement seems easier after a good stretch. Also trigger points, which are tight knots in the muscle or connective tissue, can often be relieved. For further stress reduction, some people include soft music and relaxation techniques in their stretching programs.

Stretching is also helpful for relieving muscle cramps caused by fatigue, overheating, or hormonal changes, the latter of which often occurs during pregnancy. To relieve a cramp, you need to put the contracted muscle into a stretch position. When you first stretch the muscle, it will be painful, but the cramp will soon dissipate. Massaging the stretching muscle may also help. Menstrual cramps and discomfort (dysmenorrhea) may be relieved or at least reduced through stretching. Some women find relief by leaning a hip against a wall or doing the cat stretch (on all fours arching one's back).

Stretching after a workout helps relieve and prevent muscle soreness by assisting fatigued muscles to return to their normal length. Otherwise their tendency is to return to a shortened length. Remember, workouts that require stretching may be exercise-oriented, like a basketball game, or project-oriented, such as packing and moving your belongings.

PREVENTING BACK PAIN

One of the best reasons to stay flexible is to prevent back pain. A large percentage of people (80 percent) experience back pain at some point during their lives and in most cases it can be traced to weak abdominal and spinal muscles; poor muscular endurance; inadequate flexibility in the spine, hips, and legs; and chronically poor posture.[10] Much of this pain can be prevented by keeping the correct muscles strong and flexible. Poor posture, one of the culprits of back pain, is often the result of weak, tight muscles. (Injury is also more likely under these conditions.) In addition to reducing back pain, good posture makes you look better. You may even feel more self-confident entering a room if you know that you carry yourself well.

To prevent or relieve back pain, it is helpful to understand how the spine and its supporting muscles work. The human spine is designed with three major natural curves, the lumbar, thoracic, and cervical curves (see Figure 4.1). These curves are wonderfully engineered to handle pounds of stress and the constant pull of gravity. A straight spine would not be nearly as mechanically efficient or shock absorptive. Back pain is often the result of a reduction in, or accentuation of, one of these curves. The underlying cause may be poor posture or muscle strength and flexibility imbalances. **Lordosis**, a condition in which there is excessive curvature in the lower back, occurs when the abdominal muscles are weak and the hip flexors are short (inflexible). This causes the pelvis to be pulled forward, creating a lordotic curve in the low back. (See Figure 4.2.) The reverse

problem occurs when tight hamstring muscles (back of the legs) pull the pelvis down and back, flattening the lumbar curve and rounding the low back. Either condition can result in low-back pain and referred leg pain. Sciatica, an irritation of the sciatic nerve, which runs down the leg, is often caused by problems originating in the low back.

The thoracic curve is affected when chest muscles are strengthened more than back muscles. This is most common among men who want to develop their chest muscles using the bench press, but who do not do counterbalancing back exercises. The strength imbalance results in the stronger shorter chest muscles pulling the shoulders forward, rounding the back, and increasing the thoracic curve. Rounding of the shoulders and spine may also be caused by poor posture due to a lack of attention to posture, or because an occupation requires a person to maintain a poor posture. Poor posture over many years can also result in a permanent rounding of the upper spine known as **kyphosis**. This can be prevented by periodically stretching during work hours and by performing exercises for the counterbalancing muscles.

Not only is it important to stretch and strengthen muscles that work in opposition, like the chest and the back, it is also important that both sides of the body are

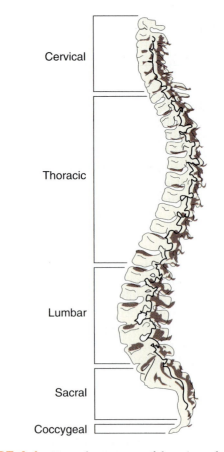

FIGURE 4.1 Normal curvatures of the spine enhance mechanical efficiency.

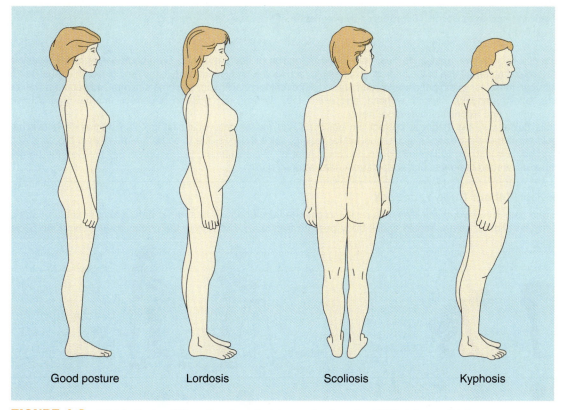

FIGURE 4.2 Which, if any, of these drawings depicts your back posture? What do you think you could do to improve your posture?

Good posture   Lordosis   Scoliosis   Kyphosis

equally strong and flexible. For example, when one hamstring muscle is stronger and more flexible than the other, the weaker, shorter one is more apt to become injured.[11] **Functional scoliosis** occurs when the spine takes on a C or an S curve because muscles are shorter on one side of the body. This can be corrected with strength and flexibility exercises as long as what is causing the imbalance is also corrected. Functional scoliosis should not be confused with **structural scoliosis,** which is the result of a structural defect such as incorrect bone formation or a short leg. Functional scoliosis can, however, lead to structural scoliosis if left unchecked. For example, carrying a heavy bookbag or purse over one shoulder results in one shoulder being lifted, which in turn causes the muscles on the opposite side of the back to shorten; in time, this can result in a permanent adaptation of the spine. To prevent this, carry loads in a centered manner (for example, in a knapsack), or carry the load on each side equally (for example, change a purse from shoulder to shoulder) plus strengthen and stretch both sides equally. Consult a specialist if you suspect you have either type of scoliosis, lordosis, or kyphosis.

The cervical curve is most often affected when the jaw or chin is jutted forward. This is a common habit among stress-ridden individuals. Take a minute to pull your chin in and release the tension in your jaw. Can you feel a difference? Relaxation, posture awareness, proper strength work, and the right flexibility exercises can help you maintain a healthy muscle balance along your spine. See Figure 4.3.

MUSCLE REFLEXES AND FLEXIBILITY

A number of different techniques can be used to stretch muscles. To understand how each kind works, it is necessary to understand the stretch reflex (myotatic reflex), the inverse myotatic reflex, and reciprocal innervation.

Stretch Reflex

Nestled in among the muscle fibers are special sensors called muscle spindles. Their job is to keep track of muscle length and the rate (speed) at which the muscle length changes. When a muscle is stretched, the spindle is stretched, and when a spindle is stretched, it sends a message to the spinal cord. The more it is stretched, or the faster it is stretched, the stronger the message. The spinal cord responds with a command to the muscle to contract when the amount or speed of the stretch is thought to endanger the muscle or, in the case of postural muscles,

FIGURE 4.3 Your back and how to care for it. (Reproduced by permission of Schering Corporation.)

Whatever the cause of low back pain, part of its treatment is the correction of faulty posture. But good posture is not simply a matter of "standing tall." It refers to correct use of the body at all times. In fact, for the body to function in the best of health it must be so used that no strain is put upon muscles, joints, bones, and ligaments. To prevent low back pain, avoiding strain must become a way of life, practiced while lying, sitting, standing, walking, working, and exercising. When body position is correct, internal organs have enough room to function normally and blood circulates more freely.

With the help of this guide, you can begin to correct the positions and movements which bring on or aggravate backache. Particular attention should be paid to the positions recommended for resting, since it is possible to strain the muscles of the back and neck even while lying in bed. By learning to live with good posture, under all circumstances, you will gradually develop the proper carriage and stronger muscles needed to protect and support your hard-working back.

How to Stay on Your Feet Without Tiring Your Back

To prevent strain and pain in everyday activities, it is restful to change from one task to another before fatigue sets in. Some people can lie down between chores; others should check body position frequently, drawing in the abdomen, flattening the back, bending the knees slightly.

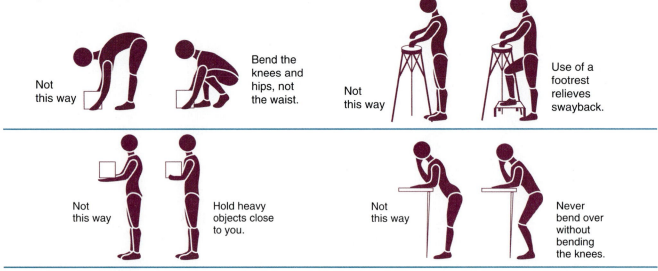

Not this way — Bend the knees and hips, not the waist.

Not this way — Use of a footrest relieves swayback.

Not this way — Hold heavy objects close to you.

Not this way — Never bend over without bending the knees.

Check Your Carriage Here

In correct, fully erect posture, a line dropped from the ear will go through the tip of the shoulder, middle of hip, back of kneecaps, and front of anklebone.

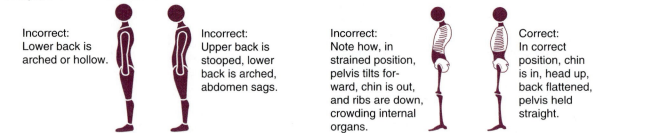

Incorrect: Lower back is arched or hollow.

Incorrect: Upper back is stooped, lower back is arched, abdomen sags.

Incorrect: Note how, in strained position, pelvis tilts forward, chin is out, and ribs are down, crowding internal organs.

Correct: In correct position, chin is in, head up, back flattened, pelvis held straight.

To Find the Correct Standing Position

Stand one foot away from wall. Now sit against wall, bending knees slightly. Tighten abdominal and buttock muscles. This will tilt the pelvis back and flatten the lower spine. Holding this position, inch up the wall to standing position, by straightening the legs. Now walk around the room, maintaining the same posture. Place back against wall again to see if you have held it.

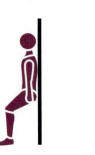

How to Sit Correctly

A back's best friend is a straight, hard chair. If you can't get the chair you prefer, learn to sit properly on whatever chair you get. To correct sitting position from forward slump: Throw head well back, then bend it forward to pull in the chin. This will straighten the back. Now tighten abdominal muscles to raise the chest. Check position frequently.

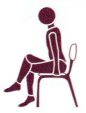 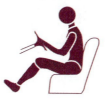 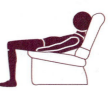

Relieve strain by sitting well forward, flatten back by tightening abdominal muscles, and cross knees.

Use of footrest relieves swayback. Aim is to have knees higher than hips.

Correct way to sit while driving, close to pedals. Use seat belt or hard backrest, available commercially.

TV slump leads to "dowager's hump," strains neck and shoulders.

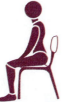 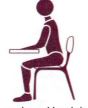 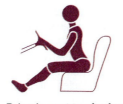 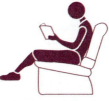

If chair is too high, swayback is increased.

Keep neck and back in as straight a line as possible with the spine. Bend forward from the hips.

Driver's seat too far from pedals emphasizes curve in lower back.

Strained reading position. Forward thrusting strains muscles of neck and head.

How to Put Your Back to Bed

For proper bed posture, a firm mattress is essential. Bedboards, sold commercially, or devised at home, may be used with soft mattresses. Bedboards, preferably, should be made of $3/4$-inch plywood. Faulty sleeping positions intensify swayback and result not only in backache but in numbness, tingling, and pain in arms and legs.

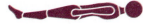 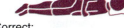 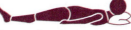 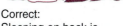

Incorrect:
Lying flat on back makes swayback worse.

Correct:
Lying on side with knees bent effectively flattens the back. Flat pillow may be used to support neck, especially when shoulders are broad.

Incorrect:
Use of high pillow strains neck, arms, shoulders.

Correct:
Sleeping on back is restful and correct when knees are properly supported.

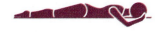 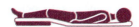 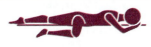

Incorrect:
Sleeping face down exaggerates swayback, strains neck and shoulders.

Correct:
Raise the foot of the mattress eight inches to discourage sleeping on the abdomen.

Incorrect:
Bending one hip and knee does not relieve swayback.

Proper arrangement of pillows for resting or reading in bed.

When Doing Nothing, Do It Right

Rest is the first rule for the tired, painful back. The following positions relieve pain by taking all pressure and weight off the back and legs. Note pillows under knees to relieve strain on spine.

For complete relief and relaxing effect, these positions should be maintained from 5 to 25 minutes.

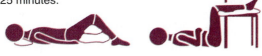 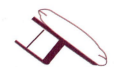

A straight-back chair used behind a pillow makes a serviceable backrest.

FIGURE 4.3 *(continued)*

Exercise — Without Getting Out of Bed

Exercises to be performed while lying in bed are aimed not so much at strengthening muscles as at teaching correct positioning. But muscles used correctly become stronger and in time are able to support the body with the least amount of effort.

Do all exercises in this position. Legs should not be straightened.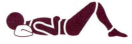

Bring knee to chest. Lower slowly but do not straighten leg. Relax.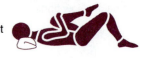

Exercise — Without Attracting Attention

Use these inconspicuous exercises whenever you have a spare moment during the day, both to relax tension and improve the tone of important muscle groups.

1. Rotate shoulders forward and backward.
2. Turn head slowly side to side.
3. Watch an imaginary plane take off, just below the right shoulder. Stretch neck, follow it slowly as it moves up, around and down, disappearing below the other shoulder. Repeat, starting on left side.
4. Slowly, slowly, touch left ear to left shoulder; right ear to right shoulder. Raise both shoulders to touch ears, drop them as far as possible.
5. At any pause in the day—waiting for an elevator to arrive, for a specific traffic light to change—pull in abdominal muscles, tighten, hold for the count of eight without breathing. Relax slowly. Increase the count gradually after the first week. Practice breathing normally with abdomen flat and contracted. Do this sitting, standing, and walking.

Bring both knees slowly up to chest. Tighten muscles of abdomen, press back flat against the floor. Hold knees to chest 20 seconds. Then lower slowly. Relax. Repeat 5 times. This exercise gently stretches the shortened muscles of the lower back, while strengthening abdominal muscles. Clasp knees, bring them up to chest at the same time coming to a sitting position. Rock back and forth.

Rules to Live By — From Now On

1. Never bend from the waist only; bend the hips and knees.
2. Never lift a heavy object higher than your waist.
3. Always turn and face the object you wish to lift.
4. Avoid carrying unbalanced loads; hold heavy objects close to your body.
5. Never carry anything heavier than you can manage with ease.
6. Never lift or move heavy furniture. Wait for someone to do it who knows the principles of leverage.
7. Avoid sudden movements, sudden "overloading" of muscles. Learn to move deliberately, swinging the legs from the hips.
8. Learn to keep the head in line with the spine when standing, sitting, lying in bed.
9. Put soft chairs and deep couches on your "don't sit" list. During prolonged sitting, cross your legs to rest your back.
10. Your doctor is the only one who can determine when low back pain is due to faulty posture. He is the best judge of when you may do general exercises for physical fitness. When you do, omit any exercise which arches or overstrains the lower back: backward or forward bends,touching the toes with the knees straight.
11. Wear shoes with moderate heels, all about the same height. Avoid changing from high to low heels.
12. Put a footrail under the desk and a footrest under the crib.
13. Diaper a baby sitting next to him or her on the bed.
14. Don't stoop and stretch to hang the wash; raise the clothesbasket and lower the washline.
15. Beg or buy a rocking chair. Rocking rests the back by changing the muscle groups used.
16. Train yourself vigorously to use your abdominal muscles to flatten your lower abdomen. In time, this muscle contraction will become habitual, making you the envied possessor of a youthful body profile!
17. Don't strain to open windows or doors.
18. For good posture, concentrate on strengthening "nature's corset"–the abdominal and buttock muscles. The pelvic roll exercise is especially recommended to correct the postural relation between the pelvis and the spine.

FIGURE 4.3 *(continued)*

when body position is about to be lost. This is called the **stretch reflex.** When a physician taps you on the knee with a rubber hammer, your patellar tendon, which is an extension of the quadriceps (thigh) muscles, is suddenly stretched. The spindles in the quadriceps feel this stretch and fire off a message. The spinal cord receives the message and sends a return message to the muscle to contract. When the quadriceps contract, your foot flies in the air. A soft knee tap receives a mild kick, a harder tap a stronger kick. This is the stretch reflex at work.

Stretching Implications

Muscle spindle activation results in muscle contraction, which hinders the ability of the muscle to stretch. While the muscle spindle will always react to a lengthening of the muscle fibers, its reaction can be minimized by moving slowly and evenly into a stretch and by holding a steady position during the stretch. Less spindle action results in more muscle relaxation, which in turn promotes muscle lengthening.

Inverse Myotatic Reflex

Another kind of sensor, the Golgi tendon organ (GTO), is located right in the tendon. GTOs are sensitive to tension. Tension is created in the tendon both when the muscle stretches and when it contracts. When muscle tension exceeds the GTO's threshold, the GTO sends a signal to the spinal cord. The spinal cord then issues a reflexive message to the muscle to relax (the **inverse myotatic reflex**). As the muscle relaxes, tension is decreased. This protective mechanism stops a contraction before the tension is great enough to rip all or part of the tendon from the bone. When a tendon injury does occur, it is usually the result of an explosive movement where the stretch to the muscle is sudden and cannot be sufficiently counteracted.

Stretching Implications

If you put a muscle into a stretch position, then hold it there long enough, the muscle tension will elicit the inverse myotatic reflex, the muscle will reflexively relax, and you will be able to stretch a little further. Similarly if you contract the muscle until you elicit the relaxation reflex, you will also be able to stretch further.

Reciprocal Innervation

When one muscle is contracting, the nervous system signals its paired muscle to relax and lengthen. For example, as your biceps flex, your triceps accommodate by relaxing and lengthening. The nervous system orchestrates the simultaneous increases and decreases in the tensions of the two muscles so well that all we consciously experience is smooth coordinated movement. Because the muscles have complementary responses, this is called **reciprocal innervation** (one reciprocates the other). When a muscle receives a message not to contract, it is said to be inhibited. Because one of the paired muscles is being inhibited in reciprocal innervation, the term *reciprocal inhibition* is also used.

Stretching Implications

During a flexibility exercise, you can help relax a muscle by consciously contracting its paired muscle. This is called active stretching.

METHODS OF STRETCHING

There are three types of stretches: static, ballistic, and proprioceptive neuromuscular facilitation (PNF). In addition, static and ballistic stretches may be performed using either an active or a passive stretching technique. PNF stretching, by definition, uses a combination of passive and active stretches. Each method of stretching facilitates flexibility in a different way.

Active and Passive Stretching

A **passive stretch** occurs when something or someone else creates a stretch in your muscles. Because an outside force is helping you stretch, this is often referred to as assisted stretching. If you are the one being stretched, it is important to relax the target muscle(s) as your partner, gravity, or another part of your body creates the stretch.

A partner creates a passive stretch by moving your muscles into a stretch position and holding you there. While the partner does the holding, you can relax and let the muscle lengthen. This works well if you have a trustworthy partner.

You can assist your own stretch by using muscles that aren't being stretched. For example, you can create a passive calf stretch by wrapping a towel around the ball of your foot and using your arms to pull your toes toward your shin. Gravity can also supply the assist. For example, a passive calf-muscle stretch is achieved when you stand on your toes on the edge of a platform and allow your heels to drop below the platform surface. Machines that put you in traction also provide a passive stretch.

In an **active stretch** you are required to contract one muscle in an effort to stretch another. This works well as long as the contracting muscle is strong enough to pull the other muscle through a full stretch. If it is not, additional stretching can be achieved by adding a passive stretch. For example, an active stretch of the hamstring is achieved by lying on your back and contracting your quadriceps muscle to pull your leg toward your head. If your quadriceps muscle is too weak to create an effective stretch, maintain the quadriceps contraction and add an assist by pulling gently with your hands. Some people also like to follow an active stretch with a passive one.

When you use active stretching, the muscle is said to move through an active range of motion (ROM). Active ROM is defined as the movement achieved in a joint through self-initiated muscle contraction. Passive ROM is the movement of the joint achieved by an outside force such as gravity or a partner.

Injuries tend to occur more often in joints that have a larger difference between passive and active ranges of motion. A good injury-prevention strategy is to maintain good active ranges of motion. This is best achieved using active stretches. Passive stretching, however, also has its merits. When muscles are too weak to pull the body part through a stretch, passive stretching can help achieve flexibility. Passive stretching may also help break through "sticking points." Both active and

To demonstrate the difference between active and passive stretching and range of motion (ROM), stand with your arms out to the sides of your body, parallel to the floor, palms forward. Pull your arms back as far as possible by contracting your shoulder and back muscles—active stretch. The distance you are able to move your arms is your active ROM. To check your passive ROM, start again, but this time have a partner passively stretch you by gently pulling your arms backward. Is there a difference between your active and passive ROMs?

passive stretching techniques can be used with the following three methods of stretching. In the discussion of PNF stretching, you will see how passive and active stretching are alternated to maximize rehabilitation of a joint.

Static Stretching

To perform a **static stretch**, move slowly into the stretch position and then hold (without moving) for a minimum of 10 seconds. Holding a stretch position "quiets" the stretch reflex and elicits the inverse myotatic reflex. This combination relaxes the muscle and allows it to stretch with little risk of injury. The stretch should be held at a point of discomfort but not pain. If you feel pain, either release the stretch and begin again, or back off until the pain is relieved. Performing a series of static stretches works even better because the GTOs' thresholds are reset at a less sensitive level following the first stretch. This allows you to stretch further before encountering resistance. Examples of active and passive static stretches are shown in the box below.

Ballistic Stretching

A **ballistic stretch** is one where you put the muscle rapidly in and out of a stretch position by bouncing or pulsing during the stretch. Ballistic stretching will improve flexibility, but there are a couple of significant drawbacks. First, the rapid lengthening of the muscle

Static and Ballistic Stretching

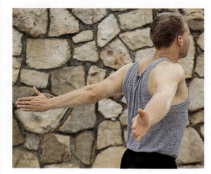

Active static stretch

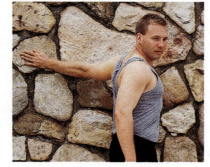

Passive static stretch (self-assist)

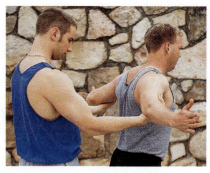

Passive static stretch (partner assist)

Advantages and Disadvantages of Static Stretching

Advantages
- Quiets the stretch reflex
- Little risk of injury
- Invokes the inverse myotatic reflex
- Causes the least muscle soreness

Disadvantages
- Only moderately prepares for ballistic motions
- Requires patience to hold the stretch

Advantages and Disadvantages of Ballistic Stretching

Advantages
- Prepares an individual for ballistic movements
- Is more motivating, less boring for some people

Disadvantages
- Higher risk of injury (small muscle or connective tissue tears)
- Invokes the stretch reflex
- Causes more muscle soreness than static stretching

elicits the stretch reflex, causing the muscle to contract—the opposite effect desired in a stretch. Second, because the movement is more forceful, it has more potential to injure the muscle and connective tissue. Thus, static stretching is generally recommended over ballistic stretching.

There is one time, however, when ballistic stretching is recommended: if you are going to be involved in an activity that requires quick explosive movements, then you need a warm-up that is specific to this. After you have warmed up and done some static stretching, you can start gently with ballistic stretching and build up to performance-level ballistic movements. To prepare a throwing arm, for example, you would warm the entire body (perhaps with a jog), do some arm circles or gentle throwing motions, stretch statically holding the arm to the front, side, and back, use a series of gentle ballistic movements to draw the arm back as if preparing to throw, and finally perform the whole throwing motion (usually with a ball), building up the speed and force of the throw. Always precede ballistic stretches with static stretches and use static stretches at the end of the workout to promote flexibility.

Passive ballistic exercises are more risky and are not recommended unless performed by a trained professional such as a physical therapist.

PNF Stretching

Proprioceptive neuromuscular facilitation (PNF) stretching was originally developed as a rehabilitation tool. PNF stretching is the most effective type of stretching, but it requires a trustworthy and patient partner, considerably more time, and can result in more muscle soreness. Static stretching is almost as effective and is usually easier to perform. PNF stretching might be something worth trying if you feel you are at a sticking point in your flexibility. Or you may want to include a few PNF stretches in a predominantly static stretching routine. There are a number of ways that PNF can be performed. Three of the most commonly used are Contract-Relax (CR), Contract-Relax-Antagonist Contract (CRAC), and Slow-Reversal-Hold-Relax (SRHR). (See the box on page 84.) These methods take advantage of the inverse myotatic reflex and reciprocal innervation to increase muscle relaxation and facilitate muscle lengthening.

DESIGNING YOUR FLEXIBILITY PROGRAM

If you are a contemplator, you are now ready to put together an individualized flexibility program. If you are already an action taker or a maintainer, this information may help you refine your program. Here are some programming guidelines:

1. Determine your flexibility needs and set goals based on these needs (Lab 4.4). There are several ways to approach this. You may want to

   a. Perform the flexibility tests provided at the end of this chapter.

   b. Keep a journal including what type of activities make you stiff and sore, when you notice a lack of flexibility, or what movements you think are being limited by inflexibility.

   c. Ask a coach or fitness specialist about sport-specific stretches that will enhance your performance and help prevent injury.

   d. Read a book on stretching. Some books include sport-specific stretching. Look for a book written by a qualified professional. (See the Suggested Readings at the end of this chapter.)

2. Select exercises that will target your goals. If you want general body flexibility, select one exercise for each major muscle group. The exercises in this text are a good way to start.

3. Determine how many repetitions of each exercise you will do and for how long you will work on each stretch.

4. Determine when you will do your flexibility exercises. Try to make it a regular time; "rituals" are the easiest to maintain. Different exercises may be done at different times of the day if they tie in to specific activities. For example, wrist flexibility exercises can precede or follow keyboard activity.

5. Warm up the joint before stretching, whenever possible. Easy ROM movements are good to get the joints "oiled up" and moving. Once you are warm, go ahead and stretch.

Experts agree that you should stretch following activity, but there is some disagreement as to the value of stretching before an activity. It has been our experience that people feel more ready for exercise after stretching. Older individuals may need more prestretching than younger individuals.

If you are generally physically inactive, it is important to start any physical activity gently. Wearing high-heeled shoes keeps the Achilles tendon in a shortened position all day; therefore, the transition from high heels to flat-soled athletic shoes must be made carefully. As we have mentioned, if you are late for an exercise class or any other vigorous physical activity, control the urge to jump right in—take the time to warm up.

Proprioceptive Neuromuscular Facilitation (PNF)

Contract-Relax-Antagonist Contract (CRAC)

Contract: Passively place the target muscle in a lengthened position using another body part, a partner, or gravity. Perform a 3-second isometric contraction of the target muscle (agonist) against a partner's resistance or an immovable object.

Relax: Release all tension for 2 seconds.

Antagonist Contract: Perform an active stretch (contraction of the antagonist) with a passive assist for 10 to 15 seconds.

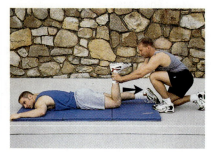
Isometric contraction

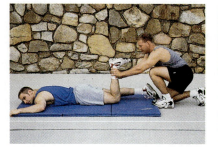
Relaxation

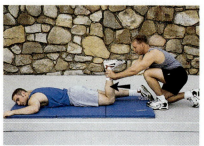
Active stretch with passive assist

Contract-Relax (CR)

Contract: Passively place the target muscle in a lengthened position using another body part, a partner, or gravity. Perform a 6-second isometric contraction of the target muscle against a partner's resistance or an immovable object.

Relax: Hold or have a partner or gravity hold, the target muscle(s) in a passive stretch for 10 to 15 seconds.

Advantages
- Most effective stretching
- Takes full advantage of physiological methods of relaxation
- Excellent tool for rehabilitation

Slow-Reversal-Hold-Relax (SRHR)

Slow: Performs a 10 to 15 second passive stretch of the target muscle using another body part, a partner, or gravity.

Reversal: Perform a 6-second maximal isometric contraction of the target muscle against the resistance of a partner or immovable object. (The muscle you stretched in the first step is contracted in this step—this is considered a reversal.)

Hold: Perform a 6-second submaximal contraction of the antagonist (muscle opposing the target muscle). This is an active stretch of the target muscle.

Relax: Perform a 10 to 15 second passive stretch of the target muscle using another body part, a partner, or gravity.

Disadvantages
- Higher risk of injury
- More delayed onset of muscle soreness (DOMS)
- More time-consuming
- Requires a partner

While there is limited evidence that stretching prior to a workout prevents injury, there is considerable evidence that good flexibility decreases injury.[12] Stretching after a workout is particularly effective for increasing flexibility because the muscles are very warm and ready to elongate.

APPLYING THE PRINCIPLES OF PHYSICAL ACTIVITY

The FIT Principle

Frequency: To improve flexibility, stretch three to seven days a week.

Intensity: Stretch to a point of discomfort, not pain. Pain is your body's way of saying that something is wrong. If you feel pain during a stretch, back off a little or relax the muscle and start over.

Time: Static Stretching: 10- to 60-second holds, 2 to 5 repetitions

Ballistic Stretching: 10- to 60-second bouts, 2 to 5 repetitions

PNF Stretching: variation dependent; refer to pages 86 to 94.

Principles of Overload and Progression

A flexibility overload is accomplished by stretching the muscle further than normal. A progressive overload is achieved by gradually lengthening the muscle over time. Too great an overload or too fast a progression may result in muscle soreness or possibly injury.

Principle of Reversibility

Flexibility can be maintained by stretching a minimum of three days a week. Flexibility is also maintained by incorporating full ROM movements into your lifestyle. Flexibility is lost by doing less than this.

Principle of Individuality

Your bone structure and ligament and tendon attachments are unique to you. Find positions and overloads that work for you. You will also have to determine how much pre-workout stretching is comfortable and necessary for you. While a good range of motion is considered healthy, no one knows for sure how much flexibility is the "right amount." For now, this will have to be a personal decision, one that depends on the types of activities you wish to be able to perform.

Principle of Specificity

You must select exercises or movements that target the joints you want to stretch. For example, stretching one shoulder will not create flexibility in the other. Stretching programs also need to be sport- or activity-specific. For example, joggers need to stretch their legs well while golfers need to stretch their backs. It is always healthy to stretch all the major muscles, but when you have limited extra time, spend it targeting the muscles you will use the most.

FLEXIBILITY EXERCISES

The following is a series of stretches for the body's major muscle groups. Pay close attention to proper stretching technique and body alignment. Also shown are common exercises that have the potential to cause injury.

Stretches That Enhance Flexibility

The exercises shown include active and passive, static, and PNF stretches. For additional stretching ideas, including sport-specific stretches, see the suggested reading list at the end of the chapter.

As with all exercises, it is important to use good technique. Keeping proper body alignment and isolating the muscle(s) you want to stretch will optimize results and minimize injuries. Hold each of the static stretches for 10 to 60 seconds. The hold times for the PNF stretches are individually labeled, as several types of PNF are used.

In the interest of brevity, each exercise is described using one side of the body. When it is appropriate, be sure to stretch both the left and right sides of the body. Photographs and descriptions of the active stretches and many passive stretches are provided along with detailed descriptions for other passive and PNF versions of the stretches. If you experience any pain during an exercise, stop at once and consult a health care provider before performing the stretch again. If you have any medical condition that may be affected by a stretching program (for example, back pain or arthritis), please consult your physician before beginning.

Stretches to Avoid

Some exercises have the potential to cause injury either soon after performing them or in the future from chronic microtrauma. In some cases such positions and stretches are used for sports competitions or aesthetic purposes (for example, dance), but they are not generally recommended for wellness-based flexibility programs. The stretching action of each of these exercises can be obtained by modifying or replacing the exercise. Some common stretches to avoid are included in the following descriptions.

Neck Rotation

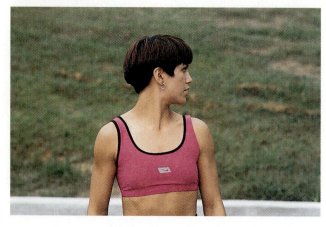

◀ Active: Rotate your head as far as you can to one side. (Look over your shoulder.) Hold. Then rotate to the other side.

Passive: Have a partner gently turn your head for you while you relax and hold it in the stretched position.

PNF: Looking straight ahead, hold your left hand against your left cheek with your elbow pointing forward and your fingers pointing behind you. Try to turn your head to the left but resist this movement with your left hand. Hold this isometric contraction for 3 seconds. Relax for 2 seconds and then turn your head as far to the right as possible. Hold for 10 seconds. CRAC

Lateral Neck Stretch

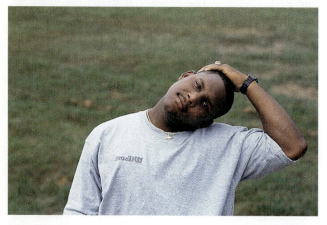

◀ Active with Passive Assist: While looking forward, use the muscles on the side of your neck to pull your ear toward the same side shoulder. To add a passive assist, gently pull your head down toward your shoulder with one hand.

Passive: Have a partner gently lay your head to the side. Or perform your own assist by gently pulling down on your head.

PNF: Place your left hand on the side of your head with elbow forward and fingers facing behind you. Try to lay your head to the left while resisting this action with your left hand. Hold for 3 seconds. Release for 2 seconds and then lay your head to the right side. Hold for 10 seconds. CRAC

Neck Flexion

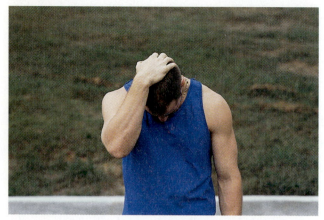

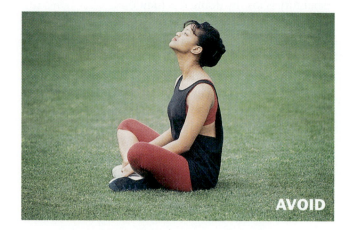

AVOID

▲ Active with Passive Assist: Using the muscles in the front of your neck, draw your chin toward your chest. Add a passive assist by gently pulling forward and down with one hand.

▲ Avoid: Hyperextending the neck places unnecessary stress on the cervical vertebrae.

Passive: Have a partner gently lower your head to your chest. Or perform your own assist by placing your hand on top of your head and gently pulling forward.

PNF: Place your hands on the back of your head. Press back against your hands (3 seconds). Relax (2 seconds) and draw your chin down toward your chest (10 seconds). CRAC

Overhead Reach

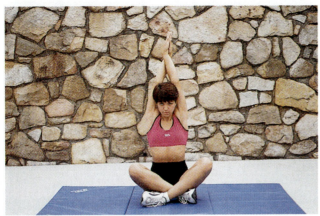

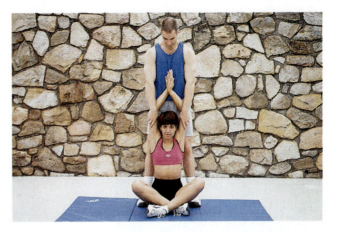

🔺 Active: Reach your arms up overhead with palms facing outward. Cross your arms so that your palms are touching. (Bend your elbows as much as needed.) Keeping your arms behind your ears, extend your elbows and reach upward.

🔺 Passive: Same as above only a partner grasps your upper arm and stretches your arms upward.

PNF: Reach your arms overhead with palms facing outward. Cross your arms so that your palms are touching. Press the palms together (3 seconds), relax (2 seconds), and stretch upward again (10 seconds). CRAC

Chest and Shoulder Stretch

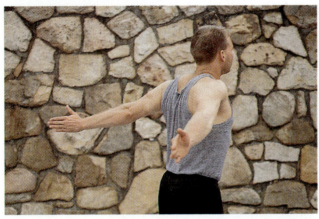

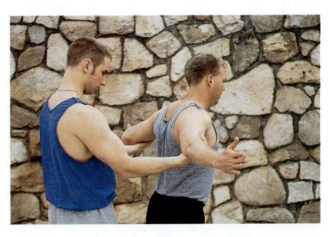

🔺 Active: Stand with your arms extended out to the sides parallel to the floor and with palms facing forward. Contract your shoulder and back muscles such that your arms are drawn backward. (Don't arch your back.) Hold.

🔺 Passive: Same position as above but have a partner grasp your arms and slowly pull them into the stretch position. Hold.

PNF: Place your hand shoulder height on a wall and turn your body away from it until you feel a stretch. In this position, press forward against the wall (3 seconds). Relax (2 seconds) and then draw your arm back using an active stretch (10 seconds). CRAC

Shoulder Hyperextension

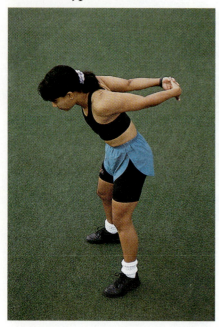

◀ Active: Stand with feet shoulder-width apart, knees bent slightly, and hands clasped behind the back. Raise your arms as high as possible and then hold.

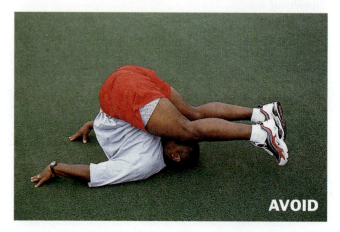

AVOID

◀ Avoid: The plow position puts the weight of the entire body on the cervical vertebrae. This is very stressful to the upper spine.

Passive: Same as active only a partner lifts your arms.

PNF: Partner performs a passive stretch. You then press down with your arms against your partner's resistance (6 seconds). Lift your arms again using an active stretch (6 seconds). Relax and finish with your partner lifting your arms in another passive stretch. SRHR

Upper Arm (Triceps) Stretch

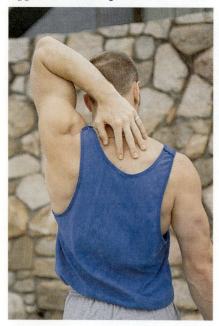

◀ Active: Stand or sit erect. Extend your left arm overhead, keeping the upper portion close to your ear. Bend the extended arm at the elbow and reach your hand, palm inward, down the middle of your back. Do not arch your back.

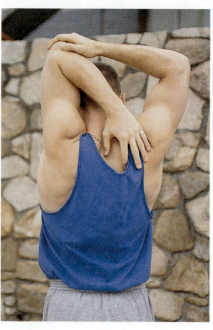

◀ Passive: Same as above only use your right arm to create a stretch by placing your right hand on your right elbow and pushing toward your back gently.

PNF: The right arm position remains the same, with the elbow close to the ear and the hand reaching down the back. Place your left hand on your lower right arm. Try to extend your right arm against the counterresistance created by your left hand (3 seconds). Relax (2 seconds) and then perform an active stretch (10 seconds). CRAC

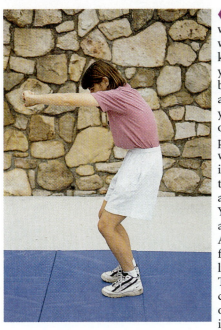

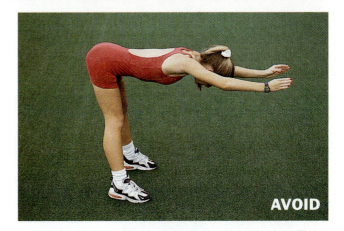

◄ Active: Stand with feet shoulder width apart and knees bent. Tuck your pelvis under by contracting your abdomen. Grasp your hands in front of your body with palms facing outward. Try to "cave in" or "hollow out" the chest and abdominal areas. Your back should appear rounded. Allow your head to follow the natural line of the curve. The same exercise can be performed on all fours in what is commonly called the cat stretch.

AVOID

◄ Avoid: The flat back position stresses the muscles and ligaments in the lower back.

Passive: Sit in a chair and lean forward, allowing your low back to stretch. You may want to provide some support during this exercise by placing your hands on your ankles or on the floor.

PNF: Lie on your back with knees bent and feet on the floor. Lift your back off the floor by contracting your buttocks (gluteal) and lower-back muscles. Hold for 3 seconds. Relax by lowering your back to the floor and then do an active stretch by drawing your knees toward your chest using your abdominal muscles. Assist the active stretch by pulling your knees to your chest with your hands. Place your hands underneath your knees to prevent putting pressure on the knee joint. Hold for 10 seconds. CRAC

BACK AND ABDOMINAL STRETCH

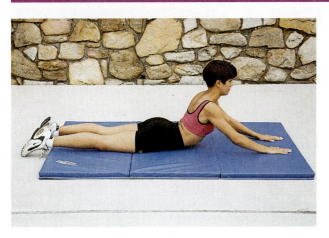

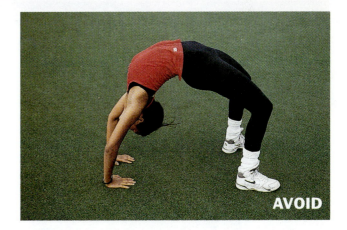

AVOID

◄ Passive: Lie in the prone position on the floor. Place your hands on the floor near your shoulders. Slowly press up creating an arch in your back. Hold briefly and lower.

◄ Avoid: Hypertension of the back is stressful to the spine.

Note: An active abdominal stretch is not included because it may be too taxing for the average person's back muscles. If you want to perform an active stretch assist by using your back muscles to help pull your torso up as you push with your arms.

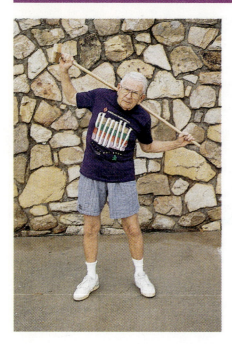

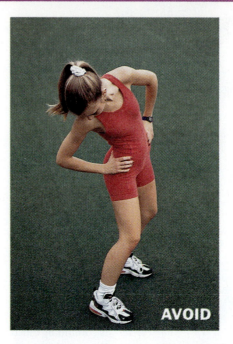

AVOID

▲ Active: Hold a wand across your shoulders and behind your head. Stand with feet shoulder-width apart and knees slightly bent. Slowly lean your shoulders and the wand directly to one side. Return to vertical and stretch the other side.

▲ Avoid: Poor alignment, pelvis rotated forward, when stretching to the side results in an arched back position that can stress the spine. To correct this exercise, pull in your abdominals and bend directly to the side: look forward to prevent twisting.

Passive: Stand with your feet shoulder-width apart, knees slightly bent, feet angled slightly outward, and the right arm on the right thigh for support. Bend directly to the side allowing gravity to pull your shoulder toward the floor. The left arm can be relaxed by your side, extended to the side, or for a more advanced stretch, extended up by the left ear. If the side stretch position is held for an extended amount of time, pressure is put on the vertebral discs, therefore controlled movement into and out of the position is recommended.

BODY ROTATION EXERCISES

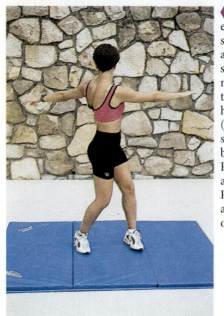

◄ Active: Stand erect with feet shoulder width apart and knees slightly bent. Arms may be extended to the side, on hips, or holding a bar (wand) along the shoulders and behind the head. Rotate to the right as far as possible. Return to center and rotate the other way.

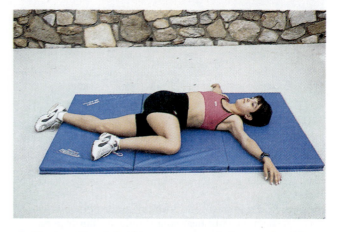

▲ Passive: Lie on the floor, arms extended out at shoulder level, the right leg extended and the left one bent. Keeping the shoulders flat on the floor, slowly lower the left knee across your body and toward the floor. Relax in this position, resting your knee on the floor if possible. Repeat to the other side.

BUTTOCKS STRETCHES

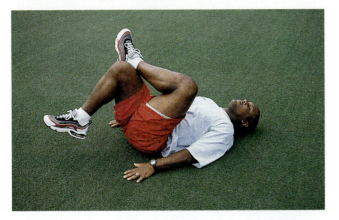

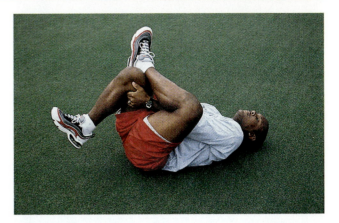

◄ Active: Lie on the floor on your back with your knees bent. Place the left foot on the right knee. Draw your right knee toward your head by contracting your right thigh (quadriceps) muscle.

◄ Passive: The same position as above but assist by placing your hands behind your right thigh and gently pulling it toward your chest.

PNF: Lie with both feet flat on the floor and tighten your buttocks (gluteal) muscles (3 seconds). Relax (2 seconds) and then proceed with the active stretch described above (10 seconds). You may assist the active stretch by pulling your leg toward you with your hands. CRAC

HIP AND THIGH STRETCHES

Thigh (Quadriceps) Stretch

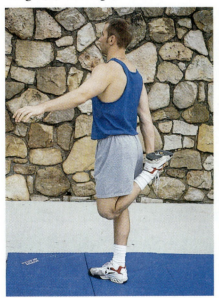

◄ Active with Passive Assist: Stand on your right leg. Bend your left leg and grasp the ankle (not the foot) with the opposite hand. The same side hand can be used as long as good alignment is maintained. An imaginary line running across the top of the pelvis should remain parallel to the floor. The left knee should remain close to the body's center line. Allow a comfortable knee bend and pull your leg gently backward by contracting the hamstring muscle on the back of your leg. (The left foot should not be forced to the buttocks.) To add a passive assist, pull gently backward with the hand holding the ankle. Maintain good posture and balance by extending your free arm, pulling in your abdominals, and looking straight ahead.

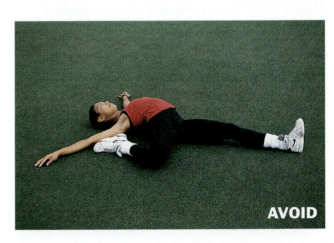

AVOID

◄ Avoid: Leaning back in the hurdler's position stresses the knee ligaments on the bent leg and may irritate your low back. To modify the exercise, move the bent knee as far from the straight leg as possible, place the bent knee at a 90 degree angle, and raise your torso and lean onto the elbow opposite the bent knee.

Passive: Kneel down on your left knee (the marriage proposal position). Move the right foot far enough forward that the right knee remains over the foot, not beyond it, throughout the stretch. Place your hands on your knee or on the floor. Press your pelvis forward and downward to create a stretch in your thigh and hip flexor muscles.

PNF: In a standing or prone lying position, bend your right knee 90 degrees. Against a partner's resistance try to extend your leg. Hold the isometric quadriceps contraction (3 seconds), relax (2 seconds), and then contract your hamstring to perform an active stretch (10 seconds). CRAC

Hip Flexor Stretches

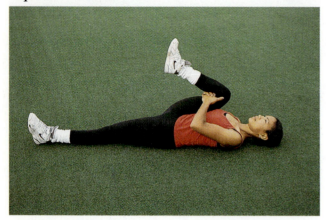

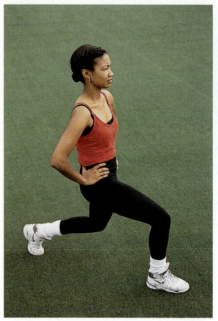

◄ Passive: Stand in a forward/back stride stance with your bent right knee over but not forward of your right ankle. Bend the left leg until the left knee touches the floor. You may wish to place a towel under this knee. Keep your body upright or place your hands on the floor to either side of your legs. Push your hips forward until you feel a stretch.

▲ Active with Passive Assist: Lie on your back with both legs extended. Draw your right knee toward your chest. Pressure may be taken off the back by using your hands as a passive assist and/or by lying on a surface (folded mat, bleacher, table, and so on) that will allow you to extend the left leg over the end and bend at the knee.

BACK OF THE LEG (HAMSTRING) STRETCHES

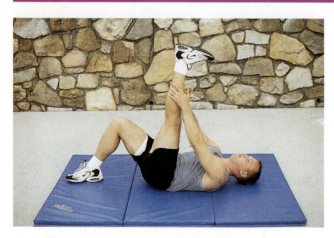

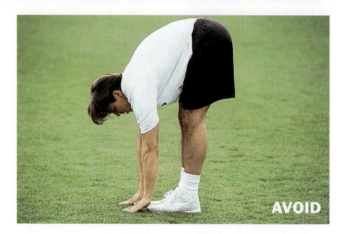

AVOID

▲ Active with Passive Assist: Lie on your back with your right leg bent and right foot on the floor and the left leg extended along the ground. Draw your left leg upward and toward your head by pulling with your thigh (quadriceps) muscles. (If you find this easy, extend your right leg.) Use your hands as a passive assist to pull your leg toward your head. If you need additional reach, loop a towel around your leg and pull on it.

▲ Avoid: The straight leg toe touch (standing or sitting) places stress on the ligaments in the lower back region.

PNF: Lie on your back with one leg extended upward and the other bent with the foot on the floor. Have a partner resist you as you try to lower your extended leg to the floor. Hold this isometric contraction (3 seconds), relax (2 seconds), then proceed with an active stretch (10 seconds). The active stretch may be assisted by using your hands or a towel wrapped around your leg to help pull the leg toward your head. CRAC

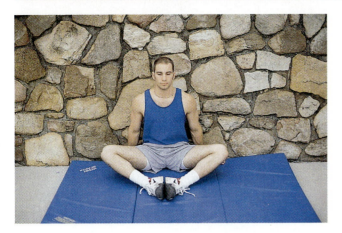

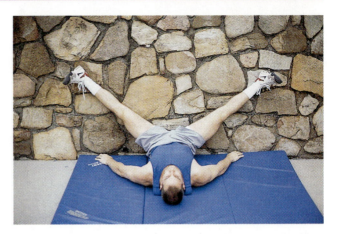

◄ Active: Butterfly or Seated Cobbler Stretch: Sit with the soles of your feet touching. Sit against a wall if you want support for your back. Using your outside thigh muscles and hip rotators pull your knees toward the floor.

◄ Passive: Wide V Wall Stretch: Put your legs in the wide V position. Now relax all your leg muscles and let gravity pull them toward the floor.

PNF: Seated Cobbler: Sit as you would for the passive stretch, but place your hands on your thighs just above your knees. Push down with your hands and up with your legs to create an isometric contraction. Hold for 6 seconds. Then relax and perform a passive stretch. CR

LOWER LEG STRETCHES

Calf (Gastrocnemius) Stretch

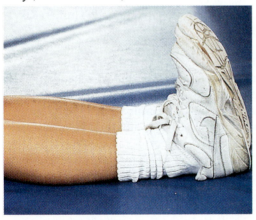

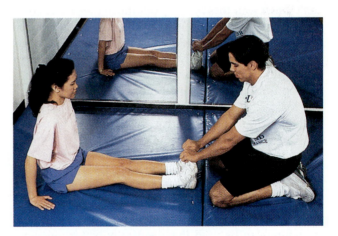

◄ Active: Sit down either in a chair or on the floor and extend your legs in front of you. Pull your toes toward your shin by contracting the muscles on the front of your shin.

◄ Passive: Same as above only pull your toes toward you using tubing or a towel or have a partner push against the bottom of your feet.

PNF: Sit on the floor with your legs extended in front of you. Point your toes as hard as you can (3 seconds), relax (2 seconds), then perform an active stretch (10 seconds). The active stretch may be assisted using a towel or exercise band to pull back on the toes. CRAC

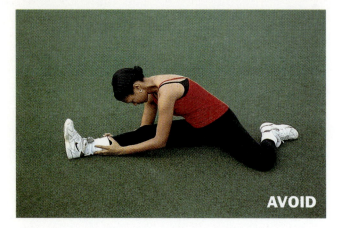

AVOID

▲ Avoid: Stretching forward in the hurdler's stretch stresses the knee ligaments of the bent leg. To modify this stretch, bring the bent leg in front of your body and place the foot by the inner thigh of the straight leg. The knee of your bent leg can be along the ground or in the air.

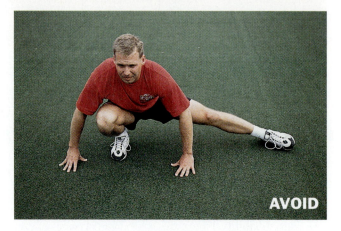

AVOID

▲ Avoid: When the knee is pushed beyond the instep, pressure is placed on knee ligaments. To correct the exercise, place the foot directly under the knee.

SUMMARY

Okay, let's face it, you're not likely to die because you can't touch your toes . . . but your life may be more comfortable if you can, especially since good flexibility helps prevent low-back pain and injury. Being flexible also lets you move more efficiently and aesthetically. As you grow older, you can maximize your independence by maintaining as much healthy joint movement as possible.

Many factors influence flexibility, but the most important factor is staying active. Stretching can be part of a warm-up and cool-down, a program of its own, or something you do periodically throughout the day. Stretches are a great way to relieve tension and relax. Static stretches are recommended for general use. Ballistic stretches are recommended only after static stretches and as a means of preparing for vigorous movement. PNF stretching can be used therapeutically or for a general flexibility workout—with a caution that it may cause more muscle soreness. Achieving flexibility and maintaining it can be done at any age, but there are advantages in starting when you are young. Make it a part of your wellness lifestyle!

SUGGESTED READING

Alter, M. J. *The science of stretching.* Champaign, IL: Human Kinetics, 1988.

Alter, M. J. *Sports stretch.* Champaign, IL: Human Kinetics, 1990.

Anderson, B. *Stretching.* Bolinas, CA: Shelter Publications, 1980.

Croce, P. *Stretching for athletics,* 2nd ed. Champaign, IL: Leisure Press, 1984.

Hardy, L., and D. Jones. Dynamic flexibility and proprioceptive neuromuscular facilitation. *Research Quarterly for Exercise and Sport* 57:150, 1986.

Kisner, C., and L. A. Colby, *Therapeutic exercises: Foundations and techniques.* Philadelphia: F. A. Davis, 1985.

Kurz, T. *Stretching scientifically. A guide to flexibility training,* 3rd ed. Island Pond, VT: Stadion Publishers, 1994.

McAtee, R. E. *Facilitated stretching: PNF stretching made easy.* Champaign, IL: Human Kinetics, 1993.

What Can I Do?

At the beginning of this chapter, you determined your stage of readiness to change with regard to flexibility. Now take out a sheet of paper and complete the corresponding section of this lab: precontemplator, contemplator, preparer, action taker, or maintainer.

Precontemplator

1. Try to identify the main reason(s) you are against becoming or not motivated to become more flexible. For some ideas, refer to the barriers listed in the Barrier Busters in this chapter.

2. Can you think of any reasons why flexibility exercises would be good for you? If necessary, review this chapter for ideas.

3. Can you think of any times when lack of flexibility limited the quality of your performance? resulted in injury? stopped you from doing something? (Keeping a daily journal for a while may help identify these items.)

4. If you have performed any flexibility tests, do your results suggest a need for change?

5. Do your answers in items 2–4 outweigh your answers in 1? If yes, what does this mean? If no, what does this mean?

6. Can you use any of the barrier-busting suggestions in this chapter to help you overcome any of the items you listed in item 1? Or can you, your instructor, or your friends think of a way to help you overcome your barriers?

7. At this point, are you willing to think about adding just one flexibility exercise to your daily routine? Maybe consider turning your head from side to side or shrugging your shoulders after a long period of studying? If you are willing to think about such a change, you are becoming a contemplator.

Contemplator

1. What are you thinking about doing to improve your flexibility?

2. What changes will this activity (item 1) bring about that are important to you? (Why are they important?)

3. Is there something you'd like to know more about? List any questions you have about flexibility in general or about specific flexibility exercises.

4. What do you need in order to consider making this change? Try to finish this statement:

   I will consider changing if . . .

   Examples

   I have a partner.

   It won't cost me any money.

   I can incorporate it into my life or workout without taking more time.

   I have a way of doing it while taking care of young children.

   (yours)_____

5. How can you overcome or accomplish the items listed above? Use the Barrier Busters within the chapter and brainstorm with friends for ideas on how to overcome your specific barriers.

6. List five to ten flexibility exercises you would consider doing on a regular basis.

7. Brainstorm, alone or with a friend, how you could fit the exercises you listed in item 6 into your schedule.

Preparer

1. What do you specifically want to accomplish? (For directions on goal setting see Chapter 2.)

   Examples

   I want to balance the flexibility between my right and left hamstrings.

   I want to develop leg and hip flexibility in order to take the stress off my lower back.

2. Which stretches will accomplish this (these) goal(s)? (See pages 86–94.)

3. Identify and experiment with ways to make stretching exercises a part of your daily routine.

   Examples

   Try stretching at different times of day, for instance, early in the morning, before and after exercise, during a work break, or after a warm bath.

   Try performing stretches in a variety of positions, such as lying on the floor, sitting in a chair, or standing, to find the most comfortable position for you.

   Add stretches to activities you are already doing.

4. Develop a stretching routine based on your answers in items 1–3. The routine may consist of smaller routines to be performed at different times of the day.

5. As a first step, select one stretch from your routine to begin performing five to seven days a week. Each week plan to add one more stretch until you are performing the entire routine.

6. What makes you think you can accomplish your flexibility goal(s)? *Or* What makes you think you can accomplish this first step?

7. Complete the following statement:

   I am going to take my first step on _____.

   date within 30 days

Action Taker

1. What are you currently doing to increase your flexibility?

2. Are your flexibility goals specifically and clearly stated?

3. Are you keeping track of your progress?

   If yes, how?

      fitness tests?

      journal?

      skill performance records?

   If no, would keeping track help to motivate you?

4. Are you receiving support or rewards for your effort?

   If yes, what kind?

   If no, why not? Can you change this?

5. Do you think you will continue? Why or why not?

6. If you were to stop, what do you think would be the major reason?

7. Is there a way to prevent this (item 6)?

8. How would you get yourself started again if you did stop?

9. Are you confident that you can reach your goals?

   If yes, why?

   If no, why not?

10. If you answered no to the above question, can you think of anything or anyone who can help you make your goal(s) possible?

Maintainer

1. For how long have you maintained your flexibility at a healthy level?

2. What are the top two reasons that make you want to continue?

3. Have you been tempted to stop? If so, what tempted you?

4. How did you convince yourself to continue?

5. Can you prevent such temptations in the future? If so, how?

6. How confident are you that you can resist temptation? What kinds of things help build your confidence? lower your confidence?

7. What kind of support do you get for your efforts?

   Examples

   Self-rewards, internal satisfaction

   External rewards, compliments from others

   Improved performance

   Higher quality of living (fewer injuries/aches)

8. How have you changed, or how have you changed the environment around you to accommodate a healthier lifestyle? Can you sustain these changes?

9. Is there anything else you need (information? support? time management?) to promote your continued maintenance?

10. If you listed something in the previous statement, can you think of a way to attain it or can you think of someone who can help you with it?

11. Are you happy with your present level of flexibility? If yes, continue what you are doing.

    If you are maintaining a healthy level of flexibility but would like to improve even more for reasons such as competition or personal achievement, you have become a contemplator of additional change. To continue, write new specific goals, establish a plan of action, set a date to begin, start, and keep good records of your progress.

Name _____   **Section**   **Date**

Sit-and-Reach Test

Note: You should perform a warm-up that includes static stretching of the lower back and posterior thighs prior to taking this test. Be sure to take this test under the same conditions each time you take it. For example, if you take it the first time before working out in the afternoon, take it again at the same time of day and do it before you exercise.

Equipment

Note: If a flexometer is available, use it. The following description assumes that one is not available..

1. Meter stick
2. Two partners
3. Pencil or pen

Directions

1. Sit with your legs extended and your feet flat against a box about 12 inches high, a folded gymnastics mat, or the feet of a person sitting opposite you.

2. Have a partner hold or place a meter stick so that the 25-centimeter mark is even with the soles of your feet. The number 1 on the meter stick should be close to you, the number 39 away from you.

3. Place one hand over the other and lean forward, gently sliding your hands down the meter stick. Use a smooth, sustained motion. Do this twice.

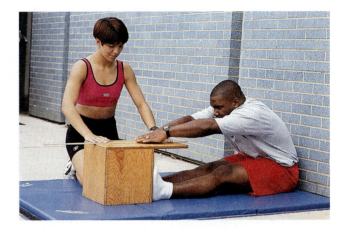

4. The measurer will note the farthest point your fingertips reach along the meter stick. (Do not count long fingernails.) Round scores to the nearest centimeter.

5. Record your highest score: _____ cm.

6. Consult the chart below to determine your fitness rating: _____ fitness rating.

	AGE (YEARS)											
Norms by age groups and gender for trunk forward flexion (cm).[a]												
Fitness Rating	**15–19**		**20–29**		**30–39**		**40–49**		**50–59**		**60–69**	
	M	**F**	**M**	**F**	**M**	**F**	**M**	**F**	**M**	**F**	**M**	**F**
Excellent	≥39	≥43	≥40	≥41	≥38	≥41	≥35	≥38	≥35	≥39	≥33	≥35
Above Average	34–38	38–42	34–39	37–40	33–37	36–40	29–34	34–37	28–34	33–38	25–32	31–34
Average	29–33	34–37	30–33	33–36	28–32	32–35	24–38	30–33	24–27	30–32	20–24	27–30
Below Average	24–28	29–33	25–29	28–32	23–27	27–31	18–23	25–29	16–23	25–29	15–19	23–26
Poor	≤23	≤28	≤24	≤27	≤22	≤26	≤17	≤24	≤15	≤24	≤14	≤23

Source: Published in the *Canadian Standardized Test of Fitness Operations Manual,* 3rd ed., 1986. Reprinted by permission from the Canadian Society for Exercise Physiology.

[a]Based on data from the Canada Fitness Survey, 1981.

Name _____ **Section** _____ **Date** _____

Quick Check Flexibility Tests

The following series of tests are pass/fail. They are quick and easy to perform. Because flexibility is joint specific, a variety of tests are provided.

If you would like to make a record of your flexibility and then check for improvement in 6–8 weeks, you can have a partner estimate or measure your present flexibility. When the measurement of an angle is called for, your partner can "eyeball" the angle, use a protractor, or use a flexometer. A simple protractor, to aid an eyeball estimate, can be made by drawing a horizontal line on a piece of paper and then subdividing it with a 90 degree line, and then breaking the 90 degrees into thirds. A simple flexometer can be made by fastening two strips of stiff paper together at one end using a paper fastener. Open or close the angle of the flexometer to match the angle of the joint. To record a score, trace the angle of the flexometer onto a piece of paper.

All the tests except the neck test require you to test both the right and left sides of your body. You may be surprised to find some differences between sides. If you do, make a note so that you can address these differences later when you put together a stretching program.

Neck Test

Stand or sit with your back straight and your face looking forward. Drop your chin to your chest. If you are able to press your chin against your hand placed at the base of your neck, give yourself a passing grade. If not, a partner can measure and record the distance between your chin and hand.

_____ pass; _____ fail, _____ inches

Shoulder Test I

Stand up straight with your arms at your side, palms facing your thighs. Raise one arm at a time forward and up overhead. Be sure your arm stays straight. If you reach 180 degrees (directly overhead) or more, give yourself a passing grade. If not, a partner can measure and record the angle between your torso and your raised arm.

Right: _____ pass; _____ fail, _____ degrees

Left: _____ pass; _____ fail, _____ degrees

Shoulder Test II

Stand up straight with your arms at your side with palms facing your thighs. Raise one arm out to the side and up overhead. Be sure your arm stays straight. If your arm is straight up by your ear, an angle of 180 degrees, give yourself a passing grade. If not, a partner can measure and record the angle between your torso and the raised arm.

Right: _____ pass; _____ fail, _____ degrees

Left: _____ pass; _____ fail, _____ degrees

Shoulder Test III

Stand up straight and attempt to touch your fingertips by reaching one hand over the same shoulder and the other hand up the middle of your back. If you can touch your hands, give yourself a passing grade. If not, have a partner measure and record the distance between your fingertips (not your fingernails).

Right arm up: _____ pass; _____ fail, _____ inches

Left arm up: _____ pass; _____ fail, _____ inches

Trunk Test

Sit in a chair with your feet flat on the floor. Place your right hand on your right shoulder and your left hand on your left shoulder. Keep your upper arms parallel to the floor and your elbows in line with your shoulder. Turn your upper body while keeping your hips square to the front. If you are able to rotate your torso 90 degrees or more (shoulders will be square to the side), give yourself a passing grade. If not, have a partner measure and record the difference between the standard of 90 degrees and how much you were able to rotate.

Right rotation: _____ pass; _____ fail, _____ degrees

Left rotation: _____ pass; _____ fail, _____ degrees

Lower Back Test

Lie on your back with both knees bent, feet off the floor, and head and lower back touching the floor. Grasp your legs underneath your knees and pull gently toward your shoulders (if you have to pull hard you fail the test). Touch both knees to their respective shoulders or lay your thighs flat along your torso with your lower back and head still touching the floor.

_____ pass; _____ fail, _____ degrees

Hip Flexor Test

Lie on your back on the floor with both legs straight. Keeping one leg straight and along the ground, draw the knee of the other leg up toward your chest. Place your hand on the back of your thigh underneath your knee and pull gently. Give yourself a passing grade if your thigh touches your torso and your other leg remains straight. If not, have your partner measure and record the angle between your torso and thigh.

Right: _____ pass; _____ fail, _____ degrees

Left: _____ pass; _____ fail, _____ degrees

Alternate Hip Flexor Test

Lie on your back on a knee-high firm surface like a folded mat, bleacher, or table. Bend your knees over the edge and put your feet flat on the floor. Draw one knee to your chest while trying to keep the opposite foot flat on the floor. If you can do this comfortably, give yourself a passing grade. If your heel lifts up, have your partner measure and record the distance between your heel and the floor.

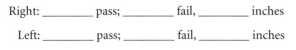

Right: _____ pass; _____ fail, _____ inches

Left: _____ pass; _____ fail, _____ inches

Hip Abduction Test

Either standing straight or lying on your side on the ground, move one leg sideways as far from the other leg as possible. If the angle between the legs measures 90 degrees or more, give yourself a passing grade. If not, have your partner measure and record the angle.

Right: _____ pass; _____ fail, _____ degrees

Left: _____ pass; _____ fail, _____ degrees

Hamstring Test

Lie on your back with both legs straight. Keeping both legs straight, lift one up and as far toward your head as possible. Give yourself a passing grade if you are able to reach a 90 degree angle (straight up) or more. If not, have your partner measure and record the angle between the floor and your raised leg.

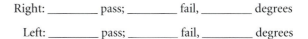

Right: _____ pass; _____ fail, _____ degrees

Left: _____ pass; _____ fail, _____ degrees

Quadriceps Test

Lie prone on the floor with your head turned to one side. Bend one knee and grasp the ankle. Without forcing it, draw your ankle toward your buttocks. Give yourself a passing grade if your heel touches your buttocks or your lower leg rests against your upper leg. If not, have your partner measure and record the angle behind your knee made by your lower and upper leg.

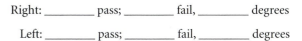

Right: _____ pass; _____ fail, _____ degrees

Left: _____ pass; _____ fail, _____ degrees

Calf Test

Sit on the floor with your legs extended straight in front of you. Flex one ankle as much as you can. Give yourself a passing grade if the angle made up of the sole of your shoe and your shin is 70 degrees or less. If not, have a partner measure and record the angle. You may want to draw a 70 degree angle on a piece of paper and have a partner hold it behind your foot so that you can more easily judge passing and failing.

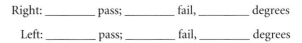

Right: _____ pass; _____ fail, _____ degrees

Left: _____ pass; _____ fail, _____ degrees

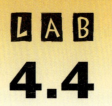

Developing Your Flexibility Exercise Program

1. Set a general goal for your program.

2. Select and organize your exercises:

Target Muscle(s)	Exercise(s)	Type of Stretch (Active/Passive/PNF)	Hold (reps/sec)

3. Determine when you will do your flexibility exercises:

4. Write one or more specific goals:

5. Use the following log to record your progress. Record the exercise, date, repetitions, and hold time for each of the exercises you list in the first column. Rep/sec = repetitions and hold time in seconds.

   Example: 2/30 = 2 repetitions held for 30 seconds each.

Exercise	WEEK OF ___		WEEK OF ___		WEEK OF ___	
	rep/sec	Circle the day of the week you stretched	rep/sec	Circle the day of the week you stretched	rep/sec	Circle the day of the week you stretched
		S M T W Th F Sa		S M T W Th F Sa		S M T W Th F Sa
		S M T W Th F Sa		S M T W Th F Sa		S M T W Th F Sa
		S M T W Th F Sa		S M T W Th F Sa		S M T W Th F Sa
		S M T W Th F Sa		S M T W Th F Sa		S M T W Th F Sa
		S M T W Th F Sa		S M T W Th F Sa		S M T W Th F Sa
		S M T W Th F Sa		S M T W Th F Sa		S M T W Th F Sa
		S M T W Th F Sa		S M T W Th F Sa		S M T W Th F Sa
		S M T W Th F Sa		S M T W Th F Sa		S M T W Th F Sa
		S M T W Th F Sa		S M T W Th F Sa		S M T W Th F Sa
		S M T W Th F Sa		S M T W Th F Sa		S M T W Th F Sa
		S M T W Th F Sa		S M T W Th F Sa		S M T W Th F Sa
		S M T W Th F Sa		S M T W Th F Sa		S M T W Th F Sa
		S M T W Th F Sa		S M T W Th F Sa		S M T W Th F Sa
		S M T W Th F Sa		S M T W Th F Sa		S M T W Th F Sa
		S M T W Th F Sa		S M T W Th F Sa		S M T W Th F Sa
		S M T W Th F Sa		S M T W Th F Sa		S M T W Th F Sa
		S M T W Th F Sa		S M T W Th F Sa		S M T W Th F Sa
		S M T W Th F Sa		S M T W Th F Sa		S M T W Th F Sa
		S M T W Th F Sa		S M T W Th F Sa		S M T W Th F Sa
		S M T W Th F Sa		S M T W Th F Sa		S M T W Th F Sa
		S M T W Th F Sa		S M T W Th F Sa		S M T W Th F Sa
		S M T W Th F Sa		S M T W Th F Sa		S M T W Th F Sa
		S M T W Th F Sa		S M T W Th F Sa		S M T W Th F Sa
		S M T W Th F Sa		S M T W Th F Sa		S M T W Th F Sa

CHAPTER 5

Muscular Strength and Endurance

Terms

- **Weight training**
- **Resistance training**
- **Muscular strength**
- **Muscular endurance**
- **Weight lifting**
- **Body building**
- **Body sculpting**
- **Strength training**
- **Muscular power**
- **Muscle fibers**
- **Motor units**
- **Hypertrophy**
- **Atrophy**
- **Anabolic steroids**
- **Static exercises**
- **Dynamic exercises**
- **Isometric**
- **Isotonic**
- **Free weights**
- **Concentric contraction**
- **Eccentric contraction**
- **Isokinetic**
- **Repetitions**
- **Sets**
- **Circuit training**

Objectives

1. Understand the importance of muscular strength and endurance as it relates to activities in your life and to injury prevention.

2. Optimize the effects of resistance exercises/activities through the application of physiological concepts of muscular strength and endurance conditioning.

3. Assess your muscular strength and endurance and set appropriate goals.

4. Establish a resistance exercise program, or plan to engage regularly in physical activities that will enhance or maintain your muscular strength and endurance.

Where Am I?

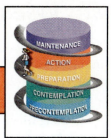

Precontemplator _____ I currently do not perform resistance exercises* and at this point I do not intend to start in the next six months.

Contemplator _____ I currently do not perform resistance exercises, but I am thinking about starting to do them in the next six months.

Preparer _____ I currently perform some resistance exercises, but not regularly.

Action Taker _____ I currently perform resistance exercises regularly, but I have begun doing so only within the past six months.

Maintainer _____ I currently perform resistance exercises regularly and have done so for longer than six months.

Select the statement above that best describes your stage of behavior change. To consider yourself an action taker or maintainer, you must be performing a minimum of eight to ten resistance exercises for the major muscle groups a minimum of twice a week, using a minimum of one set of eight to twelve repetitions to near fatigue for each exercise.[1] Setting a goal and achieving a regular habit of doing fewer exercises than this should be considered a significant personal achievement even though by definition you would fall in the category of preparer rather than action taker or maintainer. As an example, your priority may be to develop abdominal strength to relieve back strain. You may choose to delay a more complete set of exercises until you have achieved this one important goal and are confident in your ability to go further.

Resistance training for the general public is a relatively new phenomenon. It may be hard for today's college student to believe that at one time it was considered taboo for athletes other than those in competitive weight lifting, weight events in track and field, and, on a limited basis, football players, wrestlers, and boxers to train with weights.[2] Coaches feared their athletes would become muscle bound and lose flexibility and coordination. Today, science and experience have shown that resistance training enhances the physical performance of all athletes and, more importantly, enhances the health and fitness of all individuals.

Resistance training can be achieved through calisthenics and homemade equipment or through the use of weight-lifting equipment. This chapter provides exercises for both approaches so that you can work out in your home (room) or take advantage of an on- or off-campus weight-lifting facility. As you read the phrase "resistance training," picture everything from exercises in a pool to pushups and situps in your room to bench pressing in a weight room. Weight-training equipment, however, can provide a greater range of resistance and is therefore necessary when the goal is high-level muscular strength or endurance.

---

*Resistance exercises include muscular endurance and strength exercises.

WHY RESISTANCE TRAINING?

There are many excellent reasons for starting or continuing a resistance training program. Here are a few examples:

1. Becky and Joe enjoy tennis and started resistance training when they discovered it would help them hit the ball harder and play longer with less fatigue.

2. Jeremy never got involved with athletics but always envied the "jock" look. A friend invited him to try the dorm weight room, and as Jeremy's muscular physique developed, so did his self-confidence.

3. Molly started a weight-training program after she broke up with her boyfriend. It made her feel good to do something for herself and gave her a renewed sense of control over her life.

4. Jaemal's leg was badly broken in a car accident. The physical therapist suggested that he do some resistance training with his good leg in order to maintain some of the musculature in his injured leg. When the cast came off, Jaemal continued to exercise to rehabilitate his injured leg.

5. When Kristy saw her new course schedule, she knew she needed to get in shape. She was going to have to move from building to building and negotiate a campus full of hills in her wheelchair. Kristy decided to use a swimming/aquatics program to develop her upper body.

6. Patrick and Maria work summers at the Post Office. The job requires that Patrick handle 60 pounds and Maria 40. They decided to get in shape to prevent injuries and fatigue.

7. Carl, age seventy, decided he was tired of leaning on his walker and saw that some of his friends were able to walk independently after twelve weeks of resistance training. His wife Gertrude joined him when her doctor said it would help prevent osteoporosis.

Even this short list of reasons shows how muscular strength and endurance can benefit you in a variety of ways and that your reasons for exercising today may be different from the reasons you continue in five, ten, twenty, or fifty years.

HEALTH-RELATED STRENGTH AND ENDURANCE

The information that follows focuses on developing *health-related* strength and endurance. This is not meant to be a training manual for competition, although an understanding of the underlying principles and concepts is important for every level of training. For beginners, terms and principles are clearly defined and worksheets are provided for putting together a program. For athletes following a program established by a knowledgeable coach, this information will help you understand why you are doing what you are doing, and why your program is different from that of athletes in different sports, or in different positions or events in the same sport. It is also important to know how to adjust your training regimen when you are no longer in competitive athletics.

If you are a beginner or intermediate, you may feel intimidated in a weight room, particularly by well-muscled or toned individuals. The tendency is to follow any advice these individuals provide, figuring that they wouldn't look that good if they didn't know what they were doing. Unfortunately, the weight-training world is fraught with myths, drugs, and misinformation. Even a well-meaning advanced lifter can give you information that is too advanced for your present technique and condition. Find an instructor with professional training who is used to working with beginners or intermediates and start with the basics. This instructor can, in one or two sessions, also make a complicated-looking set of machines less intimidating and easy to use.

For wellness, you need enough strength and endurance to allow you to handle daily activities, leisure activities, and emergencies. If you are interested in competition, athletics, or physically challenging leisure activities, you will need higher levels of strength and endurance.

WHAT'S IN A NAME?

Weight Training and Resistance Training

For a muscle to get stronger, it must work against a greater than normal resistance. The term **weight training** is used to describe strengthening exercises, because weights have been the traditional source of resistance. But it is also possible to strengthen muscles without weights. Some machines have substituted weight plates with hydraulic or pneumatic pressure, electrical resistance, or thick rubber bands. In the pool, resistance is accomplished by pushing and pulling against the water. Polystyrene dumbbells and webbed gloves can be used to increase resistance. Exercise bands, tubing, and stretch cables have also become popular forms of resistance, especially in aerobics classes. Pressing against an immovable object like a wall, or against your own body (pressing down with your right hand while trying to press up with your left hand) also effectively creates resistance. Because all these forms of resistance can, depending on your present strength, result in muscle strength and endurance, the term **resistance training** has become a popular, more encompassing term than weight training and will therefore be the term of choice for this text.

Muscular Strength Training

Muscular strength is the amount of force that a muscle or muscle group can exert one time. You need strength to perform daily tasks such as moving furniture and appli-

BARRIER Busters

I don't have time to lift weights.

General strength and endurance can be accomplished using simple calisthenics and equipment easily made from household articles. One set (about ten repetitions) of eight to twelve exercises takes less than 30 minutes. Many other physical activities also work your muscles and help keep them toned.

If I go to a gym everyone will stare at me because I don't have any idea how to use the equipment.

Most gymnasiums offer an introductory lesson on how to use their equipment. If they don't, ask a knowledgeable friend or professional educator to assist you. You can also learn with other beginners by taking a college course from the physical education or exercise science department. If there is a strength coach on campus, you can ask for a couple of private lessons (negotiate a fee) to get you started. While you may be self-conscious in the beginning, you will find that most people at a gym are friendly, helpful, and encouraging.

Resistance training is only for the young.

Resistance training in its many forms (including weight training) is enjoyed by people as young as 90. It helps maintain bone density, muscle tissue, and muscle function—items crucial to maintaining quality of life.

I don't want big bulky muscles.

Due to physiological and hormonal differences, the vast majority of women need not worry about developing bulky muscles. Men can look forward to increases in muscle size depending on the extent of their training.

Every time I try to lift weights I get really sore or injured.

It is normal for muscles to get a little stiff when they are being overloaded or used in a new way; however, too much stiffness is a sign that you have overworked the muscles. Cut back on the amount of resistance you are using. Injuries are usually the result of starting with too much resistance, not gradual enough progression, or poor body alignment. If you have decided to exercise, or are already doing so, find a knowledgeable person who can check your program and technique.

I enjoy working out at a gymnasium but can't afford to belong to one.

Most colleges have open hours for recreational use of their weight and exercise rooms. There is either no fee, or a small student activity fee for the use of these facilities. Many dormitories now support their own equipment. If working out at a club appeals to you, see if you can trade working at the club (cleaning, answering phones, and so forth) for a membership.

Juggling school, work, and family, I find I don't have time to go somewhere and work out.

You can stay home and work out. Involve your family. You can use sim-ple calisthenics, homemade weights, and partner exercises. If you can afford it, there are also a number of homestyle weight machines and free weights available for purchase.

If I'm not strong enough to do something, I can always get help.

There is some truth to this; however, there are a number of situations in which you are alone, or where it is nice to be self-sufficient. In an emergency you may be alone, or have others depending on you, and not have enough time to get help. Well-timed, strong movements in self-defense can ward off a would-be attacker, and in the event of an accident a strong body is less likely to be hurt as badly as a weak one. On a more day-to-day level, being able to do things like shovel snow, change a flat tire, and move your own belongings can not only allow you to be more independent, but also save you money.

If my muscles get tired, I can always rest.

This may often be true; however, muscular endurance will allow you to do more in a shorter amount of time and add to the enjoyment of the activity. Getting the leaves raked in four hours is nicer than taking two days because of frequent rests. A certain amount of endurance is also needed to enjoy recreational activities like hiking and cycling.

---

ances, picking up a child, pushing a car out of a ditch, opening a jar, or putting your bike on the roof rack. Many sports require strength as well. It helps you to kick, throw, or hit a ball with speed, to jump high or far, to climb a rope, or to lift a dance partner. Yet basic strength is something many Americans need to improve and maintain. By the age of 70 almost one-third of men and two-thirds of women can't pick up as little as ten pounds.[3] Even if you are strong when you are younger, an inactive lifestyle coupled with aging can diminish your strength. You can't just get fit and put it away like money in the bank; you have to keep working at it.

Strength gains are maximized by working against a heavy resistance. However, it is very difficult and not always wise to perform maximum lifts. Strength training is generally practiced using submaximal loads, relatively high (but not maximum) levels of resistance that can be lifted for a low number of repetitions. A variety of weight-lifting regimens are used by weight lifters. For an overview of some of these "systems," see the box on the next page.

1. **Isometric**—iso = equal, metric = measurement. Muscle length doesn't change during contraction.

2. **Isotonic**—iso = equal, tonic = tension. Muscle tension doesn't change during movement through a range of motion.

3. **Isokinetic**—iso = equal, kinetic = motion. The speed of the muscle flexing or extending doesn't change over a range of motion.

4. **Multiple Set System**—More than one set with a rest period between sets. When performing three to five sets, this may be called the bulk system. (One set is called the single set system.)

5. **Split System**—Various muscles are worked on alternate days; the split may be (a) upper- and lower-body muscles, or (b) chest, shoulders, and back alternated with arms, legs, and abdominals.

6. **Light to Heavy System**—Multiple sets with an increase in resistance with each set. As the load becomes heavier the number of repetitions often decreases.

7. **Heavy to Light System**—Opposite of light to heavy system.

8. **Pyramid System**—A multiple set system in which you begin with a light load, work up to a heavy load, and then back down to a light load. It can also be done heavy to light to heavy.

9. **Tonnage System**—A system in which numbers of repetitions and sets can vary but the total amount of weight lifted (tonnage) stays the same.

10. **Circuit System**—Movement through a series of stations performing one set at each station, often with timed exercise periods and breaks. May repeat circuit multiple times (sets). May be called the aerobic system when breaks are very short. (Not aerobic enough to replace regular aerobic exercise.)

11. **Superset System**—Performing back-to-back sets (no break) of two exercises, one each working opposing muscles (for example, biceps/triceps), or two exercises that work the same muscle.

12. **Cheat System**—Breaking strict form of the exercise in order to recruit additional muscles so that heavier lifts can be performed. Breaking form can be dangerous. This system should be used only on rare occasion by highly experienced lifters who are preparing for competition.

13. **Blitz**—A variation of the split system in which only one body part is trained per session, using a number of different exercises.

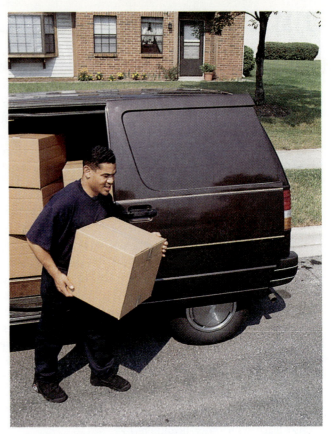

Activities that require your muscles to maintain a certain level of force for an extended period of time require isometric contraction of those muscles.

Depending on your fitness level, heavy workloads can be achieved using simple calisthenics, free weights (barbells and dumbbells), or weight machines.

Muscular Endurance Training

Muscular endurance is defined as the ability to (1) exert a submaximal force repeatedly, and/or (2) maintain a submaximal force for an extended period of time. The first part of this definition describes repetitive muscular contractions such as those you would use to mow the lawn, walk up three flights of stairs, row a boat, or hike down a canyon. This kind of endurance is developed using light to moderate resistance for a moderate to high number of repetitions. The second part of the definition describes isometrically held contractions—contractions in which muscles are exerting a force but not moving. "Hiking out" on a sailboat (leaning out to balance the boat holding on to a rope) requires isometrically held contractions of both the abdominals and arm muscles. So does carrying a suitcase, box, or bag of groceries. Any time body position needs to be maintained in a fixed position, isometric contractions are occurring. Often both kinds of muscle endurance are required at the same time. For example, during a push-up, the arm muscles exert the submaximal force repeatedly (part 1 of the definition) while the abdominals, buttocks, and leg muscles perform isometric contractions to maintain body position (part 2 of the definition).

Weight Lifting, Body Building, and Body Sculpting

Weight lifting and body building are competitive sports; they require strength far beyond that needed for wellness. **Weight-lifting** contests involve several types of lifts in which the objective is to lift as much weight as possible each time. You may have seen Olympic athletes perform clean and jerks (lift to shoulder height and then press overhead with a split step) and snatches (lift the bar from the ground to overhead in one motion). Power lifters compete with the bench press, squats, and dead lift (lift the bar from the ground going from a squat position to a standing position). Weight lifters win based on the total amount of weight they are able to lift.

Body building is a contest of muscle size, symmetry, and definition. Winners are able to pose with confidence, showing off their strengths and minimizing their weaknesses. Body builders train with heavy weights to develop muscle definition and high numbers of repetitions with lighter weights to develop muscle size. Gender differences prevent most women body builders from achieving the same muscle size increases as men (see pages 111–112) so their workouts and competitions stress body proportions and symmetry more than size. **Body sculpting** is the process of developing a well-proportioned physique. Body sculpting is part of body building but may also be a noncompetitive activity for people who want to tone and shape their muscles.

Athletics and Weight Training

Athletes in sports other than weight lifting, body building, and body sculpting use special weight-training programs as a way to improve their motor skills (for example, jumping, throwing) and to prevent injury. Whether you play a sport competitively or recreationally, it is ex-

citing to see the difference a good resistance training program can make.

Again a note of caution: although a lot can be learned from professional athletes, care must be taken not to follow blindly what they do. These athletes have been gifted with a body that can handle higher than normal physical stress. And by the time we see these athletes and hear about their programs, they have been training for a number of years. Performing an advanced program without the proper progressions and a high fitness level can be dangerous. By learning the basic principles and concepts that underlie all resistance training, you will be able to recognize, select, or create a program that best fits your fitness, wellness, and recreational needs.

THE STRENGTH-ENDURANCE CONTINUUM

Muscular strength and endurance are closely related, yet distinct, components of physical fitness. Their relationship can be described as a continuum, with maximum strength to the far left and maximum endurance to the far right (see Figure 5.1). Far-left activities would include things like weight lifting, football blocking, and pushing a car out of a ditch while far-right activities would include marathon running, the Tour de France (cycling), and swimming the English Channel. Notice that as you approach the middle of the continuum, there is no clear-cut place where strength leaves off and endurance begins. This is because many activities develop and require a certain degree of both strength and endurance. Wellness, or health-related resistance programs, fall in this middle part of the continuum because their goal is moderate gains in both strength and endurance.

The same exercise (or activity) can be a strength workout for one person and a muscular endurance one for someone else. For example, the push-up test requires one to do as many push-ups in a row as possible. A person who can do only one push-up is performing a maximum effort (1 RM). This is a strength test. However, for

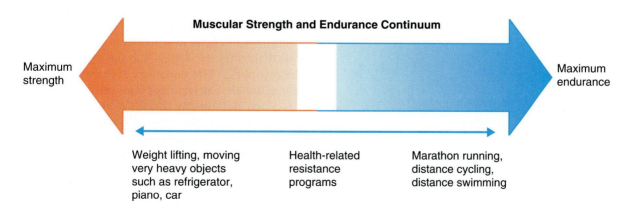

FIGURE 5.1 Most health-related resistance programs aim for a blending of muscular strength and endurance rather than emphasizing either maximum strength or maximum endurance.

someone who can do fifty in a row, this is a muscular endurance test. Daily activities such as washing windows or cutting grass emphasize muscular endurance more than strength. But, again, fitness level must be considered. An inactive elderly person, or someone recovering from an injury, may find these activities physically taxing and require frequent breaks. These individuals are performing short bouts of difficult work—a recipe for strength gain.

The phrase **strength training** is often used as a general term to describe both strength and endurance exercises, but you can see that one could easily lose any distinction between strength and endurance—instead it should be reserved for activities that fall toward the left of the continuum.

To understand better how to put together a resistance training program that meets your needs, it is helpful to know how muscles work and how they respond to different kinds of exercise. The next section will discuss muscle anatomy and physiology and relate the importance of this information to resistance training.

HOW MUSCLES WORK

Muscle Physiology

The connective tissue surrounding the center (belly) of a muscle tapers off to form one or more muscle tendons at each end. The tendons attach to bones on opposite sides of a joint. When the muscle contracts, its tendon(s) are pulled in toward the belly of the muscle bringing the attached bone(s) with them. Figure 5.2 shows how flexion of the biceps muscle pulls the lower arm bone (ulna) to the upper arm bone (humerus) together. This pulling action cannot be reversed into a pushing action. To extend your arm, the triceps muscle and its tendons (which cross the elbow joint and attach to the backside of the lower arm bones) must contract and pull the bones apart. The human body is designed with many pairs of opposing muscles. When one muscle or set of muscles flexes, the other muscle or set of muscles relaxes and extends.

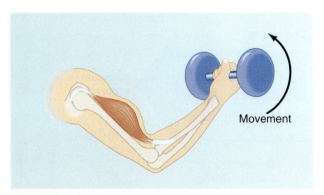

FIGURE 5.2 When a muscle contracts it *pulls* on the bones to which it is attached. (S. Powers and E. Howley. *Exercise physiology: Theory and application to fitness and performance.* Debuque, IA: Wm. C. Brown 1994.)

Fitness Implications

To achieve good body symmetry, opposing muscles should both be exercised. Imbalances can result in injury, loss of flexibility, or poor posture. For example, individuals who fail to work the upper back as hard as the chest muscles will find that the stronger chest muscles pull the shoulders forward into a rounded posture. Similarly, an imbalance between a strong calf muscle and a weaker tibialis anterior (muscle in the front of the lower leg) can contribute to an irritation called shinsplints. Back problems related to strength and flexibility imbalances are discussed on pages 76–77. For a list of opposing muscle groups, see page 120.

Muscle Fibers

Inside the previously mentioned connective tissue, each muscle is made up of bundles of **muscle fibers** (cells). These bundles, called fasciculi (or fascicles), give the muscle form and structure. The fibers inside the fasciculi are arranged in different ways according to the function of the muscle. Muscles that need to move bones through wide ranges of motion have fasciculi with fibers running longitudinally because this allows for maximum contraction (contracting to about one-half its length). The longer the fibers, the greater the contraction and the resulting movement of the bones. The calf muscle (gastrocnemius) is a good example of this kind of muscle structure. Other muscles have fasciculi with fibers running diagonally. These fibers are shorter but also more plentiful. The more fibers in a muscle, the greater its capacity for strength. The second arrangement allows for more fibers in a given area, and thus will provide more strength. The compromise is a loss of fiber length, resulting in a smaller range of motion. The thigh (quadriceps) muscle is an example of diagonally arranged fibers. Fibers in fasciculi can be arranged in several different ways, providing for various combinations of range of motion and strength.

Inside each fiber in the fascicula are smaller strands called myofibrils. Inside each myofibril are even smaller protein strands called myofilaments. There are two kinds of myofilaments, the thicker myosin and thinner actin. See Figure 5.3 for muscle structure.

The myosin and actin myofilaments are arranged in units called sarcomeres, which line up end to end to form the myofibril. (The sarcomere segments are what give skeletal muscle a striated appearance.) A sarcomere contracts when the myosin and actin fibers slide over one another. To picture this, place two combs (one with thicker teeth than the other) facing each other. Slide the thicker teeth between the thinner teeth about a quarter of an inch. This is how the myosin (thick teeth) and actin (thin teeth) look when the sarcomere is at rest. Now slide the combs toward each other, overlapping the teeth even more. This is what happens during a contraction. When energy (ATP) is available and the nerve signal to contract

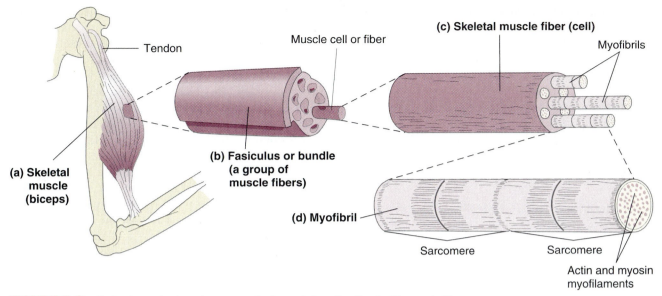

FIGURE 5.3 Skeletal muscle tissue is composed of muscle bundles (fasciculi), muscle fibers (cells), myofibrils, and myofilaments (actin and myosin).

arrives, myosin reaches out with hairlike arms, attaches to special sites along the actin, and pulls the two filaments past one another. Myosin can release and reattach further along the actin and continue to pull until the desired contraction is achieved. The combination of many sarcomeres contracting allows for the great contractibility of muscle tissue. The sliding of the actin and myosin is called the Sliding Filament Theory.

Fitness Implications

Resistance training, which is primarily anaerobic, increases the amount of energy, ATP and PC, that can be stored directly in the muscle fiber. This energy can then be used to fuel contractions. Resistance training also raises the muscles' tolerance to lactic acid. With more stored energy and a higher LA tolerance, muscles can perform more work (contractions) before experiencing exhaustion.

The Motor Unit

The nervous system serves as the communication link between the brain and the muscles. When a decision for action is made, the message is sent from the brain (or spinal cord) to the muscles via nerve fibers called motor neurons. Think of the motor neuron as a sophisticated electrical wire. The wire splits (branches) and enters a number of fasciculi. It passes through the elastic connective tissue that covers and binds the fasciculi together, then splits again, sending a branch out to each intended muscle fiber. One motor neuron may innervate just a few muscle fibers or hundreds with an average of 150 fibers.[4] One motor neuron and the fibers it innervates is called a **motor unit.** When a motor unit contracts, all of the

fibers in the unit contract. Small motor units are necessary for precise, delicate work such as that performed by the eye muscles. Large motor units are found in muscles used for heavy work such as the quadriceps (thigh). The strength of a contraction is determined by the number and size of the fibers recruited, not by how hard the individual fibers contract. According to the all-or-none law, a muscle fiber contracts either 100 percent or not at all. The strength of a contraction is orchestrated by recruiting the correct number and type of fibers. The nervous system "recruits" more motor units (groups of muscle fibers) for a strong contraction than for a gentle one. Occasionally the nervous system is "faked out"— when you think something is going to be heavy and it turns out to be light, too many motor units are recruited and the resulting contraction is inappropriately strong. Do you remember what happened the first time you picked up one of those styrofoam fake rocks?

The human potential to recruit muscle fibers fully is glimpsed in the rare cases where average persons under conditions of extreme emergency perform feats like lifting a car off another person. In these unusual and fascinating cases, these individuals are somehow able to recruit more motor units than normally humanly possible.

Fitness Implications

Strategies for maximizing fiber recruitment have been devised to develop the muscle more fully. If you fatigue the initially recruited fibers, additional fibers will be recruited. This occurs when you perform (1) a high number of consecutive repetitions, (2) more than one set of repetitions, or (3) two exercises in a row that work the same muscle. In the latter case, the second exercise may be a simple body position change (for example, widening the hand set on a bar during a bench press) or may be a completely different exercise (for example, leg extensions and leg squats). The second exercise works the muscle in a slightly different way, thereby recruiting fresh fibers.

Free weights (barbells, dumbbells) recruit more muscle fibers than machine weights because of the need to balance the bar as well as move it. For "wellness" purposes, the increased fiber recruitment that free weights cause is not significant; plus weight machines offer safety and convenience.

Slow Twitch and Fast Twitch Fibers

Muscle fibers are not all alike. Like people, they have specialized talents and preferred working conditions. The two basic fiber types are slow twitch (ST) and fast twitch (FT). Slow twitch fibers work best under aerobic conditions and are often referred to as Type I, red, or slow oxidative (SO) fibers. ST fibers contract more slowly than FT but are capable of sustaining low to moderately intense contractions over much longer periods of time. For example, ST fibers are the primary suppliers of energy for the muscle tone needed to sustain posture and the energy needed to run a marathon. While a marathon is intense in an overall sense, the muscle contractions are of moderate intensity, repeated many thousands of times. People gifted with a high percentage of ST fiber tend to gravitate toward aerobic activities.

Fast twitch fibers, alias Type II, white, and fast-glycolytic (FG), are so named because they have great speed and contractibility. Explosive anaerobic movements like sprinting and a badminton smash depend on FT fibers. These fibers, rich in stored energy, can react quickly but only for a short time. Individuals with a high percentage of FT fibers are genetically predisposed toward anaerobic activities.

There are two kinds of FT fibers, FTa (Type IIa) and FTb (Type IIb). FTa fibers possess some of the oxidative (aerobic) properties of ST fibers and some of the anaerobic properties of FTb fibers. FTb have higher concentrations of stored phosphocreatine (PC) and glycogen, both of which can be rapidly broken down to produce ATP in the absence of oxygen. All three (ST, FTa, and FTb) have some aerobic and some anaerobic capabilities, but ST have the most aerobic and least anaerobic capability. FTa are somewhere in the middle and FTb have the least aerobic but the most anaerobic capability.

All the fibers in one motor unit are the same type, but within a muscle there can be motor units of different types. The percentages of FTa, FTb, and ST vary from person to person and to some extent from muscle to muscle on one person. The numbers of fibers and percentages of slow and fast twitch are established by the time you are about eight years old.[5] Most people's muscles are in the middle, half FT and half ST.[6] This means that most of us are genetically built to be equally capable

of aerobic and anaerobic work, but not necessarily outstanding at either. Elite endurance runners have a high proportion of ST and FTa fibers, while elite sprinters have a high proportion of FT and a small proportion of ST fibers.[7,8]

A muscle biopsy can be taken to determine a person's percentages of fast and slow twitch fibers. Much like a geological core sampling of the earth, scientists insert a hollow cylindrical "needle" into the muscle and pull out a "core" sample of tissue to analyze. Although this is a fascinating research technique and helpful to elite athletes, the idea of having muscle extracted does not appeal to most people. A fast or slow time on a 100-meter dash is a much easier test for the curious layperson. Speed events favor FT fibers and endurance events ST fibers, but there are also numerous sport and activities that fall in the middle, and as a result require a more equal mix of fibers to sustain both aerobic and anaerobic activity.

Two other terms that can be explained in terms of muscle fibers are the "kick" and "hitting the wall." Ever wonder why a distance runner can still sprint at the end of the race? This final "kick" is the result of unused energy in the FT fibers. Researchers found that after running 30 kilometers (13.6 miles) their thirty subjects had depleted their ST fibers but still had energy available in their FT fibers.[9] When athletes run 400-meter races they often talk of "hitting the wall." This describes the discomfort they feel as their bodies deplete the anaerobically generated and stored energy of the FT fibers and start to depend on aerobically generated energy which takes longer to supply.

Fitness Implications

Aerobic and muscular endurance conditioning will improve the ability of ST fibers to generate and use energy. This is the kind of program you would want to improve your hiking stamina. Speed and strength conditioning will enhance FT fibers. This would be the program you would need to improve your ability to sprint or change directions quickly. Resistance training can increase the size of fibers but not the number or type. FTa however, appear to be somewhat trainable, developing in the direction of the most training.[10]

Muscle Fuels

In Chapter 2, you learned about the three metabolic systems, ATP–PC, aerobic glycolysis, and the lactic acid system. The fuel source for muscle contraction varies with the intensity and volume of the program. Very intense short exercise bouts (1 to 30 seconds) depend on the stored energy available through the ATP–PC system. This system can be trained through a resistance program that emphasizes strength and power. The lactic acid system becomes the major source of energy for movements that last between 30 seconds and about 3 minutes. This carbohydrate-burning system produces ATP for energy with a simultaneous buildup of lactic acid. As the lactic acid concentration increases, so does exercise discomfort and the ability of the muscle fibers to contract. The result is growing fatigue and finally exhaustion. Think about how you feel toward the end of an all-out sprint (to get to an exam on time or catch a train). Your legs start to feel heavy, maybe even burn, and finally you can't take another step.

Fitness Implications

A training regimen that uses a moderate to high intensity and a few to a moderate number of repetitions trains the lactic acid system. Stop-and-start sports, such as basketball, soccer, and racquetball, depend heavily on this system. High-number repetition, low-resistance exercises draw energy from both the lactic acid system and aerobic glycolysis. Even though the aerobic system is involved, the resulting training effect from resistance work is significantly less than the training effect from aerobic conditioning. Circuit weight-training programs in which you move through a series of weight machines with only a short break between exercises show average increases in VO$_2$max of only about 4 to 8 percent compared to 15 to 20 percent with aerobic training.[11] Lower-fit individuals may, however, see more improvement in their initial training. Resistance training is not a substitute for aerobic training for increasing aerobic capacity.

GENDER DIFFERENCES

Absolute and Relative Strength

There are many differences between men and women, but muscle tissue strength is not one of them. Regardless of gender, muscle tissue creates a force of 3 to 8 kilograms per square centimeter of cross section.[12] So why is the average man stronger? Simply put, he has more muscle. When men and women of the same size and conditioning level are compared, more of the man's weight is attributable to muscle. Interestingly, men have a higher percentage of their muscle in their upper body than women. This may help explain why greater strength differences are found between genders in the upper body as compared to the lower body.

When discussing strength and gender, it is important to differentiate between absolute strength and relative strength. Absolute strength refers to the actual amount of weight or resistance a person handles. If a large person and a small person both lift 100 pounds, both have an absolute strength of 100. If Maria lifts 80 pounds and Jason lifts 160 pounds, Jason has twice as much absolute strength. The majority of research evidence indicates that an average woman's absolute strength is not as great as an average man's. In total body strength, the average

woman is about 63.5 percent as strong as the average man.[13] Similar differences in absolute strength are found between highly conditioned male and female athletes.

Relative strength compares two people's strength with an adjustment made for differences in muscle mass. For example, if Jason, who lifted 160 pounds, has twice as much muscle as Maria, who lifted 80 pounds, their relative strength would be the same. A smaller muscle may lift less actual poundage compared to a larger muscle, but in relative terms they are equally strong. This puts a nice spin on the phrase "you are really strong for your size." When strength is expressed relative to lean body mass or muscle cross-sectional area, the difference in strength between the genders in many, but not all, instances disappears.[14]

Hypertrophy and Strength

An increase in muscle size is called **hypertrophy,** a decrease **atrophy.** Hypertrophy is the result of an increase in fiber size and not an increase in the number of fibers. Until fairly recently, it was widely accepted that men's muscles hypertrophied more than women's muscles and that this was probably due to hormonal differences. Circumference measures (tape measurements around the girth of a muscle) supported this idea. Men's circumferences increased to a greater extent than women's.

Then CAT scan technology enabled scientists to measure muscle independent of other tissues. CAT scan studies have resulted in a surprising, new conclusion. The magnitude of cross-sectional muscle growth was equal in men and women who participated in comparable heavy resistance training programs.[15] Men and women hypertrophy at the same rate. Why then, are men's muscles bigger? First, both genders have roughly the same number of muscle fibers per muscle, but women's muscle fibers are smaller than men's. This size difference may be due to considerably lower levels of testosterone and other growth hormones. When, with training, you increase the size of a small muscle 5 percent and a large muscle 5 percent, you get a greater absolute difference in size with the large muscle. Women's muscles hypertrophy like men's, but because they have less mass the percentage gain is less noticeable. Second, body composition changes can cause circumference measures to be misleading. Women have more fat than men between muscle fibers. When some of this fat, which is less dense than muscle, is lost at the same time that muscle size is gained, little or no difference in muscle circumference will occur. It is even possible to lose circumference and gain strength.

Interestingly, the amount a muscle will hypertrophy varies from one person to the next and from one muscle to another on one person. Jason may find, for example, that his shoulders hypertrophy a lot but his chest does not respond to the same extent. This is believed to be tied to a genetic predisposition.

A small percentage of women have larger amounts of hypertrophy. This may happen when a woman has[16]

- A higher than normal resting testosterone, growth hormone, or other contributing hormone level
- A greater hormonal response than normal to a resistance training program
- A lower than normal estrogen-to-testosterone ratio
- A genetic disposition to develop a large muscle mass
- The ability to perform a more intense resistance training program

A woman who experiences more hypertrophy than she wants can modify her program to minimize this effect. But in general women do not excessively hypertrophy and although the rate of hypertrophy is the same between genders, there is still some question as to whether women will hypertrophy to the same extent as men with long-term training. Muscle size is not the only factor that contributes to strength. Strength increases are also the result of enhanced neuromuscular efficiency, which means that greater numbers of motor units are recruited in a more coordinated fashion. Long-term strength gains in women may be due more to neural adaption than increases in muscle size.

Transient Hypertrophy

When you perform resistance exercises, the muscles temporarily enlarge. This "pumped-up" effect is called *transient hypertrophy* and is caused by an accumulation of water in the muscle. Normally the amount of fluid that moves out of the blood, across the capillary membranes, and into the muscle tissue and muscle cells is balanced by an equal return of fluid into the blood. Resistance exercises temporarily upset this homeostatic state, resulting in an accumulation of fluid (mostly water) in the interstitial and cellular spaces of the muscle. This condition, called edema, causes the muscle to be larger than normal or appear "pumped up." When you stop working out, the muscle will stay enlarged for a short period of time and then return to its normal size. Within several hours, the fluids will return to the blood and homeostasis is restored. To obtain accurate body measurements, take them before you work out or several hours after exercising. Transient hypertrophy is much more apparent in men than in women because of their greater muscle size.

Training Implications

Women respond to the same training programs as well or better than men; therefore there is no need for special programming for women. It may be that when women respond better to a program, it is because they have more room for improvement in the beginning. This would be especially true for upper body strength. Women, compared to men, generally require less absolute resistance (weight) to work out owing to absolute strength differences, but the actual exercise regimen can be the same. Sport-specific or aesthetic goals may affect program design, but this is true independent of gender. The higher percentage of fat in women's muscles mentioned earlier does not affect trainability of the muscles. Women can tone and shape muscles to the same extent as men but some of the muscle definition will be hidden by the additional fat required for a woman's health.

Women can, and should, enjoy the benefits of resistance training. Female super models, astronauts, military personnel, and athletes are examples of high-profile women whose careers depend on good muscular strength and tone. The important message, however, is that every woman can benefit from increased muscular strength and endurance. Because of physiological and hormonal gender differences the vast majority of women *need not worry about developing "bulky" muscles,* while most men can look forward to this training benefit. Both genders can enjoy the benefits of muscle symmetry, tone, and definition as well as increased strength.

Resistance training provides additional benefits for women who carry and deliver a child. Strong muscles help a pregnant woman maintain good posture and handle the extra weight as her abdomen expands and her center of gravity moves away from the spine. There is also some evidence that muscular endurance and strength may lead to easier births and a faster recovery.[17] Strong abdominal muscles may also result in less stretching of the skin and therefore fewer stretchmarks.

The Effects of Anabolic Steroids on Muscles

Anabolic steroid pills and injections, synthetic versions of the male hormone testosterone, can increase muscle strength and growth, but they can also destroy your wellness. The body maintains a delicate balance of chemicals and hormones. When you pump in extra hormones without medical supervision, you upset the natural balance and the side effects can be deadly. The desire, especially among young men, to have large, strong muscles makes the use of anabolic steroids very seductive, despite the numerous unhealthy side effects outlined in the box on page 113.

Steroids are not the only drug that strength seekers abuse. Human growth hormone (HGH), which doctors use to promote growth in individuals whose pituitary glands do not produce enough, are used by abusers to promote muscle and bone growth and heal tendons and ligaments. When the natural growth rate is accelerated in this way, there is tremendous opportunity for long-range, irreversible problems including gross deformities and cardiovascular disease. Side effects also include acromegaly (giantism), premature bone closure, muscle and ligament laxity, goiter (thyroid enlargement), decreased sex drive and/or impotence, and menstrual disorder.

Anabolic Steroids:
A Threat to Mind and Body

Raising a Red Flag

Although controlled studies on the long-term outcome of mega dosing with anabolic steroids have not been conducted, extensive research on prescribed doses for medical use has documented the potential side effects of the drug, even when taken in small doses. Moreover, reports by athletes and observations of attending physicians, parents, and coaches do offer substantial evidence of dangerous side effects.

Some effects, such as rapid weight gain, are easy to see. Some take place internally and may not be evident until it is too late. Some are irreversible.

The Dangers

... to Men

Males who take large doses of anabolic steroids typically experience changes in sexual characteristics. Although derived from a male sex hormone, the drug can trigger a mechanism in the body that can actually shut down the healthy functioning of the male reproductive system. Some possible side effects:

- Shrinking of the testicles
- Reduced sperm count
- Impotence
- Baldness
- Difficulty or pain in urinating
- Development of breasts
- Enlarged prostate

... and to Women

Females may experience "masculinization" as well as other problems:

- Growth of facial hair
- Changes in or cessation of the menstrual cycle
- Enlargement of the clitoris
- Deepened voice
- Breast reduction

... and to Both Sexes

For both males and females, continued use of anabolic steroids may lead to health conditions ranging from merely irritating to life-threatening. Some effects are

- Acne
- Jaundice
- Trembling
- Swelling of feet or ankles
- Bad breath
- Reduction in HDL, the "good" cholesterol
- High blood pressure
- Liver damage and cancers
- Aching joints
- Increased chance of injury to tendons, ligaments, and muscles

Special Dangers to Adolescents

Anabolic steroids can halt growth prematurely in adolescents. Because even small doses can irreversibly affect growth, steroids are rarely prescribed for children and young adults, and only for the severely ill. The Office of the Inspector General in the U.S. Department of Health and Human Services has gathered anecdotal evidence that preteens and teens taking steroids may be at risk for developing a dependence on them and on other substances as well.

The Threat of AIDS

People sometimes take injections of anabolic steroids to augment oral dosages, using large-gauge, reusable needles normally obtained through the black market. If needles are shared, users run the risk of transmitting or contracting the HIV infection that can lead to AIDS.

The Psychological Effects

Scientists are just beginning to investigate the impact of anabolic steroids on the mind and behavior. Many athletes report "feeling good" about themselves while on a steroids regimen. The downside, according to Harvard researchers, is wide mood swings ranging from periods of violent, even homicidal, episodes known as "roid rages" to bouts of depression when the drugs are stopped.

The Harvard study also noted that anabolic steroids users may suffer from paranoid jealousy, extreme irritability, delusions, and impaired judgment stemming from feelings of invincibility.

NIDA Anabolic Steroids, DHHS Publication No. (ADM) 91-1810. To obtain printed copies of this report, please call or write the National Clearinghouse on Alcohol and Drug Information, P.O. Box 2345, Rockville, MD 20852.

As you will read in Chapter 14, most of the drugs that are being abused today were initially developed for medical purposes or discovered in pursuit of a medical treatment. Steroids are synthetic versions of testosterone that were developed to treat problems like kidney disease, severe burns, some muscle diseases, and breast cancer. Physicians prescribe steroids in small, controlled doses and watch their patients very carefully for side effects. Steroid abusers use doses 20 to 100 times stronger and are therefore at much greater risk of dangerous side effects. Used properly, steroids and HGH enhance wellness; used improperly, they tear it down. This is a case where too much of a good thing becomes dangerous.

TRAINING YOUR MUSCLES

Static and Dynamic Training

There are two types of exercises for muscles: static and dynamic. Just as it sounds, a **static exercise** is performed without movement. **Dynamic exercises** are the opposite; they involve moving through a range of motion. Dynamic movements dominate our daily activity but they are often performed in combination with static ones. For example, your arm muscles use dynamic contractions to pick up a bag of groceries but static contractions to hold it while you walk (dynamically) into the house. Archery provides another excellent example: you pull back the string dynamically but hold a static contraction while finalizing your aim.

Strength gains tend to be specific to the type of training the muscle receives. If you want dynamic strength, it is best to train dynamically and for static strength to train statically.[18] Static strength is especially important for postural muscles, and static strength exercises are important in rehabilitation, when the muscle is weak in one specific position. Most people want dynamic strength because this is what most activities require.

Static strength may be achieved using isometric contractions (exercises). During an **isometric** contraction, the muscle fibers contract but the length of the muscle does not change. The muscles involved are unable to change length because the bones they are attached to are working against an immovable object. For example, when you stand in a doorway and push against the frame with both hands, your arm muscles contract but, because the door frame won't budge (normally!), your arms can't straighten. Some people use isometric exercises to relieve tension, especially at times when dynamic exercises are not appropriate, such as when riding in a car or sitting at a desk. For more information about isometric strength, see Activity 5.1.

Dynamic strength can be developed using either isotonic or isokinetic contractions (exercises). An **isotonic** contraction is one in which the tension in the muscle stays the same throughout the range of motion. When this name was selected, it was meant to describe typical movements such as the one used in the bench press. It was believed that the tension remained the same in a muscle as long as the weight of the object being moved stayed the same. We now know that the tension in the muscle varies during the movement. The reason: our bones and muscles work together in a leverage system, which means that in certain positions we have more mechanical advantage. No doubt you have experienced how much more difficult it is to lift a box up off the floor than to pick it up off a 12-inch stool. The box weighs the same, but you have a mechanical advantage in the second position, so it "feels" lighter. Like the chain with the weak link, you can lift only the amount of weight your muscles can handle at their weakest point in the range of motion. This weak point is often referred to as the "sticking point." De-

---

Activity 5.1
Sample Isometric Exercises

Neck and Arms

Interlock your fingers and place them on the back of your head. Press your head backward while pressing forward with your hands.

Inner Thighs and Arms

Place your palms against the insides of your knees. Press your knees inward while pressing outward with your arms.

Outer Thighs, Chest, and Arms

Place palms of your hands against the outside of your knees. Press your hands inward while pressing outward with your thighs.

Upper Back, Shoulders, and Fingers

Hold your hands in front of your chest (elbows bent) with one palm facing inward and the other outward. Clasp your fingers. Pinch your shoulder blades together as you try to pull your hands apart. Do not let go your fingers.

Chest and Arms

Clasp your hands with palms facing inward. Hold your hands at chest height. Press one hand against the other.

Arms and Shoulders

Sit up straight on a chair. With your arms at your sides, grasp the edges of the chair seat. Pull upward against the chair.

Abdominals, Arms, Chest, Hip Flexors

Sit in a chair (or car seat) and place your hands palm side down on your thighs. Push down with your hands while you try to lift up with your legs. You may find it easier to do one leg at a time.

Upper Back, Arms, Shoulders

While sitting in a car (not driving) place the palms of your hands against the roof of the car. Press your arms upward. (This can also be done by having a partner's hands or your own hand take the place of the roof of the car.)

---

signers and manufacturers were intrigued: Would it be possible, they wondered, to design a machine that could vary resistance to match the human strength curve?

This discovery revolutionized weight-training equipment. Universal and Nautilus were the first to build weight machines that could compensate for human strength differences during a lift. Pulleys, levers, and cams were, and still are, used to vary the resistance, increasing resistance when you are in a "strong" position and easing up on the resistance when you are in a "weak" position. These machines are called, naturally, "variable resistance" machines. The idea behind these machines is sound, but it should also be noted that these machines are designed around an average person's strength curve. As an individual, you may be strong or weak in a slightly different position than the machine adjusts for. Many of these machines are also built for the average male body. Cushions may need to be strategically placed to keep a smaller person properly positioned.

Free weights (barbells and dumbbells) provide a constant resistance and have therefore been named "constant resistance" or "fixed resistance" exercises. It is technically incorrect to call both constant and variable resistance training isotonic training, although the term is widely used for both. In variable resistance training, "equal tension" (the definition of isotonic) is not maintained.

Dynamic contractions can also be described according to the lengthening or shortening of the muscle fibers. When the muscle is shortening, it is said to be in a **concentric contraction;** when it is lengthening, an **eccentric contraction.** Flexing your arm requires the biceps muscle to shorten and is therefore a concentric contraction. When your arms slowly lower the weight (as opposed to letting the weight fall with the pull of gravity), the biceps muscle fibers slowly lengthen in an eccentric contraction.

Sometimes concentric contractions are referred to as positives and eccentric contractions as negatives. Negatives can be performed using heavier loads than positives because you are slowing the weight's descent as opposed to pushing it up against gravity. Eccentric weight training requires one or more partners to help raise the weight to the starting position. Research is mixed on eccentric training but generally shows that it is effective but not significantly more effective than concentric training.[19] It has also been found to cause more delayed muscle soreness, especially for the first couple of weeks. Eccentric training is not popular for these reasons, but there are two ways it can be helpful in a basic fitness program. First, weights should always be raised *and* lowered with control. Second, eccentric contractions can be used when an individual is incapable of even one concentric contraction. For example, a person who cannot do a pull-up can train the pull-up muscles by performing negatives. The individual can use a chair or partner to position herself above the bar and then slowly relax the arms. Training with eccentric contractions (negatives) will eventually enable the individual to do concentric contractions (positives) such as pull-ups.

Isokinetic contractions exert force through a range of motion at a designated speed. Special machines have been built on which the speed of movement is preset. On a regular machine or barbell, the harder you bench press, the faster the machine and weights fly up—not so with isokinetic equipment. Its ability to adjust the resistance to match your effort has earned it the name of "accommodating resistance." No matter how hard you push or pull against the machine, you cannot exceed the set speed. The biggest advantage to this type of training is that you have control over the force of effort at every point during the movement. This is especially helpful with rehabilitation where the load needs to vary according to (accommodate) the strengths and weaknesses of the injured muscle(s). Before isokinetic equipment was available, a physical therapist had to make a "best guess" about how much resistance a recovering muscle could handle at its weakest point. Isokinetic machines provide resistance to however much force is applied; thus, even at its weakest point the working muscle's capability will be matched, not exceeded. This allows for safe strength and endurance conditioning while preventing re-injury.

Isokinetic machines work only concentric contractions. When the biceps muscle pulls the machine upward, the triceps muscle is required to pull the machine back down. Because eccentric contractions are not used, less delayed muscle soreness is experienced. Water exercises are somewhat similar. The more you push against the water, the more it resists you and you must exert a force against the water with every movement.

Finally, even though isokinetic and variable resistance exercises can more effectively challenge the strong points in the strength curve, they are no more effective than fixed resistance exercises in their ability to strengthen the weak point. Although each of these three types of resistance training has advantages and disadvantages, all three are effective ways to increase strength and endurance.

APPLYING THE PRINCIPLES OF PHYSICAL ACTIVITY

The FIT Principle

Frequency as a First Step

Resistance training performed two to three times a week with a 48-hour rest between workouts is recommended for moderate improvements in strength and endurance. Twice a week is a minimum for developing strength. Once a week will maintain strength if the workout is performed at the same intensity you trained at to achieve that strength. The 48-hour rest between workouts allows muscle tissue to recover and rebuild at greater strength. If moderate to heavy resistance training of the same muscle is performed every day, muscles may actually start to weaken. Individuals who train four to seven days a week are usually working different muscle groups on consecutive days so that the rest break is maintained. This is called a split program. The workout is usually split by working the upper body one day and lower body the next.

Intensity: Adding Resistence

When developing strength, intensity is increased by adding resistance and maintaining or lowering repetitions. For developing endurance, the resistance is also increased, but this is done more gradually in order to continue using a high number of repetitions. Endurance intensity can also be increased by performing more consecutive repetitions.

Time: Duration of the Workout

The length of the workout is influenced by the number of **repetitions** of an exercise and the number of **sets** of repetitions performed. Depending on the focus of the workout (strength or endurance), the number of repetitions usually falls between one and twenty and the sets between one and five. Between each set is a rest break. Short breaks (10 to 30 seconds) allow only partial recovery and are therefore used to develop endurance. Longer breaks (1 to 3 minutes) allow for greater recovery and are used to space strength exercises that require more maximal efforts. Therefore, the overall duration of the workout depends on the number of exercises in the program, the number of repetitions and sets, and the length of the breaks. Usually a general-fitness weight-training program consisting of one to three sets of ten to twelve exercises can be completed in 30 to 60 minutes.

Mode

Activities such as tennis, golf, simple calisthenics, washing the car, and cleaning the house can help build and maintain muscular endurance. Strength is built through calisthenics or activities that are challenging enough that you can do only about six to ten repetitions or through a resistance training program like weight training.

Principle of Progressive Overload

According to ancient legend, Milos, a famous Greek athlete, strength trained by lifting a young bull onto his shoulders. As the bull grew, so did Milos' strength. Milos was putting to work the principles of progression and overload. He gradually added weight over time (progression), lifting more than he was accustomed to (overloading) each time. You can achieve a progressive overload by adding resistance to your workout whenever it begins to feel "easy." Baechle and Grove[20] offer the "2 × 2" rule of thumb for weight training: when you can lift two more repetitions than normal for two workouts in a row, increase the weight. If your goal is to perform between eight and twelve repetitions, the new resistance should put you back down around eight. You will find that you have to add more weight (5 to 10 pounds) to large-muscle exercises such as leg squats than to small-muscle exercises (1 to 5 pounds) such as the arm curl.

Overloading, or increasing intensity, is accomplished by increasing the load (weight) in dynamic exercises, increasing the force exerted against an immovable object in isometric exercises, and increasing the force exerted through a range of motion in isokinetic exercises. Shorter rest breaks between sets also increase overload because the muscle fibers are not able to recover fully before the next lift. Endurance overloads are achieved by increasing the number of sets and repetitions and decreasing the length of breaks.

Principle of Specificity

It appears that muscle cells are narrow-minded. If you train using dynamic contractions and then test your strength using an isometric test or vice versa, the research says you'll be disappointed more often than not. Isometric training shows improvement when tested for isometrically, but not when it's tested dynamically.[21] (If, however, isometrics are done at enough joint angles, dynamic strength does improve.) Similarly, dynamic strength gains are evident on dynamic strength tests but not on isometric strength tests.[22]

Exercise technique and form play an important role in specificity. If muscles other than the target muscle (or muscle group) are allowed to be used during an exercise, less training of the targeted muscle occurs. If you are performing an arm curl with a bar, you must not let your back arch to aid the arm muscles. Poor form such as this not only undermines specificity, it can also lead to injury.

Principle of Reversibility

Change works both ways. When muscles are challenged, they get stronger; when muscles are inactive or face less rigorous activity than normal, they grow weaker. Muscle atrophy is very subtle and may go unnoticed for a long period of time—then suddenly you'll notice you've gone "soft." Don't let it sneak up on you. Keep active and, if possible, exercise regularly. Once you have developed strength, you can maintain it with as little as one or two weekly workouts.

Principle of Individuality

The army recruiters are right, "Be all that you can be." Just be sure to place a special emphasis on the word *you*. People are different—mentally, emotionally, and physically. The rate and potential to which you will develop strength and endurance will naturally be different from someone else's. As you've learned, fiber type percentages vary, the ability to hypertrophy varies, neuromuscular efficiency varies, and so will training progress. Different programs work for different people. Individualize your program and try not to judge your progress on the basis of someone else's. Each of us has a tremendous untapped potential—the key is to develop it according to *your* needs on *your* timeline.

MANIPULATING RESISTANCE TRAINING PROGRAM VARIABLES

At the beginning of the chapter, we introduced the idea of a continuum between strength and endurance. It is now time to look at how repetitions, sets, breaks between sets, and resistance can be combined to design programs along the continuum. Innumerable combinations of these variables will work. The six discussed here are (1) a strength program, (2) an endurance program, (3) a general fitness program, (4) a power program, (5) a hypertrophy program, and (6) a circuit resistance training program. A summary of guidelines for the first three programs, using dynamic exercises, appears in Table 5.1.

Strength Program

Dynamic Strength

The greatest amount of weight (load) that a person can lift, push, or pull one time is referred to as one repetition max, or 1 RM. It is not advisable for a beginner to work with maximal loads, nor do advanced lifters use maximal loads all of the time. There has been a lot of research done trying to establish what the best load and number of repetitions is for maximal strength gains. There is still some debate, and it has become evident that more than one program works, but a good basic rule is to use one to six repetitions. These one to six repetitions are performed to the point of voluntary exhaustion. This means that you use a weight that you can lift up to six times but cannot lift seven times. This is referred to as one set of 6 RM. Multiple sets (two to five) are recommended for optimum strength gains. A beginner should start with lighter loads, more repetitions, and one set until technique is mastered.

A program that emphasizes strength uses and develops the ATP–PC and lactic acid energy systems. The ATP–PC system can produce energy very quickly for short bouts (1 to 3 seconds) of exercise, but once used, takes several minutes to recover. Breaks should therefore be 2 to 3 minutes long between sets. Because most of the sets take more than 3 seconds, the lactic acid system is also involved. Both types of FT fibers are recruited. (Because all three fiber types are involved in every movement, some ST fibers will also be recruited, but they play a minor role in this type of workout.)

Different sets can all use the same resistance or they can be of increasing or decreasing amounts of resistance. One popular strength/general fitness program is the De-Lorme system, in which the first set is done using 50 percent of 10 RM, the second at 75 percent of 10 RM, and the third at 100 percent of 10 RM, where 10 RM is the maximum amount of weight you can lift ten times.

Example

Able to bench press 80 lb, 10 times.

1st set = 40 lb (50 percent of 80), 10 repetitions

2nd set = 60 lb (75 percent of 80), 10 repetitions

3rd set = 80 lb (100 percent of 80), 10 repetitions

Isometric Strength

Isometric strength training is particularly helpful for developing strength in one position. Isometric contractions of maximal force held for a duration of 30 seconds (one hold of 30, two of 15, and so on) will result in strength gains. The strength, however, is limited to the joint angle used in the exercise and a carryover of about 20 degrees in both directions. If you want to be stronger through a full range of motion, you must exercise at several joint angles. For example, to strengthen your biceps through a ROM you can perform isometric contractions at 150 degrees, 120 degrees, 90 degrees, 60 degrees, and 30 degrees.

Isometric training has several advantages. It requires little or no equipment, which means it can be done while traveling or at home, or as a break during the workday. The exercises can be performed alone or with an exercise partner. They can be very helpful for getting past the sticking point in dynamic exercise or for stabilizing a position such as good standing posture. One drawback to isometric exercises is the dramatic rise in both diastolic and systolic blood pressure during maximal muscle contractions.[23] For this reason, hypertensive individuals should consult a physician before using isometric contractions. Motivation may also be difficult to maintain because there is no visual feedback, such as a stack of weights moving. Motivation is crucial because submaximal forces (especially those less than two-thirds of maximum) result in significantly less strength development. Furthermore, without special equipment you can't tell whether your force production has improved.

Muscular Endurance Program

Muscle endurance is developed using lighter weights for a high number of repetitions. There is no upper limit on the number of repetitions, but the fact that strength training also increases endurance suggests that limiting the number to ten to twenty may be more efficient. Here is an example of how strength affects endurance: if a person's maximum lift is 100 pounds, then 50 pounds is 50 percent of 1 RM. If, however, maximum strength is increased to 150 pounds, 50 pounds represents only 33 percent of 1 RM. More repetitions at 33 percent can be performed than at 50 percent, therefore the strength gain is an endurance gain.

The exception to the ten- to twenty-repetition guideline would be for athletes interested in "extreme" en-

TABLE 5.1 ■ Program Summaries for Strength, General Fitness, and Endurance

	Strength	General Fitness	Endurance
Reps:	1–6	8–12 (15)	12–20+
Load:	80–100 percent 1 RM	70–80 percent 1 RM	20–70 percent 1 RM[a]
Sets:	4–10 primary muscles 1–3 assisting muscles	1–3	2–3
Breaks:	2–3 min	30–90 sec	30–60 sec for 12–20 repetition sets 2–3 min for >20 repetition sets
Energy:	ATP–PC/LA	LA	LA/Aer.Gl.
Fiber:	FT (a + b)	FT (a + b)	FTa/ST

[a]The low end of this range refers to muscle endurance that is built during aerobic activities such as the leg toning that occurs while jogging. The low load is matched with a very high number of repetitions.

durance training. For example, a tri-athlete (swimming, running, cycling) must train for very high endurance in all muscle groups. Both ST and FTa fibers are involved in endurance exercises.

General Fitness Program

After a thorough review of the research literature, the American College of Sports Medicine[24] makes the following recommendations for resistance training for the average healthy adult: a minimum of eight to ten exercises involving the major muscle groups should be performed a minimum of twice a week. A minimum of one set of eight to twelve repetitions to near fatigue should be completed for each exercise. This minimum standard will produce about 70 to 80 percent of the improvement reported for programs using additional frequencies of training and combinations of sets and repetitions.[25] Multiple sets will result in greater gains, but these smaller gains must be weighed against increasing the length of the workout, which results in higher dropout rates.

Power Program

Muscular power can be achieved by manipulating the amount of the resistance and the speed with which it is moved. Power is often equated with strength but is in fact a combination of strength and speed. The strongest person is not necessarily the most powerful. A person who can move a 200-pound object from floor to overhead in 4 seconds is stronger but less powerful than someone who can move a 150-pound object in 2 seconds. How can this be? Let's look at the numerical formula. Power equals the amount of work that can be done in a unit of time or power = work ÷ time. Since work equals force × distance, substitute this in the formula and you get:

power = work (force × distance) ÷ time

The force is the amount of resistance. The distance in our example is about 10 feet and the time is 2 or 4 seconds. As you can see below, person 2 is more powerful than person 1.

Person 1: force (200 lb) × 10 feet ÷ 4 seconds = 500 ft-lb/sec

Person 2: force (150 lb) × 10 feet ÷ 2 seconds = 750 ft-lb/sec

This does not mean that powerful people aren't strong; some powerful athletes can move heavy resistances very quickly. What it does mean is that a person has to give up some strength to maximize power.

Power training can be strength-related or speed-related, and the conditioning program varies depending upon the desired outcome. For example, a football lineman needs strength-related power in order to push a 200- to 300-pound opponent around. The lineman will have to give up a little hitting strength to have the speed necessary to move quickly against the opponent. A softball player who wants a powerful throw needs some strength but will train with more moderate resistances to emphasize speed. Lighter resistances allow you to train speed because they can be moved more rapidly through a range of motion than can heavier resistances.

Hypertrophy Program

If you desire muscle size, hypertrophy, you must train in a way that causes one set of muscle fibers to become fatigued so that additional fibers are recruited. This is achieved with a high volume of sets and repetitions. Multiple sets (two to five) of eight to fifteen repetitions are generally recommended. (Body builders may use as many as seven sets with fifteen to twenty repetitions.) The lactic acid system is the major supplier of energy. Primarily FT fibers are recruited.

Circuit Resistance Training Program

Circuit training means to move from one exercise into the next with little to no break between exercises. Circuits can be designed for muscular strength and endurance, or cardiorespiratory endurance, or a combination of the two. Circuit resistance training (CRT) emphasizes muscular endurance and may provide some aerobic benefit (particularly for those with low cardiovascular fitness), but it is not a substitute for aerobic exercise. CRT is often used in health clubs where a line of weight machines is set up and participants simply follow the line, performing either on their own or to instructions from a tape recorder about when to set the resistance, start, stop, and move to the next station. Usually eight to fifteen repetitions are performed in 15 to 30 seconds at each station. CRT has some distinct advantages.

If you are using machines, it is relatively quick and easy to perform. It takes about 1 minute per station to set the weight, get in position, and perform the repetitions, which means a twelve-exercise circuit can be completed in under 15 minutes. Two sets can be performed in 30 minutes. You can complete a warm-up, 20 minutes of aerobic work, 30 minutes of resistance work, and a cool-down all in a one-hour workout. CRT is excellent for moving large numbers of people through a facility. If it is properly designed, once you have started, you will be able to move from one machine to the next without waiting.

A circuit can also be performed with free weights. This requires a fair number of weight changes in a short amount of time but is, despite the inconvenience, a good way to work out. If you plan to do two sets, fewer weight changes are required if you perform both sets of an exer-

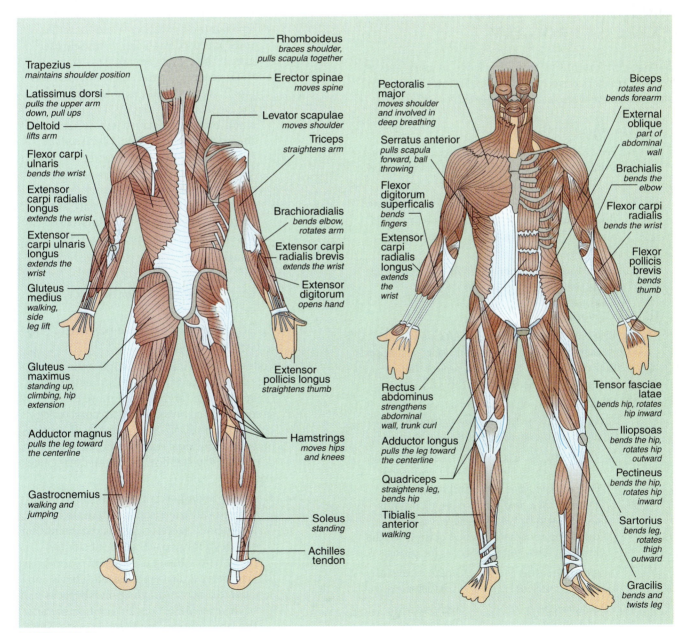

FIGURE 5.4 Muscles of the body.

cise (with the appropriate break between sets) before moving on to the next. You should still plan more time if you are doing a free-weight circuit.

Mini-circuits consisting of only three or four exercises can also be performed. By the time you complete one rotation of the circuit, at least 2 to 3 minutes (probably 5 to 6) will have passed. Thus, when you start the circuit for a second time, the original muscle will have had a 2- to 3-minute break—the break needed for strength workouts. The biggest advantage to mini-circuits is that they allow you to perform a demanding strength workout in a short amount of time. Several mini-circuits may be used in a workout. Mini-circuits can also be used for a general fitness program, but there is no additional benefit.

DESIGNING A RESISTANCE EXERCISE PROGRAM

Now it's time to put all this knowledge to work and set up your resistance exercise program. Follow this series of steps using the worksheets as indicated.

I. Assess your needs.

    A. Assess your present levels of strength and endurance using any or all of the tests provided in labs at the end of this chapter.

    B. Think about the types of activities you like to do and determine what muscles are involved and whether the contractions are static or dynamic.

    C. Based on A and B, write down some general goals (Lab 5.5).

II. Select your exercises (Lab 5.5).

    A. Based on your general goals, decide which muscles you need to work and select exercises that target them. Select equipment that is available and cost-effective for you.

    B. Organize your selected exercises onto a log sheet (Lab 5.5) using one, or a combination of more than one, of the following systems:

        1. Opposing Muscles System: This system is based on the belief that body symmetry and muscle balance are important. For every muscle worked, the opposing muscle will also be worked. Here is a list of opposing muscles and their action; see the muscle chart (Figure 5.4) for locations.

gastrocnemius	ankle extension
tibialis anterior	ankle flexion
quadriceps	leg extension
hamstring	leg flexion
erector spinae	trunk extension
abdominals	trunk flexion
iliopsoas	hip flexion
gluteus maximus	hip extension
extensor carpi ulnaris	forearm extension
flexor carpi radialis	forearm flexion
triceps brachii	elbow extension
biceps brachii	elbow flexion
latissimus dorsi	pulls arms down
trapezius/deltoid triceps	pushes arms overhead
pectoralis major/ triceps	pushes arms away
rhomboids/biceps	pulls arms in

        2. Large-Muscle/Small-Muscle System: In this system, large-muscle exercises precede small-muscle exercises when the small muscle is used in the large-muscle exercise. If these exercises are performed in the reverse order, the small-muscle exercise is fatigued and less able to assist in the large-muscle exercise. The loss of small-muscle assistance will decrease the load you can handle, which will in turn decrease the training effect on the large muscles. Since many resistance exercises do not involve both large and small muscles, this system applies only to some exercises. Here are some examples of small-muscle/large-muscle exercise pairs:

Lunges, squats, or leg press before heel raises

Lat pull-down, seated or bent-over row before biceps curl

Bench press, or overhead press before triceps extensions

Following the same logic, single-muscle activities should follow multi-muscle activities (smaller versus larger sets of muscles), such as squats or leg press before leg curls or leg extension. Similarly, back exercises should precede abdominal exercises because the abdominals help stabilize the trunk during back exercises.

        3. Upper Body/Lower Body: In this system, upper-body exercises are alternated with lower-body exercises, an arrangement that ensures a muscle will get a substantial break before being used again. Good body symmetry is also emphasized. This is considered a demanding regimen because half of the exercises under this system involve the large muscles of the lower body. This

Sample Weight-Training Program

Performed in order, this program alternates upper and lower body exercises, places large muscle and multimuscle exercises before small or single-muscle exercises, and places the back exercise before the abdominal exercise.

Bench Press (Pectorals, Deltoids, Triceps)	10 reps/2 sets
Leg Press (Quads, Hamstrings, Gluteals)	10 reps/2 sets
Lat Pull (Latissimus Dorsi, Rhomboids, Deltoids)	10 reps/2 sets
Leg Flexion (Hamstring)	10 reps/2 sets
Seated Row (Rhomboids, Deltoids)	10 reps/2 sets
Leg Extension (Quadriceps)	10 reps/2 sets
Arm Curl (Biceps)	10 reps/2 sets
Curl-Ups (Abdominal)	20 reps/2 sets
Heel Raises (Gastrocnemius)	10 reps/2 sets
Arm Extension (Triceps)	10 reps/2 sets

can be true but is not always true of other systems.

4. Circuit Resistance Training (CRT): As described earlier in the chapter, series of exercises are performed one after another with very short breaks between exercises. If you work out at a facility, the number and order of exercises in the circuit may be predetermined. If you are laying out the circuit, you can use some of the systems described earlier to determine the order of exercises. In a predetermined circuit, you can also skip exercises or add exercises if the facility is not too crowded and you can easily leave and reenter the circuit.

III. Decide where on the continuum (Lab 5.5) you wish to work. Which of the following do you wish to emphasize?

A. Muscular strength
B. General fitness
C. Muscular endurance

IV. Based on your answer to the previous question, determine and record on the log sheet (Lab 5.5) the:

A. Number of repetitions
B. Number of sets
C. Length of breaks

V. Determine the frequency of your workouts and record on your selected exercise list (Lab 5.5) which days of the week you will train. Remember, a split routine must be used if you choose to work out on two consecutive days.

VI. Determine your resistance for each exercise and record it on your exercise log (Lab 5.5). If you are just starting out in a general fitness program, it is probably easiest to use trial and error to find a weight that you can lift at least eight times but not more than twelve. Be sure to warm up first, either with light loads and stretching or with 3 to 5 minutes of cardiovascular work and some stretching.

VII. Set more specific goals (Lab 5.5) now that you have more information concerning your present ability and your desired outcome. Write down your goals on your exercise log. Be sure that your goals are specific and reasonable. Include your target level (desired gains expressed as additional weight or repetitions to be lifted or as the total amount you wish to lift) and a date by which you'd like to reach your goal.

VIII. Start your program and keep track of your progress on your exercise log (Lab 5.5).

Adapting Equipment and Programs for People with Disabilities

Resistance training is an excellent activity for individuals with physical disabilities. Equipment can be adapted to accommodate wheelchairs, to provide easier gripping for those with hand grip limitations, and to establish movement plans for the blind. For more information concerning a specific disability, contact an adaptive physical education teacher, appropriate foundation, experienced club owner, or other specialist. Two excellent books on resistance training and fitness conditioning with a disability are listed at the end of this chapter in the Suggested Reading list.

Safety and Technique Pointers for Resistance Training

1. Breathe properly. Holding your breath is dangerous. When the glottis covers the windpipe, pressure can build up in the chest cavity. This situation, called the Valsalva Maneuver, can result in blacking out during exercise.

2. Control your movement. All resistance training should be performed with smooth, even movements. Even when acceleration is used in lifts, the movement should be fluid.

3. Work through a full range of motion (ROM). This promotes strength and flexibility at every point in the exercise.

4. Do *not* lock out a joint. As you reach the end of a full range of motion, stop just short of locking out the joint.

5. Isolate the target muscle(s). Work only the muscle or muscle group for which the exercise is designed. Poor body alignment or technique results in the recruitment of other muscles. When this happens, the extra muscles help bear the load and the target muscle(s) is (are) not properly overloaded. The poor alignment can also cause injury.

6. Concentrate. Stay focused throughout the exercise. This encourages good technique, high motivation, and safety.

7. Use strict exercise form. This results in proper, safe, effective lifts that isolate the proper muscle(s).

8. Eat a balanced, nutritious diet. You need sufficient carbohydrates to fuel your workout. Most Americans eat too few complex carbohydrates and too many fats and proteins. Amino acids and other supplements are not necessary when a balanced diet is followed. Please see Chapter 6 for more information.

Safety Tips Specific to Free Weights

1. Always work with a partner—never lift alone. People have died, strangled by a weight bar, when the weight they were bench pressing overcame them and they had no partner to rescue them. This usually happens in a basement or garage where no one can see that they are in trouble. Other injuries such as strains and sprains can also be prevented by working out with a partner.

2. Be sure that your partner is positioned correctly, can handle the weight you are lifting, and is paying attention throughout the lift.

3. Use locking devices to secure weights on the bar. Because weights have to be changed frequently, some people become lazy and don't use the locks. If a lift is performed unevenly, weights can shift suddenly, resulting in injury to the lifter, the spotter, or a spectator if the weights fall off the bar or the bar is dropped.

4. Load and unload weights evenly from each end of the bar. If you pull the weight off one end of a bar on a narrow stand, the weight left on the other end will cause that end of the bar to fall to the ground.

RESISTANCE TRAINING EXERCISES

There are many different ways to approach resistance training—weight machines, exercise bands, homemade weights, water exercises, and partner exercises, for example. The following is a sampling of exercises for the major muscle groups of the body. Two exercises will be pictured for each of the major muscles or muscle groups. The first will be an exercise performed on a weight machine. Most campuses have these available to all students, not just athletes, and weight machines provide a safe and easy way to create a conditioning overload. The machines available to you may look slightly different than the ones pictured in this book, but the basic action of the machine will be the same. A qualified instructor at your facility will be happy to assist you with the equipment and show you the correct technique for each piece. The second exercise described is one you can perform without formal equipment. Some students are uncomfortable at a weight room or do not have one available at the time they want to exercise. For these reasons, this second set of exercises can be done in the privacy of your home or dorm room. These exercises may provide less available resistance when compared to weight-training equipment, but they can often provide adequate resistance for general fitness. Before performing any of the following exercises, be sure to warm up and stretch your muscles. Also be sure to breathe during each exercise. For moderate to heavy resistances, breathe out during the work phase (lifting, pushing, pulling) and breathe in during the recovery phase. On lighter resistance exercise, you can maintain the breathing pattern just described or simply concentrate on normal breathing.

1. Ankle Extension Using a Machine
Muscles Involved: Gastrocnemius, Soleus

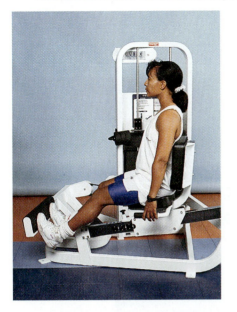

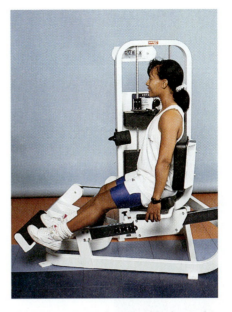

🔺 Position: Sit with your back firmly against the back pad. Place your feet on the foot plate (or bar) and adjust the seat until your legs are extended but slightly bent. Place your feet parallel and shoulder width apart. For additional benefits, perform this exercise with your heels angled slightly outward or inward.

🔺 Action: Extend your ankles by pushing your toes against the foot plate. Slowly lower the weight. Do not use the rest of your legs during this exercise; move only at the ankle and toe joints.

2. Ankle Extension (Toe Raise) with Homemade Materials
Muscles Involved: Gastrocnemius, Soleus

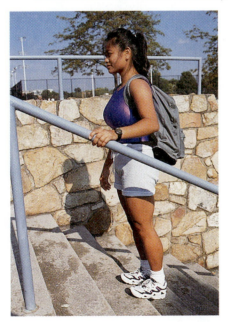

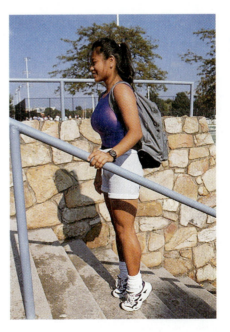

🔺 Position: Stand on a stair so that the balls of your feet are on the stair but your heels extend back off the stair. The railing can be used for balance. Place your feet parallel and shoulder width apart for a basic toe raise. Toe raises with the heels angled slightly outward or inward will further increase the amount of calf muscle trained.

🔺 Action: Rise up on your toes. Lower down, allowing the heels to go below the height of the stair. Additional resistance can be obtained in the exercise by wearing a weighted vest, or holding books, or other homemade weights such as backpack or gallon jugs filled with water or sand.

1. *Leg Extension with a Machine*
Muscles Involved: Quadriceps

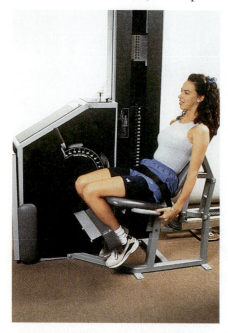

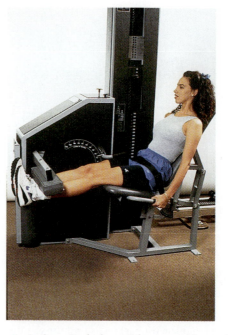

◆ Position: Sit with your back straight and against the back of the chair. If this is not possible, adjust the machine or add an extra cushion behind your back. Place your lower legs behind the padded ankle bars. Hold on to the hand grips on the sides of the seat.

◆ Action: Push the weight upward by straightening your legs, together or one leg at a time. Do not lock your knee joints. Exhale as you lift the weight and inhale as you slowly lower the weight.

2. *Isometric Wall Sit*
Muscles Involved: Quadriceps, Gluteals, Hamstrings

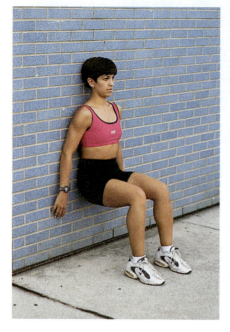

◆ Position: Stand with your back against a wall. While pressing your back against the wall, move your feet away from the wall and slide down into a sitting position with your thighs parallel to the floor. Your feet should be far enough away from the wall to create a right angle in the knee joint. Toes should point forward and feet should be shoulder-width apart.

Action: Hold this sitting position for 10 to 30 seconds. Breathe normally throughout.

1. Leg Curl with a Machine
Muscles Involved: Hamstrings

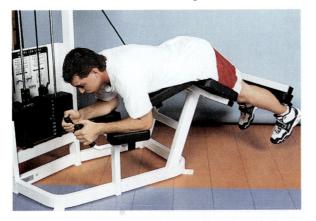 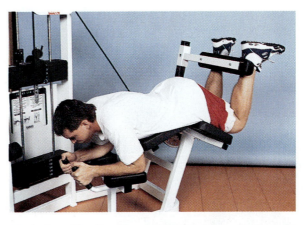

🔺 Position: Lie down (prone) on the machine bench (pad). Some benches have a bend at the hips to help prevent low back involvement. To further protect your back, keep your head and shoulders flat on the bench or if provided, place your forearm on rests below the pad. Place the back of your ankles underneath the leg/ankle pads. Grasp the sides of the pad or use hand grips, if available.

🔺 Action: Flex (bend) your knees and draw the leg/ankle pads toward your buttocks. Exhale when pulling the weight up, inhale while slowly lowering it down.

2. Leg Curl with a Partner
Muscles Involved : Hamstrings

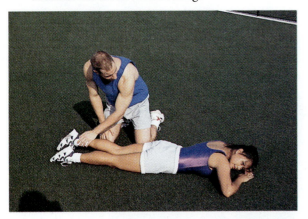 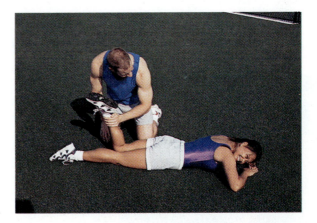

🔺 Position: Lie prone on the floor or other sturdy flat surface. Have a partner kneel or stand next to you facing your feet and place his or her hands on the back of one of your ankles.

🔺 Action: Bend your knee, drawing your foot toward your buttocks while your partner provides enough resistance against you to make it challenging but not impossible to move your leg through the full range of motion. (If you do not have a partner available, you can use an exercise band or ankle weight.)

MUSCULAR STRENGTH AND ENDURANCE   **125**

1. Hip Adductor with a Machine
Muscles Involved: Adductors, Pectineus, Gracilis

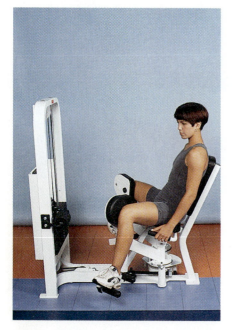 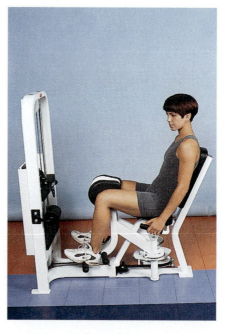

⬥ Position: Sit down with your back against the pad. Place your legs so that the machine pads rest against your inner thighs. Hold on to the hand grips to stabilize your body. Start with your legs apart.

⬥ Action: Pull your legs together against the resistance. Exhale as you pull, inhale as you slowly return your legs to their starting position.

2. Inner Thigh Pull with or without an Exercise Band
Muscles Involved: Adductors, Pectineus, Gracilis

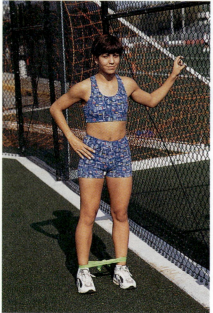 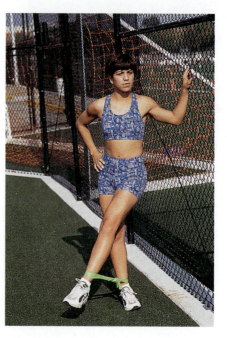

⬥ Position: Stand straight and sideways to something sturdy you can hold on to for balance (a doorjamb will work). If you are using an exercise band, loop the band around your ankles or make a loop with the band around your inside ankle and a sturdy post.

⬥ Action: Keeping your weight on the leg farthest from your support object, lift the working leg slightly forward and as far across the front of your other leg as possible. Be sure to maintain good back alignment throughout the exercise. This exercise can also be done lying on your side.

1. Hip Abductor with a Machine
Muscles Involved: Gluteus maximus, Piriformis

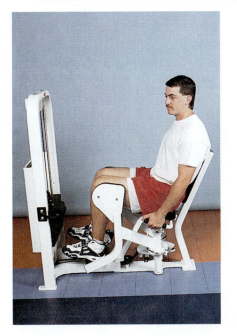

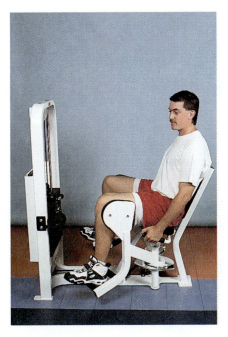

▲ Position: Sit with your back against the pad. Place your legs such that the leg pads are touching the outside of your thighs. Place your feet on the foot plates. Hold on to the hand grips to stabilize your body. Start with your legs together.

▲ Action: Push the leg pads apart, separating your legs into as wide a straddle as comfortably possible. Slowly bring them back together. This exercise can also be performed lying on your side.

2. Outer Thigh Leg Raise with or without an Exercise Band
Muscles Involved: Gluteus maximus, Piriformis

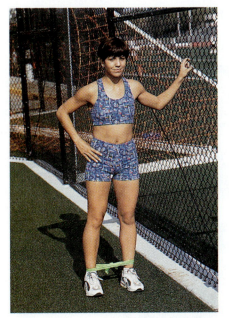

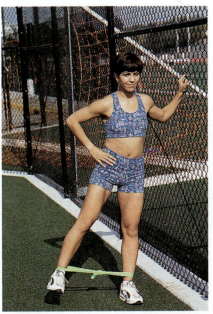

▲ Position: Stand sideways to a sturdy object and hold on for balance (a doorjamb will work). If you are using an exercise band, loop the band around your ankles or tie the band around the post of a sturdy object and stand sideways in the loop. Hold on to something for balance.

▲ Action: Put your balance on your inside leg (closest to hand support). Keep your outside leg straight and lift it directly to the side as high as possible. Slowly lower it. Be sure to maintain good back alignment throughout the exercise. This exercise can also be done lying on your side.

1. Leg Press with a Machine
Muscles Involved: Gluteus maximus, Quadriceps, Hamstrings, Gastrocnemius, Soleus

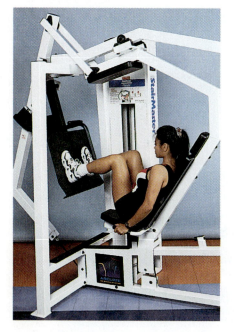

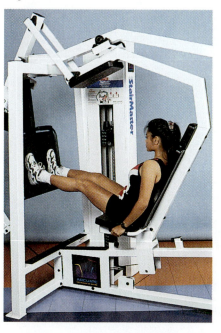

◆ Position: Adjust the seat so that when your feet are on the foot plates your knee joint creates a right angle. Sit with your back flat against the pad and hold on to the hand grips on the sides of the seat.

◆ Action: Push the weight by straightening your knees. Do not lock the knee joints. Exhale during the lift, inhale as you slowly lower the weight. Extending the ankles (pointing the toes) at the end of the push adds the equivalent of the calf extension (toe raise) exercise described earlier. This exercise can also be performed lying on your side.

2. Leg Squat with Optional Free or Homemade Weights (also may be performed without weights)
Muscles Involved: Gluteus maximus, Quadriceps, Hamstrings, Gastrocnemius, Soleus

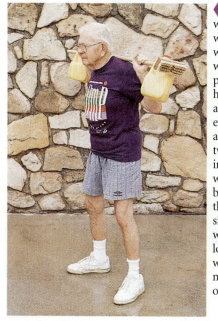

◆ Position: Stand with your feet a little wider than shoulder width apart. If you wish to use weights, position a bar behind your neck and along your shoulders either by taking it off a rack or by having two spotters lift it into position. If working with dumbbells, simply hold them at your sides. Homemade weights such as gallon jugs filled with water or food cans may be used in place of dumbbells.

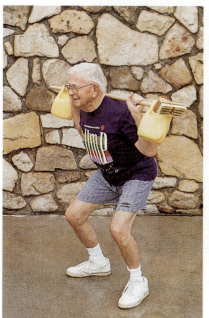

◆ Action: Squat down by bending your knees to about 90 degrees. As you squat, sit back as though you are trying to sit on a chair behind you. Keep your back straight and bend forward at the hips for balance. Keep your head up by focusing on a point about 1 foot above eye level. As you straighten your legs, exhale. Be sure to maintain muscular control throughout the movement.

Abdominals Introduction

The rectus abdominis is a long muscle that attaches to the pubic bone at one end and the ribs at the other. The whole muscle will contract during any abdominal exercise, but some exercises tend to emphasize the upper two-thirds of the muscle while others emphasize the lower third. The oblique muscles run from the ribs to the pelvic girdle on an angle. When they contract, they twist (or rotate) the trunk with respect to the pelvic girdle. The transversalis is the deepest of the muscles. It lies underneath both the rectus abdominis and the obliques. Its primary function is postural; practicing good posture by keeping your abdomen lifted and pulled in is the best way to keep this muscle toned. This muscle is often referred to as the transverse abdominal muscle because the fibers run across the body.

Curl-ups are the exercise of choice because they are much easier on the lower back and just as effective as sit-ups. In a curl-up, your head and shoulders follow a natural curl as you lift until your shoulder blades come off the floor.

Placing the hands behind the head or neck can be stressful to the neck if the head is pulled forward by the arms pressing the chin to the chest. For this reason, many exercise leaders do not use this position. In properly executed curl-ups, the arms remain passive and the abdominal muscles do all the pulling.

The position with the arms near or behind the head is good in two situations. First, some individuals can clearly maintain good technique and handle the weight of the arms in this position. Second, some individuals experience neck fatigue prior to abdominal fatigue and like to rest their head in their arms to relieve the neck muscles.

To concentrate on the oblique muscles, you have to twist before curling. A common error is to sit or curl up and then twist. The oblique muscles can be exercised using a twisting curl-up by hanging from a bar and drawing your knees up to one side of your chest and then the other or by using the appropriate adjustment (for example, rotated sit position) on an abdominal curl machine.

Strengthening the lower third of the abdomen and not straining the back is a challenge. The majority of people experience back pain sometime in their lives—pain that is often caused by a lack of abdominal strength and leg/hip flexibility. Some exercises seem as though they would increase abdominal strength but in fact can cause lower back pain.

Double leg lifts are one such culprit. A double leg lift requires the abdominal muscles to lift about one-half the body's weight. If the abdominal muscles are too weak to lift both legs, the hip flexors come to the rescue, particularly the iliopsoas. The problem is that the iliopsoas attaches to the spine in the lower back region. When it contracts, it pulls against the lower spine. When the iliopsoas is handling a lot of weight such as in a double leg lift, it pulls the lower back up off the floor, often resulting in lower back pain. Plus, leg lifts that strengthen the hip flexors (iliopsoas and others) fail to do the one thing you set out to do—strengthen the abdomen. Only individuals who possess very strong abdominals and who can keep the lower back on the floor should lift both legs.

Many exercises fall into the "double leg lift" category: straddling the legs six inches off the floor, sitting and pushing both legs out, scissoring at a low angle, and others. Exercises that are better for the majority of the population are single leg lifts, bicycling the legs, or reverse curls (curling the legs and hips toward the chest). Strengthening the abdominals will help support the spine and decrease susceptibility to back pain. Following is the standard curl-up with, and without a resistance machine.

ABDOMINALS I

1. Abdominal Curl with a Machine
Muscles Involved: Rectus abdominis, Obliques, Transversalis

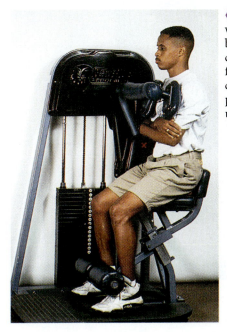

◀ Position: Sit with your ankles behind the padded curl bars, arms folded across your chest, and the upper pad on your upper chest.

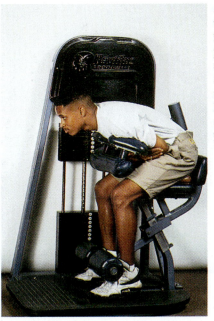

◀ Action: Contract your abdominal muscles and pull your body into a curl position. Slowly return to an upright position. Exhale during the curl and inhale as you straighten up.

2. Curl-Up

Muscles Involved: Rectus abdominis, Obliques, Transversalis

Position: Lie flat on your back with your knees bent, feet flat on the floor and shoulder-width apart. Arms may be at your sides, across your chest, or by your head.

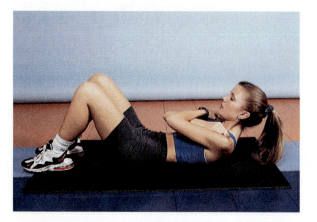

🔺 Action: Lift your upper body up off the floor while pressing your lower back into the floor. Be sure to "curl" your neck and torso naturally—do not try to force your neck into a tight curl. Roll back down to the floor. Beginners can relax between curl-ups; more advanced individuals can curl down until their shoulder blades touch and curl up again.

2. Twisting Curl-Up

Muscles Involved: Obliques, Rectus abdominis

Position: Lie on your back on the floor with your knees bent, feet flat on the floor, and arms either alongside your body, across your chest, or near your head. Rotate your torso to one side while leaving your hips flat on the floor.

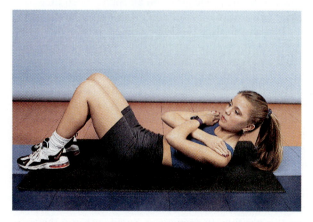

🔺 Action: Curl straight up just as you would for a regular curl-up.

ABDOMINALS II

---

1. Twisting Curl with a Machine

Muscles Involved: Obliques, Rectus abdominis

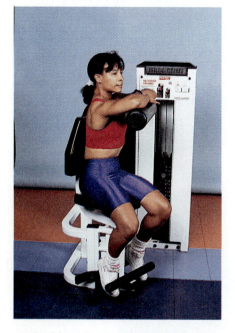

🔺 Position: Same as the regular curl but with the seat turned to one side.

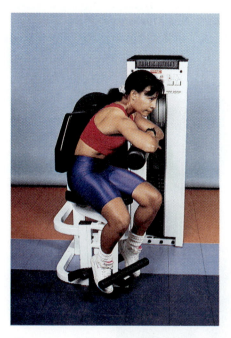

🔺 Action: Curl the body forward as in a regular curl.

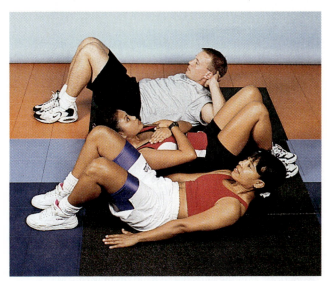
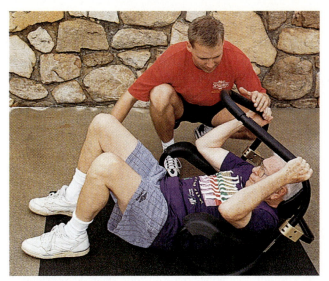

Arm placement can make curl-ups progressively more difficult. With your arms at the sides of your body, your abdominal muscles are lifting only the weight of your head and trunk. When you cross your arms over your chest, your abdominals must lift the weight of your arms, trunk, and head. When you move your arms up by your head, they represent even more resistance because they are away from your center of gravity. Additional resistance can be obtained by doing the curl-up on an incline board, holding a weight on your chest, using a weighted curl-up bar, or placing your feet on a chair.

Back Introduction

Strength and flexibility are very important to maintaining a healthy back. Flexibility exercises are provided in Chapter 4. The following exercises are for strengthening the back muscles. As with any exercise, if you feel pain you should stop using the exercise until you have discussed it with your physician. If you have back pain now or any other health condition that might affect your back, consult with your physician before trying these exercises. Abdominal strength is an integral part of back care. Strong abdominal muscles provide support for the trunk and take pressure off your back, so be sure to include exercises from the abdominal section in your healthy back plan.

BACK I

1. ***Upper Back with a Machine***
   Muscles Involved: Trapezius, Erector spinae, Rhomboids, Deltoids

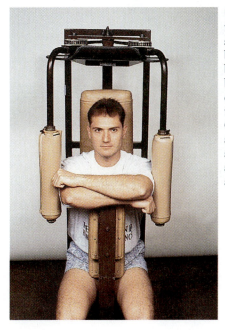

◀ Position: Sit in the machine by straddling the bench. Place your back against the back pad (use an extra pad or adjust the seat as needed). Cross your arms and place the outer side of your upper arms against the arm pads.

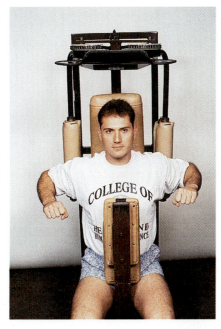

◀ Action: Press back with your arms as far as possible while drawing your shoulder blades together. Exhale as you push back; inhale as you slowly return to your starting position.

2. Seated Row with an Exercise Band

Muscles Involved: Trapezius, Erector spinae, Rhomboids, Deltoids

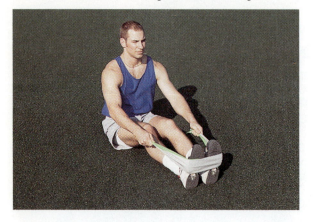 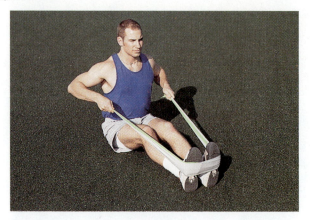

🔺 Position: Sit on the floor with your feet and legs extended in front of you. Hold on to the ends of an exercise band and loop the middle of the band around the soles of your feet. Sit up straight with your arms extended. Shorten the band enough that there is some tension at this time.

🔺 Action: Pull the ends of the band up toward your armpits, keeping your elbows up and out to the side. Use only your arm and upper back muscles; do not allow movement at the hips.

BACK II

1. Back Extension on a Machine

Muscles Involved: Erector spinae, Gluteus maximus

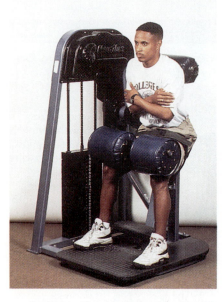 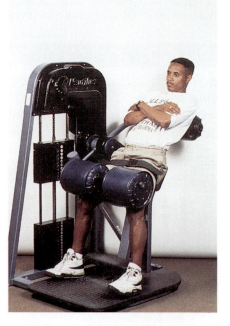

🔺 Position: Sit with the back pad on your upper back. Adjust the seat height as needed. Place your thighs behind the leg pads and put on the seat belt. Cross your arms and sit tall with your chest lifted.

🔺 Action: Push back against the upper back pad. Exhale as you press backward; inhale as you slowly return to your starting position.

2. *Prone Lift (no equipment)*
Muscles Involved: Erector spinae, Gluteus maximus

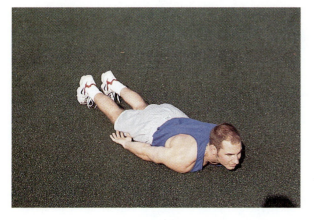

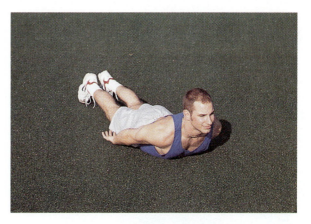

➤ **Position:** Lie prone on the floor or a mat, arms down by your sides.

➤ **Action:** Lift your shoulders and trunk up off the floor, hold for several seconds, and then lower. Breathe normally throughout.

BACK III

1. *Lat Pull-Down with a Machine*
Muscles Involved: Latissimus dorsi, Erector spinae, Deltoids, Biceps brachii, Pectoralis major, Trapezius, Rhomboid

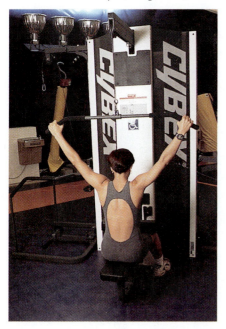

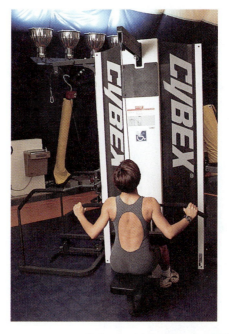

➤ **Position:** Grasp the bar with your hands shoulder-width apart and palms facing downward. Draw the bar down as you sit on the seat or kneel in front of the machine. Secure your ankles under the bar provided or if needed have a partner hold down your shoulders. Arms should be extended at this time.

➤ **Action:** Pull down with both arms until the bar is in front of (or behind) the base of the neck. Exhale as you pull down; inhale as you extend your arms. For variation, you can narrow or widen your grasp on the bar. (If you use a triangular bar, grasp it with your palms facing inward. Pull down in front of your chest.)

2. *Pull-Up (Optional Partner Assist)*
Muscles Involved: Latissimus dorsi, Deltoids, Biceps

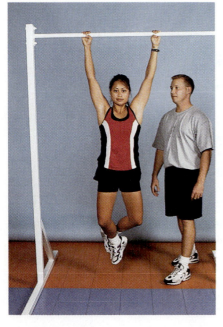

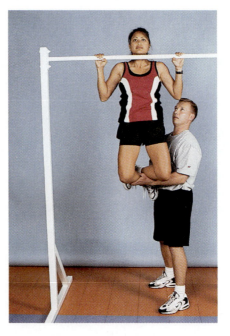

🔺 Position: Grasp a bar with your hands shoulder width apart with palms facing away from your body. Hang with straight arms.

🔺 Action: Pull your body upward until your chin is above the bar. Lower slowly. If you can't do a pull-up, have a partner assist you or place a chair where you can lightly assist yourself by pushing with your legs.

BACK, SHOULDERS, AND ARMS

1. *Shoulder Press (Overhead Press) with a Machine*
Muscles Involved: Trapezius, Deltoids, Triceps

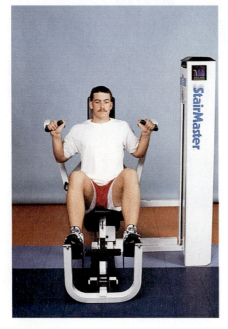

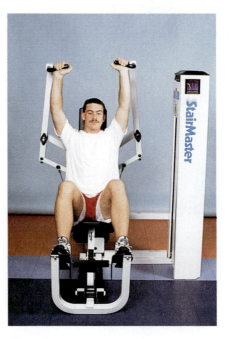

🔺 Position: Sit up straight with your back against the pad. Grasp the handles with your palms facing inward or to the front. Adjust your sitting position or the machine until your shoulders are underneath your hands. Maintain a straight back posture.

🔺 Action: Press your arms upward until they are fully extended. Exhale when lifting the weight; inhale as you slowly lower it.

2. *Shoulder Press with Homemade or Free Weights*
Muscles Involved: Trapezius, Deltoids, Triceps

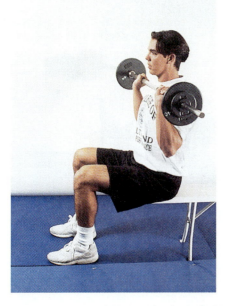 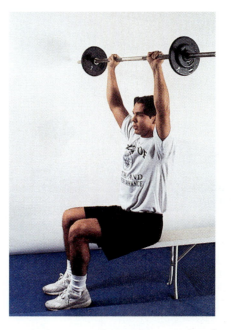

🔺 Position: Stand or sit with a barbell, dumbbells, or home-made weights (canned goods, milk jugs looped over a broom-stick, etc.) held at shoulder height. If working with a bar, use an overhand grip with hands a little more than shoulder-width apart. Keep your back straight and your feet on the floor.

🔺 Action: Press the weight upward, making sure to maintain back alignment throughout the exercise. Exhale during the overhead press; inhale as you lower the weights.

CHEST AND SHOULDERS I

1. *Bench Press with a Machine*
Muscles Involved: Pectorals, Deltoids, Triceps

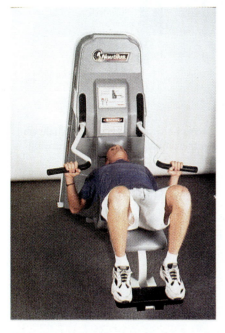 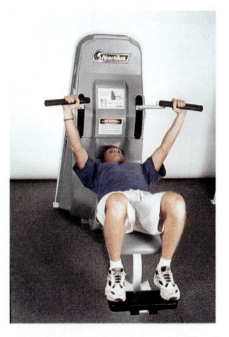

🔺 Position: Lie on a bench with your knees bent and feet either flat on the floor or up on the bench so that your lower back is relaxed (not arched). Adjust your position so that your shoulders are under the hand grips. Grasp the handles with your palms facing your feet.

🔺 Action: Press the weight upward until your arms are fully extended but your elbows are not locked. Exhale as you press upward; inhale as you lower the weight slowly.

2. *Push-Up*
Muscles Involved: Pectorals, Deltoids, Triceps

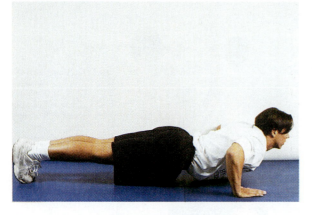 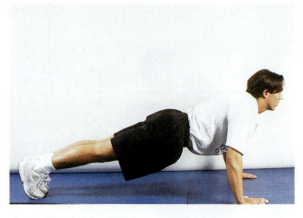

⬆ Position: For a regular push-up, brace yourself on your toes and hands with your hands shoulder-width apart and your back and hips straight. Lower your body until your chest is about 3 inches off the floor. (For a modified push-up, rest your knees on the floor.)

⬆ Action: Push up to the starting position. Be sure to breathe out as you push up.

CHEST AND SHOULDERS II

1. *Chest Press with Machine*
Muscles Involved: Pectoralis major, Deltoids

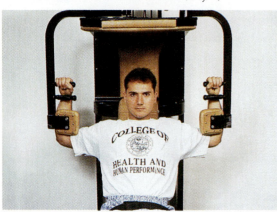 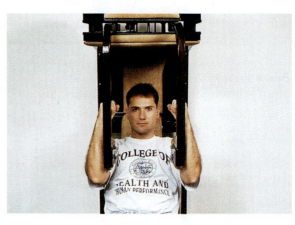

⬆ Position: Sit on the seat with your back against the pad. Place your forearms against the pads. If available, grasp the hand grips.

⬆ Action: Pull your arms in toward each other. Exhale when bringing your arms together; inhale when slowly returning them to the starting position.

2. Lateral Curls (Flies) with Homemade or Free Weights
Muscles Involved: Pectoralis major, Deltoids

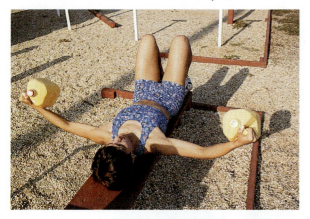

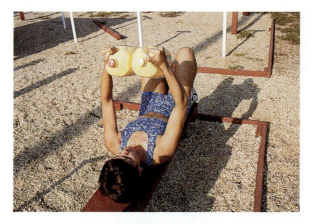

🔺 Position: Lie down on your back on a bench or other raised flat surface. Bend your knees and place your feet flat on the floor or on the bench so that your lower back is flat and relaxed. Hold a dumbbell (or soup cans or other homemade weights like milk jugs) in each hand. Start with your hands and weights together directly over your chest with your arms extended and elbows slightly bent. Lower your arms out to the side until your arms are even with your body.

🔺 Action: Pull your arms back up to the starting position. Exhale as you raise your arms; inhale as you lower them. Maintain slight elbow flexion throughout.

UPPER ARMS I

1. Arm Flexion (Biceps Curls) with a Machine
Muscles Involved: Biceps brachii, Brachialis (close grip only)

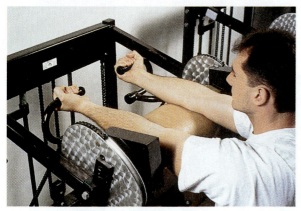

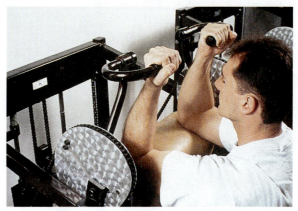

🔺 Position: Sit in the machine. Extend your arms over the pads in front of you. With palms up toward the ceiling grasp the hand grips or bar.

🔺 Action: Bring your hands toward your chest by flexing your elbows. Exhale when pulling up; inhale while slowly lowering the weights. Do not lock out your elbow joints; maintain a slight elbow bend.

2. *Arm Flexion (Biceps Curl) with Homemade or Free Weights*
Muscles Involved: Biceps brachii

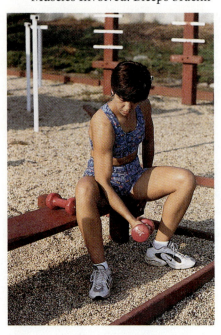 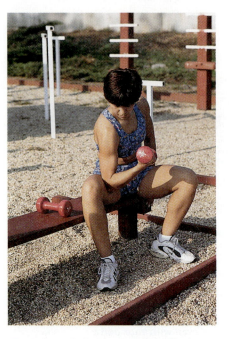

🔺 Position: Hold a weight in one arm. Sit on a bench and anchor the elbow of your working arm next to your body and on your upper leg. Spread your legs apart enough to allow the weight to be lowered between your knees. Extend your arm fully but do not hyperextend your elbow.

🔺 Action: Raise the weight by flexing your elbow and drawing it toward your chest. Exhale as you draw the weight upward; inhale as you lower it.

UPPER ARMS II

1. *Arm Extension (Press) with a Machine*
Muscles Involved: Triceps

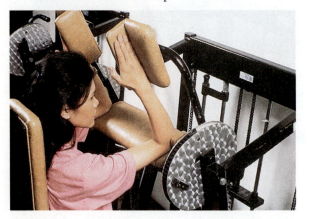 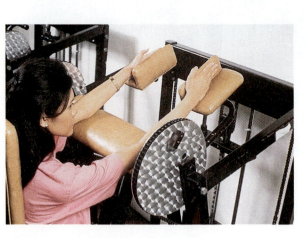

🔺 Position: Sit in the arm extension machine. Place your elbows on the pads in front of you. Face your palms toward each other and place the little finger of each hand on the hand pads.

🔺 Action: Extend your arms by pressing forward and down. Exhale as you press down; inhale as you allow the bar to come up. Maintain your elbow anchors; do not allow them to lift off the pads.

2. Dips
Muscles Involved: Triceps, Deltoids

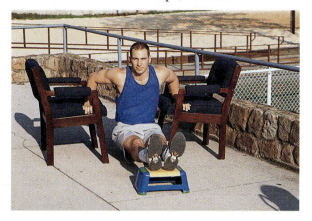

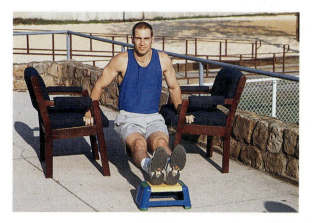

➤ Position: Using chairs: Place one hand on each seat of a sturdy chair, with your fingers pointing forward. Support yourself on straight arms with your buttocks between the chairs. Extend your legs forward (or for more difficulty put them up on a stool or third chair). A stair may be used in place of the chairs. Bend your arms, lowering your body until your elbow joints create right angles.

➤ Action: Press upward until your arms are fully extended. Exhale on the way up; inhale on the way down.

SUMMARY

One version of Milos legend claims that he came across a wedge stuck in a tree trunk and, determined to demonstrate his strength, attempted to remove it with his bare hands. But just as he freed the wedge, his fingers became caught in the trunk. Alone and trapped, he most unfortunately became dinner for a wild animal. The moral: (1) for wellness one need only attain strength, not prove it, and (2) never attempt feats of strength alone!

Attaining good muscle endurance and strength will allow you to do more with less fatigue and less risk of injury. You may also find that increasing your muscular strength and endurance will improve your physical performance. You might be the one hitting the ball harder at the picnic softball game, going the distance on the charity walk-a-thon, or finishing a physically demanding project with energy to spare.

SUGGESTED READING

American College of Sports Medicine. The recommended quantity and quality of exercise for developing and maintaining cardiorespiratory and muscular fitness in healthy adults. *Medicine and Science in Sports* 22(2):265–274, 1990.

Baechle, T. R., and B. R. Groves. *Weight training steps to success.* Champaign, IL: Leisure Press, 1992.

Bartels, R. L. Weight training. *The Physician and Sportsmedicine* 20:233–234, 1992.

The best workout: Free weights vs. machines, *University of California Berkeley Wellness Letter* 9:6, 1993.

Bodybuilding for the nineties, *Nutrition Action Health Letter* 19:1, 5–7, 1992.

Fleck, S. J., and W. J. Kraemer. *Designing resistance training programs,* 2nd ed. Champaign, IL: Human Kinetics, 1997.

Gettman, L. R., and M. L. Pollock. Circuit weight training: A critical review of its physiological benefits. *The Physician and Sportsmedicine* 9:44–60, 1981.

Lockette, K. F., and A. M. Keyes. *Conditioning with physical disabilities.* Champaign, IL: Human Kinetics, 1994.

Miller, P. D., ed. *Fitness programming and physical disability.* Champaign, IL: Human Kinetics, 1995.

Strength training, *Mayo Clinic Health Letter* 8:2–3, 1990.

Wilmore, J. H., and D. L. Costill. *Training for sport and activity,* 3rd ed. Champaign, IL: Human Kinetics, 1993.

Behavioral Lab 5.1

What Can I Do?

At the beginning of this chapter, you determined your stage of readiness to change with regard to muscular strength and endurance. Now take out a sheet of paper and complete the corresponding section of this lab: precontemplator, contemplator, preparer, action taker, or maintainer.

Precontemplator

1. Try to identify the main reasons you are against or not motivated to become stronger or build more muscle endurance.

   For some ideas, refer to the barriers in the Barrier Busters feature on page 105.

2. Can you think of any reasons why muscular strength and endurance exercises would be good for you? See page 104 for ideas.

3. If you have taken any strength or endurance tests, do the results support a need for change?

4. Can you think of any times when lack of strength or endurance has limited your performance? Resulted in injury? Stopped you from doing something? (A journal might be helpful.)

5. Do your answers in numbers 2, 3, and 4 outweigh your answers in number 1?

6. Can you use any of the "barrier busting" suggestions to eliminate the items you listed in number 1?

7. Will you think about adding just one strength or endurance exercise to your daily routine?

Contemplator

1. What are you thinking about doing to improve your strength and/or endurance?

2. What changes will this activity bring about that are important to you? (Why are they important?)

3. Is there something you'd like to know more about in order to move ahead? If yes, where do you think you could get the information? For example, instructor, books, pamphlets by professional organizations.

4. What do you need in order to consider making this change? Try to finish this statement:

I would consider changing if . . .

   I had a partner and time to do it.

   It wouldn't cost me any money.

   (yours) _____

5. How can you overcome or accomplish the items listed above?

6. Which strength and endurance exercises or activities do you think you would like to do?

7. Where would you consider performing the exercises you listed in number 6? For example, at home, in the dorm, at a club, and so forth.

8. When do you think you could best fit resistance exercises into your schedule?

Preparer

1. What do you specifically want to accomplish?

2. What type of activities/exercises will accomplish this goal? (For programming ideas see page 32–33.)

3. Brainstorm ways that you can experiment with the resistance activities/exercises you listed in number 2 to find the best medium and combination for you.

   Examples
   Try using a resistance machine, exercise bands, free weights, water exercises, and so forth.

   Experiment with dynamic and isometric exercises.

4. Put together a trial resistance training program using the exercises you identified in numbers 2 and 3.

5. As a first step, identify one or two resistance exercises from your trial program to start doing three times a week, and establish an order and timeline

for adding the other exercises—such as one new one every week or every other week.

6. Now that you have a plan, what kinds of things might tempt you to put off starting a strength and endurance program?

7. What strategies can you use to eliminate or neutralize these temptations?

8. What makes you believe you can accomplish your goal(s)? *Or* What makes you believe you can accomplish this first step?

9. If your first step doesn't work for you, what will you do?

10. Complete the following statement:

    I am going to take my first step on _____ .

    date within 30 days

Action Taker

1. What are you currently doing to develop muscular strength and/or endurance?

2. Are you keeping track of your progress?

    If yes, how?

    > fitness tests?
    >
    > journal?
    >
    > log sheet?
    >
    > body measurements?

    If no, would it help motivate you to keep a record of your progress?

3. What positive results or rewards are you experiencing as a result of your actions?

4. Are you receiving support for your effort? If yes, what kind? If no, why not? Can you change this?

5. Do you think you will continue?

6. If you were to stop, what do you think would be the major reason for stopping?

7. Is there a way to prevent this (item 6)? (barrier busting in advance)

8. How would you get yourself started again if you did stop?

9. Are your muscular strength and endurance goals specifically and clearly stated? And are they reasonable?

10. Do you believe that you can reach your goals? If yes, why? If no, why not?

11. If you answered no to the above question, can you think of anything or anyone who could help you? How can you bolster your confidence? What resources do you have available?

12. What strategies are you presently using, or would you like to use to decrease the temptation to stop and increase your confidence to continue?

Maintainer

1. For how long have you maintained your muscular strength and endurance program?

2. What are the top two reasons that make you want to continue?

3. Have you been tempted to stop? If so, what tempted you?

4. How confident are you that you can resist temptations to stop your resistance program? If your confidence level is low or has changed, can you identify why? How can you bolster your confidence?

5. How do you convince yourself to continue when you are tempted to stop or skip a day? (What strategies do you use?)

6. How can you prevent temptations from occurring?

7. Are you at a level of muscular fitness you are happy with or do you wish to continue to improve? If you want further improvement go to number 8, if not, go to number 9.

8. Do you know how to set a new progressive overload? If no, do you know someone who can help you?

9. Do you receive support for your efforts? If yes, what kind? Internal (self)? External (from others)? If no, can you think of ways to develop support?

10. How have you changed or how have you changed the environment around you to accommodate a healthier lifestyle?

11. Is there anything else you need (information? support? time management?) to promote your continued maintenance?

12. If you listed something in the previous statement can you think of a way to attain it or can you think of someone who can help you with it?

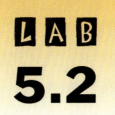

Curl-Up Test

This is the Robertson Modified Curl-Up Test. Because its norms were developed from testing college physical education majors it may indicate higher standards than are needed for health-related fitness. At this time the authors are unaware of college-age norms for the regular student body.

Equipment

1. Mat with a 3-inch wide line running across it. If you use 1½-inch athletic tape this can be achieved with two strips of tape. If the tape is placed 3 inches in from the edge of the mat, you will be able to feel for the edge of the mat with your fingers during the test. Or, for the same effect, you can tape something like a yardstick on the far side of the line.

2. Stopwatch

3. Pencil and paper

Directions

1. Lie on your back with your knees bent 90 degrees, arms straight and parallel to your trunk, fingers pointing toward your feet and touching the near side of the line. Your palms should be flat on the floor.

2. Keeping your hips, heels, and fingertips in contact with the floor, curl up until fingertips simultaneously reach the far side of the 3-inch line. Your shoulder blades must touch down between curl-ups. Breathe normally throughout the curl-up. Curl-down.

3. Practice this curl-up technique five times.

4. When you are ready, your partner will start the stopwatch and time you for 1 minute.

5. Your partner should count correct curl-ups aloud. If you hear a number repeated, you need to correct your technique.

6. At the end of the test, your fingertip position should be rechecked. If you have moved (fingertips not touching the near side of the line), your score is not valid.

   _____ correct number of curl-ups performed

7. Stretch your legs and abdominal muscles.

8. Check the norm table to find your fitness level.

   _____ fitness level

Preliminary Norm Table Based on Physical Education Majors' Scores (Northern Illinois University)

Performance Level	SCORE	
	Male	Female
Excellent	103–118	98–115
Good	87–102	80–97
Average	69–86	60–79
Below Average	53–68	42–59
Poor	37–52	23–41

Source: Reprinted with permission from the *JOPERD (Journal of Physical Education, Recreation, and Dance),* August 1993, pp. 62–66. *JOPERD* is a publication of the American Alliance for Health, Physical Education, Recreation and Dance, 1900 Association Drive, Reston, VA 22091-1599.

Name _____ **Section** _____ **Date** _____

Push-Up Test

Equipment

1. Partner
2. Mat or towel (for knees during modified push-ups)
3. Pencil or pen

Directions

1. Warm up and stretch, especially arms and chest.

2. Decide whether you will be performing regular or modified push-ups. (Regular push-ups are performed on hands and toes, modified push-ups are performed on hands and knees.) The norms for modified push-ups are based on a female population, whereas the norms for regular push-ups are based on a male population. (Either gender may perform either test as long as it is understood that so far no norms have been compiled for females doing regular push-ups and males performing modified push-ups.)

3. To begin this test, lie on your stomach, legs together. Position your hands under your shoulders with fingers pointing forward. On the start signal push up from the mat, fully extending your elbows, and then lower down until your chin touches the mat. Your chest and abdomen should not touch the floor. You must maintain a straight body alignment at all times. Your partner will count only correctly completed push-ups.

4. There is no time limit on this test. Perform as many correct push-ups as you can without taking a break. The test will be stopped when you strain forcibly or are unable to maintain correct technique over two repetitions.

5. Record the number of correct push-ups you complete.

   _____ push-ups Circle one: Regular Modified

6. Consult the norms below and record your fitness level. (Fill in an "X" if there are no gender-appropriate norms for the test position you selected.)

   _____ fitness rating

7. Stretch your arms and chest muscles to prevent soreness.

Norms by Age Groups and Gender for Push-Ups[a]											
	AGE (YEARS)										
Fitness Rating	**15–19**		**20–29**		**30–39**		**40–49**		**50–59**		**60–69**	
	M	**F**	**M**	**F**	**M**	**F**	**M**	**F**	**M**	**F**	**M**	**F**
Excellent	≥39	≥33	≥36	≥30	≥30	≥27	≥22	≥24	≥21	≥21	≥18	≥17
Above Average	29–38	25–32	29–35	21–29	22–29	20–26	17–21	15–23	13–20	11–20	11–17	12–16
Average	23–28	18–24	22–28	15–20	17–21	13–19	13–16	11–14	10–12	7–10	8–10	5–11
Below Average	18–22	12–17	17–21	10–14	12–16	8–12	10–12	5–10	7–9	2–6	5–7	1–4
Poor	≤17	≤11	≤16	≤9	≤11	≤7	≤9	≤4	≤6	≤1	≤4	≤1

Source: Published in the *Canadian standardized test of fitness operations manual,* 3rd ed., 1986. Reprinted by permission from the Canadian Society for Exercise Physiology.

[a]Based on data from the Canada Fitness Survey, 1981.

Source: Bishop, J. G. *Fitness through aerobics,* 3rd ed. Scottsdale, AZ: Gorsuch, Scarisbrick Publishers, 1995, p. 167. Reprinted by permission of Allyn & Bacon.

Weight Training— Muscular Endurance Test

The following is a test for muscular endurance. In this particular test endurance is measured using 20 RM or the amount of weight you can lift twenty times but not twenty-one times. Muscular endurance can be achieved (to varying degrees) using fewer or greater than twenty repetitions but to compare yourself with this test's results, you have to use 20 RM. To prevent soreness and possible injury, perform this test after 6 to 8 weeks of regular resistance training.

Equipment

1. Resistance equipment for the following four exercises: biceps curl, bench press, leg press or half-squat, and hamstring curl
2. Scale in pounds
3. Paper and pencil

Directions

1. Using trial and error, determine your 20 RM for each exercise. Rest for several minutes between attempts. Increase or decrease the weight until you can perform only twenty repetitions.
2. Calculate your muscular endurance/body weight ratio for each exercise. To do this divide the weight for 20 RM by your body weight in pounds.

   Examples

   A 130-lb woman with a 20 RM of 135 lb for the leg press would have a muscular endurance/body weight ratio of 1.04.

   $$\frac{135 \ (20 \ RM)}{130 \ (wt/lb)} = 1.04$$

A 180-lb man with a 20 RM of 280 lb for the leg press would have a muscular endurance/body weight ratio of 1.56.

$$\frac{280 \ (20 \ RM)}{180 \ (wt/lb)} = 1.56$$

3. Check the muscular endurance/body weight ratio charts below and determine your muscular endurance category. Both the examples in Step 2 would receive "good" ratings.

Muscular Endurance/Body Weight Ratio

Women

Biceps Curl	Bench Press	Hamstring Curl	Muscular Endurance Category
≥ 0.32	≥ 0.50	≥ 0.38	Excellent
0.23–0.31	0.42–0.49	0.31–0.37	Good
0.15–0.22	0.35–0.41	0.23–0.30	Average
0.12–0.14	0.27–0.34	0.15–0.22	Fair
< 0.12	< 0.27	< 0.15	Poor

Leg Press or Half-Squat	Muscular Endurance Category
≥ 1.15	Excellent
1.00–1.14	Good
0.88–0.99	Average
0.77–0.87	Fair
< 0.77	Poor

Source: From B. L. Johnson, and J. K. Nelson. *Practical measurements in physical education.* Minneapolis: Burgess, 1986. Reprinted by permission of Allyn & Bacon.

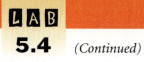

Men

Biceps Curl	Bench Press	Hamstring Curl	Muscular Endurance Category
≥ 0.50	≥ 0.76	≥ 0.40	Excellent
0.43–0.49	0.70–0.75	0.33–0.39	Good
0.37–0.42	0.60–0.69	0.27–0.32	Average
0.30–0.36	0.50–0.59	0.20–0.26	Fair
< 0.30	< 0.50	< 0.20	Poor

Leg Press or Half-Squat	Muscular Endurance Category
≥ 1.66	Excellent
1.50–1.65	Good
1.33–1.49	Average
1.16–1.32	Fair
< 1.16	Poor

Results

Date: _____

Body Weight: _____

Exercise	20 RM	Ratio	Muscular Endurance Category
Biceps Curl	_____	_____	_____
Bench Press	_____	_____	_____
Hamstring Curl	_____	_____	_____
Leg Press or Half-Squat	_____	_____	_____

Developing Your Strength and Endurance Program

■ Set one or more general goals for your program:

■ Select your exercises based on the muscles they work and decide when and how you will perform each exercise. Use the following headings to organize this information. Use another sheet of paper if necessary.

Muscle(s) Worked   *Exercise*   *Equipment*   *Days of the Week*

■ Indicate where on the continuum your goals place you. This will help you determine the number of repetitions and sets to put in your workout.

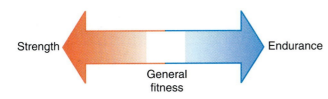

Strength   Endurance

General
fitness

■ Use the daily log on the next page to organize your exercises and record your progress.

■ Set specific goals:

DAILY LOG

Exercise		Date								
		/	/	/	/	/	/	/	/	/
	wt									
	reps									
	sets/brk									
	wt									
	reps									
	sets/brk									
	wt									
	reps									
	sets/brk									
	wt									
	reps									
	sets/brk									
	wt									
	reps									
	sets/brk									
	wt									
	reps									
	sets/brk									
	wt									
	reps									
	sets/brk									
	wt									
	reps									
	sets/brk									
	wt									
	reps									
	sets/brk									
	wt									
	reps									
	sets/brk									
	wt									
	reps									
	sets/brk									

CHAPTER 6

Striving for Wellness with Proper Nutrition

Terms

- Recommended dietary allowances (RDAs)
- Nutrients
- Calorie
- Empty calories
- Saturated fat
- Monosaccharide
- Disaccharide
- Soluble and insoluble fiber
- Amino acids
- Complete and incomplete proteins
- Strict vegetarians
- Mega dose
- Free radical
- Antioxidant
- Osteoporosis
- Carbohydrate loading

Objectives

1. Understand the basic nutrients and how they are important to wellness.

2. Be able to explain the food pyramid and national dietary guidelines.

3. Understand what it means to have a balanced diet.

4. Identify sources of dietary fat and reduce excessive fat.

5. Learn how to reduce intake of sugars and increase consumption of fruits and vegetables.

6. Learn a few reasons why vitamin supplementation might be necessary.

7. Understand the facts and fallacies about osteoporosis.

8. Initiate and maintain a healthy diet.

Where Am I?

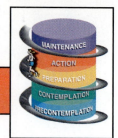

Precontemplator _____ I do not keep my dietary fat consumption below 30 percent, I do not eat five servings of fruits and vegetables daily, and I do not intend to start.

Contemplator _____ I do not keep my dietary fat consumption below 30 percent and I do not eat five servings of fruits and vegetables daily, but I am considering doing so in the next few months.

Preparer _____ I do not or I do not consistently keep my dietary fat consumption below 30 percent and I do not eat five servings of fruits and vegetables daily, but I plan on changing my diet within the next thirty days.

Action Taker _____ Yes, I do keep my dietary fat consumption below 30 percent and eat five servings of fruits and vegetables daily, but I have done so for less than six months.

Maintainer _____ Yes, I have been keeping my dietary fat consumption below 30 percent and have been eating five servings of fruits and vegetables daily for more than six months.

Before you begin this chapter, do a personal nutrition assessment by completing Lab 6.2. Then answer the above staging questions on dietary fat and fruits and vegetables, and determine which stage best fits your current behaviors. In the action or maintenance stages, the percentages of calories in your diet that come from fat must be below 30 percent and you must be consuming at least five fruit and/or vegetable servings each day.

Obviously, there is more to eating healthy foods than reducing dietary fat and consuming adequate amounts of fruits and vegetables. The Stages of Change Model in this chapter focuses on reducing dietary fat and consuming at least five fruits and vegetables because most individuals need to make these changes. In addition, lowering fat and eating ample fruits and vegetables are closely related to other important aspects of a nutritious diet that are discussed in this chapter, such as having a low cholesterol level and getting enough vitamins.

As you read the chapter you will see that many other important nutritional practices are discussed in detail, and you will be encouraged and taught how to make changes in all aspects of proper nutrition.

Never before has there been more emphasis on the importance of proper nutrition. Every day the media report the results of yet another scientific study that has evaluated a certain food or drink that we consume too much or too little of. We are bombarded with such a wealth of information about nutrition and disease that it is easy to get confused.

Much of the media information is in the form of advertisements that encourage us to buy certain products. Unfortunately, this information is one of the primary sources of knowledge we use in deciding which foods to eat. Food producers are quick to promote the benefits and hide the not-so-healthy aspects of their products, and unless consumers are aware of correct nutrition principles, it is highly unlikely that they will consume a healthy diet.

Many of the activities in this chapter involve reflecting on the completed dietary analysis and discovering ways you can increase your wellness when it comes to nutrition.

MAKING WISE FOOD CHOICES

We tend to select the same kinds of foods every time we visit the grocery store. From a broad perspective, our diets contain very little variation. Today's busy schedules may cause us to depend more on drive-up windows, microwaveable foods, single-serving prepackaged meals, home deliveries, and room service. Thanks to birthday parties and other celebrations, we learn at a very young age to associate good times with sweet, high-fat food. As children, we discover that traveling often means eating fun foods that may lack nutritional value but provide convenience and great taste.

Other factors that determine what we eat are the time of day, the cost of food, our religious beliefs, what our parents eat, and what food looks like. Far too often, the overall nutritional quality of our diets is determined by our environment rather than by sound principles of nutrition.

With the exception of the very poor and the chronically ill, people with nutritional deficiencies in this country are rare; yet six of the ten leading causes of death in the United States are associated with what we eat.[1] None of these killers (coronary heart disease, stroke, cancer, diabetes, arteriosclerosis, and liver disease) is related to nutritional deficiencies; however, each can be caused by poor food choices or by overeating. Indeed, improper diet and overeating were partly responsible for 71 percent of all deaths in the United States in 1988. In the industrialized world, approximately 35 percent of the adult population is obese, and current estimates indicate that over 50 percent of adults in the United States are overweight.[2] The wellness lifestyle requires careful attention to both the quality and the quantity of the foods we eat.

EATING A BALANCED DIET

To help us improve the quality of our diets, the U.S. Department of Agriculture introduced the food pyramid (Figure 6.1). It replaces the traditional classification of four basic food groups and demonstrates the relative quantity of the foods we should eat in order to provide optimal nutrition. The food pyramid includes six food groups, each representing an important aspect of a balanced diet. The fats, oils, and sweets group sits on the top of the pyramid and is to be consumed in smaller quantities than any of the other groups. These items should be used sparingly because of the detrimental health effects of consuming a diet high in fat and simple sugars. Close inspection of the pyramid shows that fats and sugars occur naturally in many foods or are added in processing; thus, foods not appearing in the fats and sugars group may still be high in fat and sugar and should also be used sparingly.

The milk, meat, fruit, and vegetable groups each require two to four servings per day. The wide base of the pyramid contains the breads and cereals group, foods that should form the basis of a healthy diet. This group represents most of the sources of complex carbohydrates and requires six to eleven servings per day. Table 6.1 can provide you with an idea of how much is in a serving of each of the food groups.

The selection of only one or two foods from each group does not guarantee a balanced diet. A potato chip from the fats and oils group will be nutritionally different from a boiled potato from the vegetable group. Although both are made from grains, a doughnut is very

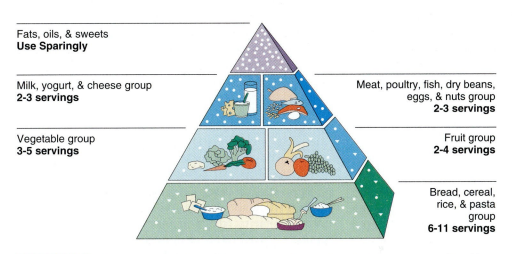

Fats, oils, & sweets
Use Sparingly

Milk, yogurt, & cheese group
2-3 servings

Meat, poultry, fish, dry beans, eggs, & nuts group
2-3 servings

Vegetable group
3-5 servings

Fruit group
2-4 servings

Bread, cereal, rice, & pasta group
6-11 servings

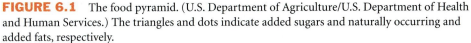

FIGURE 6.1 The food pyramid. (U.S. Department of Agriculture/U.S. Department of Health and Human Services.) The triangles and dots indicate added sugars and naturally occurring and added fats, respectively.

TABLE 6.1 ■ What's in a Serving?

Food Group	Serving Size
Fats, Oils, and Sweets (use sparingly)	• 1 tablespoon butter, margarine, oil, ketchup, mayonnaise • 1 tablespoon salad dressing
Milk, Yogurt, and Cheese (2–3 servings)	• 1 cup milk or yogurt, 1½ oz natural cheese, or 2 oz processed cheese • ½ cup cottage cheese
Meat, Poultry, Fish, Dry Beans, Eggs, and Nuts (2–3 servings)	• 4 to 5 oz cooked lean meat, fish, or poultry • 1 to 1½ cups cooked dried beans • 1 egg • 2 tablespoons peanut butter • ¼ cup nuts • 3 oz tuna
Vegetables (3–5 servings)	• 1 cup leafy green vegetables • ½ cup chopped raw vegetables • ½ cup cooked vegetables
Fruits (2–4 servings)	• one banana, apple, or orange • ½ grapefruit • ¾ cup fruit juice • ½ cup canned fruit • ¼ cup dried fruit
Breads, Cereals, Rice, and Pasta (6–11 servings)	• 2 slices bread • ½ cup dense cereal (such as granola) • ¾ cup cooked rice • 3 or 4 crackers • bagel, hamburger bun • 1 cup cooked cereal or pasta • 2 waffles or pancakes • 1 oz ready-to-eat cereal

Source: U.S. Department of Agriculture. *The hassle-free guide to a better diet.* Washington, D.C.: U.S. Government Printing Office, 1980.

different from a bagel, while plain zucchini in a salad will have much less fat than fried zucchini. Choosing a variety of foods from within each group will help to ensure a balanced diet.

As research continues to reveal new relationships between diet and disease, the food pyramid will likely undergo further modification. As changes do occur, we should be willing to make the appropriate changes in our diets.

The National Research Council and the National Academy of Sciences have established nutritional standards for vitamins and minerals for various population groups. These standards are known as the **recommended dietary allowances (RDAs)** and provide guidelines that represent the average level of nutrition needed for healthy living. A substantial safety margin is included in these guidelines, so that even if a person fails to attain the RDA for a particular vitamin, the chances of experiencing health problems related to vitamin deficiencies are very unlikely. The RDAs are an important part of determining just how many vitamins and minerals we consume on any given day. Later in this chapter, we will show you how to read nutrition labels and determine the level of vitamins and minerals consumed in each food serving.

NUTRITION BEGINS
WITH NUTRIENTS

All foods are made up of six different **nutrients:** fats, carbohydrates, proteins, vitamins, minerals, and water. Nutrients are defined as the constituents of food that sustain us physiologically. Because each nutrient provides a specific function and interacts with the other nutrients to keep the body functioning properly, lack of any one nutrient may impair vital bodily processes. Recommended allowances for important nutrients are shown in Table 6.2.

Protein, fats, and carbohydrates are energy sources our bodies need to perform all physiological functions; however, fats have much more energy than do proteins or carbohydrates. Each gram of dietary fat has nine calories of energy whereas carbohydrates and proteins each have four calories of energy per gram. A **calorie** is a measure of the amount of energy or heat required to raise the temperature of one gram of water one degree Celsius. Because this unit of measure is so small, the kilo-

calorie is the standard unit of measure used when referring to the amount of energy a food contains. For simplicity, the prefix "kilo" is dropped, leaving just "calories" or "Kcal" as the standard unit of measure. Foods that have very little if any nutritional value with the exception of providing calories found in simple sugars are said to provide **empty calories.** Soft drinks, artificial fruit drinks, and candy are examples. From a nutritional perspective, these foods are indeed "empty."

Nutrition experts believe that fats should provide no more than 30 percent of the calories our bodies use. Carbohydrates should account for 58 percent of the energy we consume, with simple sugars accounting for only 10 percent of this amount (or 5.8 percent of total energy), while the calories received from protein should not exceed 12 percent of the total daily energy requirement. This ratio of fats, carbohydrates, and protein is chosen because scientific evidence suggests that specific diseases can be avoided by following these guidelines. As you might expect, the typical American diet does not match this ratio.

TABLE 6.2 ■ Recommended Dietary Allowances for Some of the More Important Nutrients

	Simple and Complex Combined (%)	Complex (%)	Simple (%)	Protein (%)	Fat (%)
Men 15–24 yr	58	48	10	12	30
Men > 24 yr	58	48	10	12	30
Women 15–24 yr	58	48	10	12	30
Women > 24	58	48	10	12	30
Pregnant women	58	48	10	12	30
Lactating women	58	48	10	12	30

	Saturated Fat[a] (%)	Cholesterol (mg)	Fiber[b] (g)	Calcium (mg)	Iron (mg)
Men 15–24 yr	10	< 300	20–35	1,200	10
Men > 24 yr	10	< 300	20–35	800	10
Women 15–24 yr	10	< 300	20–35	1,200	15
Women > 24	10	< 300	20–35	800	15
Pregnant women	10	< 300	20–35	1,200	30
Lactating women	10	< 300	20–35	1,200	15

Source: Food and Nutrition Board, National Academy of Sciences—National Research Council.
Recommended dietary allowances. Washington, D.C.: U.S. Government Printing Office, 1989.

Notes: See Appendix A for detailed RDA information.

[a]Total daily consumption of fat should not exceed 30 percent of caloric intake and no more than 10 percent of the total amount should come from saturated fats.

[b]Fiber is considered complex carbohydrates.

FATS: FINDING THE PROPER BALANCE

Fat is a necessary component of proper nutrition because of its various functions. Dietary fat gives foods a distinct flavor and texture. We need dietary fat, but all too often we consume too much. Currently, 38 percent of the calories consumed in a typical American diet come from fat. Some experts suggest that the figure should be as low as 20 percent. The generally accepted guidelines state that no more than 30 percent of all the calories consumed in one day should come from fat.

The basis for these guidelines comes from research that has linked diets high in fat to a number of diseases and conditions. Obesity is perhaps the most common condition associated with the consumption of fat. Fat is high in calories, and those who consume more calories than they expend will store the extra energy in the form of body fat.

Body fat acts as an efficient storehouse of energy. It helps to insulate and protect vital organs and tissues and even gives shape to our bodies. Body fat also provides storage for several fat-soluble vitamins.

Although some body fat is necessary, obese individuals are more susceptible to hypertension, stroke, high blood cholesterol, osteoarthritis, cancers of the breast, colon, and uterus, and non-insulin-dependent diabetes. Excessive body fat is also the leading cause of heart disease. There is a close relationship between the amount of dietary fat a person consumes and the amount of body fat a person possesses.

In a recent study, a positive relationship between the amount of fat people ate and the amount of body fat they possessed was demonstrated.[3] Eating a diet high in fat may lead to increased body fat even if a person exercises and does not overeat. Only 3 calories are required to store 100 calories of fat, whereas 23 to 27 calories are used to digest and store 100 calories of carbohydrates. It appears that dietary fat requires less energy to be stored than do carbohydrates; thus, diets high in fat may result in greater fat storage. The health risks associated with diets high in fat are typically dependent on the amount of dietary fat and the type of fat.

Fats are compounds made by combining fatty acid and glycerol to form glyceride. A triglyceride is a fat that has three fatty acids attached to one glycerol. The fatty acids that make up triglycerides are either saturated, monounsaturated, or polyunsaturated. The difference between these fatty acids is based on the number of chemical bonds they have. If a fat has all the hydrogen atoms it can hold, it is said to be **"saturated."** If there is room for one hydrogen atom, it is called monounsaturated, and if there is room for more than one hydrogen atom, the fat is polyunsaturated. Other types of fats include phospholipids and sterols, which include cholesterol.

Saturated Fat

Saturated fats have all the hydrogen atoms they can hold and are considered stable, whereas unsaturated fats lack hydrogen atoms and tend to spoil with time. To avoid spoilage, manufacturers process unsaturated fats by adding hydrogen atoms. Look at the nutritional label on most processed foods and you will find partially hydrogenated vegetable oil as an ingredient. This substance is a mono- or polyunsaturated fat that has become saturated through processing; it has become a saturated fat. Saturated fats have been singled out as being directly related to elevated blood cholesterol, stroke, and coronary heart disease. By reducing the amount of saturated fat in one's diet, it is possible to achieve a 10 to 20 percent decrease in total blood cholesterol. When dietary cholesterol is reduced, the amount of total blood cholesterol does not always decrease. The liver converts saturated fat into cholesterol, so when dietary cholesterol is reduced, the liver uses saturated fats to produce cholesterol. Therefore, the amount of cholesterol in the bloodstream is thought to be more closely related to the amount of saturated fat in one's diet than to the amount of cholesterol consumed.

As a general rule of thumb, fats that are saturated are solid at room temperature. A cube of margarine is solid at room temperature, but tends to melt at warmer temperatures. The fat on meat is solid until it is cooked, at which time some of it melts and drips off.

Saturated fats taste good, they act as thickeners, and they are relatively inexpensive to use in processed foods. Animal products are the primary source of saturated fats. Animal foods high in saturated fats include red meat, pork, lard, bacon, sausage, hot dogs, veal, lamb, luncheon meats (except turkey and chicken), cheese, whole milk, butter, and cream. Saturated fats are generally found only in animal products with the exception of coconut oil and palm oil, which are also widely used in processed foods. Doughnuts and other fried foods are fried in saturated fats. Since the 1980s, many of the major fast-food restaurants that served french fries and foods fried in animal fat have switched to preparing their foods in vegetable oils containing only a fraction of the amount of saturated fats found in lard or animal-based cooking oils. The average consumption of saturated fat accounts for 15 percent of total daily calories; experts recommend that saturated fats account for no more than 10 percent of the calories a person consumes on any given day. How does your intake of saturated fat compare? Many individuals could cut their consumption of saturated fats in half and still consume too much.

If you cook with oils or like fried foods, there is a way to continue some of your eating patterns without eliminating all the foods you like to eat. Choose those oils that contain small amounts of saturated fats, but remember that all oils are 100 percent fat and cooking oils

I don't have time to cut up all those vegetables.

Try frozen vegetables. They're easier to prepare and can be just as good for you as fresh vegetables because they are frozen right after they are picked so that vitamins are locked into the food.

Fresh fruits and vegetables cost too much.

Look for sales on canned and frozen fruits and vegetables, and stock up.

I really don't like fruits and vegetables.

Try adding some variety to your diet by trying just one new fruit or vegetable each week. If you give yourself an opportunity to experiment, you will probably acquire a taste for some of the new foods you try. Also, don't forget that fruit juice counts as a serving of fruit.

But I like high-fat foods.

Go ahead and enjoy that bowl of ice cream, your favorite cookies, or your dad's famous fried chicken. Just don't do it too often.

Everyone around me eats high-fat foods, so if I want to eat with others, I have to eat that kind of food, too.

If your family or friends eat high-fat foods regularly, offer to make dinner and then serve a low-fat, tasty meal.

I know my diet isn't the best, but it's what I've always known and it seems to work for me.

Changing a lifetime of eating habits takes time. Make small changes one at a time.

---

are a major source of fat in our diets. Margarine and butter are both 100 percent fat, although margarine is only 20 percent saturated fat whereas butter is 67 percent saturated. Just because an oil is promoted as being 100 percent vegetable oil does not mean that it is low in saturated fats and cholesterol. Tropical oils such as coconut or palm kernel oil contain more saturated fat than beef fat or lard. Though all vegetable oils are cholesterol free, the amount of saturated fat they contain can affect long-term health. If you must cook with oil, your wisest choices may be oils containing polyunsaturated or monounsaturated fats.

Polyunsaturated and Monounsaturated Fats

These fats come from various vegetable oils including safflower oil, olive oil, and sunflower oil. Evidence suggests that they may actually help lower the level of blood cholesterol by helping the body get rid of excessive, newly formed cholesterol. The average person consumes too much monounsaturated and too little polyunsaturated fat. Simply reducing the amount of saturated fat in a person's diet can help bring about a diet with the correct balance of fats.

Fat Substitutes: A Peek at the Future

Walk down the aisles of your supermarket and you'll get a glimpse of the future: foods made with fat replacers. For instance, there are now dozens of ice cream clones with the taste and texture of real ice cream, but with little or no fat. To approximate the creamy texture of ice cream (or salad dressing or mayonnaise), food manufacturers are constantly experimenting with different combinations of proteins, carbohydrates, and fats to develop tasty, safe, imitation fats (substances used to reduce food's fat and calories while maintaining the texture provided by fat).

The most popular substitute is Olestra, an imitation fat made from fat. The taste, texture, and "mouth feel" of Olestra are very similar to real fats. Because of the tight molecular structure of this product, the human body is unable to digest it. Since it is not digestible, it contains no usable calories and is considered calorie free. To determine the safety of Olestra, a panel of independent government and industry experts pored over each of the 150 separate animal and human studies that have evaluated the safety of regular consumption of foods containing Olestra. The group agreed that the data provided a reasonable certainty that there is no danger in consuming foods that contain Olestra, but long-term studies could prove otherwise.

Adapted from U.S. Food and Drug Administration, *Olestra and other fat substitutes,* FDA Backgrounder BG95-18; November 28, 1995.

MENU ALTERNATIVES

A more healthful diet doesn't have to leave you feeling hungry or deprived. Below, we've transformed two days' worth of standard American meals and snacks. The Typical meals, with familiar foods and reasonable portions, derive more than 40 percent of their calories from fat, an amount that's usual for many Americans. The Prudent meals substitute low-fat dressings, spreads, and dairy products, bring on fresh fruits and vegetables, and go for high-fiber grains. They are still familiar, filling, and tasty, and they meet the goals set by the Government's Dietary Guidelines for Americans. The ideal meals make additional changes in the same direction, reaching the ideal levels of fat and carbohydrate advised by our experts. Here, fat is dramatically reduced, yet the essence of familiar American meals remains intact. For all meals, total calories are in a range appropriate to the average man; women would likely have smaller portions. Both days' menus provide close to or more than the U.S. RDA for all nutrients, with one exception: Typical meals on Day Two are slightly low in zinc and vitamin C.

DAY 1

Typical	Prudent	Ideal
BREAKFAST		
2 scrambled eggs in 1 tsp. butter 2 slices white toast with 1 tsp. butter, 1 tsp. jam 4 ounces orange juice 1 cup lowfat (2%) milk Coffee or tea	1 egg yolk, 2 whites scrambled in 1 tsp. soft margarine 2 slices whole-wheat toast with 1 tsp. soft margarine, 2 tsp. jam 8 ounces orange juice 1 cup lowfat (1%) milk Coffee or tea	3-egg-white Spanish omelet (tomato, peppers and onions) in 1 tsp. soft margarine 2 slices whole-grain toast with 1 tsp. soft margarine, 2 tsp. all-fruit preserves 1 cup strawberries 1 cup skim milk Coffee or tea
LUNCH		
Ham sandwich 3 ounces regular ham on white bread with 1 tbsp. mayonnaise, lettuce 1/3 cup potato salad 1 ounce tortilla chips	Ham sandwich 3 ounces extra-lean ham on whole-wheat bread, 1 tbsp. fat-free mayonnaise, lettuce, tomato 1/2 cup German potato salad 1 ounce pretzels	Turkey sandwich 2 ounces turkey breast on whole-grain bread, 1 tbsp. cranberry sauce, lettuce 1/2 cup three-bean salad and 1/2 cup carrot-raisin salad 1 ounce whole-wheat pretzels
SNACK		
1 ounce peanut brittle	4 fig bars	1 small bran muffin
DINNER		
4 ounces meat loaf with 1/4 cup mushroom gravy Lettuce and tomato with 1 tbsp. regular blue-cheese dressing 1 biscuit 1/2 cup broccoli with 2 tbsp. cheese sauce 1/2 cup vanilla ice cream	3 ounces lean meat loaf with 1/4 cup tomato sauce Mixed greens and tomato salad with 1 tbsp. low-calorie blue-cheese dressing 2 slices French bread with 1 tsp. soft margarine 1/2 cup steamed broccoli with 1 tsp. soft margarine 1/2 cup vanilla ice milk with 1 sliced fresh peach	1 cup spaghetti with 2 ounces extra-lean ground meat, 1/2 cup spaghetti sauce Mixed greens and tomato salad with 1 tbsp. fat-free blue-cheese dressing 1 whole-wheat roll with 1 tsp. soft margarine 1/2 cup broccoli with garlic sauteed in 1/2 tsp. olive oil 1/2 cup nonfat ice cream with 1 cup fresh fruit salad
LATE SNACK		
1 cup lowfat (2%) milk 2 small chocolate chip cookies	1 cup lowfat (1%) milk 6 vanilla wafers	1 cup skim milk 6 graham-cracker squares
TOTALS		
2239 calories 11 grams of fiber 777 milligrams of cholesterol	2211 calories 23 grams of fiber 353 milligrams of cholesterol	2230 calories 37 grams of fiber 116 milligrams of cholesterol

47% — (16%), 16%, 37%
52% — 30%, (8%), 18%
61% — 21%, (4%), 18%

Total fat Saturated fat Protein Carbohydrate

DAY 2

Typical	Prudent	Ideal
BREAKFAST		
1 cup corn flakes 4 ounces apple juice 1 cup lowfat (2%) milk Coffee or tea	1 cup wheat-flake cereal 1 banana 4 ounces orange juice 1 cup lowfat (1%) milk Coffee or tea	1 cup bran-flake cereal 1 cup blueberries 1 orange 1 cup skim milk Coffee or tea
MORNING SNACK		
1 glazed doughnut	1 small blueberry muffin; 1 tsp. margarine	1 bagel; 2 tsp. soft margarine; 1 tsp. jam
LUNCH		
Tuna sandwich 3 ounces oil-packed tuna, 2 tbsp. mayonnaise on white bread with lettuce 1/2 cup macaroni salad 1 ounce corn chips 1 slice apple pie	Tuna sandwich 2 ounces water-packed tuna, 2 tbsp. cholesterol-free mayonnaise on whole wheat bread with lettuce, tomato 1/2 cup pasta salad 1 ounce tortilla chips 1 baked apple	Tuna sandwich 2 ounces water-packed tuna, 2 tbsp. light mayonnaise on thickly sliced whole-grain bread with lettuce, tomato 1/2 cup cucumber-onion salad and 1/2 cup tortellini-vegetable salad 1 ounce no-oil tortilla chips 1 apple
SNACK		
1/2 cup frozen yogurt	1/2 cup lowfat frozen yogurt	1 cup lowfat frozen yogurt with 1/2 cup fresh fruit salad
DINNER		
Baked 1/2 chicken breast and chicken drumstick with skin 1/2 cup french fries 1/2 cup canned green beans 1/2 cup chocolate pudding (2%) milk	Baked 1/2 chicken breast and chicken drumstick without skin 1 cup mashed potatoes with lowfat (1%) milk, 1 tsp. soft margarine 1/2 cup steamed green beans with 1 tsp. soft margarine 1/2 cup chocolate pudding (1%) milk	1/2 baked chicken breast without skin 1 baked potato with 2 tbsp. half-and-half sour cream topping 1 cup stir-fried vegetables with garlic in 1 tsp. oil 1/2 cup chocolate pudding (skim milk)
TOTALS		
2588 calories 9 grams of fiber 284 milligrams of cholesterol	2199 calories 20 grams of fiber 182 milligrams of cholesterol	2217 calories 36 grams of fiber 127 milligrams of cholesterol

42% — (11%), 19%, 39%
49% — 31%, (6%), 20%
64% — 18%, (3%), 18%

Total fat Saturated fat Protein Carbohydrate

Dietary Fat: Visible and Hidden

Some dietary fats are often difficult to detect. (See Table 6.3.) Many processed foods include large amounts of fat, but because the fat is "cooked" into the food, its presence is not easily detected. Advertisers may employ considerable deception in the marketing of food products that are high in fat. For example, a package of lun-

Activity 6.1 Cutting the Fat in Your Diet

Take a look at the foods you listed in your nutritional analysis (Lab 6.2). Which foods that you ate are high in fat? List those foods in the left-hand column below.

High-Fat Foods

_____

_____

_____

_____

_____

_____

_____

Low-Fat Alternatives

_____

_____

_____

_____

_____

_____

_____

Review the suggestions found in the Menu Alternatives on the opposite page. Then, for each of the high-fat foods you listed above, provide a suitable low-fat alternative—use a substitute food or change your cooking methods.

cheon meat can boldly state that the contents are 95 percent fat free. This actually means that 95 percent of the weight of the meat contains no fat, when in reality, the amount of calories from fat may be very high. This is analogous to a half ounce of butter being stirred into a 10-ounce glass of water. The resulting product is 95 percent fat free by weight; however, because water contains no calories, the drink actually provides 100 percent of its calories in the form of fat. Remember, fat content can be displayed by weight or calories. Of the total weight of a glass of 2 percent milk, 2 percent of the weight comes from fat; however, 32 percent of the calories come from fat. To determine the fat content of the foods you eat, you should always read the label.

As a rule, any food that looks or tastes greasy has a lot of fat. The fat may leave a shine on your fingers or an oily stain on the table or napkin. These foods include all fried foods, potato chips, and most crackers, cheeses, pastries and cookies, and pizza. Other high-fat foods include salad dressings, butter, margarine, sour cream, cheese spreads, most dips, and cream soups. Usually there are more calories in the dressing that tops a salad than there are in the rest of the salad. A salad starts out as a wonderfully healthy food, but when a generous helping of regular dressing is poured on, it becomes a high-fat food. Most snacks are also high in fat. Although it may sound healthier than some other choices, just one individual fruit snack pie has over 475 calories and is 79 percent fat.

Do you have to stop eating all these foods for the rest of your life? The answer is no. Most individuals need to reduce the amount of total fats and saturated fats in their diets. Reducing fats can be accomplished by eating fewer of the foods that are high in fat, especially those high in saturated fats. It is not necessary to eliminate all high-fat foods from your diet. Granted, a reduction in the amount of many foods may be required, but even a doughnut can be worked into a healthy food plan occasionally. The following are several practical ways to reduce the amount of fat we consume.

Prepare meatless main dishes, or those containing small amounts of meat.

Eat no more than seven ounces of meat, seafood, and poultry a day.

Use skinless chicken and turkey.

Eat more fish, but bake or broil it instead of frying.

Use lean cuts of meat, trim all visible fat, and throw away any fat that cooks out.

Eat no more than four egg yolks a week, including those used in cooking.

Bake, broil, roast, barbecue, or stew foods instead of frying them.

Cook stews and gravies a day early, refrigerate, then discard the fat that has risen to the top.

Limit yourself to five to eight teaspoons of fat or oil a day for cooking, baking, and salads.

Drink fortified skim milk and eat cheeses made from low-fat milk.

Substitute low-fat or no-fat alternatives for high-fat dressings and sauces.

TABLE 6.3 ■ Fat Content of Commonly Eaten Foods

		PERCENTAGE OF TOTAL CALORIES FROM FAT			
Food	Fat (g)	Total % of Calories from Fat[a]	Saturated %	Mono %	Poly %
Domino's Pepperoni Pizza (two slices)	18	35.2	9	7	2
McDonald's Big Mac	26	46.8	9	16	1
Burger King Whopper	36	52.8	12	13	13
Taco Bell soft taco	12	48	5	trace	1
Egg, whole, raw	5.01	64	19	25	8
Butter (Tbs)	11.4	100	67	31	4
Margarine, regular, hard (Tbs)	11.0	100	20	45	32
Cheese, cream (1 oz)	9.9	90	57	25	3
Cheese, cheddar (1 oz)	37.5	74	47	20	2
Cheese, cottage (1 cup)	10.1	39	25	11	
Milk, whole (1 cup)	8.2	49	30	14	2
Skim milk (1 cup)	1.0	6	4	1	trace
Frankfurter (2 oz)	16.6	82	33	40	3
Fish sticks (1 oz)	3.4	39	10	18	10
Tuna, canned, oil-packed (3 oz)	6.9	38	8	10	17
Tuna, canned, water-packed (3 oz)	2.1	7	trace	trace	trace
Ground beef (3 oz)	19.2	65	25	28	3
Chicken breast, fried, flour-coated (7 oz)	17.4	36	10	14	8
Potato (baked)	0.06	1	trace	trace	4
Potato chips (1.5 oz)	13.0	61	16	11	31
Ice cream, vanilla, regular (1 cup)	22.5	48	28	14	2
Apple (raw, unpeeled)	0.5	6	1	trace	2

Source: Information summarized from *Nutritive value of foods,* rev. Washington, D.C.: U.S. Government Printing Office, 1981.

Notes: Trace: less than 0.5% of fat.

[a]Includes undifferentiated fats.

CARBOHYDRATES

Carbohydrates are the primary source of energy for all human metabolism. During physical activity, carbohydrates are the primary suppliers of energy as long as the body has sufficient stores. You will recall that each gram of carbohydrate provides 4 calories of energy. The energy released in one gram is the same, whether it comes from sugar, potatoes, or milk. When carbohydrate stores are depleted, our bodies turn to fats and proteins for the required energy. An overall shortage of carbohydrates will result in the metabolism of fat and protein, resulting in decreased muscle mass and body fat. Shortages of carbohydrates occur only during periods of fasting, crash diets, or during prolonged periods of intensive endurance-type physical activity.

Several groups of nutrients are classified as carbohydrates: simple carbohydrates, or sugars; complex carbohydrates, or starches; and fiber. Experts recommend that at least 58 percent of our total daily caloric intake should come from carbohydrates. The average diet comes close to this amount, except that the ratio of complex carbohydrates, sugars, and fiber is not in line with nutritional standards deemed necessary for optimal health. In this section, you will have an opportunity to compare your nutritional analysis to both the recommended ideal and the typical American diet.

Carbohydrates are vital to health and optimal functioning. Fiber, a form of complex carbohydrate that absorbs water and aids in digestion, acts as a softening agent in the digestive tract, serving as a natural laxative. A recent study of the use of fat as a source of energy found that fat is in essence burned in a carbohydrate furnace. Without carbohydrates, fat cannot be used for energy and simply remains on the body, which suggests that weight-loss diets should contain adequate amounts of carbohydrates.

Simple Carbohydrates

Simple carbohydrates are one of the largest sources of dietary calories. Almost 25 percent of the average daily caloric intake comes from simple carbohydrates. Taste is one of the biggest factors in determining which foods we eat, and because foods with sugar taste good, we tend to eat a lot of them. A simple sugar molecule is called a **monosaccharide;** a **disaccharide** is composed of two sugar molecules. Glucose, fructose, and galactose are monosaccharides and are the basic building blocks of all other carbohydrates. Two monosaccharides combine to produce a disaccharide. White table sugar, for example, is a disaccharide containing one molecule of glucose and one of fructose. The average person consumes two and a half times the recommended amount of simple carbohydrates. In just one year, the typical American consumes 130 pounds of refined sugars. Most individuals need to cut their consumption of simple sugars by half if they are to approximate the recommended daily intake of simple sugars.

For people who are very physically active, the consumption of high amounts of simple carbohydrates may actually decrease the body's ability to meet high demands for energy. Calories can be easily attained by eating foods loaded with simple sugars; however, foods with refined sugars typically do not contain essential vitamins and minerals. Without the proper vitamins and minerals, the body cannot use the available stores of energy. When this happens, all of the processes that require energy slow down or stop. People who consume diets high in simple sugars may experience persistent fatigue and weakness. Thus, diets high in simple sugars may, in extreme cases, lead to malnutrition.

The simple sugars found in processed foods are difficult to detect unless you know what to look for. Refined sugars used in packaged foods include high-fructose corn syrup, honey, sucrose, corn syrup, cornstarch, dextrose, sorghum, and maltose.

Naturally occurring sugars are found in fruits, vegetables, honey, and milk. Foods with large amounts of nutrients and low numbers of calories are said to be nutrient dense, as opposed to the "empty calorie" foods we discussed earlier. Even though some naturally occurring foods are very sweet to the taste, they generally contain large quantities of other nutrients, making nutrient-dense foods an ideal source of energy. All naturally occurring fruits and vegetables are nutrient dense. By reducing the amount of calories that come from such empty-calorie foods as candy, most snacks, sodas, and alcohol, and consuming more fruits and vegetables, you can achieve a more well-balanced diet and lower your health risks.

Following are some guidelines for reducing the amount of sugar in your diet:

Buy cereals that are low in sugar and don't add sugar to them.

Buy fruit canned in its own juice rather than in sweetened juices or syrup.

Read food labels and cut back on foods that list any type of sugar as one of the first three ingredients.

Cut back on the amount of sugar you use in recipes. Often the amount of sugar can be cut by as much as half without affecting the taste or texture.

Gradually reduce the amount of sugar you add to tea and coffee, with the goal of eventually drinking them without sugar.

Replace soda, the number one source of dietary sugars, with unsweetened fruit juices or water.

Cut back on other major sources of sugar: pastries, cookies, cakes, and pies.

The development of sugar substitutes has expanded the sales of popular soft drinks, gums, candies, and other high-sugar products. Nutrasweet, Equal, saccharin, and cyclamate are just a few of the more popular artificial sweeteners. They mimic the chemical structure of sugars in such a way that our tastebuds tell us they taste sweet. Some are made of proteins and can be up to 300 times sweeter than sugar, so only extremely small amounts are used. Since protein has about 4 calories per gram and only a small portion is needed, soda sweetened with sugar substitutes typically has only 1 or 2 calories. Another sweetener, called Sunette, provides no calories because it is not broken down by the body. The advent of sugar-free foods has greatly facilitated the ability of diabetics to control their blood sugar and allowed many people the opportunity to eat their favorite sweet foods without consuming sugar.

Complex Carbohydrates

With the exception of some fiber, all carbohydrates ultimately are broken down into glucose. Complex carbohydrates are simple sugars that have been connected to form long complex chains. These are sometimes referred to as starches. Many popular diets recommend that starchy foods such as cereals, rice, pasta, potatoes, legumes, and breads be avoided because of their high caloric content. These diets are entirely based on anecdotal experience and have no scientific basis for the recommendations.

Because starchy foods come from plants and are low in fat, they contain fewer calories than most other foods. Individuals who make these complex carbohydrates the main portion of their diets have decreased cardiovascular disease, obesity, cancer, and diabetes, and may even have fewer cavities. Research indicates that a healthy diet should obtain at least 45 percent of its calories from complex carbohydrates. That's almost double current levels of consumption. Although most individuals eat a generous portion of complex carbohydrates, the toppings often used on these foods may offset their nutritional value. For example, a baked potato is a highly nutritious food, but when it is topped with butter, salt, chili, cheese, creamy dressings, or sour cream, it no longer qualifies as a wise nutrition choice. The same principle applies to pasta, rice, and breads.

Fruits and vegetables are another important source of carbohydrates and have recently emerged as heroes of a healthy diet. There is strong evidence that a diet rich in fruits and vegetables reduces the risk of certain cancers. Diets containing large quantities of fruits and vegetables, especially cruciferous vegetables such as broccoli and cauliflower, offer significant protection against cancers of the lung, colon, breast, cervix, esophagus, oral cavity, stomach, bladder, pancreas, and ovaries. It is believed that this protection is caused by several factors: cruciferous vegetables are good sources of antioxidants (substances that inhibit reactions promoted by oxygen); several seem to contain other specific anticancer compounds, and dietary fiber can be found in all of them. Researchers feel that a level of protection is provided by consuming five to seven servings of fruits and vegetables per day. This is more than double the current average intake. If you adopt a diet that contains adequate fruits and vegetables, your overall consumption of fats will decrease while the amount of dietary fiber you consume increases. Refer to Activity 6.2 to assess your current consumption of fruits and vegetables.

Fiber

Some experts believe that fiber should be classified as the seventh basic nutrient. Fiber (or roughage) is a general term for food substances that our bodies fail to digest completely. Fiber actually consists of complex chains of carbohydrates that are broken down by bacteria and enzymes that humans lack. Plant matter like grass and wood are types of fiber, and contain large amounts of energy in the form of carbohydrates. This food source is only good for energy if the chains can be broken. Cattle, termites, beavers, and many other animals are able to digest and exist on this type of fiber. The human need for dietary fiber concerns another role fiber plays in the digestive process.

Fiber can be classified into two basic types, soluble and insoluble. Every plant food contains both kinds of fiber to some degree. The National Cancer Institute recommends that we eat 20 to 35 grams of fiber a day.[4] The average American diet contains less than half this recommended amount.

Activity 6.2
Taking Inventory: Fruits and Vegetables

Review your nutritional analysis (Lab 6.2) for the number of servings of fruits and vegetables you consumed each day of the three-day assessment. (One fruit = 1 serving; ½ cup vegetables = 1 serving.) Record the number of each below:

Day 1

Number of servings of fruits: _____

Number of servings of vegetables: _____

Total fruit and vegetable servings: _____

Day 2

Number of servings of fruits: _____

Number of servings of vegetables: _____

Total fruit and vegetable servings: _____

Day 3

Number of servings of fruits: _____

Number of servings of vegetables: _____

Total fruit and vegetable servings: _____

Add the totals above and divide by 3 to determine your average daily consumption. How does your diet compare with the recommended five to seven servings of fruits and vegetables a day? How does it compare with the average American's consumption of two to three servings a day?

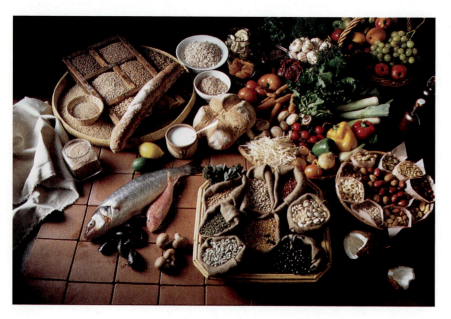

A balanced diet of foods high in nutrients serves as a valuable source of energy and also plays a preventative role.

Soluble Fiber

Soluble fiber was thrown into the national spotlight after several studies found that oat bran (a good source of soluble fiber) was found to reduce blood cholesterol levels. Soluble fiber dissolves in water or is broken down in the large intestine. A summary of several clinical trials, published in the *Journal of the American Medical Association,* determined that eating oat bran cereal and oatmeal every day can lower blood cholesterol levels 2 to 3 percent. Other studies found that there is moderately strong evidence that diets containing other high soluble fiber foods such as strawberries, Brussels sprouts, beans, and lentils can also reduce blood cholesterol.

Soluble fibers include gels and pectins that dissolve in water. Once dissolved, this mixture thickens and adds bulk to the contents of the stomach, which slows the emptying of the stomach and provides a sense of fullness, thus decreasing the sensation of hunger and perhaps aiding in the control of body weight. This gel also slows the digestion of sugars from the small intestine, lowers insulin requirements, and decreases elevated levels of blood pressure among diabetics.[5] Perhaps most important, soluble fiber binds with cholesterol-containing compounds in the intestine and reduces cardiovascular risk by lowering the level of blood cholesterol. Corn bran, apples, pears, prunes, oranges, sweet potatoes, dried beans, and other fruits, vegetables, and legumes are good sources of soluble fiber (see Table 6.4).

Insoluble Fiber

Insoluble fiber is that part of the foods we consume that is not digested. Rather, this fiber remains in the digestive tract and adds bulk to the intestinal contents. The added bulk increases the speed at which foods pass through the intestines. This increase has been shown to have several

---

TABLE 6.4 ■ Foods High in Fiber

Food Item	Serving Size	Fiber (g)
Fruits		
Apple, with skin	1	4.0
Avocado	¼ cup	2.5
Banana	1	2.3
Cantaloupe	½	2.0
Orange	1	3.8
Peach	1	13
Raisins	½ cup	2.5
Strawberries	½ cup	15
Grains and Cereals		
Bread, whole wheat	1 slice	2.5
Bread, mixed grain	1 slice	14
Oatmeal, cooked	½ cup	3.0
Tortilla, corn	1	0.9
Legumes		
Garbanzo beans, cooked	½ cup	4.9
Kidney beans, cooked	½ cup	4.6
Vegetables		
Beans, green, cooked	½ cup	2.0
Broccoli, cooked	½ cup	2.1
Carrot, raw	1	1.8
Cauliflower, cooked	½ cup	2.3
Corn, cooked	½ cup	4.6
Peas, green, cooked	½ cup	3.5
Potato, baked with skin	1	15.0
Spinach, cooked	½ cup	3.5
Tomato, medium	1	1.8

Source: U.S. Department of Agriculture. *The hassle-free guide to a better diet.* Washington, D.C.: U.S. Government Printing Office, 1980.

health benefits. Because the stool is softer and moves more quickly, constipation is prevented. Constipation results in increased abdominal pressure, which is one of the major causes of hemorrhoids. A soft stool can prevent hemorrhoids. Most laxatives sold today include insoluble fiber in their ingredients. In particular, cellulose (wood) is added to many of these products. However, a diet rich in complex carbohydrates will contain enough fiber to prevent most cases of constipation.

The added bulk of fiber prevents intestinal contents from becoming compacted, which can obstruct the appendix and lead to appendicitis. A soft stool may also prevent diverticulitis, a condition in which the intestine bulges out into "pockets" that can become infected and rupture. A soft stool helps keep the intestinal wall flexible and gives it tone.

Colon cancer is the second most common cancer in the United States and the second leading cause of cancer death. In countries in which people consume low-fat and high-fiber diets, the risk of colon cancer is 80 to 90 percent lower than the U.S. rate. Experts believe that insoluble fiber stimulates the production of mucus secreted from the intestinal wall. This helps provide a protective barrier between cells of the intestinal wall and any cancer-causing agents that may reside in the stool. Because the transit time for digesting food is decreased, the amount of exposure any cancer-causing agents might have with the intestinal wall is greatly reduced. For those persons who fail to consume adequate amounts of dietary fiber, the risk of colon cancer is clearly increased. Foods high in fiber generally contain both soluble and insoluble fiber. We know that whole grains, beans, wheat bran, and most fruits and vegetables with their skin are rich sources of fiber, but what types of foods are low in fiber?

The more a food is processed, the less fiber it usually contains. White bread made from bleached flour, white rice, french fries, potato chips and pretzels, pancakes, refined sugars, fruit drinks, candies, meats, and high-fat foods contain very little fiber. The processing technique used to bleach flour removes all nutrients except the carbohydrates. After processing, some vitamins and minerals may be replaced to make the food "enriched."

Evaluate the labels found on bread products; if the product contains wheat flour, chances are it is made from bleached white flour and contains very little fiber. Instead, choose foods that have not been highly processed. All fruits and vegetables contain some amount of fiber. A high-starch diet will not only allow you to get proper amounts of complex carbohydrates, but a secondary benefit may be a big increase in the amount of dietary fiber.

Most Americans consume ten to thirteen grams of dietary fiber every day. As with the quantity of fruits and vegetables, recommended levels of fiber intake are double the amount typically consumed. This much fiber is typically consumed by the average vegetarian, so for nonvegetarians, it is important to increase slowly the amount of fiber we consume. Gradually add fiber-rich foods over a period of several weeks. Gastrointestinal problems can occur when large amounts of fiber are consumed in a short period of time.

Rather than count individual grams, a better method to ensure proper intake is to consume a diet high in fruits, vegetables, and grains. For additional tips on how to increase the amount of dietary fiber, see the following list. If your diet is low in fiber, introduce it gradually over a period of four to six weeks, with these tips:

Eat ¼ to ½ cup whole-grain cereal every day.

Buy bread that lists "whole wheat" or "stone-ground wheat" as its first ingredient.

Whenever you can, eat unpeeled fresh fruits and vegetables.

Add brown rice, millet, bulgur, or barley to soups, stews, and casseroles.

To make higher fiber breads, muffins, or other baked goods, substitute whole-wheat flour for some or all of the white flour.

Cook with recipes that include bran and other good sources of fiber.

Substitute brown rice for white rice.

Snack on popcorn instead of potato chips and pretzels.

Read labels. Look for whole-grain breads, macaroni, egg noodles, and cereals.

PROTEINS: THE BODY'S BUILDING BLOCKS

The word *protein* comes from the Greek, meaning "of prime importance." Like carbohydrates and fats, protein contains carbon, oxygen, and hydrogen and can be converted to energy. Protein, however, is the only energy-containing nutrient that has nitrogen. Our bodies are 12 to 15 percent protein, with most of this found in muscle. Structural proteins are the primary components of muscle, hair, skin, nail, tendons, and ligaments. Globular proteins are responsible for almost 2,000 enzymes that control metabolism, insulin production, blood cell formation and function, antibodies, cell growth, and repair. Of all the recommendations for proper nutrition, only the guideline for protein is close to the average dietary rate consumption. The typical American consumes the recommended level of protein; however, some people think that large amounts of protein are good for them, believing that if a little is good, then a lot will be better.

Excessive protein is converted to fat, not muscle, with the excess nitrogen being excreted in the urine, causing strain on the kidneys. Excess protein can also cause the body to excrete large amounts of valuable calcium, further taxing the kidneys. There is some evidence that too much protein can contribute to heart disease and osteoporosis and accelerate growth of tumors.

All proteins, whether they come from plants or from animals, are composed of smaller protein subunits called **amino acids.** In all, twenty amino acids are required by the human body, of which eleven can be produced by the body itself. These eleven are called nonessential amino acids; the other nine, which must be obtained through diet, are called essential. Essential amino acids are similar to some vitamins in that they are required for normal body functioning but must be acquired through a balanced diet. Specific foods that contain all nine of the essential amino acids are called **complete proteins.** Examples include meat, fish, poultry, eggs, milk, and cheese. Essential amino acids are found in most plants and animals, whereas foods that cannot provide all the essential amino acids are **incomplete proteins**.

There is considerable support from food producers and the media for increased protein consumption for individuals who are engaged in strength training or weightlifting activities. A multitude of high-protein drinks, mixes, foods, and concoctions are being purchased by body builders and strength trainers in the hope of increasing muscle mass. The body of research on this topic suggests that the protein requirements for those who are trying to gain muscle mass do not exceed the recommended level of 0.8 g/kg/day.

How Much Protein Should I Consume?

To calculate how much protein you need, divide your body weight in pounds by 2.2, which converts pounds to kilograms. The RDA for protein is 0.8 grams per kilogram of body weight per day. Multiply your body weight in kilograms times 0.8 and the number you end up with is the number of grams of protein you need for one day. For example, a typical woman who weighs 120 pounds will require 44 grams of protein.

$$\frac{120 \text{ lb}}{2.2} \times 0.8 \text{ g} = 44 \text{ g}$$

An average man weighing 154 pounds will require 56 grams of protein per day.

$$\frac{154 \text{ lb}}{2.2} \times 0.8 \text{ g} = 56 \text{ g}$$

These amounts are quite small when you consider that one fast-food hamburger has 23 grams of protein, over half the daily requirement for women. One glass of milk has about 9 grams and one roasted chicken breast has 58 grams. People consume too much protein and should cut back. However, pregnant women or mothers who are currently nursing infants are encouraged to increase protein consumption an extra 20 to 30 grams a day.

At rest, the primary sources of energy for our bodies come from carbohydrates and fats; however, 2 to 5 percent of the body's resting energy comes from protein. This amount can go as high as 10 to 15 percent during moderate and intense levels of physical activity. Without the proper amounts of carbohydrates, the body will break down protein to attain the required energy. Some starvation diets severely limit the number of calories, which forces the body to begin breaking down the protein found in muscle. People who are athletic or very physically active may find that the best way to preserve muscle mass is to consume the recommended amount of protein along with a high-carbohydrate diet.[6]

On Being a Vegetarian

There are various degrees of vegetarian diets, with **strict vegetarians** or "vegans" being the most restricted. Vegans refrain from eating any animal product, including milk, meat, and poultry or egg products. All dietary protein is derived from plant foods, which requires careful meal planning in order to acquire all the essential amino acids. As you might have guessed, vegans have no problems consuming the recommended amounts of fruits, vegetables, and complex carbohydrates. Dietary fat is low, and sources of saturated fat are confined to some plant sources and oils. In fact, vegetarians have lower blood cholesterol, lower blood pressure, lower body fat, and reduced rates of coronary heart disease and have been shown to have lower mortality rates than nonvegetarians.[7]

Lactovegetarians exclude eating meat and eggs, but do consume dairy products, while lacto-ovo-vegetarians include eggs in their diets. These more liberal levels of vegetarianism include at least one high-protein food source, which means there is little difficulty getting proper quantities of amino acids in the diet.

Close inspection of the food pyramid reveals that the recommended diet is slowly migrating more toward a vegetarian diet, and as research continues to clarify the role of diet and health, it is likely that the next set of dietary guidelines will suggest even greater emphasis on plant foods.

In order for the body to make protein, all the needed amino acids must be present simultaneously. A vegetarian diet that consists of incomplete proteins should be carefully planned in order to supply the necessary amino acids. The plant foods are classified into four basic food groups: grains, legumes, seeds and nuts, and vegetables. By combining foods from at least two of these groups, incomplete proteins complement each other by supplying all the necessary amino acids for protein formation. One food combination that forms complementary proteins would be peanut butter and bread.

VITAMINS: ESSENTIAL COMPONENTS

Even though our bodies require only small amounts of vitamins to maintain good health, failure to eat a variety of foods can result in insufficient supplies of vitamins, which can lead to fatigue and disease. The various processes of the body cannot complete their functions without specific enzymes and substances that are formed from vitamins. These processes lead to the formation of hormones, enzymes, antibodies, and tissues and are vital to the production of blood coagulation (clotting) and energy. Without vitamins, these processes are impaired and deficiency diseases can result. Today, deficiencies are rare in developed countries because consumption of a variety of foods almost guarantees that all the required vitamins will be obtained. A diet that contains only 1,200 calories but includes a variety of foods is sufficient to supply all of the vitamins and minerals needed by the average individual. Table 6.5 contains a list of sources and functions of each vitamin.

Water-Soluble and Fat-Soluble Vitamins

The required vitamins are classified by the way they are processed in the body. Vitamins C and the B complex vitamins can dissolve in water and are considered *water-soluble vitamins.* Because they dissolve in water, they cannot be stored for extended periods of time, so that any amount that is not required for some chemical process is excreted in the urine. Large doses of these vitamins do not pose any specific health dangers because excesses are simply removed by the kidneys and excreted. Vitamins A, D, E, and K, however, are *fat soluble,* do not dissolve in water, and are stored in fat inside the body. These vitamins remain in the body until the fat is mobilized to supply needed energy, at which point the vitamins are released to be used in processes or to be stored again. Daily consumption of these vitamins is not vital, because they are stored. Large doses of vitamins A and D can result in an accumulation inside fat stores, which can easily reach toxic levels.

A table of the recommended dietary allowances for all vitamins and minerals can be found in Appendix A. These guidelines provide a flexible range of recommended nutrient levels for seventeen population groups based on age and gender. They establish an average level of nutrition and include a safety margin, so that a diet that includes only two-thirds the RDA is still likely to provide good health. The RDA guidelines vary according to age, gender, size, health status, activity level, and environment.

Should You Take Vitamin Supplements?

Despite the plenitude of naturally occurring vitamins in the wide selection of foods available for consumption, 40 percent of Americans insist on taking a daily nutrient supplement. Some surveys report that 33 percent of Americans take supplements in excess of ten times recommended levels. Traditionally, many Americans believe that vitamin supplements are a necessity for healthy living. Supplement manufacturers have aggressively marketed not only the products themselves, but also the idea that supplements are necessary for people of all ages. It would appear from the advertisements that young and old, male and female, and even pets should be using supplements.

Although there is some discussion among nutrition experts concerning vitamin supplementation, most agree that healthy people who consume a balanced diet do not need to supplement. Those who should be taking daily supplements include:

People with a medically determined requirement for a specific vitamin

Pregnant and lactating women

People who eat erratic diets or have unusual lifestyles, such as alcoholics or drug abusers

People participating in medically supervised low-calorie diets

Elderly people who do not get regularly balanced meals

Newborn infants (vitamin K is given to prevent excess bleeding)

Even if you do fall into one of these categories, most likely supplementation will not produce any dramatic changes in health. It is not surprising that vitamin supplementation has failed to show any benefit for those who already consume a balanced diet. When a vitamin supplementation exceeds ten times the recommended amount for that vitamin, the dose is considered a **mega dose.** Mega doses of vitamin A and vitamin D should be limited to five and two times the recommended amounts respectively, with mineral mega dose levels set at three times the RDA. To better understand the roles of separate vitamins, researchers are currently evaluating the effects of specific vitamins on cancer, colds, heart disease, and aging. Scientists report detecting significantly lower rates of cancer and heart disease among people who have consumed greater than average quantities of vitamins C, E, and A (or beta carotene). Of all the required vitamins, only these three have the ability to reduce premature cell destruction caused by oxygen.

Oxygen, which liberates energy from carbohydrates and fats, is usually transformed into water (H_2O) and carbon dioxide. Occasionally an atom of oxygen loses one too many electrons during its processing and becomes an electron-hungry scavenger. These altered atoms, called **free radicals,** try to take an electron from another atom or structure. When the free radical finds and takes the needed electron, the atom from which the electron was taken becomes the next free radical and is left with a shortage of electrons until it, too, can locate another atom and remove one of its electrons. This cycle of stealing electrons continues throughout the body, causing damage to lipids, proteins, cell walls, and more important, DNA.

Experts believe that free radicals may be responsible for premature aging, heart disease, and cancer. This chain of stealing electrons continues until either the free radical

TABLE 6.5 ■ Vitamins: A Brief Overview

	Vitamin	Common Sources	Why Your Body Needs It	Possible Effects of Mega Dosing
Fat Soluble	A	Eggs, cheese, butter, fortified milk, carrots, spinach, cantaloupe, green vegetables	Maintenance of eyes, vision, skin, linings of mouth, throat, nose; aids the immune system	Loss of appetite, headaches, nausea, diarrhea, itching skin, liver damage
	D	Fortified milk, egg yolk, tuna, sunlight on skin	Useful in the formation of bones and teeth; helps the body absorb calcium	Deposits of calcium in the blood and kidneys, weakness, vomiting
	E	Vegetable oils, nuts, whole grains, olives, green vegetables	Maintains and protects cell membranes, aids in the formation of red blood cells	May cause increased levels of blood cholesterol
	K	Green leafy vegetables, cereals; body produces half the recommended amount	Assists in blood clotting, helps maintain bone metabolism	No serious side effects have been documented
Water Soluble	Vitamin B1 (Thiamin)	Whole-grain and enriched breads, pork, oatmeal, peas	Helps convert carbohydrates into other usable forms of energy	Few cases of side effects have been reported
	Vitamin B2 (Riboflavin)	Nuts, dairy products, meat, eggs, whole-grain and enriched cereals	Helps release energy from carbohydrates, proteins, and fats, maintains mucous membranes	None reported
	Vitamin B3 (Niacin)	Meat, fish, poultry, whole grains, enriched breads, green leafy vegetables, beans	Essential for growth and formation of hormones; facilitates energy release	Flushing of skin (hot flashes), nausea, vomiting, changes in the metabolism of glycogen and fatty acids
	Vitamin B6 (Pyridoxine)	Vegetables, meats, whole-grain cereals, peanuts, potatoes	Aids in the metabolism of proteins and formation of red blood cells, helps the body use fats	Skin disorders, irritability, mental depression
	Vitamin B12	Eggs, milk, liver, beef, shellfish	Maintains normal function of the nervous system and is required for the formation of red blood cells	None reported
	Folacin	Dark green leafy vegetables, wheat germ, beans and peas	Works with B12 to produce hemoglobin; useful in DNA synthesis	Reduction of zinc absorption; possible kidney damage
	Vitamin C	Broccoli, spinach, citrus fruits, tomatoes, potatoes, peppers, other fruits and vegetables	Promotes healthy gums, capillaries, teeth, aids in absorption of iron, aids in healing wounds	Diarrhea, abdominal cramps, kidney stones, stomach ulcers from digesting supplements in pill form

Source: Food and Nutrition Board, National Academy of Sciences—National Research Council. *Recommended dietary allowances.* Washington, D.C.: U.S. Government Printing Office, 1989.

meets another free radical, at which time the two become stable, or a free radical meets an **antioxidant.** Today, there is increasing interest in vitamins A, E, and C, which are capable of acting as antioxidants. In short, antioxidants can prevent or slow down the chain of free radicals long enough for two free radicals to meet. It is believed that without antioxidants, a buildup of free radicals may accumulate and cause tissue damage and destruction.

Special antioxidant vitamin supplements are now available over the counter; however, the research that evaluated the beneficial effects of diets high in these vitamins evaluated the health of people who ate a variety of *foods* high in these vitamins, not the diets of those who took vitamin supplements. Therefore, it is not known whether the supposed benefits of antioxidants come from the vitamins themselves or from the foods in which the vitamins are found. The health-promoting benefits of supplementation with extra amounts of vitamins A, E, and C are at best obscure. Moderation in all things should be the guiding force behind all dietary modifications. A diet high in fruits and vegetables not only follows the recommendations of the food pyramid, but also may provide a proven safe level of the antioxidants.

MINERALS

You will recall that vitamins were primarily involved in activating chemical processes in the body without becoming assimilated into the final product of the processes. Minerals perform some of the same types of functions, except that they do become incorporated within the chemical structures of many of the products and reactants produced by the various chemical processes and thus require continual replenishment. Minerals provide internal structure in teeth and bones. They are extremely important in muscular contraction, neural activity, and maintaining heart rhythm and acid-base balance of the body, and are vital components of enzymes and hormones that control metabolic processes. Many of the reactions needed to break down fats, proteins, and carbohydrates are entirely dependent on minerals.

Most people pay little attention to their consumption of the proper amounts of minerals. Fortunately, deficiencies of most minerals are rare. Minerals are classified according to the amounts found in our bodies. Those present in the body in large quantities (more than 5 grams) and that have known physiological functions are called *macrominerals.* Some minerals are needed in quantities of less than 100 mg a day. These are called *trace minerals.* (See Table 6.6.)

Macrominerals, which can be found in water, soil, and most plant foods, account for 60 to 80 percent of all inorganic material in the human body. These include calcium chloride, magnesium, phosphorus, potassium, sodium, and sulfur. Owing to the relative abundance of minerals in foods and the fact that people need only small quantities of minerals, illnesses and diseases due to

TABLE 6.6 ■ Classification of Macro and Trace Minerals	
Macro	**Trace**
Calcium	Arsenic
Chloride	Boron
Magnesium	Chromium
Phosphorus	Cobalt
Potassium	Copper
Sodium	Fluoride
Sulfur	Iodine
	Iron
	Manganese
	Molybdenum
	Nickel
	Selenium
	Silicon
	Vanadium
	Zinc

mineral deficiencies are rare. Only a few threats to overall health are related to mineral deficiencies or excesses. The only macrominerals that may pose serious threats to health and wellness are calcium, iron, and sodium. (See Table 6.7.)

Calcium

Calcium provides the primary structural support for bone. The quantity in which it is laid down as bone determines to a large extent how strong the bone will be. The RDA for adolescents and young adults is 1,200 mg of calcium, which is about the amount in four 8-ounce glasses of milk. More than 75 percent of adults consume less than the daily requirements, and about 25 percent of all women in the United States consume less than 300 mg of calcium on any given day.[8] When there is a lack of dietary calcium, the body draws on its calcium reserves found in bone. With time, the condition of **osteoporosis** may set in as the bone loses its mineral mass and becomes progressively brittle and porous.

One out of three women over fifty will eventually suffer a vertebral fracture, which can cause the spine to collapse and lead to a loss of height as well as stooped posture. Thinning of the bones also causes more than 300,000 hip fractures a year, making an older woman's risk for a debilitating bone break in the upper leg equal to the risk of breast, uterine, and ovarian cancer combined. Osteoporosis afflicts twenty-four million Americans and is responsible for one and a half million bone fractures annually. This figure is expected to double in just twenty-five years because of the aging of the population.

Prevention of osteoporosis is easily accomplished if a few relatively simple lifestyles are adopted early in life.

TABLE 6.7 ■ Common Minerals: A Brief Overview

Mineral	Common Sources	Why Your Body Needs It
Calcium	Milk and milk products, fortified orange juice, green leafy vegetables	Maintains teeth and bones, aids in blood clotting, nerve impulse, and muscle contraction
Phosphorus	Milk, cheese, cereal, legumes, meats	Required for bone and teeth formation; regulates the release of energy
Potassium	Meats, milk, fruits, vegetables, grains, legumes	Promotes regular heartbeat, aids in muscle contraction, controls water balance
Sodium	Salt	Helps regulate blood pressure and water balance
Fluorine (trace)	Water containing fluoride, fish, tea	Aids in the formation of solid bone and teeth
Iodine (trace)	Iodized salt, seafood, sea salt	Helps the thyroid function properly and maintains normal body metabolism
Iron (trace)	Red meats, egg yolks, legumes, nuts, dried fruits, enriched grain products	Forms part of hemoglobin, which carries oxygen to the tissues
Zinc (trace)	Meat, poultry, eggs, milk, whole grains	Helps in synthesis of proteins, RNA, and DNA

Source: U.S. Department of Agriculture. *The hassle-free guide to a better diet.* Washington, D.C.: U.S. Government Printing Office, 1980.

From birth to around age thirty-five the body deposits bone mass in quantities determined by a number of lifestyle factors such as diet, smoking, exercise, alcohol consumption, and other nonmodifiable factors. After this age, no further deposition is possible; in fact, bone mass gradually decreases over time. If the amount of bone mass is sufficiently large when it peaks at age thirty-five, the gradual loss of bone mineral in subsequent years will not be enough to cause osteoporosis. In short, the years before the age of thirty-five are critical to the prevention of osteoporosis. Women older than thirty five can only slow the rate at which bone mass is lost, thus delaying the onset of osteoporosis.

Prevention and Treatment of Osteoporosis

Much of the risk of osteoporosis is preventable. There are three main methods currently being used to treat and prevent the disease. The first is exercise. The force that muscle imparts on bone during contraction has been shown to stimulate the deposition of bone mineral. This relationship was noted several years ago when the bone density of the right and left arms of tennis players were compared. The bone mass of the right arms of right-handed tennis players had significantly more bone mass

than did the left arms of the same people. Subsequent research has shown that any weight-bearing exercise can increase bone mass in persons under the age of thirty-five and help maintain bone mass in persons over age thirty-five.

Weight-bearing activities are those types of physical activities that require participants to support and transfer their own body weight. Walking, jogging, weight training, and most other physical activities except swimming and bicycling require the participant to resist gravity and support body weight. The physical force placed upon the bones is the main cause of the bone deposition.

It may surprise you to learn that too much exercise can also lead to bone loss and osteoporosis. Among women athletes who train intensely and reduce their body mass and body fat to the point that the normal menstrual cycle ceases, there is a significant decrease in the hormone estrogen, which is associated with decreases in bone density. Without estrogen, any positive effects of weight-bearing activities are negated. Many women athletes are in their bone-forming years, when the deposition of bone mass should proceed without impedance. Typically, when the intensity of the activity is reduced and body fat levels return to more normal levels, the menstrual cycle and calcium metabolism return

Osteoporosis Fact and Fallacy

Myth: Although osteoporosis can cause a great deal of pain and disability, it won't kill you.

Fact: As many as 20 percent of all people who suffer a hip fracture die within a year, usually because of complications such as pneumonia or blood clots in the lung that are related either to the fracture itself or to being confined to bed.

Myth: Osteoporosis in men is extremely rare.

Fact: No one will argue about osteoporosis being largely a woman's disease. Women lay down 10 to 25 percent less bone on their skeletons than men during their early development and are therefore more prone to fractures when they lose bone as a natural consequence of aging. With the average life span for men increasing, the incidence of osteoporosis in men is expected to rise, currently one out of five osteoporosis victims is male.

Myth: You finish building bone when you stop growing (for most people, at about age eighteen).

Fact: More and more evidence has been coming to light that you can continue to add bone mass to your skeleton until your thirties.

Myth: Since the calcium in calcium-fortified foods like certain brands of orange juice and cereal does not occur in those foods naturally, it is not very well absorbed.

Fact: The calcium in foods like juice and cereal might not necessarily be as well absorbed as the calcium in, say, milk, but those foods are still reasonable sources of the mineral.

Laboratory-produced calcium carbonate pills (or antacids like Tums that contain calcium carbonate) are among the most concentrated sources of calcium.

Myth: Since menopause dramatically increases the rate at which women lose bone mass, all women who have stopped menstruating should be consuming more calcium than the rest of the population.

Fact: The loss of bone is sped up dramatically for the first five to ten years after the onset of menopause because of a dramatic decrease in estrogen, a hormone that improves calcium absorption and reduces the amount of calcium excreted in the urine. Thus all women not on estrogen replacement therapy are advised by the National Osteoporosis Foundation to up their daily calcium intake goal by 50 percent from 1,000 to 1,500 milligrams. But for women who are on estrogen replacement therapy, 1,000 milligrams of calcium a day is considered enough.

Myth: There are few known risk factors for osteoporosis.

Fact: There are many risk factors for the disease such as early menopause (before age forty-five), insufficient exercise, a thin, small body frame, European or Asian background (people of African descent are less likely to suffer from the condition), and taking medications that can impact negatively on bone mass (such as thyroid medication or high doses of cortisone-like drugs).

Courtesy of National Dairy Council®.

---

to normal. But levels of bone mass may never be as high as they could have been.

A second method to treat and prevent osteoporosis is the consumption of adequate dietary calcium. Both calcium that comes naturally from foods and calcium from supplements can be very beneficial. The RDA of calcium for college-age adults is 1,200 mg for both men and women. More recent findings lean toward raising the RDA for calcium from 1,200 mg to 1,500 mg for women who are postmenopausal. It is not difficult to attain the required amount of dietary calcium if careful planning and proper food selection are practiced. Adequate supplies of vitamin D assist the metabolism of calcium, whereas excessive consumption of meat, alcohol, coffee, and salt and the use of tobacco can greatly reduce the body's ability to absorb calcium. In these cases, even if there is sufficient dietary calcium, the body may still be deficient for failing to successfully absorb what is available.

The third and most effective method of treating and preventing osteoporosis in women is the use of estrogen in hormone replacement therapy. Women who have had their ovaries removed or who are postmenopausal no longer produce enough estrogen to protect against bone mineral depletion.

Iron

Although iron is the most abundant trace mineral, 30 to 50 percent of women fail to consume sufficient quantities. Lack of dietary iron, failure to absorb the iron that has been consumed, and regular menstrual bleeding are the main reasons why women can be iron deficient. Much of the body's iron supply is lost due to bleeding. In athletes, some iron is rendered unusable when red blood cells are destroyed by becoming crushed in the tissues of the feet after sustained jogging or jumping on hard surfaces. The destroyed blood cells are excreted through the urine; a small amount of iron can also be lost through sweat.

Iron plays a vital role in the oxygen-carrying capacity of the blood and muscles. Hemoglobin, a protein found in the red blood cells that carry oxygen, requires 80 percent of the body's supply of iron. Short-term deficiencies of iron are not detrimental because the body has some limited supplies of iron reserves. However, when a recurring deficit of iron continues for an extended period of time, all iron reserves and hemoglobin become depleted, reducing the oxygen-carrying capacity of the blood.

Women with low levels of iron may suffer from *iron deficiency anemia.* Low iron levels decrease the amount of functioning hemoglobin, which diminishes the oxygen content of the blood. General sluggishness, loss of appetite, susceptibility to infection, shortened attention span, impaired learning abilities, and a reduced capacity for sustaining even mild exercise are symptoms of iron deficiency anemia.

Iron is found in two forms, one coming from plants and the other from animal sources. Only 2 to 10 percent of the iron that comes from plant foods is absorbed by the body, whereas 10 to 35 percent of the iron derived from animal foods is absorbed. The RDA for iron takes into consideration the different absorption rates of the two forms of iron. Even though the RDA for iron should be sufficient for most individuals, many women fail to consume adequate amounts. To make matters worse, diets that include excessive caffeine may further reduce the amount of iron that is absorbed. Men and women require 10 and 15 milligrams of iron respectively. Red kidney beans, vegetables, Cream of Wheat, and all lean beef products are good sources of iron. Those who do not consume adequate amounts of iron from food may want to take a daily iron supplement. The nutrition assessment lab at the end of this chapter will assist you in determining whether or not you should take a calcium or iron supplement.

Sodium

The mineral sodium has been given special attention ever since it was implicated as one of the major causes of some forms of hypertension (high blood pressure). Recommended daily levels of sodium consumption range from 1,100 to 3,000 milligrams a day. Salt contains about 40 percent sodium by weight, so that a teaspoon of salt includes 2,000 milligrams of sodium, about the right amount a person should consume each day. The typical diet, however, contains two to three times this amount. The known serious side effects of consuming large amounts of sodium include those diseases caused by hypertension, including strokes, and heart and kidney disease.

Only 5 to 10 percent of people are salt-sensitive, meaning that high amounts of dietary sodium can be responsible for elevated levels of blood pressure. It is difficult to determine who is sensitive, so experts suggest that because virtually all Americans consume excessive sodium, encouraging the reduction of sodium by the entire population will include those 5 to 10 percent of individuals who are adversely affected by it.

Most of the sodium we consume can be found in processed foods. Canned soup, cheese, chips, dried or smoked meats, prepared vegetables, pickles, and even chocolate pudding contain large amounts of sodium. One bacon, egg, and cheese biscuit contains 1,215 milligrams—the recommended intake for an entire day.

Most fast foods have large amounts of salt added to them before they ever reach the table. High sodium levels are further increased when table salt is added. Following are some basic guidelines for reducing the amount of sodium you consume.

Don't salt food before tasting it.

Use very little table salt or none at all.

Try seasoning foods with sodium-free spices such as pepper, allspice, and garlic.

Processed foods have the highest amounts of sodium—try to eat natural foods instead.

Avoid smoked meats, including bacon, sausage, and ham.

Reduce intake of canned and instant soups or look for low-sodium varieties.

Read labels of all foods for sodium content and choose low-sodium products.

WATER: THE MOST VITAL NUTRIENT

All of the metabolic processes of the body are conducted in an environment that contains water. Our bodies are about 60 percent water by weight and use water for a variety of functions. This nutrient found inside and around all tissues provides the main ingredient of the various body fluids. Blood and lymph, which are vital parts of the circulatory and immune systems, are dependent on a constant supply of water. All of the freely movable joints are surrounded by a water-based, synovial fluid that acts as a lubrication to reduce friction between bones. Water is also important in the digestion of food, removal of wastes, sensation of balance and movement, and control of body temperature.

Without water, the systems of the body can stop functioning in just one or two days, depending on weather conditions. Therefore, it is important to provide our bodies with a constant supply of water. Much of the water we obtain comes from fluids we drink and the foods we eat. Fruits contain up to 80 percent water, whereas foods such as bread, cheese, meats, vegetables, and butter contain lesser amounts. Some of the by-products of the metabolism of foods are carbon dioxide and water. For example, the breakdown of 100 grams of fat, proteins, and carbohydrates produces 107, 100, and 55 grams of water, respectively. This is not nearly enough water to supply the body with adequate amounts.

Water is lost through sweat, urine, feces, and evaporation in the lungs. To maintain a proper balance between water loss and water need, a good rule to remember is to drink eight cups of fluid a day. This will, of course, vary according to a person's body size, the temperature, and the amount of exercise a person is doing.

During periods of decreasing water levels, we thirst. Thirst is a good indicator of the need for additional water. However, under conditions of vigorous exercise or illness, thirst may not accurately represent our body's actual water needs, and special efforts should be made to ensure that larger than normal quantities of water are consumed. In hot and humid climates, conditions such as heat stroke and heat exhaustion are more common; many people do not realize that their need for water can be five to six times greater than normal under such conditions. Exercising in these environments can further increase water demands. Maintaining proper water balance is relatively quick and easy to do if fluids are consumed regularly throughout the day.

CURRENT TRENDS IN EATING

Americans have become accustomed to being on the move and spending their time and energies in areas other than preparing and serving food. Why slave over a hot stove to cook a nice dinner and then have to wash the dishes when a complete meal with all the trimmings can be delivered to your home with just one quick phone call? We have drive-through windows, twenty-minute deliveries, microwaveable foods, and instant everything.Much of the tendency toward quick meals and eating out may be attributed to the increase in the number of two-income homes. When both parents work full time, there is less time and energy for meal preparation. Two major eating trends have developed over the past years: consumption of more fast foods and increased snacking.

Fast Food

One out of every five Americans eats at a fast-food restaurant daily, and from 1970 to 1980 the number of fast-food outlets more than quadrupled. Fewer and fewer families sit down together and have meals at home.[9,10] The nutritional value of diets containing a large proportion of fast foods has come under close scrutiny from nutrition experts. Their concerns focus on the high amounts of fat, sodium, and protein and the low levels of fiber and complex carbohydrates.

Much of the success of fast-food establishments is based upon the taste, price, and atmosphere the restaurant can provide. Fast food is fun and tasty and doesn't require any preparation or dish washing.

Foods that taste good sell. As children we learn to eat according to our tastes and don't start making health-related food choices until later in life. Because we tend to eat according to taste, most fast foods contain large amounts of fat and sodium. One extra crispy chicken wing is 66 percent fat. The typical fast-food meal of a cheeseburger, fries, and shake contains over 1,200 calories and consists of about 45 percent fat.

Is it possible to get a nutritionally balanced meal from fast food? Yes, but it takes some effort. Because of customer demand, most restaurants now serve a wider variety of foods, including whole-wheat bread and rolls,

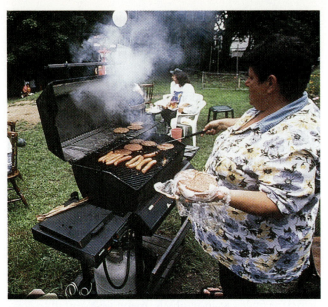
Traditional eating habits often mean foods high in fat.

lower-fat meats, low-fat milk products, salads, pasta, and plain baked potatoes. It is becoming increasingly clear to customers that what they want is what they get. If everyone stopped eating triple-patty bacon-cheeseburgers, restaurants would stop serving them.

Selecting appropriate foods is the only way to get a balanced diet from fast food. Eating an occasional high-fat fast-food meal will not result in an improper diet. However, regularly eating doughnuts for breakfast, a taco and onion rings for lunch, and pizza for dinner is not a wise idea. To help you make healthy fast-food choices, nutritional tables of the foods served by several of the most popular fast-food restaurants are included in Appendix B. Look closely at the foods you eat and try to choose healthier items the next time you have fast food.

Snacking

We consume more of our calories between meals than ever before. Smaller, more frequent meals are replacing the traditional three meals a day. Eating small amounts of food many times throughout the day poses no threats to health if we make wise food choices. The problem with snacking is that the nutritional quality of the most common snack items is very low. On the other hand, a diet that consists of three large, nutritionally poor meals is just as bad as spending the entire day nibbling on the more popular snack foods. Many popular candy bars have over 250 calories and are over 40 percent fat. None of the most popular snack foods would qualify as a healthy snack, but they sure taste good.

The important thing to remember is that our health is based on the amount of nutrients eaten in a whole day. A high-fat snack in the afternoon will make little difference nutritionally if the rest of a daily diet is balanced and full of nutrient-dense low-fat foods. So go ahead, have a snack. Just be sure to control the overall quality of your diet.

FOOD LABELS: TRUTH AND DECEPTION

The FDA now requires all food manufacturers to provide easy-to-understand nutritional information labels on products to which one or more additional nutrients have been added, or for which some nutritional claim has been made.[11] These labels contain information about the number of servings per container, calories per serving, grams of carbohydrate, fat, and protein, and additional information on the percentage of the RDA of seven other essential vitamins and minerals. The purpose of the labels is to provide consumers with enough information so that healthy food choices can be made.

With a few exceptions because of size or food type, food packages must, by law, show how their product will fit into a 2,000-calorie food plan that includes no more than 65 grams of fat, which is around 30 percent of the total calories. Figure 6.2 shows an example of the food labels.

One of the terms used on these labels is Daily Values, which is a combination of Daily Reference Values and Recommended Daily Intakes. The bottom section of the labels shows how much fat, saturated fat, cholesterol, sodium, carbohydrates, and fiber that persons who consume about 2,000 and 2,500 calories a day ought to consume. For example, a college-age woman who consumes around 2,000 calories a day should consume less than 65 grams of fat per day. The top of the label shows the same nutrients except that the percentages listed represent how much of the total daily amount a serving of that food can provide. Figure 6.2 has some additional information to assist you in understanding the nutritional information listed on the labels.

A simple rule to remember is that 1 gram of fat contains 9 calories. The grams of fat are listed on all food products. By multiplying the number of fat grams by 9 and dividing this number by the total calories per serving you get the total percent of fat calories for the food. For example, if a food label lists a total of 100 calories per serving and there are 6 grams of fat in each serving, you can determine the percent of calories that come from fat by multiplying 6 (grams of fat) times 9. This equals 54 calories of fat. Fifty-four divided by the total calories per serving (100) equals 0.54 or 54 percent. Any food that is 54 percent fat should either be avoided or be used very sparingly.

Food labels also include claims from manufacturers about the various health promotion qualities of the product. In the past, these words were not regulated so that any food could claim to reduce heart disease or be new and improved or lite. The FDA has stepped in to help protect the consumer. Following is a list of the more

---

Serving Size

Is your serving the same size as the one on the label? If you eat double the serving size listed, you need to double the nutrient and calorie values. If you eat one-half the serving size shown here, cut the nutrient and calorie values in half.

Calories

Are you overweight? Cut back a little on calories! Look here to see how a serving of the food adds to your daily total. A 5'4", 138-lb. active woman needs about 2,200 calories each day. A 5'10", 174-lb. active man needs about 2,900. How about you?

Total Carbohydrate

When you cut down on fat, you can eat more carbohydrates. Carbohydrates are in foods like bread, potatoes, fruits and vegetables. Choose these often! They give you more nutrients than **sugars** like soda pop and candy.

Dietary Fiber

Grandmother called it "roughage," but her advice to eat more is still up-to-date! That goes for both soluble and insoluble kinds of dietary fiber. Fruits, vegetables, whole-grain foods, beans and peas are all good sources and can help reduce the risk of heart disease and cancer.

Protein

Most Americans get more protein than they need. Where there is animal protein, there is also fat and cholesterol. Eat small servings of lean meat, fish and poultry. Use skim or low-fat milk, yogurt, and cheese. Try vegetable proteins like beans, grains and cereals.

Vitamins & Minerals

Your goal here is 100% of each for the day. Don't count on one food to do it all. Let a combination of foods add up to a winning score.

Nutrition Facts

Serving Size 1/2 cup (114g)
Servings Per Container 4

Amount Per Serving

Calories 90 　　　Calories from Fat 30

　　　　　　　　　　　　　　% Daily value*

Total Fat 3g	**5%**
Saturated Fat 0g	**0%**
Cholesterol 0mg	**0%**
Sodium 300mg	**13%**
Total Carbohydrate 13g	**4%**
Dietary Fiber 3g	**12%**
Sugars 3g	
Protein 3g	

Vitamin A	80%	• Vitamin C	60%
Calcium	4%	• Iron	4%

*Percent Daily Values are based on a 2,000 calorie diet. Your daily values may be higher or lower depending on your calorie needs:

		Calories	2,000	2,500
Total Fat	Less than		65g	80g
Sat Fat	Less than		20g	25g
Cholesterol	Less than		300mg	300 mg
Sodium	Less than		2,400mg	2,400 mg
Total Carbohydrate			300g	375g
Fiber			25g	30g

Calories per gram:
Fat 9 • Carbohydrate 4 • Protein 4

More nutrients may be listed on some labels.

Total Fat

Aim low: Most people need to cut back on fat! Too much fat may contribute to heart disease and cancer. Try to limit your **calories from fat**. For a healthy heart, choose foods with a big difference between the total number of calories and the number of calories from fat.

Saturated Fat

A new kind of fat? No — saturated fat is part of the total fat in food. It is listed separately because it's the key player in raising blood cholesterol and your risk of heart disease. Eat less!

Cholesterol

Too much cholesterol — a second cousin to fat — can lead to heart disease. Challenge yourself to eat less than 300 mg each day.

Sodium

You call it "salt," the label calls it "sodium." Either way, it may add up to high blood pressure in some people. So, keep your sodium intake low — 2,400 to 3,000 mg or less each day.*

*The AHA recommends no more than 3,000 mg sodium per day for healthy adults

Daily Value

Feel like you're drowning in numbers? Let the Daily Value be your guide. Daily Values are listed for people who eat 2,000 or 2,500 calories each day. If you eat more, your personal daily value may be higher than what's listed on the label. If you eat less, your personal daily value may be lower.

For fat, saturated fat, cholesterol and sodium choose foods with a low % **Daily Value**. For total carbohydrate, dietary fiber, vitamins and minerals, your daily value goal is to reach 100% of each.

g = grams (About 28 g = 1 ounce)
mg = milligrams (1,000 mg = 1 g)

FIGURE 6.2　How to read food labels. (Food and Drug Administration. *How to read the new food label*, 1993.)

common claims and the conditions the FDA has required producers to comply with in order to use the words. These terms now appear on foods. Here are some of the meanings:[12]

More:	Has 10 percent more of Daily Reference Values (DRV) or Reference Daily Intakes (RDI) in reference to protein, vitamins, minerals, dietary fiber, or potassium; has 4 percent more of DRV in reference to complex carbohydrate or unsaturated fat.
Free:	Product contains little or no fat, saturated fat, calories, sugar, cholesterol, or sodium.
Low:	May be used on foods that can be eaten frequently without a person's exceeding the dietary guidelines:

Low fat: 3 grams or fewer per serving.

Low saturated fat: 1 gram or less per serving.

Low sodium: 140 milligrams or less per serving.

Very low sodium: fewer than 35 milligrams per serving.

Low cholesterol: no more than 20 milligrams per serving.

Low calorie: no more than 40 calories per serving.

Less:	Contains at least 25 percent less sodium, calories, fat, saturated fat, or cholesterol than the original product.
Reduced:	Contains at least 50 percent less sodium, fat, saturated fat, or cholesterol than the original product.
Lean:	Provides fewer than 10 grams of fat, fewer than 4 grams of saturated fat, and fewer than 95 milligrams of cholesterol per serving.
Extra lean:	Provides fewer than 5 grams of fat, fewer than 2 grams of saturated fat, and fewer than 95 milligrams of cholesterol per serving.
Light/lite reduction:	Contains 33.3 percent fewer calories and a minimum reduction of more than 40 calories per serving; if more than 50 percent of calories come from fat, fat must be reduced by at least 50 percent.

Additional Terms

Source of:	Provides at least 10 to 19 percent of the daily value for a particular nutrient.
Enriched:	Some of the nutrients lost in food processing have been added back into the product.
Imitation:	If a food does not meet FDA standards of identity, or if it is not as nutritious as the

product it resembles or is a substitute for, it must be labeled "imitation." Substitute products that are not nutritionally inferior do not have to carry this label.

Percent fat free:	These foods must be low fat or fat free to begin with. This is the percentage of the food's weight that is fat free.

Food manufacturers are required to list all of the ingredients included in the product. These items are listed in order, with the ingredient making up the largest percentage of the product being listed first. You may have noticed that many of the ingredients on processed food labels look as if they belong on a chemistry exam. There are thousands of artificial additives in the foods we eat.

OPTIMAL NUTRITION FOR EXERCISE

Optimal nutrition is defined as having a diet that contains enough nutrients for tissue repair, maintenance, and growth without an excess of energy intake. Everyone should get optimal nutrition, but there is no "one" diet that is optimal for everybody. For individuals who participate in long-duration physical activities or who compete in athletic competition, basic nutritional needs are essentially the same as those of nonathletes. But depending on the sport and the duration of the activity, some athletes may need to alter their diets to provide additional nutrients.

For example, those individuals who participate in endurance physical activities such as jogging, cycling, hiking, and swimming must replenish energy stores with carbohydrates. Energy for activity is stored as glucose in the bloodstream and glycogen in muscles and the liver. When activity is prolonged, these stores are gradually depleted until all available glucose and glycogen is depleted.

Endurance athletes call this "hitting the wall." Fatigue sets in, performance decreases, and the athlete experiences weakness and dizziness. In extreme cases a person can collapse and even slip into a coma. To prevent this from happening during training and competition, athletes practice **carbohydrate loading.** This consists of gradually reducing the amount of physical activity four days before the event and consuming a diet of at least 70 percent carbohydrates. When activity has been reduced and large amounts of glucose are entering the bloodstream, the body tends to overcompensate the amount of glucose that should be metabolized so that two to three times the normal amount of glucose is stored.

All this energy cannot help a person go any faster than normal, but it can help an athlete maintain a level of intensity for a longer period, which results in faster overall times. Carbohydrate loading is only recommended for persons participating in high-intensity endurance activities that last a minimum of eighty minutes and are continuous.[13]

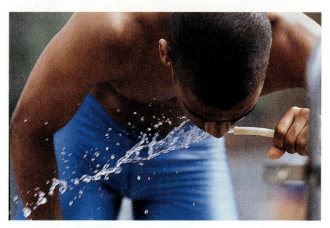

Water is one of our body's most vital nutrients, particularly for people with active lifestyles.

Consumption of adequate amounts of water is also critical to having an active lifestyle. In hot weather, an athlete can lose 2 to 3 liters of sweat an hour, all of which must be replaced. Despite the advertising and marketing claims of the makers of the various sports drinks, they provide no advantage over consumption of water for the person who needs fluid replacement. In cases of long-term exercise such as long-distance running and cycling, however, there may be some benefit from drinking a fluid that contains some glucose and minerals. The glucose may be used for additional energy during the long hours of energy expenditure, and the added minerals may help by speeding up the absorption of the water. Normally, however, a balanced diet contains all of the minerals needed for any form of physical activity.

There is little research that demonstrates the need for extra protein, amino acids, or powder protein drinks for persons doing resistance-type training (weightlifting). Again, a balanced diet will provide adequate nutrition for all activities.

GUIDELINES FOR HEALTHY EATING

In 1989, the U.S. Department of Agriculture and the Department of Health and Human Services gathered the best-known nutrition experts to produce a set of dietary guidelines that summarized all the current nutrition information. By following these guidelines, you will attain optimal nutrition and reduce the risk of several diseases.

1. **Eat a variety of foods.** Use the six food groups found on the food pyramid as a guide, and choose the appropriate number of servings from each group.

2. **Maintain a healthy body weight.** Excess body weight increases the risk for diabetes, heart disease, cancer, and other diseases. Weight loss should not exceed 2 pounds a week. Proper weight loss must

include two components: (a) some reduction in the number of calories consumed, and (b) an increase in the amount of energy expended in endurance-type physical activity.

3. **Consume a diet low in fat, saturated fat, and cholesterol.** Heart disease and some cancers are related to diets high in fat. Saturated fats and cholesterol are specifically linked to increased risk of heart disease. Recommended levels of saturated fat are only 10 percent of daily caloric intake, and cholesterol consumption should not exceed 300 milligrams a day (one egg has 250 milligrams).

4. **Eat plenty of vegetables, fruits, and grain products.** These foods contain fiber, vitamins, and minerals and are low in fat and high in complex carbohydrates. They help reduce our risk of various types of cancer.

5. **Use sugars in moderation.** This guideline suggests our need for more complex carbohydrates and fewer simple sugars. Rather than consume the average amount of sugar (54 pounds per year), we should eat only about one-third that amount. The rest of our carbohydrates should come from complex carbohydrates.

6. **Use salt and sodium in moderation.** To help reduce the risk of high blood pressure, many Americans could benefit by cutting back on the amount of sodium they consume.

7. **If you drink alcohol, do so in moderation.** Alcohol can be addictive and is related to many health problems, not to mention its detrimental effects on society. It is associated with various forms of cancer and with accidents. Moderation means no more than two drinks a day for men and no more than one drink a day for women (women cannot metabolize alcohol as easily as men).

MAKING LONG-TERM DIETARY CHANGES

Assessment

The first step to attaining optimal nutrition is to evaluate your current nutritional status. A nutrition assessment provides you with information about the healthy and "not so healthy" aspects of your diet.

Lab 6.2 is a complete three-day diet analysis. You can calculate it by hand or use nutritional computer software. The assessment should be completed before you decide what aspect of your diet to modify. From the assessment you will be able to determine whether each of the foods from the different levels of the food pyramid were represented in your diet and how many servings of each you consumed. Were the total calories from fat less than 30 percent? Do you eat enough fiber and drink enough water? The assessment will also provide you with information about sugar and sodium intake as well as alcohol consumption.

From the analysis you will likely discover that your diet meets the recommended requirements for at least some of the nutrients. Identify those areas of your diet where you may need to improve and list them in order of their importance to you. It may be helpful to review the last section of Chapter 1, which includes various methods that can be used to modify behavior. These methods apply to dietary interventions as well. Then find the stage of readiness to change that best describes you and complete the corresponding questions at the end of the chapter.

Your Plan of Action

It is not enough to know that you should make dietary changes. Your nutrition knowledge must be put into action and your daily diet should represent a balanced approach to healthy eating. When altering your diet, keep in mind the following suggestions.

Don't try to do too much at one time. The smaller the change, the longer it is likely to last. Rather than reconstructing your entire diet, select one small portion of your diet that needs modifying and focus your efforts on changing just that part, allowing yourself time to adjust your tastes and habits. Make changes gradually. A good example of this concept is a process that can be used to switch from drinking whole milk to 1 percent or skim milk. Instead of switching straight from whole to skim, try 2 percent for a while, or mix a half gallon of whole with a half gallon of 2 percent until you have grown accustomed to the taste. Then move from 2 percent to 1 percent to skim. This may take weeks to accomplish, but the change will likely be permanent.

Plan ahead for the foods you will eat. Home is the best place to effectively alter eating habits. By planning menus, preparing shopping lists, making extra for another meal, and cooking in advance, many of the last-minute "what should I eat?" decisions can be made properly.

Dine out wisely. Maintaining healthy eating behaviors is much more difficult in restaurants. Serving sizes are larger and you don't always have control over the way your food is cooked. Butter comes in mounds, salad dressings are used liberally, and it is often very difficult to determine just how much fat a food might have. Ask questions about how foods are cooked and how they will be served. Most restaurants will be eager to meet your requests. Ask that salad dressing be served on the side so that you can measure the amount you want. Cheese, mayonnaise, butter, and gravy should also be served separately so you can avoid them or use them sparingly. Carefully select foods that will provide a balanced meal. Avoid fried foods and fatty meats.

One good strategy is to limit the number of times you eat out at restaurants. If you must eat out, make sure

the other meals of the day are low in fat so that you can compensate for having a high-fat restaurant meal. Pass on the steak and fried potatoes and choose a meal that contains less fat. All these little food choices make a large difference in the amount of fat eaten at restaurants.

Ethnic restaurants provide an intriguing variety of foods. However, you must choose carefully here as well. A taco salad with all the fixings has as much fat as ten glazed doughnuts. If you think the food you are eating must contain a lot of fat, you are probably right. Select foods that are not fried or sautéed in oils. If you do not know enough about a food to determine whether it is high in fat, ask your server what it contains and how it will be prepared.

Analyze your favorite dishes. You don't have to abstain from your favorite dishes. Instead, reduce the amount or the number of servings or substitute your favorite for a low-fat brand. For example, low-fat or nonfat ice creams and frozen yogurts are growing in popularity and make great desserts.

SUMMARY

Ideal nutrition is clearly related to good health and reduced disease; unfortunately, the overall quality of the typical American diet is far from ideal. Taste preferences and tradition are but a few reasons why the typical daily consumption of fats and simple sugars is too high and that of fruits and vegetables is too low. Some individuals also struggle to get the proper amounts of calcium, iron, and sodium. Although research continues to refine our knowledge of proper nutrition, consumers should be cautious when making food and supplement selections based on claims of big benefits. Sound advice would be to use the food pyramid as your guide to a healthy diet.

SUGGESTED READING

Ballentine, C. L. Hunger is more than an empty stomach. *FDA Consumer,* February 1984.

Belasco, W. J. *Appetite for change.* New York: Pantheon, 1989.

Brody, J. *Jane Brody's nutrition book.* New York: Bantam, 1987.

Connor, S., and W. Connon. *The new American diet.* New York: Simon and Schuster, 1989.

Donkersloot, M. *The fast food diet: Quick and healthy eating at home and on the go.* New York: Simon and Schuster, 1991.

Garrison, R. H., and E. Somer. *The nutrition desk reference,* rev. ed. New Canaan, CT: Keats Publishing, 1990.

Jacobson, M. F., L. Y. Lefferts, and A. W. Garland. *Safe food: Eating wisely in a risky world.* Los Angeles: Living Planet Press, 1991.

Behavioral Lab 6.1

What Can I Do?

The following lab is designed to help you make healthy eating a part of your everyday life. At the beginning of this chapter, you determined your stage of readiness to change to a healthy diet. Now complete the corresponding section of this lab: precontemplator, contemplator, preparer, action taker, or maintainer.

Precontemplator

1. Try to identify the main reasons you are against eating or not motivated to eat healthy foods. For some ideas, refer to the barriers listed in the Barrier Busters on page 155.

2. Can you think of any reasons why establishing a healthy diet would be good for you? If necessary, review this chapter for ideas.

3. If you have done any nutrition assessments, do the results support a need for change?

4. Do your answers in items 2 and 3 outweigh your answers in item 1?

5. Can you use any of the Barrier Busters in this chapter to eliminate the items you listed in item 1?

6. In your opinion, which of your barriers is the biggest one to overcome? Why?

7. Of all the benefits of a healthy diet, which one appeals to you the most? Why?

8. If you were going to make one change to make your diet healthier, what would you do?

Contemplator

1. What are you thinking about doing to improve your diet?

2. How would your life be different if you did what you mentioned in item 1?

3. There are many reasons why changing your diet is hard to do. List as many of these barriers as you can. For example: I like the taste of high-fat foods.

4. Which of the barriers you named in item 3 is the hardest one for you to overcome?

5. What can you do differently to overcome this barrier?

6. Eating a healthy diet has many benefits. List some of them.

7. Which of the benefits you identified in item 6 appeals to you most? Why?

Preparer

1. What do you specifically want to accomplish? (For directions on goal setting, see Chapter 2.)

2. What foods are you currently eating that are part of a healthy diet?

3. List five of your favorite high-fat foods. List five low-fat foods you could use as substitutes.

4. List three ways you could cook differently to reduce the fat content in your diet.

5. What type of actions will accomplish the goal you identified in item 1?

6. What is the first step you need to take to accomplish your goal(s)?

7. What makes you think you can accomplish this first step? What makes you think you can accomplish your goal?

8. Complete the following statement:

   I am going to take my first step on _____ .

   date within 30 days

Action Taker

1. What are you currently doing to keep your diet low in fat and high in fruits and vegetables?

2. Are your nutrition goals specifically and clearly stated?

3. Are you keeping track of your progress?

If yes, how? For example, nutrition assessments, journal, log sheet. If no, would it help motivate you to keep a record of your progress?

4. Are you receiving support or rewards for your effort?

    If yes, what kind? If no, why not? And can you change this?

5. Do you think you will continue? Why?

6. If you were to stop, what do you think would be your major reason for stopping?

7. Is there a way to prevent this (item 6)?

8. How would you get yourself started again if you did stop?

Maintainer

1. How long have you maintained your proper nutrition program?

2. What are the top two reasons that make you want to continue?

3. Have you been tempted to stop? What tempted you?

4. If you have relapsed, list the reasons why you think you did and what you did to get back on track.

    Reasons: _____

    How I Got Back on Track: _____

5. Write down a few things you can do to prevent relapse in the future.

6. Are you at a level of healthy eating that you are happy with, or do you wish to continue to improve?

7. If you wish to improve your eating habits, how are you going to keep track of your improvement?

8. What kind of support do you get for your efforts? These may be some type of self-reward, internal reward, or external reward.

9. How have you changed or how have you changed the environment around you to accommodate a healthier lifestyle? (*Example:* I am careful when I shop for food or eat out. I eat more salads and I avoid fast-food restaurants.)

10. Is there anything else you need to promote your continued maintenance? For example, information, support, time management.

11. If you listed something in item 10, can you think of a way to attain it, or can you think of someone who can help you with it?

Name _____   Section   Date _____

Completing a Dietary Analysis

Nutrition Analysis by Hand

To complete this lab you will need a calculator, the food nutrition tables in Appendix B, and multiple copies of the following food tally chart.

We will analyze your diet over a three-day period. One of the three days should be a Saturday or Sunday, because most people eat differently on those days.

Step 1

Using the food tally chart, write down all the foods and the number of servings you eat during a consecutive three-day period. Include everything you eat. Remember to write it down as soon as possible; it's easy to forget. If the food you eat has a label, use it to record the information listed across the top of the tally chart. If your food does not have a label, use the food nutrition tables in Appendix B. For example, if you eat an orange, look up "orange" in the table and record the required information. If a food you eat is not on the table, find a food that is similar and use it instead. If you need more food tally charts, make a photocopy of the one in this book.

Step 2

Once your food tally chart is complete, add each column and record the total at the appropriate space on the bottom of the chart. Add the total grams of fat, carbohy-drates, and proteins. To determine what percentage of your diet comes from fat, you must convert total grams of fat to calories. To do this, multiply total grams of fat by 9 and divide by the total number of calories consumed. For example, if you ate a total of 310 grams of fat and consumed 6,800 calories in three days, the percentage of your total calories that came from fat would be

$$\frac{310 \text{ g} \times 9 \text{ cal/g}}{6800} = 41\%$$

Do the same to determine the total number of calories from saturated fat, carbohydrate, and protein. Remember that 1 gram of fat has 9 calories per gram, carbohydrate 4 calories per gram, and protein 4 calories per gram. For fiber, cholesterol, and sodium, simply sum the total number of grams or milligrams of each.

Step 3

The last row of the food tally chart shows the recommended total for each nutrient. Compare your results to what is recommended. Then return to the beginning of this chapter to complete the Where Am I? feature and learn more about how nutrition impacts wellness.

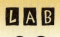

Food Tally Chart

Food	Servings	Calories	Protein (g)	Fat, total (g)	Saturated fat (g)	Carbohydrate (g)	Cholesterol (mg)	Sodium (mg)
Actual totals[a]			g / %	g / %	g / %	g / %		
Recommended totals			≤15%	≤30%	7–10%	≥55%	≤300 mg	≤3,000 mg

Date _____   Day: M T W Th F S S

[a]Total the values in each column. Protein and carbohydrate provide 4 calories per gram; fat provides 9 calories per gram. For example, if you consume a total of 270 grams of carbohydrate and 2,000 calories, your percentage of total calories from carbohydrate would be (270 g × 4 cal/g) ÷ 2,000 cal = 54%.

CHAPTER 7

Understanding Body Composition

Objectives

1. Understand the differences between lean body weight and fat weight.

2. Distinguish between essential and nonessential body fat.

3. Learn the dangers of obesity.

4. Comprehend the health risks associated with the different body shapes.

5. Learn how to measure and evaluate body shape and body fat.

6. Calculate ideal body weight.

Terms

- Essential fat
- Nonessential fat
- Amenorrhea
- Subcutaneous
- Percent body fat
- Lean body weight
- Obesity
- Overweight
- Android
- Gynoid
- Muscle wasting
- Body mass index

Your knowledge of body composition gained from this chapter will improve your understanding of how to control your body weight, the subject of Chapter 8. Because the material in these two chapters is so closely related, the Where Am I? and What Can I Do? features relevant to body composition are only presented in Chapter 8.

Next time you visit a crowded location, take a few minutes and observe the different sizes and shapes of people. Some are tall and thin, others are short and heavy, and still others are somewhere between these two extremes. Body length and shape are determined primarily by the genes we inherited from our parents. If our mother and father had skinny thighs, we also tend to have skinny thighs. Those who have inherited body shapes characterized by large, heavier upper bodies have greater health risk than people who have thin upper bodies. Because body shape is a good indicator of health risk, several methods have been developed to assist us in determining whether or not we have additional risk.

Health risks are also associated with the composition of our bodies. All of our body's tissues can be classified as either fat or lean body weight. The amount of fat and lean body tissue we possess is largely determined by heredity, the quantity of food we eat, and the amount of physical activity we undertake. Those who are regularly physically active and do not overeat tend to have less body fat. If too much of your body weight is fat, the risk of several life-threatening diseases increases.

Knowing how much you weigh is not enough to find out whether you have too much or too little body fat. You need to learn what percent of your body is fat and what percent is lean body weight. This chapter will help you determine the composition and shape of your body and assist you in calculating what your ideal body weight should be.

TYPES OF BODY FAT

Body fat (sometimes called adipose tissue) can be classified into two groups: essential fat and nonessential fat. Approximately 5 percent of the body weight of males and 12 percent of the body weight of females is **essential body fat.** This is the minimum percent of body fat we should possess. Essential fat acts as padding and provides energy and building material for the kidneys, brain, bone marrow, spinal cord, heart, and many other organs. Without at least this much fat, our bodies will not function properly. **Nonessential fat** is any body fat that is more than what we need for normal physiological function. As we will discuss later in the chapter, an excessive amount of nonessential fat is unhealthy.

The difference in the amount of essential body fat between men and women is due to the extra fat requirements of the breasts, uterus, and other gender-specific female organs. Women need more essential body fat than men because of the demands of childbearing. Gender-specific differences in body fat can be easily seen in the way men and women deposit fat. Men usually store fat in the abdomen, chest, and back, whereas women deposit fat in the hips, thighs, and breasts. Men typically have broad shoulders and narrow hips and tend to be more muscular. Women have subtle curves that make them appear noticeably different from males. These gender differences in body shape are due primarily to the storage of body fat.[1]

Women who are extremely thin can have levels of body fat below the amount that is essential. Cross-country runners, dancers, gymnasts, and women with eating disorders like anorexia often have less than essential amounts of fat. Many of these develop **amenorrhea,** a condition that occurs when normal menstruation ceases. This state of infertility affects estrogen production and calcium absorption and will continue as long as body fat levels are below the essential level. A major health risk for these individuals is the decrease in bone density that occurs when calcium absorption is reduced. This condition can lead to osteoporosis in later life. When body fat is regained, and an essential level of fat is stored, menstruation restarts, estrogen flows, and calcium absorption will increase. In both men and women, essential body fat represents a threshold that should be maintained to ensure good health.

Some body fat is considered **subcutaneous** (sub = below, cutaneous = skin) because it is found just below the skin. By pinching yourself you can feel the subcutaneous fat. A pinch of the skin on the back of your hand will not find very much body fat; however, the body fat found on the abdomen is easily felt when you pinch a small section of the stomach. The rest of our body fat surrounds our abdominal organs or is deposited in muscle. Figure 7.1 illustrates the location of abdominal subcutaneous fat. Fat that is located in muscle (intramuscular fat) will supply additional energy for long periods of sustained physical activity.

The storage of fat is our body's way of saving excess energy for later use. Fat storage becomes detrimental, however, when the quantity of fat becomes so large that normal bodily functions are impaired.

FUNCTIONS OF BODY FAT

The fat we have in our bodies has three main functions: storage of energy, padding, and shape. Each gram of fat we consume has nine calories. Every gram of fat stored in the body also contains nine calories that can be expended in muscle contraction or other metabolic functions. The amount of energy we carry in the form of stored fat is substantial. The average man has approxi-

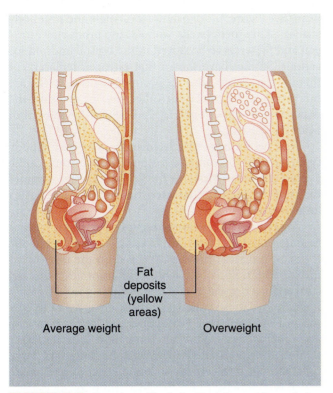

Fat deposits (yellow areas)

Average weight   Overweight

FIGURE 7.1 Location of body fat. Fat is located beneath the skin and around the organs.

mately 21 pounds of fat or 10,500 grams. That is equal to about 95,000 calories or the amount of energy needed to run 1,100 miles. The average woman carries about 33 pounds of fat or 138,000 calories that could supply enough energy to run 1,600 miles.[2]

Fat is the most efficient means we have of storing energy. Without it, we would have to eat constantly to maintain energy levels and proper body functioning. Individuals who have become stranded in remote areas without food have been able to survive prolonged periods of starvation because they had sufficient energy stores in the form of body fat.

Fat that is deposited between our skin and muscles and around many of the organs in our bodies provides a layer of padding to protect against accidents and trauma. Even the bottoms of the heels contain small pads of fat that absorb shock as we walk. Fat does not contain as much water as muscle and acts to insulate our bodies from extreme temperatures. On cold days, people with very little body fat must maintain their body temperature by contracting muscle through physical activity or shivering, or they must put on more layers of clothing than a person with higher amounts of body fat.

PERCENT BODY FAT

If you could weigh just the portion of your body that is fat, you could detect the percentage of your body's total weight that comes from fat. This is what is meant by **per-**

cent body fat or fat weight. The portion of your body that is not fat is considered **lean body weight.** This includes skin, muscle, hair, bone, blood, other organs, and all other nonfat tissues in our bodies. Lean body weight and fat weight constitute 100 percent of our total body weight. The use of "percent" in measuring body composition is independent of how much a person weighs, so that a man who weighs 220 pounds and a woman who weighs 130 pounds could both have the same percent body fat. Body weight is a poor indicator of health risk, but the amount of fat a person carries can affect his or her health.

OBESE OR OVERWEIGHT? NEITHER IS A HEALTHY OPTION

Obesity is defined as the accumulation of body fat greater than 25 percent of total body fat in men and 32 percent in women. Obesity has also been defined as having body weight of 20 percent greater than the ideal body weight as determined by height and weight tables.

According to the National Center for Health Statistics, 34 million Americans (33 percent of all adults) are 20 percent or more over their ideal body weight.[3] People this much overweight are usually also considered clinically *obese*. It is rare for individuals to be obese from childhood to adulthood. Most adults are not overweight at the age of 20, but as the years pass, 65 percent of all adults will exceed their recommended body weight and most will become obese.[4]

The term **overweight** does not consider body composition but is used to describe a person who is more than 10 percent above the ideal body weight. Ideal body weight can be determined by using a weight and height chart. By definition, a large, muscular person who exceeds ideal body weight figures by 10 percent could be considered overweight even though he or she may be very lean. It is also possible for a person to have a weight close to the ideal amount and still have excess body fat. The term *overweight* only provides a rough estimate of body composition and should not be used to determine weight-loss goals.

Excess body fat is caused by many different factors, including genetics, excess food consumption, and sedentary living. A lifestyle that leads to obesity may result in the development of serious health conditions, including both physical and psychological problems.

BODY FAT DISTRIBUTION

Some people have more of their fat deposited in and around the abdominal areas than on their hips or thighs. This type of fat deposition is characteristically labeled the **android,** or apple, body shape. The barrel-shaped

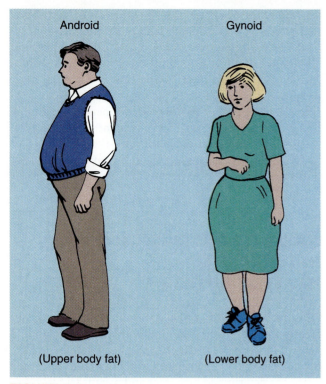

Android	Gynoid
(Upper body fat)	(Lower body fat)

FIGURE 7.2 The gynoid body type is characterized by body fat being stored in the hip and thigh areas. The android body type stores excess fat in the trunk and abdominal areas and is a higher health risk.

upper body resembles an apple and is the predominant location for fat storage among males.

The body shape more common among females is the **gynoid**, or pear, body type. This body type is characterized by the deposition of fat on the hips and thighs. The pear body type has a slender upper body and small breasts, so that the entire body resembles the shape of a pear. (See Figure 7.2 for examples of apple and pear body shapes.) After menopause, women stop producing estrogen and fat tends to be stored in the typical android locations. Studies have shown that estrogen replacement therapy for women who are postmenopausal or who are not producing estrogen for other reasons can slow the deposition of upper body fat and reduce the amount of heart disease risk.[5]

Few people have strictly an android or gynoid body type. Indeed it is common for men to have some of the gynoid characteristics and for women to have some of the apple or android characteristics. Most people have a little of both.

Recent research into the causes of premature death among individuals who are obese has demonstrated differences in disease prevalence based on the location of the stored fat. The obese who suffer from heart disease, stroke, cancer, and diabetes tend to have predominantly upper body fat. Several explanations are given as to why the android body type is at higher risk for heart disease and other diseases. First, abdominal fat cells are larger than fat cells located elsewhere in the body. The large cells have an intolerance for blood sugars and insulin, which is conducive to the development of diabetes. Second, excessive insulin can interfere with normal kidney function, resulting in high blood pressure, which is one of the primary risks of heart disease.

Third, abdominal fat cells have high levels of fat-mobilizing enzymes that facilitate the removal and storage of fat. The rapid release and storage of fat from the android locations cause the level of blood cholesterol to increase, which in turn increases cardiovascular disease risk. Among active people, the fat released from fat cells is quickly taken up by muscle cells and used for energy. Because android fats are easily released to the bloodstream, body fat can be easily gained and lost. Over a hol-

The waist-to-hip ratio may be an indicator of an individual's risk for a heart attack.

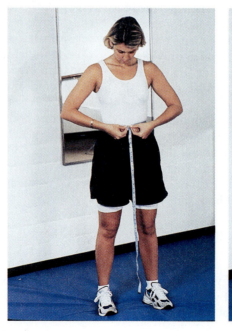
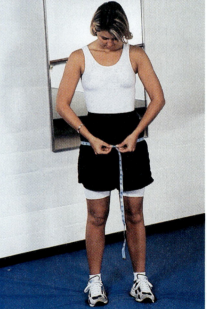

iday, one might gain five pounds of fat, but with a little exercise and a few weeks' time, the extra weight can easily disappear.

By contrast, fat located in the gynoid body locations seems to resist efforts for removal. In fact, it is possible that exercise and dietary restriction may not be able to remove some forms of fat. It is important to realize that everyone is created differently and that it is not only unrealistic, but often impossible for some people to attempt to attain what society deems the perfectly proportioned body shape.

Measuring Body Shape

To measure the amount of fat in the upper and lower body areas and to determine which body shape you have, a ratio of the circumference of the waist and the circumference of the hip is used. The waist-to-hip ratio is used primarily to determine risk of heart disease. See Lab 7.1 for instructions on how to calculate your waist-to-hip ratio and to determine whether you have an android, gynoid, or neutral body type.

A high waist-to-hip ratio does not mean that you will have a heart attack. It simply means that there is an increased number of heart attacks among persons who have high ratios.

HEALTH CLASSIFICATIONS FOR BODY FAT

As discussed earlier, body fat is usually measured and discussed as the percentage of total body weight that is fat weight. Health classifications for the percentage of body fat for both men and women are shown in Table 7.1.

Most often, society dictates the current trends in physical appearance, placing a strong emphasis on the

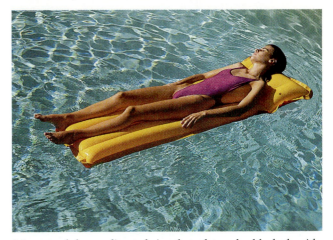

Many people have a distorted view that relates a healthy body with thinness.

outward appearance of the body. Clothing designers, manufacturers, and retailers depend on models to sell their fashions and set the latest trends. The fashionable body type for women is tall and extremely thin, while men are expected to be lean and muscular. Popular body types are generally unrealistic for the vast majority of Americans, yet people exert tremendous effort trying to attain the fashionable look. Of course, the ideal body composition for appearance depends on individual preference, but it should be realistic, keeping in mind the importance of maintaining the proper amount of body fat. Unrealistic ideals can lead to negative self-image and eating disorders.

When the amount of body fat falls into the lean category, it usually means one of several things: the person is ill or has an eating disorder; participates in long-duration endurance-type activities on a regular basis; or has been on a very low-calorie, restricted diet. Regardless of the cause, very low levels of body fat are associated with insufficient energy intake and muscle wasting. When food consumption fails to provide sufficient levels of energy and nutrients, the body is able to convert muscle protein into energy. The conversion that removes protein from muscles and weakens them is referred to as **muscle wasting.** Fatigue, eating disorders, amenorrhea, and loss of bone mass among women are also related to low levels of body fat.

Optimal body fat is the level of body fat at which the health risks associated with too much and too little body fat are minimized. The pursuit of wellness includes reaching and maintaining this optimal level.

As the percentage of body fat reaches the slightly overfat and fat levels, there is a gradual, ongoing increase in the amount of risk for cancer, heart disease, and diabetes. Once the amount of body fat exceeds optimal levels, the risk of disease increases with each added percent of body fat. Just because a person is classified as overweight does not mean that he or she is suddenly at risk, but the farther a person's body fat moves away from optimal levels, the greater risk he or she experiences.

TABLE 7.1 ■ Health Classifications for Percent Body Fat		
	PERCENT BODY FAT	
Classification	**Women**	**Men**
Excessively lean	<8	<5
Lean (high performance)	8–17	5–9
Healthy	18–25	10–20
Moderately Overfat	26–32	21–25
Obese	>32	>25

Source: Wilmore, J. H., et al. Body composition: A round table. *Physician and Sportsmedicine* 14:152, 1986. Reproduced with the permission of McGraw-Hill, Inc.

EXCESSIVE BODY FAT AND POOR HEALTH

Implications for Physical Well-Being

If everyone were at ideal weight there would be 25 percent less coronary heart disease and 35 percent fewer pulmonary disorders and strokes. The importance of obesity as a health problem is clear. As body fat increases, so do disease and the risk of premature death.[6]

High blood pressure is three times more common among those who are obese. This is even true for school-aged children who are just becoming obese. Obese children and adults may have greatly elevated levels of blood cholesterol and other blood fats.[7] High levels of cholesterol are one of the main predictors of heart disease; indeed, obese people have significantly higher rates of heart disease.[8,9] Obese people also suffer from diabetes at a rate three times higher than that for people of normal weight. Some forms of diabetes can be eliminated through weight loss.[10] Obese men have higher rates of colon, rectal, and prostate cancer, and women suffer from higher rates of gallbladder, breast, cervical, uterine, and ovarian cancer. Because of the added health risks associated with obesity, people who are at least 40 percent overweight have premature death rates nearly twice those of average-weight individuals. Overall, obese people have an overall premature death rate one and a half to two times higher than that of people of normal weight.[11]

Implications for Psychological Well-Being

Society promotes the idea that thin is in. Beauty has evolved to include the physical characteristic of thinness. Because of strong societal pressures to be thin, obese people often suffer from feelings of guilt, depression, low self-esteem, and anxiety. Obese adolescents may suffer the brunt of this burden because they lack a well-developed self-concept and tend to receive verbal and physical abuse from adolescent peers who also lack self-esteem and many times fail to demonstrate kindness and understanding.[12]

Obese children and adults often suffer from social isolation and prejudice because of society's lack of compassion and understanding of obesity. In a country that associates beauty, intelligence, and success with thinness, being overweight also has emotional and social consequences; it is not uncommon for overweight adults to experience psychological stress, reduced income, and discrimination both on the job and in their personal lives.

ASSESSING RISK OF OBESITY

There are many ways to assess body fatness. Some methods are more accurate than others, some more costly, and some much more difficult to conduct.

Cellulite Fact and Fiction

What Is It?

Cellulite is the same kind of fat as that stored throughout the body, except it has a dimpled appearance or cottage-cheese look. It is deposited in areas of the body where the skin is slightly less tight. This fat gets trapped in the connective tissues that attach your skin to the underlying muscle. The dimpled areas appear where the skin is more firmly attached to the muscle. They can occur anywhere in the body but are more common in the hips, buttocks, and thighs. Differences in skin thickness and arrangement of connective tissues explain why women get cellulite more often than men. Another difference between cellulite and other stored fat is that cellulite is slow to free up the energy stored in its fat cells, making fat loss difficult.

Can I Get Rid of It?

Skin elasticity, connective tissue arrangement, and fat deposition location are all very much controlled by genetics. If you really want to know whether you will get cellulite, take a look at your parents. Chances are your body types will be very similar. Since you cannot change your heredity, will diet and exercise reduce cellulite? The answer is no. More important, there is *no* cream, tea, or pill that can make it go away. The only thing you will lose with these products is your money. To truly be happy and healthy, eat a balanced low-fat diet, exercise regularly, and accept yourself for who you are.

Body Mass Index

One method to determine risk of having too much body fat is the measurement of body mass. The **body mass index** (BMI) is a technique that involves dividing body weight (in kilograms) by height squared (meters²) and comparing this figure to a table of calculated risk. (See Activity 7.1.) BMI is based on the concept that weight should be proportional to height. Although this method does not evaluate the amount of body fat, it is more accurate than height/weight tables because it is dependent on age and gender.

BMI is fairly accurate for people who do not have a lot of muscle weight. Obese status is generally considered for men who have a BMI above 28 and women above 32. The American College of Sports Medicine has stated that a BMI of 21–23 is ideal for women and 22–24 is desirable for men. When the BMI exceeds 27.8 for men, or 27.3 for women, there is significantly increased risk for cardiovascular disease. High BMIs have been related to hypertension, high levels of blood cholesterol and triglycerides, and low levels of HDL (good) cholesterol. Other studies have found strong relationships be-

Instructions

With a partner measure your height in inches and your weight in pounds. Before calculating your own BMI read through the following example:

Example

For a woman who is 66 inches tall and weighs 128 pounds, use the following calculations:

weight (pounds) = ____128____

height (inches) = ____66____

$$BMI = \frac{weight \times 705}{(height \times height)} = \frac{128 \times 705}{(66 \times 66)} = \frac{90,240}{4,356} = 20.71$$

BMI = ____20.72____

Insert your own weight and height here:

weight (pounds) = _____

height (inches) = _____

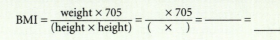

$$BMI = \frac{weight \times 705}{(height \times height)} = \frac{\times 705}{(\quad \times \quad)} = \frac{}{} = \underline{\quad}$$

BMI = _____

Risk Evaluation

Locate your BMI number and associated risk on the table according to your age and gender.

Some risk means that you may be susceptible to health risks associated with having too little body weight. These include osteoporosis, infertility, eating disorders, and, if you smoke, diseases associated with smoking. (Smokers tend to fall below desirable weight ranges more than the general population.)

High risk means that you have a significantly increased risk of early mortality due to diseases of the heart, cancer, and diabetes.

People who have a desirable BMI have the lowest risk of early disease and death.

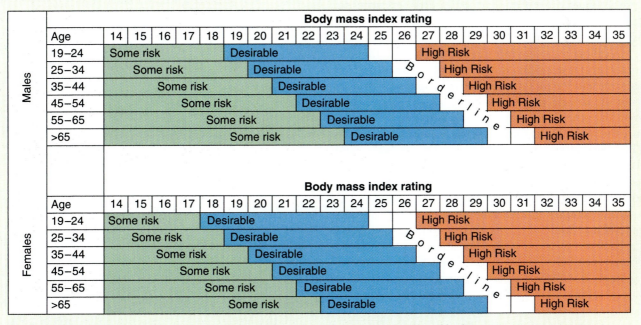

Body mass index and risk of chronic disease. (Adapted from E. Jequier. Energy, obesity, and body weight standards. *American Journal of Clinical Nutrition* 45:1035–1047, 1987.)

tween high BMIs and cardiovascular disease. The BMI is useful in determining risk of overfatness for large populations, but it fails to distinguish fat from lean body weight. The best way to determine body composition is to measure the percentage of fat in total body weight.

Measuring Body Fat

There are now dozens of methods to assess body composition. Hydrostatic weighing, skinfold measuring, and bioelectric impedance are among the more common methods.

Hydrostatic Weighing

Hydrostatic (underwater) weighing is considered one of the more accurate indirect ways to measure body composition. The person to be weighed sits on a platform attached to a scale. The platform is lowered into the water until the person is totally submerged. After the person exhales as much air as possible, a weight measurement is taken. Since fat floats, a fatter person will weigh less under water than a lean person. The person's underwater weight is adjusted to account for any air left in the lungs after full exhalation and any gas trapped in the gastrointestinal tract. Finally, an estimate of fat is computed.

This process is fairly costly in both time and facilities. It requires expensive equipment and well-trained technicians. Although you do not have to be a swimmer to participate, this procedure does not work well with individuals who are uncomfortable underwater. If you are comfortable in water and wish to be underwater weighed, check with the physical education department at a university or college or with a local sports medicine center. Most places charge a fee for this service.

Skinfold Method

Using calipers, this technique measures skinfolds at specific sites to estimate percentage of body fat. It's important to test the exact sites, to measure each site at least three times, and to take measurements at approximately the same time of day, because the amount of water in the body changes during the day. It is a little less accurate than underwater weighing, but it still provides a very useful measurement.

A caliper is used to measure the thickness of the subcutaneous fat in several different places. The technician uses one hand to pull the skin and subcutaneous fat away from the muscle with his or her thumb and forefinger. With the other hand, he or she uses the caliper to measure the width of the pinched fat. (See photo in Lab 7.2.) The measurements from the different sites are added and this sum is put into a formula. Although some formulas use only one site, some three, and some six or more, scientists prefer to use the multiple-site formulas for accuracy and then recommend the most predictive sites for general use. Some of the most commonly used sites are the back of the arm, the area just above the hip, the abdomen, just below the shoulder blade, and the front of the thigh. Because it is easier to train technicians to measure skinfolds than to perform underwater weighing, this test is widely used. When a fee is charged for this service, it is usually quite small. The test takes only a few minutes to complete. You can also use Lab 7.2 to do the measurements with a partner.

Bioelectric Impedance

A third method of analyzing body composition uses a body analyzer or impedance machine. This machine sends a small, harmless, electrical impulse through the body. A computer records both the time the impulse takes to travel through the body and the amount of resistance the impulse encounters. The computer uses these data to compute your percent body fat. Because this method depends on total body water values, it is important to be at an appropriate level of hydration each time you are tested. Working out before the test or retaining

water because of menstruation or other conditions can throw off the accuracy of this test. Some universities, hospitals, and health clubs have these machines available. The test takes only 10 or 15 minutes and is often accompanied by a computer readout that details your percent fat, recommended weight, and how to attain it. Some professionals still question the accuracy of this test, although others believe it to be as accurate as the skinfold technique when subsequent tests are performed at a similar hydration level.

CALCULATING IDEAL BODY WEIGHT

For years people have been counseled to attain their ideal weight. How healthy your ideal body weight is depends on how much of it is fat, where on your body it is located, and whether you have weight-related medical problems.

By now, it should be clear that ideal body weight and socially fashionable weight are not the same. Many of today's female models have great difficulty maintaining the body size required by fashion; hence, many live with eating disorders and near-starvation dietary restrictions. In determining ideal body weight, two underlying principles should guide your actions: (1) always consider the amount of body fat; (2) strive to achieve and maintain at least a healthy percent body fat of 9 to 20 percent for men and 18 to 25 percent for women.

Determining ideal body weight requires some subjective decision making on your part. There is some variation in the amount of body fat a person can have and still be above essential levels and below levels where increased risks begin to accumulate. For example, a 20-year-old woman could have a percentage of body fat between 17 and 25 percent and still avoid most of the health risks associated with being overly fat. To achieve and maintain a level of body fat below 17 percent, however, a woman would have to engage in daily, strenuous physical activity. This high performance level of activity requires the expenditure of large amounts of energy. Endurance athletes and fitness buffs may be able to maintain this level of body fatness, but if this level of physical activity ceases, weight gain is sure to result. Athletes and nonathletes alike may gain weight when marriage, sedentary employment, or childbearing bring new commitments that leave less time for exercise.

Two methods for calculating your healthy/ideal weight are presented here. One method uses height, but assumes that ideal body weight includes 15 to 19 percent body fat for men and 18 to 22 percent body fat for women. The other requires the measurement of the percentage of body fat.

Ideal Body Weight from Height

When measurement of body fat is not possible, ideal body weight can also be estimated from height.[13] These calculations are based on average, medium-boned men and women. The formulas for estimating a target weight based on height involve multiplying your height in inches by 3.5 (for women) or 4.0 (for men) and subtracting 108 (for women) or 128 (for men). If you are large boned you should add 10 percent to the final figure. Women are considered to have large bones if their dominant wrist (the wrist supporting the hand you write with) has a circumference larger than 6½ inches. Men are large boned if their dominant wrist measures more than 7 inches.

Ideal Body Weight from Percent Body Fat

If you are able to have your percent body fat measured, you can use a more accurate method for finding your ideal weight. This method involves determining your current lean body weight and then adding to that the percentage of body fat you would like to maintain. Because this method takes into account your current per-

cent body fat, it gives a more accurate figure for what is ideal for you as an individual. Refer to Activity 7.2 to calculate your ideal body weight based on your known percent body fat.

Try calculating your ideal weight both ways and see how they compare. If there is a lot of discrepancy and you have been able to use the body fat method, use that figure since percent body fat is directly incorporated in the calculation. Remember, ideal weight is an individual decision and must be realistic, so carefully consider your lifestyle, health status, cultural and social values, and personal desires when you decide what level of body fat you would like to strive for.

Several factors can affect your body composition. It is possible to reduce the amount of body fat simply by increasing the amount of muscle weight you possess. Proper weight-control programs include a considerable amount of exercise. By participating in physical activity you can eliminate energy stored in excess fat and increase

Activity 7.2 Determining Ideal Body Weight Based on Percent Body Fat

Example: A woman weighing 160 pounds has a current percent body fat of 29 percent. After evaluating her fitness goals she decides that a desirable amount of body fat is 19 percent.

1. Current body weight × current percent body fat = pounds of fat

   $160 \times 0.29 = 46.4$ lb

2. Current weight – pounds of fat = lean body pounds

   160 lb $- 46.4$ lb $= 113.6$ lb

3. Lean pounds ÷ (1.0 – desired percent body fat) = ideal weight

   113.6 lb $\div (1.0 - 0.19) =$ ideal weight

   113.6 lb $\div (0.81) = 140.2$ lb

You can see from these calculations that her ideal body weight is 140 pounds. Subtracting this from her current weight (160 lb – 140 lb = 20 lb) shows that the amount of fat she needs to lose is 20 pounds.

Now use the following directions to help you determine your ideal weight:

1. Considering your current level of body fat and your personal fitness objectives, determine your desired percent body fat. Use Table 7.1 introduced earlier in this chapter as a guide, and try to be realistic.

2. Determine how many pounds of fat your body currently contains by multiplying your current body weight by your current percent body fat.

   _____ × _____ = _____
   current body weight   current % body fat   lb of fat

3. Calculate lean body pounds by subtracting your pounds of fat from your current body weight.

   _____ – _____ = _____
   current weight   pounds of fat   lean body pounds

4. Compute ideal body weight by using this formula:

   _____ ÷ _____ = _____
   lean pounds   (1.0 – desired percent body fat)   ideal weight

lean body weight. Be sure to check your weight and your body composition regularly as you strive to attain your ideal weight.

SUMMARY

A major threat to good health and wellness is excessive body fat. Though it is necessary to have some fat, too much can contribute to the risk of heart disease, diabetes, and cancer. All the components of the human body can be classified as either lean body weight or fat. The amount and location of body fat can be measured using height and weight charts or by indirect estimation of total body fat using skin calipers, hydrostatic weighing, or bioelectric impedance, among other methods. Once the amount of body fat is known, it is possible to calculate ideal body weight. Individuals who have body weights at or near ideal tend to be somewhat protected from the diseases associated with excessive body fat.

SUGGESTED READING

Bruch, H. *Eating disorders.* New York: Basic Books, 1973.

Katch, F. I., and W. D. McArdle. *Nutrition, weight control, and exercise,* 3rd ed. Philadelphia: Lea & Febiger, 1988.

What Is Your Body Shape?
Calculating Waist-to-Hip Ratios

Directions

With a partner, look at the photos on page 182 to see how the waist and hip measures are taken. Stand with your feet together and arms slightly raised. Use a tape measure to measure the distance all the way around the smallest diameter at the waist. Make sure the tape is horizontal all the way around. This is the waist measurement. The hip is measured in the same fashion except at the largest circumference around the hips. Measure each diameter accurately to at least the nearest millimeter or one-sixteenth of an inch.

Calculation

To calculate the ratio simply divide the waist measurement by the hip measurement:

ratio = _____ ÷ _____ = _____
     waist   hip
   measurement   measurement

Determine Your Risk

Using the graph for men or women below, locate your age and plot your ratio. Your risk is indicated by the different zones labeled in the graph.

Your risk level: _____

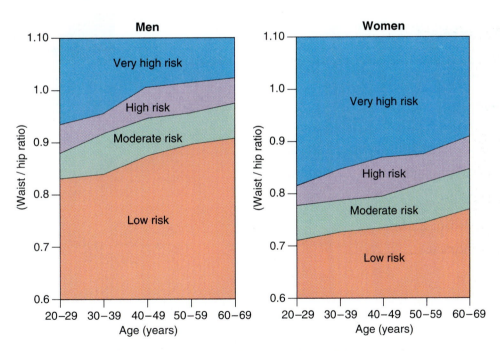

Waist-to-hip ratio and risk of chronic disease. (From G. A. Bray and D. S. Gray. Obesity: Part 1—Pathogenesis. *Western Journal of Medicine* 149:429–441, 1988. Reprinted by permission of the *Western Journal of Medicine*.)

Measuring Body Fat Using the Skinfold Method

For this lab you will need to work with a partner. Your instructor will demonstrate where and how to measure the various skin folds. Follow the instructions to help you measure the amount of body fat your partner has. Then have your partner do the same for you.

The three skinfold sites for men are the triceps, chest, and subscapula; women's sites include the triceps, abdomen and suprailium (just above the hip).

To measure the skinfold, softly pinch a skinfold between the thumb and forefinger. While holding the skinfold, use your free hand to open the calipers and place the jaws of the calipers over the skinfold. The tips of the calipers should be one-half inch from your fingers. Allow the calipers to close on the skin and read the measurement (see photo). Release the calipers and allow the skin to resettle, then repeat the measure two more times; use the average of the three measures. Record the average value for each site. Once you have completed the three measures add up the three scores. With the sum of three sites you can refer to the accompanying tables to determine your percent body fat. Be sure to use your age and the table for men or women on the next two pages accordingly.

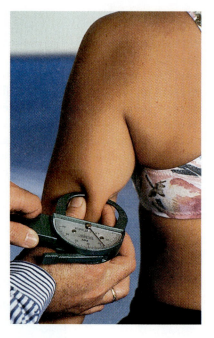

Skinfold Measures

Measure the triceps just above the top of suprailium and the suprailium just above the top of the pelvic bone.

Men	*Women*
Triceps: _____	Triceps: _____
Chest: _____	Suprailium: _____
Subscapula: _____	Abdomen: _____

Sum of three skinfolds: _____

Your percentage body fat: _____

Your body fat classification: _____

Percent Fat Estimate for Women: Sum of Triceps, Abdomen, and Suprailium Skinfolds

	Sum of Skinfolds (mm)	AGE TO LAST YEAR								
		18–22	23–27	28–32	33–37	38–42	43–47	48–52	53–57	>57
Essential	8–12	8.8	9.0	9.2	9.4	9.5	9.7	9.9	10.1	10.3
	13–17	10.8	10.9	11.1	11.3	11.5	11.7	11.8	12.0	12.2
	18–22	12.6	12.8	13.0	13.2	13.4	13.5	13.7	13.9	14.1
	23–27	14.5	14.6	14.8	15.0	15.2	15.4	15.6	15.7	15.9
High performance	28–32	16.2	16.4	16.6	16.8	17.0	17.1	17.3	17.5	17.7
	33–37	17.9	18.1	18.3	18.5	18.7	18.9	19.0	19.2	19.4
	38–42	19.6	19.8	20.0	20.2	20.3	20.5	20.7	20.9	21.1
Good fitness and health	43–47	21.2	21.4	21.6	21.8	21.9	22.1	22.3	22.5	22.7
	48–52	22.8	22.9	23.1	23.3	23.5	23.7	23.8	24.0	24.2
	53–57	24.2	24.4	24.6	24.8	25.0	25.2	25.3	25.5	25.7
	58–62	25.7	25.9	26.0	26.2	26.4	26.6	26.8	27.0	27.1
	63–67	27.1	27.2	27.4	27.6	27.8	28.0	28.2	28.3	28.5
Marginal fitness and health	68–72	28.4	28.6	28.7	28.9	29.1	29.3	29.5	29.7	29.8
	73–77	29.6	29.8	30.0	30.2	30.4	30.6	30.7	30.9	31.1
	78–82	30.9	31.0	31.2	31.4	31.6	31.8	31.9	32.1	32.3
	83–87	32.0	32.2	32.4	32.6	32.7	32.9	33.1	33.3	33.5
Obese	88–92	33.1	33.3	33.5	33.7	33.8	34.0	34.2	34.4	34.6
	93–97	34.1	34.3	34.5	34.7	34.9	35.1	35.2	35.4	35.6
	98–102	35.1	35.3	35.5	35.7	35.9	36.0	36.2	36.4	36.6
	103–107	36.1	36.2	36.4	36.6	36.8	37.0	37.2	37.3	37.5
	108–112	36.9	37.1	37.3	37.5	37.7	37.9	38.0	38.2	38.4
	113–117	37.8	37.9	38.1	38.3	39.2	39.4	39.6	39.8	39.2
	118–122	38.5	38.7	38.9	39.1	39.4	39.6	39.8	40.0	40.0
	123–127	39.2	39.4	39.6	39.8	40.0	40.1	40.3	40.5	40.7
	128–132	39.9	40.1	40.2	40.4	40.6	40.8	41.0	41.2	41.3
	133–137	40.5	40.7	40.8	41.0	41.2	41.4	41.6	41.7	41.9
	138–142	41.0	41.2	41.4	41.6	41.7	41.9	42.1	42.3	42.5
	143–147	41.5	41.7	41.9	42.0	42.2	42.4	42.6	42.8	43.0
	148–152	41.9	42.1	42.3	42.4	42.6	42.8	43.0	43.2	43.4
	153–157	42.3	42.5	42.6	42.8	43.0	43.2	43.4	43.6	43.7
	158–162	42.6	42.8	43.0	43.1	43.3	43.5	43.7	43.9	44.1
	163–167	42.9	43.0	43.2	43.4	43.6	43.8	44.0	44.1	44.3
	168–172	43.1	43.2	43.4	43.6	43.8	44.0	44.2	44.3	44.5
	173–177	43.2	43.4	43.6	43.8	43.9	44.1	44.3	44.5	44.6
	178–182	43.3	43.5	43.7	43.8	44.0	44.2	44.4	44.6	44..8

Source: Adapted from A. S. Jackson, and M. L. Pollock. Practical assessment of body composition. *Physician and Sportsmedicine* 13(5):88 (table 8), 1985. Reproduced with the permission of McGraw-Hill, Inc.

Percent Fat Estimate for Men: Sum of Triceps, Chest, and Subscapula Skinfolds

	Sum of Skinfolds (mm)	AGE TO LAST YEAR								
		<22	23–27	28–32	33–37	38–42	43–47	48–52	53–57	>58
Essential	8–10	1.5	2.0	2.5	3.1	3.6	4.1	4.6	5.1	5.6
	11–13	3.0	3.5	4.0	4.5	5.1	5.6	6.1	6.6	7.1
	14–16	4.5	5.0	5.5	6.0	6.5	7.0	7.6	8.1	8.6
	17–19	5.9	6.4	6.9	7.4	8.0	8.5	9.0	9.5	10.0
High performance	20–22	7.3	7.8	8.3	8.8	9.4	9.9	10.4	10.9	11.4
	23–25	8.6	9.2	9.7	10.2	10.7	11.2	11.8	12.3	12.8
	26–28	10.0	10.5	11.0	11.5	12.1	12.6	13.1	13.6	14.2
	29–31	11.2	11.8	12.3	12.8	13.4	13.9	14.4	14.9	15.5
	32–34	12.5	13.0	13.5	14.1	14.6	15.1	15.7	16.2	16.7
	35–37	13.7	14.2	14.8	15.3	15.8	16.4	16.9	17.4	18.0
	38–40	14.9	15.4	15.9	16.5	17.0	17.6	18.1	18.6	19.2
Good fitness and health	41–43	16.0	16.6	17.1	17.6	18.2	18.7	19.3	19.8	20.3
	44–46	17.1	17.7	18.2	18.7	19.3	19.8	20.4	20.9	31.5
	47–49	18.2	18.7	19.3	19.8	20.4	20.9	21.4	22.0	22.5
	50–52	19.2	19.7	20.3	20.8	21.4	21.9	22.5	23.0	23.6
	53–55	20.2	20.7	21.3	21.8	22.4	22.9	23.5	24.0	24.6
	56–58	21.1	21.7	22.2	22.8	23.3	23.9	24.4	25.0	25.5
	59–61	22.0	22.6	23.1	23.7	24.2	24.8	25.3	25.9	26.5
	62–64	22.9	23.4	24.0	24.5	25.1	25.7	26.2	26.8	27.3
	65–67	23.7	24.3	24.8	25.4	25.9	26.5	27.1	27.6	28.2
	68–70	24.5	25.0	25.6	26.2	26.7	27.3	27.8	28.4	29.0
	71–73	25.2	25.8	26.3	26.9	27.5	28.0	28.6	29.1	29.7
	74–76	25.9	26.5	27.0	27.6	28.2	28.7	29.3	29.9	30.4
Marginal fitness and health	77–79	26.6	27.1	27.7	28.2	28.8	29.4	29.9	30.5	31.1
	80–82	27.2	27.7	28.3	28.9	29.4	30.0	30.6	31.1	31.7
	83–85	27.7	28.3	28.8	29.4	30.0	30.5	31.1	31.7	32.3
	86–88	28.2	28.8	29.4	29.9	30.5	31.1	31.6	32.2	32.8
	89–91	28.7	29.3	29.8	30.4	31.0	31.5	32.1	32.7	33.3
Obese	92–94	29.1	29.7	30.3	30.8	31.4	32.0	32.6	33.1	33.4
	95–97	29.5	30.1	30.6	31.2	31.8	32.4	32.9	33.5	34.1
	98–100	29.8	30.4	31.0	31.6	32.1	32.7	33.3	33.9	34.4
	101–103	30.1	40.7	31.3	31.8	32.4	33.0	33.6	34.1	34.7
	104–106	30.4	30.9	31.5	32.1	32.7	33.2	33.8	34.4	35.0
	107–109	30.6	31.1	31.7	32.3	32.9	33.4	34.0	34.6	35.2
	110–112	30.7	31.3	31.9	32.4	33.0	33.6	34.2	34.7	35.3
	113–115	30.8	31.4	32.0	32.5	33.1	33.7	34.3	34.9	35.4
	116–118	30.9	31.5	32.0	32.6	33.2	33.8	34.3	34.9	35.5

Source: Adapted from A. S. Jackson, and M. L. Pollock. Practical assessment of body composition. *Physician and Sportsmedicine* 13(5):87 (table 7), 1985. Reproduced with the permission of McGraw-Hill, Inc.

CHAPTER 8

Controlling Body Weight

Objectives

1. Understand the prevalence and seriousness of being overweight or obese.

2. Understand how excessive body fat can affect health.

3. Be able to explain the energy balance and set point theories of weight gain.

4. Explain how genetics, metabolism, and adiposity can contribute to obesity.

5. Be able to describe and identify eating disorders.

6. Outline an appropriate weight-loss and weight-maintenance strategy.

7. Distinguish a healthy weight-loss program from a fad or get-rich-quick program.

8. Explain why a program of diet and exercise is the best method to lose weight and maintain weight loss.

Terms

- Energy balance theory
- Age onset obesity
- Set point theory
- Metabolism
- Resting metabolic rate
- Anorexia nervosa
- Bulimia
- Very low calorie diet
- Weight cycling
- Spot reducing

Stages of Change

Where Am I?

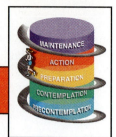

Precontemplator _____ I do not have a healthy level of body fat, and I do not intend to change it.

Contemplator _____ I do not have a healthy level of body fat, and I am considering reducing it.

Preparer _____ My body fat level is too high, but I intend to begin reducing it in the next month.

Action Taker _____ My body fat level is in an acceptable range, but it has been for fewer than six months.

Maintainer _____ My body fat level is in an acceptable range, and it has been for more than six months.

To help you make long-term weight control a part of your life, you will need to determine your current percent body fat. Lab 7.2 shows you how to do this. After you have determined your current level of body fat, use the staging questions above to identify the stage that best describes your current weight-control behavior. To be in the action or maintainer stages, your body fat must be below 32 percent for females and 25 percent for males.

If you could change anything about the way you look, what would you choose? Many people are concerned about their age, others don't like their hair or muscles, but the number one feature that distresses our society is body weight. Fifty-six percent of men and 78 percent of women are unhappy with their current weight, and if the price tag for weight loss is any indication, most adults are not afraid to spend money to lose those extra pounds.[1] Our battles with body weight support the $33 billion weight-loss industry. Thigh creams, liquid drinks, diet pills, fashion diets, and commercial weight-loss programs all drive an industry that has flourished in profits and floundered in results.

More often than not the drive to be thin is fueled by vanity and the desire to possess the socially accepted body type. The current trend is the lean, fit look that is characterized by low levels of body fat and toned mus-

cles. Although efforts to acquire the fit look are improvements over the past when most women were striving for the ultra-thin look, many individuals have become obsessed with the desire to have the fitness look. It is estimated that fewer than one-half of women who diet actually need to lose weight, and even with the numerous health risks associated with excess body fat, only one out of ten women diets for health reasons.[2] Unrealistic expectations about body weight and shape can cause eating disorders, diet anxiety, and added health risk. In this chapter you will discover why proper body weight is important to good health and learn how to sort out the fact from the fiction as we strive to reach and maintain an ideal body weight.

Americans are the most overfat people in the world, with one-quarter of the population considered to be clinically obese.[3] At any given time, 24 percent of adult

194

men and 40 percent of women in the United States are practicing some type of weight-loss method. Almost one-quarter of the adult population is currently trying to maintain weight loss. These figures emphasize two disturbing facts: (1) many U.S. adults are overweight and (2) weight-loss methods are rarely successful.[4]

WHY DO WE STORE FAT AND GAIN WEIGHT?

The **energy balance theory** of weight gain suggests that extra fat is stored when more energy is consumed than is expended. During the holidays when food is plentiful and physical activity is often replaced with more sedentary activities, the amount of calories expended does not keep up with food intake and many people gain weight. It is no wonder that New Year's resolutions are often centered on weight loss. The theory of weight loss is fairly simplistic: we must use more calories than we consume. (See Figure 8.1.)

The only way to supply the body with energy is to eat, but there is a big difference in the amount of energy contained in different types of foods. As discussed in Chapter 6, one gram of fat contains nine calories, whereas an equal amount of protein or carbohydrates contains only four. A diet high in fat will contain more calories than a leaner diet and may lead to excessive body weight. Infants have more body fat than any other age group, because their level of activity is low and their food consumption is usually high in fat and calories. As they become more active, energy expenditure exceeds intake, and as they begin using the stored fat for energy, their percent body fat begins to drop.

Between the ages of twenty and sixty the percent body fat in men typically increases from 15 percent to 25 percent, whereas women will see body fat increase from 20 percent to 32 percent. During this same time period, physical activity and muscle mass decrease while food intake either stays constant or increases.[5] Changes in diet, exercise, metabolism, and body composition all contribute to the increase in body fat with increased age. Some refer to this phenomenon as **age onset obesity.** However, age does not have to be associated with weight gain; there are many ways to avoid the added body fat and the health risks typically associated with aging.

A second popular theory that might explain why we gain weight is the **set point theory.** It is believed that the body has a preference for a certain weight (its "set point") and defends that weight against weight loss and weight gain. Part of the rationale for this theory is that after dieting and weight loss, body weight typically returns to the prior weight within a relatively short period of time.

Proponents of this theory contend that the set point is partly established by genetics and that our body weight is therefore somewhat predetermined. The only effective way to lower the set point and the amount of body fat in the body is to make physical activity a permanent component of daily life. Neither energy balance nor the set point theory completely explains why fat is gained, but there is strong evidence suggesting that the best way to control body weight is with calorie restriction and regular exercise.

Although there are no simple explanations of why we gain or lose weight, much is known about how we store and expend excess energy. Genetics, lifestyle, and environment play major roles in how we store fat and how much energy we expend at rest. An understanding of these factors can assist us in effectively controlling body weight.

Metabolism

Energy expenditure is determined by two main factors: metabolism and physical activity. **Metabolism** is the sum of all vital body processes by which food, energy, and nutrients are made available to and used by the body. Total body metabolism is composed of resting metabolic rate (RMR) and energy required to digest and use food and perform physical movement. **Resting metabolic rate,** the largest component of metabolism, represents the energy required to maintain vital functions. If the average adult were to sit or sleep for twenty-four hours continuously, he or she would expend about 1,650 calories during that time period. This is the amount of energy required to maintain life; it makes up about 55–75 percent of all expended energy.

The energy used to digest food accounts for 5 to 15 percent of total daily energy expenditure. Many of the complex molecules found in food must be broken down or converted to other substances before they can be used by the body. The actual caloric content of one gram of

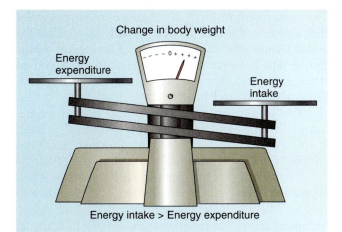

FIGURE 8.1 The theory of energy balance helps explain body weight. When energy intake exceeds expenditure, a person gains body fat. Body fat is lost when expenditure exceeds intake.

Activity 8.1
Calculating Your Resting Metabolic Rate

The World Health Organization has developed a table that can assist you in approximating your resting metabolic rate. Though these are only estimates, the table will provide you with sufficient information to prepare an accurate weight-loss program. Body weight should be measured in kilograms. To convert weight in pounds to kilograms, divide body weight in pounds by 2.2. Then use the appropriate equation in the table below to determine resting metabolic rate.

Age in Years	Equation to Use
Women	
10–17	$(12.2 \times weight) + 746$
18–29	$(14.7 \times weight) + 496$
30–60	$(8.7 \times weight) + 829$
over 60	$(10.5 \times weight) + 596$
Men	
10–17	$(17.5 \times weight) + 651$
18–29	$(15.3 \times weight) + 679$
30–60	$(11.6 \times weight) + 879$
over 60	$(13.5 \times weight) + 487$

Example: A 20-year-old woman who weighs 145 pounds would have a resting metabolic rate of 1,466 calories per day. First, convert pounds into kilograms:

145 lb ÷ 2.2 = 66 kg

Then, look on the table for the appropriate formula for a 20-year-old woman.

$(14.7 \times 66 \text{ kg}) + 496 = 1,466$ calories per day

Now determine your resting metabolic rate. First, convert your body weight in pounds to kilograms:

$$\underset{\text{weight in lb}}{_____} \div 2.2 = \underset{\text{weight in kg}}{_____}$$

In the table above, find the equation that corresponds with your age. Then solve the equation.

The result is your resting metabolic rate, or the minimum number of calories you burn each day.

World Health Organization. *Energy and protein requirements: Report of a joint FAO/WHO/UNO expert consultation,* Technical Report Series 724. Geneva: World Health Organization, 1985. Reprinted by permission.

protein is really 5.6 calories, but by the time it is absorbed and made available for metabolism, only four calories remain.[6] The type of food you eat can have some impact upon the energy expenditure you use to digest the food. For example, simple sugars are most easily digested and proteins and complex carbohydrates require the most energy for digestion. (See the box on calculating your resting metabolic rate to determine the amount of energy you spend at rest.)

Have you ever known an inactive person who could eat large quantities of food and still maintain ideal body weight? These exceptional individuals have abnormally high metabolic rates that may have been inherited or be the result of a hyperactive thyroid. They are able to expend large amounts of energy without the use of exercise. Both behavior and genetics can affect metabolic rate. The more muscle a person possesses, the higher his or her metabolic rate because every pound of muscle requires thirty to sixty calories per day just for maintenance. Metabolic rates decrease with age, but this decrease is likely owing to reductions in muscle mass that occur with sedentary living. Women have lower metabolic rates than do men.

When a person loses weight and gains it back repeatedly, metabolic efficiency may be increased, meaning fewer calories are required to maintain body functions. Weight becomes harder to lose and easier to gain back. Resting metabolism is also affected by stimulants such as caffeine and nicotine. It is well known that smokers have lower levels of body fat than do nonsmokers because of the stimulation of nicotine. Coffee and other caffeine-containing substances also increase the amount of energy the body uses at rest. Many of the pills or drink mixes marketed as weight-loss aids contain fairly large doses of caffeine, which stimulates the body into burning more energy than normal. However, stimulants are not without harmful side effects.

Genetics

The most recent research in the area of obesity suggests that a genetic disorder may be partially responsible for added weight gain in some people.[7] This genetic condition is rare, however, and researchers are quick to note that genetics usually play only a small role in the overall cause of obesity. (See Figure 8.2.)

Studies have shown that identical twins have the same body shape and body fat and that overfeeding them as infants results in similar weight gains for each. Even adopted children are inclined to resemble their biological parents in weight rather than their adoptive ones, suggesting a genetic cause to some body fat.[8] Children of parents who are obese have a greater likelihood of also becoming obese, but except in rare cases, no one genetic factor is completely responsible for the weight we gain. Children with obese parents tend to share similar eating and exercise habits.

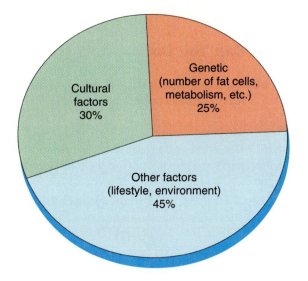

FIGURE 8.2 Factors that are responsible for individual differences in body fat. (Data from C. Bouchard, L. Perusse, C. LeBlanc, et al. Inheritance of the amount and distribution of human body fat. *International Journal of Obesity* 12:205–215, 1988.)

The greatest causes for obesity are the environmental, cultural, and lifestyle factors that influence what and how we eat and whether or not we participate in regular physical activity. Advertising and marketing campaigns are very effective in selling foods and lifestyles conducive to obesity. Many of the most popular foods in our society are very high in fat.

Obesity is also caused by lack of physical activity. Our high-tech world has minimized the amount of physical activity we experience in daily living. This results in an energy imbalance and weight gain.

ONLY THE OVERFAT NEED TO LOSE WEIGHT

In Chapter 7, several methods were used to determine ideal body weight. Of these methods, the most accurate involved the measurement of percent body fat. Current levels of body fat should be compared to desired levels, and weight-loss goals should be based on eliminating the difference between these two levels. Thus, ideal body weight is based on body composition rather than total body weight or body shape and on the attainment of optimal health rather than some arbitrary desire to be a certain weight.

Even though a body fat level may not be high enough for a person to be considered obese, even smaller amounts of fat can be associated with physical disease and psychological and social distress. Unfortunately, many normal-weight or thin women are striving to lose additional body fat even though they may be damaging their bodies both physically and emotionally.

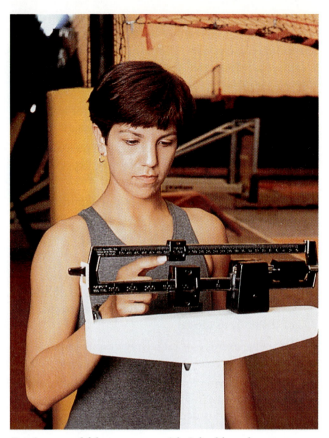

Keeping a watchful eye on your weight is healthy as long as your goals are realistic and appropriate for your body type.

EATING DISORDERS

Individual perceptions of body fatness and strong environmental and peer pressures can cause some people to believe they are overfat when in reality they are not. Poor self-concept and unrealistic weight-loss goals can lead to eating disorders and even death in extreme cases.

Anorexia Nervosa

Some individuals start to diet and then can't stop. They look in the mirror and see a fat person when in reality they are thin. This condition is characteristic of a disease called **anorexia nervosa,** which is widespread among American women. It is estimated that between one and three million Americans suffer from the disease. Men can also suffer from it, but the cases of men with anorexia nervosa are thought to be relatively few at this time.[9]

Anorexia nervosa is often associated with life-threatening weight losses and denial of weight loss by the dieter. Gradual self-starvation and use of exercise as a way to expend calories begin to cause malnutrition and nutrient deficiencies. Body fat levels become so low that anorexics take on a skeletal appearance and the internal organs that are normally supported by fat begin to sag and can gradually stop functioning.

Not known among most college-age students is the fact that 15 to 20 percent of anorexics die as a result of self-inflicted starvation.[10] The American Psychiatric Association has developed a list of criteria to identify those who are anorexic.

1. Inordinate fear of gaining weight and/or becoming fat despite being significantly underweight

2. Absence of at least three consecutive menstrual cycles when they would normally be expected to occur

3. Unwillingness to maintain a minimal normal body weight for the person's age and height

4. Weight loss that leads to body weight 15 percent or more below normal

5. Disturbed and unrealistic perceptions of body weight, size, or shape; feeling of being fat although emaciated and possibly perceiving one specific part of the body as too fat

6. Excessive exercise or exercising despite physical injury

7. Rituals involving food, rigid dieting, maintenance of rigid control in lifestyle. Security is often found in control and order[11]

The causes of anorexia are complex, but a few general patterns have emerged from the research. A genetic cause may be present, because anorexia has been documented among sets of sisters. Anorexia is also common among women who were raised by domineering mothers and among women who feel extreme cultural pressure to be thin. Most become obsessed with body size and are preoccupied with becoming thinner through starvation and exercise. The psychological nature of anorexia makes it very difficult to find any one cause of the disease. Much like alcoholics, people who suffer from anorexia deny that they have a problem and go to great lengths to hide the problem, which makes them less likely to admit to needing treatment.

Treatment involves hospitalization and medications to stimulate appetite. To ensure long-term compliance with normal eating behaviors, most treatment programs include extensive nutritional and psychological counseling. If you know anyone suffering from anorexia, do everything possible to get him or her to a professional; it is difficult for an anorexic person to make positive changes without outside help.

Bulimia

Bulimia, another eating disorder, is characterized by eating regular or large meals and then intentionally emptying the food out of the stomach by self-induced vomiting or use of laxatives. The lining of the throat and esophagus can become damaged from repeated contact with stomach acids during regurgitation. Other dangers include

erosion of tooth enamel, electrolyte imbalances, and a host of psychological problems including altered mood states, depression, and anxiety. Surprisingly, people suffering from bulimia usually look healthy. Most try to hide their binge-and-purge behavior, and many do so for long periods of time. Surveys report that 2 to 8 percent of adolescents and college-age women suffer from bulimia. The disease also affects men, but much more rarely. The following list indicates common characteristics of bulimics.

1. Constant concern with body weight

2. Regular, secret eating characterized by binging (rapid consumption of large quantities of food in a short time)

3. Loss of control over eating behavior while eating binges are in progress

4. At least two eating binges a week for at least three months

5. Frequent purging after eating, using techniques such as self-induced vomiting, laxatives, or diuretics, often accompanied by frequent fasts, strict dieting, or excessive physical activity

Bulimia develops over time as young women find that purging allows them to eat large amounts of food and not worry about gaining weight. The appeal to begin this practice comes from the need to maintain a fashionable body shape and size while still enjoying a healthy appetite. With practice, bulimics can purge without much effort. The biggest danger of the disease occurs when the individual finds himself or herself in a vicious cycle of binging, purging, and feeling guilt and remorse for his or her lack of self-control, only to soon lose control and begin binging again. Some bulimics become so involved in the practice of purging that they eventually lose control of the purging process and are unable to refrain from purging. At that point, their bodies reject any food they consume.

Like anorexics, bulimics need immediate psychological and medical attention. Treatment is similar to that for anorexia, but usually does not require hospitalization. Extensive counseling and behavior control are practiced and monitored.

SAFE AND SUCCESSFUL WEIGHT-LOSS STRATEGIES

Successful weight loss requires control of food consumption and energy expenditure. Energy balance is the key to reaching ideal body weight. Consuming more or fewer calories than you expend will determine whether or not you gain or lose weight. To lose weight you can change the number of calories you eat, change the number of calories you burn, or, most effectively, do both.

Exercise

Use of muscle during physical activity requires energy. One way to burn off a lot of calories quickly is to run hard for an hour. The average 155-pound adult would expend 1,220 calories if he or she could run hard for one hour. Realistically, most 155-pound adults could not run hard for one hour and would probably suffer serious injury if they pushed themselves that hard. The intensity of this activity would quickly discourage even the most fit from using exercise as an effective weight-loss method.

In order to successfully use exercise to control body weight, the intensity of the activity needs to be low enough to allow the person to continue exercising for 20 to 60 minutes and not cause injuries. The activity should be aerobic in nature, because as discussed in Chapter 3, aerobic exercises use large muscle groups and therefore expend more energy per minute. The level of intensity should range from 60 to 75 percent of maximum, and the activity should be conducted at least six or seven times a week. Several kinds of exercise meet these exercise guidelines. Table 8.1 shows several such activities and the number of calories they expend per hour. A person who weighs 158 pounds could do aerobics for just one-half hour and expend over 220 calories. Walking and cycling do not use as many calories, but their low intensity makes them particularly appealing to many adults.

Perhaps the most important aspect of using physical activity as part of weight control is to do some form of regular exercise every day. A complete lifestyle modification is required to make exercise a daily habit. We all take time to sleep, eat, and relax; regular physical activity should be part of our daily lives as well. In addition, there are other things we can do during the day to increase our energy expenditure. Taking the stairs instead of the elevator, parking the car far from the entrance and walking the remaining distance, and doing yard and housework all require energy and can help reduce body fat and increase muscle.

Exercise Stimulates Metabolism

The lower one's metabolic rate, the more difficult it is to control one's weight. Metabolism is the sum total of all chemical reactions in cells of the body. For every decade of life after age thirty, there is a decrease in metabolism. That means that with age our bodies burn fewer calories in the course of a day. Exercise helps prevent decrease in two ways: (1) through the maintenance and increase of muscle mass that occurs with regular exercise and (2) by causing an increase in the resting metabolic rate after the exercise session is completed.

Muscles require energy for maintenance, even if no exercise is done. The more muscle mass a person has the higher his or her metabolic rate will be. Physically active adults experience fewer decreases in metabolism with increased age.

After an exercise session, there is a slight increase in metabolism. Researchers are not sure how long this postexercise increased metabolism lasts, but it expends about 15 calories for every 100 calories expended in physical activity. For example, if you just completed 60 minutes of tennis and expended 420 calories, you could also expect to burn an additional 63 calories (420 calories × 0.15 = 63 calories) in increased metabolism. This may not seem like much, but over several days it all adds up. In order to keep metabolic rates high and maintain muscle mass, exercise must be part of daily life.

Another benefit of aerobic exercise is the increased rate at which fat is utilized. After 20 minutes of aerobic activity your body gets 50 percent of its fuel from fat, while anaerobic exercise uses only carbohydrates for fuel. Aerobic exercise has a definite advantage over anaerobic activities when it comes to effectively controlling weight.[12]

Proper Diet

Calorie control is of vital importance in successful weight-loss programs. Most often, dieting consists of dramatic changes in diet through either drastic calorie restriction or total elimination of certain foods. This change in diet usually results in weight loss, but the newly adopted diet restrictions are quickly replaced with old habits and the weight quickly returns. Because

TABLE 8.1 ■ Calories Expended in Various Activities

Activity	Calories per Hour[a]	Average Calories Used	Activity	Calories per Hour[a]	Average Calories Used
Sleeping	65	520 (for 8 hr)	Aerobic dancing (med.)	445	222 (for ½ hr)
Watching TV	80	80 (for 1 hr)	Running in place or skipping rope (50–60 steps/min)	510	255 (for ½ hr)
Driving a car	100	50 (for ½ hr)			
Dishwashing by hand	135	67 (for ½ hr)	Downhill skiing	595	1,190 (for 2 hr on slope)
Bowling	190	190 (for 1 hr)	Swimming, 5.5 min/220 yd	600	300 (for ½ hr)
Washing and polishing car	230	230 (for 1 hr)	Hill climbing	600	300 (for ½ hr)
Dancing (waltz, rock, fox-trot)	250	105 (for 5 dances; 25 min)	Touch football	600	300 (for ½ hr actual play)
Walking, 25 min/mile	255	127 (for ½ hr)	Soccer	600	600 (for 1 hr)
Baseball (not pitching or catching)	280	560 (for 2 hr)	Snow shoveling, light	610	306 (for ½ hr)
Weight training	300	150 (for ½ hr)	Jogging, 11 min/mile	655	327 (for ½ hr)
Swimming, 11 min/220 yd	300	150 (for ½ hr)	Cross-country skiing, 12 min/mile	700	2,800 (for 4 hr)
Walking, 15 min/mile	345	172 (for ½ hr)	Basketball, full court	750	750 (for 1 hr)
Volleyball, badminton	350	350 (for 1 hr)	Squash, racquetball	775	775 (for 1 hr)
Gardening	390	780 (for 2 hr)	Martial arts (judo, karate)	790	395 (for ½ hr)
Calisthenics	415	207 (for ½ hr)	Running, 7.5 min/mile	800	400 (for ½ hr)
Bicycling, 6 min/mile	415	207 (for ½ hr)	Ice hockey, lacrosse	900	900 (for 1 hr)
Tennis	425	425 (for 1 hr)			

Source: Reprinted by permission of the author from C. Kuntzleman, *Diet free!* Spring Arbor, MI: Arbor Press, 1981.

[a]The bigger and more vigorous you are, the more calories your body uses for a given activity. The calories listed here are for the average, 158-pound adult. You will lose 1 pound for every 3,500 calories of exercise, as long as you eat the same amount of food.

human nature is difficult to change and long-term habits are hard to break, most diets fail.

In Chapter 6, you estimated your total caloric intake per day. Lab 8.2 at the end of this chapter will help you determine how many calories you expend every day. Your actual energy expenditure should equal your caloric intake if you are neither gaining nor losing weight. With this information, you can prepare a personal weight-loss program. Reduce total daily caloric intake by no more than 500 calories a day, or by 1,000 calories a day if your present diet exceeds 3,000 calories. Weight loss should be

gradual to be long-lasting. Relatively small reductions in total caloric intake are easier to maintain for long periods of time. Everyone should consume a minimum of 1,200 calories every day.

Try the following hints for reducing your caloric intake:[13]

1. Eat planned meals with emphasis on ease of preparation and easy access.

2. Eat fiber-rich foods. These are bulky and will help make you feel full.

3. Eat fresh vegetables and fruits whenever possible. Canned and frozen foods are usually higher in sugar and salt.

4. Chew slowly so that the meal lasts longer even though you are eating less.

5. Try to eat 75 percent of your calories at breakfast and lunch.

6. Eat low-fat meats whenever possible. Poultry (except duck and goose) and fish are good low-fat replacements for meat. Red meat is generally quite high in fat despite advertising to the contrary.

7. Limit the number of times you eat out. This will keep you from eating foods you ordinarily wouldn't consume. When you do eat out, choose foods prepared simply, without butter, salt, or fattening sauces.

8. Write down everything you eat. Awareness is half the battle.

9. Keep fattening foods out of the house. This helps eliminate temptation.

10. Allow yourself an occasional treat during the week, or daily if necessary, so that you aren't tempted to binge.

11. Pick one or two areas to improve in at one time. Gradual changes in lifestyle are easier to accept than radically new ones. In other words, don't try to break two favorite habits at the same time, such as drinking soda and eating chocolate; take them one at a time.

As previously stated, Americans currently consume 36 to 43 percent of calories from fat. Accepted health standards suggest that total fat consumption not exceed 30 percent of total daily calories. For dietary purposes, total fat consumption should be closer to 20 percent of total caloric intake. As you now know, dietary fat has a greater influence on body fat than do carbohydrates and protein. It is stored as fat more easily and requires less energy to digest than do carbohydrates. Over 25 percent of the energy in complex carbohydrates is required for digestion, whereas fat is easily digested and efficiently stored.

Reduction in the amount of dietary fat not only brings fat consumption within healthy limits, but makes a significant reduction in total daily calories. Reduce the amount of fat in your diet and you will lose weight and be healthier.

Realistically, few people are willing to regularly consume a diet that contains only 20 percent fat. Such a diet consists mostly of fruits, vegetables, breads, grains, low-fat milk products, and other complex carbohydrates. There is little room for fatty meats or high-fat processed foods. The food pyramid presented in Chapter 6 reveals that we should consume a minimum of five servings of fruits or vegetables every day. Dieters may wish to consume more than this minimum amount.

A diet that relies less on meats and processed foods can greatly reduce fat intake. Complete elimination of high-fat foods is not required, but reduction in the amount of fat may make a big impact on body weight. Creamy sauces, fast foods, fried foods, and dairy products are high in fat, as are most processed foods. As we have discussed, the best way to determine the fat content of the foods you eat is to read the labels.

Very Low Calorie Diets

Of the 33 percent of U.S. adults who are obese, 66 percent are considered mildly obese and can successfully lose weight through low-fat dieting, changing behaviors, and exercising regularly.[14] Obese people with body mass indexes of greater than 30 kg/m^2 may have more

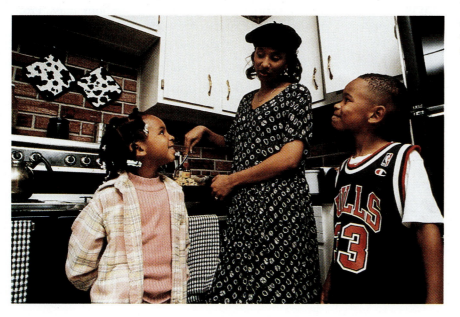

Dietary habits usually begin when growing up. Your favorite recipes, healthy or not, are often those you picked up at home.

success engaging in extreme dietary restriction. Such diets are called **very low calorie diets** (VLCDs) because they limit total caloric intake to between 400 and 800 calories. These diets are medically supervised, with the person checking into a hospital or care facility. For these individuals, traditional diet reduction and exercise programs may have been ineffective or too slow. Patients on VLCDs typically lose between 3 and 5 pounds a week, with total weight loss after sixteen weeks averaging around 40 to 45 pounds. Initial weight loss is mostly water and glycogen; as weight loss slows, lost weight comes mainly from fat and some protein and metabolic rates drop by 20 percent.[15]

This rapid weight loss quickly lowers health risks and improves overall health; unfortunately, about half of all patients do not complete the program. Those who do finish lose about 85 percent of their excess body fat, but despite team efforts from dietitians, physicians, psychologists, and exercise physiologists only 5 to 20 percent are able to maintain ideal weight for longer than 18 months.[16] Although the odds of successfully completing the program and maintaining ideal body weight are about one in four, for many very obese people the hope of reaching and maintaining ideal body weight is worth the effort.

Even if an obese person has a high body fat level, VLCDs may not be appropriate. Patients must have tried traditional weight-loss methods and failed, and they must be free from any serious medical conditions. If you are interested in learning if you qualify for a VLCD, contact your physician.

Yo-Yo Dieting

Perhaps one reason why so many individuals are almost constantly attempting to lose weight is due to yo-yo dieting, also known as **weight cycling.** Yo-yo dieting refers to the phenomenon of successfully losing weight only to gain it back within a few months, followed by renewed dieting, another weight gain, and so on. It is possible to gain and lose the same ten pounds many times throughout one's life. Researchers believe that there may be some health risks associated with weight cycling, the largest health risk being premature heart disease. Based on a long-term study of 3,000 residents of Framingham, Massachusetts, researchers evaluated the connection between repeated weight gain and loss with heart disease and death. The participants with the greatest weight fluctuation had a 25 to 100 percent increase in risk of heart disease and other causes of death.[17]

However, more recent research has failed to show a relationship between yo-yo dieting and increased health risks.[18] Most experts agree that until more is known about yo-yo dieting, any concerns about increased health risk are premature. In the meantime, it is wise to lose weight gradually, just one-half to one pound a week, which will keep you off the dieting roller coaster and give you the chance to change your lifestyle so that the weight stays off.

The American College of Sports Medicine has reviewed all of the scientific research conducted in the area of successful weight loss and maintenance. They state that a desirable weight-loss program is one that

1. Provides a caloric intake no lower than 1,200 calories in order to get a properly balanced diet
2. Includes foods acceptable to the dieter from the viewpoints of sociocultural background, usual habits, taste, cost, and ease of acquisition and preparation
3. Provides a negative caloric balance
4. Includes the use of behavior modification techniques
5. Includes endurance exercise of at least 5 to 7 days a week, for 20 to 30 minutes, at a minimum intensity of 60 percent of maximum heart rate
6. Provides that new eating and physical activity habits be continued for life in order to maintain the achieved lower body weight

Diet and Exercise: The Recipe for Successful Weight Loss

In a classic study of weight-loss methods, William Zuti and Lawrence Golding compared the effects of exercise, diet restriction, and exercise and diet restriction combined, on weight reduction.[19] Figure 8.3 demonstrates that the total amount of weight lost by exercise and by diet restriction is essentially the same, and if you just exercise or just restrict your diet, you will probably lose weight. However, the composition of the lost weight varies considerably. Notice that the group that dieted lost just as much lean body mass as fat and that the exercise group lost twice as much fat and actually gained lean body mass. The group that both dieted and exercised lost the most body fat while gaining lean body mass. From this and other studies we know several important facts about effective weight-control methods:

1. Exercise can reduce body fat.
2. Exercise can build muscle.
3. Diet restriction alone will decrease both body fat and muscle.
4. Diet and exercise combined result in weight loss from reduced body fat.

The most effective weight-loss programs include a balanced diet, with some reduction in the number of calories consumed. Reduction of the amount of dietary fat is enough to significantly reduce total caloric intake. Successful programs also incorporate regular aerobic physical activity. Such programs will reduce body fat, not muscle, and will likely result in long-term weight loss as

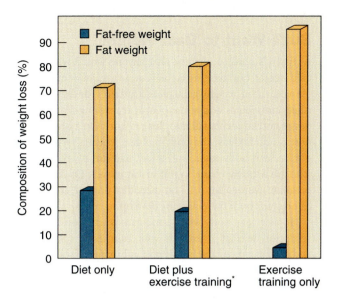

FIGURE 8.3 The composition of weight loss is partially determined by the use of diet, diet and exercise, and exercise alone. Exercise tends to save lean body mass when weight is lost. *Diets were generally very low or low-calorie (400–1000 kcal per day). (Data from W. A. Zuti and L. A. Golding. Comparing diet and exercise as weight reduction tools. *Physician and Sportsmedicine* 4:49–53, 1976.)

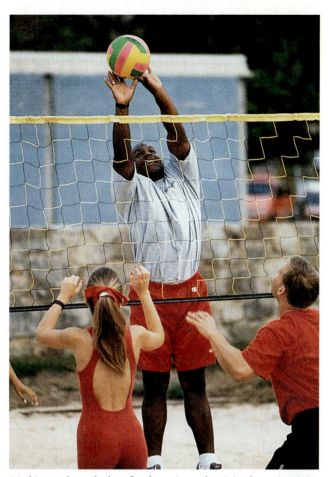

Nothing replaces the benefit of exercise and activity for maintaining a healthy body weight.

long as the exercise remains a part of daily lifestyle. In short, any weight-control method that does not include both diet and exercise will likely produce some short-term weight loss, but with the passage of time, weight will be gained or even increased above pre weight-loss levels.

During the first week of a weight-loss program you may experience rapid weight loss. This initial weight loss is mostly from water. Commercial weight-loss programs use this fact in their marketing strategies by guaranteeing clients that they will lose five pounds in the first week or have their money refunded.

Between the first and third day of dieting, over 70 percent of weight loss is from water, and 25 percent is from fat. Every gram of carbohydrate stored in your body requires three grams of water for storage. When the carbohydrates are used for energy, the water is released into your sweat, urine, and exhaled breath. Thus the early stages of weight loss utilize all available stores of carbohydrates for energy, releasing the stored water and causing rapid decreases in body weight. Once the initial depletion of extra carbohydrates is finished, loss of body weight slows considerably as the composition of the weight loss gradually changes from mostly water to mostly fat. After seven to nine days, try to keep weight loss at a steady ½ to 1 pound per week. This may seem like a small loss, but most of it will be lost body fat. Remember that gradual weight loss is easier to maintain than rapid weight loss. Don't get discouraged if your weight remains constant from time to time. Continue exercising and watching your diet and you will begin to lose again.

RECOGNIZING DIET FACT AND FICTION

In today's diet-crazed society, there is an overabundance of fiction about the effectiveness and safety of many popular weight-loss programs. The entire weight-loss business is exactly that—a business—and because money drives the system, there is potential for abuse, misuse, and deceit. Some commercial weight-loss products, however, are safe and effective when combined with lifestyle change and the adoption of health-promoting behaviors.

New diets appear regularly. Someone decides to lose weight by eating or not eating a specific food or by eating foods on certain days or times of the year. He or she may or may not exercise, but one way or another loses some weight. This person tells the good news to someone else who tries it, who then tells another and another until it has gained some level of popularity. The grapefruit diet, the Dolly Parton diet, and the Beverly Hills diet are just a few of the scores of diets that have been popular in recent years. Most diets have not been evaluated scientifically to determine whether or not they work, so that the average person is left to judge for him- or herself.

Unbalanced Diets

Some fad diets stress one type of food. You have learned that it is important to get foods from all the food groups in order to get all the essential nutrients. Lack of necessary nutrients can leave you fatigued, depressed, and irritable. The popular high-protein diets are usually low in carbohydrate and fat. When your body does not have sufficient quantities of carbohydrates and fats, it uses protein for energy. Nitrogen is a by-product of the protein energy cycle, and too much nitrogen can be toxic. In an effort to clear the body of excess nitrogen, the kidneys combine it with water to make ammonia, which is excreted in the urine. (It can also be sweated out in small amounts.) When a lot of protein is consumed, the body has to work hard to clear the nitrogen. Large quantities of water are needed for this process. High-protein diet plans usually tell you to drink an additional six to eight glasses of water per day. Few people can drink sixteen glasses of water a day, and often the result is dehydration. If the diet is continued, the dehydration can become severe enough to lead to kidney failure and death. Even if you don't dehydrate, the low level of carbohydrate will probably make you feel irritable, sick, and fatigued. High-protein diets may also encourage high meat and dairy food consumption, which can lead to an unhealthy diet full of saturated fats.

Finally, watch out for any "all you can eat" approach to dieting. On any diet, if you eat more calories than you expend, you will gain weight.

Weight-Loss Myths

There are many good diet books and diet plans, but a tremendous number of fad diets violate the most fundamental rules of good nutrition. Someone makes a lot of money on them when they first come out, and then they fade into anonymity when everyone finds out they don't work. Weight-loss fad diets and phony weight-loss programs are easy to spot because they often

1. Promise quick and easy weight loss
2. Sound too good to be true
3. Require the use of a substance that has a secret ingredient
4. Require you to use only their foods or products
5. Do not include a balanced diet or require you to mix certain foods together to get a special effect
6. Claim that you can eat all you want
7. Don't encourage exercise

If you are thinking about purchasing a weight-control product or program with any of these features, you should reconsider.

Most fad diets depend on your not caring what kind of weight you lose. As we've discussed, in the beginning stages of a diet, weight loss is primarily from water.

But I Want to Gain Weight

At first it's hard to imagine that anyone would want to gain weight, but there are actually quite a number of people who need weight-gain diets. Certainly undernourished individuals and some people recovering from illnesses and accidents fall into this category. On a brighter note, so do athletes and body builders who are trying to put on lean body mass, and a few, like sumo wrestlers, who are actually trying to put on fat as well. Of course, pregnant women must be on diets that provide enough calories for both them and the developing fetus.

To gain lean body weight, increase your calorie consumption so that it exceeds your calorie expenditure and do resistance exercises. If you only eat extra calories and don't exercise, you will store the extra calories as fat. Pregnant women are the exception to this rule. A pregnant woman's weight gain involves eating more calories than daily activity expends, but the extra calories are used to sustain the higher metabolic rate of the mother and for the growth and development of the baby. Roughly speaking, a pregnant woman needs to consume an extra 300 calories per day, which usually happens automatically because of the mother's increased appetite.

Weight gain for the average person will require adding additional calories in a way that maintains the recommended balance of carbohydrate, protein, and fat. A common mistake is to increase protein intake without a corresponding increase in carbohydrates. The body ends up with an excess of protein and too few carbohydrates for normal body functioning. Some experts suggest a 700–1,000 calorie a day increase, provided the calorie content comes from a variety of foods. Increase in muscle (lean body mass) is most easily accomplished through progressive resistance exercises like weight training. Some lean body mass gains may be obtained through aerobic-type endurance exercises if the individual has been previously sedentary, although as a whole, aerobic exercise is not an effective way to significantly increase muscle tissue. If you are serious about gaining body weight, increase your caloric intake by at least 700 calories a day and begin a rigorous resistance training program. Chapter 4 contains information to help you get started on your program.

Some of the more popular fad diets include plastic wrappings or rubber suits to trap in heat to sweat off pounds, saunas, diet pills, waist and thigh belts, vibrating machines, and toning tables. A recent gimmick is the weight-loss spray. This product's ads claim that when it is sprayed into the mouth, it suppresses appetite and you will eat less. Thigh creams are promoted as a weight-loss lotion that, when applied to your thighs, will cause the fat to dissolve and disappear. Unfortu-

I don't have time to exercise to help control my body fat.

Lack of time is a common problem when trying to exercise. Successful weight control and maintenance probably will require a lifestyle change and a hard look at your use of time.

I dislike low-fat foods.

If you don't like the taste of low-fat foods, don't completely drop your old diet. Change just one food at a time.

Exercise makes me sweaty and uncomfortable.

Vigorous exercise is not for everyone. Try walking, gardening, or a round of golf. Don't think of it as exercise; think of it as time to play.

I've always eaten a lot and feel deprived when I can't.

If you can't control your appetite, eat fruit and vegetables. You can eat a lot and not gain weight.

I never stick with anything. Why should healthy eating be any different?

Is your self-confidence low? Make your goals easy to reach until you are ready for a more ambitious plan of attack.

nately, the only thing that disappears is your $29.99. Don't get drawn into a fad diet.

WEIGHT MAINTENANCE

Studies of the long-term success rate of most diets conclude that only 5 percent of dieters reach and maintain their target weight for more than one year.[20] Dieting provides temporary success for most individuals, yet people continue to diet even though failure has been a constant result.

For most people, exercise is not enjoyable and requires a drastic change in lifestyle to develop and maintain a schedule of regular physical activity. Unfortunately, many people have the idea that exercise is like a prescription designed to help our bodies recover from illness (in this case, overweight). When the "illness" has subsided and we have lost weight, we stop using the prescription. Discontinuing exercise after weight loss inevitably leads to weight gain.

Once you have reached your ideal body weight, the biggest mistake you can make is to stop exercising and resume your former eating habits. Maintaining a healthy weight is like doing a handstand. Watch gymnasts stand on their hands and you will see slight adjustments being made with the fingertips and wrists the whole time they are upside-down. Balance is dynamic, not static. In order to keep your weight and body composition in balance, you need to be aware of your body's needs and activity level and adjust your intake accordingly.

Eating and Exercising for Long-Term Weight Control

The first lesson in this usually occurs in the late teens when you hear yourself remarking, "I haven't changed my diet at all and suddenly I'm gaining weight." This is probably because you are done growing and don't need as many calories. It may also reflect a change in lifestyle. Whenever you become more or less physically active you need to adjust your diet accordingly. Imagine the different caloric needs of a teenager, a nursing mother, a construction worker, a business executive, and an elderly person. Some of the critical adjustment periods occur during and after pregnancy, around middle age, and at retirement. Listening to your body, adjusting your dietary intake, and maintaining a regular exercise regimen can keep you on balance throughout your life. Here are a few tips to help you maintain the body weight you have worked so hard to attain.

1. *Learn to Enjoy Exercise.* Learn a new sport, try cross training, alternate activities throughout the week, but don't stop exercising.

2. *Try Not to Buy Bigger Clothes.* You may have to in the short term for comfort, but consider losing the extra weight instead.

3. *Know Your Hunger Triggers.* Time of day, the smell of food, stress, boredom, grocery shopping, and advertisements are triggers that can make us want to eat. Successful weight maintenance requires conscious identification and control of hunger triggers. Learn to eat because you are hungry, not because it's noon.

4. *Social Support Groups.* Social support can help you learn new ways to cope with weight control and will give you the extra confidence you need to be successful. Immediate family members and close friends can supply some of the best support and morale.

5. *Expect to Relapse.* Expect an occasional dietary relapse, but don't give up when it happens. The sooner you get back to your weight-control plan, the sooner you'll lose those few extra pounds and be back in control of your lifestyle.

SUMMARY

Despite increases in physical activity and an improved overall diet, Americans are more overweight now than ever before. Obesity directly contributes to several diseases and other health conditions. It is caused by a combination of three interrelated factors: cultural influences, genetics, and lifestyle, and no one theory can explain why individuals gain and lose weight. Increased social and emotional pressures can force some individuals to become victims of equally dangerous eating disorders. Successful weight loss and maintenance require a lifelong commitment to healthy eating and regular physical activity.

SUGGESTED READING

Bennion, L. J., E. L. Bierman, J. M. Ferguson, and the Editors of Consumer Reports Books. *Straight talk about weight control: Taking the pounds off and keeping them off.* Yonkers, NY: Consumers Union, 1991.

Kano, S. *Making peace with food.* New York: Harper & Row, 1989.

Ornish, D. *Eat more, weigh less: Dr. Dean Ornish's life choice program for losing weight safely while eating abundantly.* New York: HarperCollins, 1993.

Behavioral Lab 8.1

What Can I Do?

The following lab is designed to help you make controlling your body weight a part of your everyday life. At the beginning of this chapter, you determined your stage of readiness to change with regard to controlling body weight. Now take out a sheet of paper and complete the corresponding section of this lab: precontemplator, contemplator, preparer, action taker, or maintainer.

Precontemplator

1. Precontemplators have many reasons for wanting to reduce their body fat. Following are listed several reasons why people are resistant to change. Which of these items best describe your reasons for not wanting to change?

_____ I don't have enough self-control to alter my diet.

_____ I have tried too many times unsuccessfully and I don't want to try again.

_____ I hate exercising and dieting.

_____ I don't have time to exercise.

_____ My family is all overweight and I feel I am unable to do anything about my weight.

_____ Every time I lose weight, I gain it back. So why try again?

_____ I am content the way I am.

_____ Other reasons _____

2. You completed several activities in Chapter 7 that would help you determine whether you need to change your body composition. Do the results support a need for change?

3. Can you think of any reasons why learning to control your body weight would be good for you? (See page 184 for some ideas.)

4. Do your answers in items 2 and 3 outweigh your answers in item 1?

5. Can you use any of the Barrier Busters in this chapter to eliminate the items you listed in item 1? Which ones?

6. In your opinion, which of your barriers is the biggest one to overcome? Why?

7. Of all the benefits of a healthy body composition, which one appeals to you the most? Why?

8. If you were going to make one change to make your body composition healthier, what would you do?

Contemplator

1. What are you thinking about doing to improve your body composition?

2. What changes will this action (item 1) bring about that are important to you? Why are they important?

3. What barriers might keep you from making this change?

4. Review the Barrier Busters found on page 205 in this chapter. How can these help you overcome your barriers?

5. What do you need in order to consider making a change? Try to finish this statement:

I would consider changing if . . .

Examples: I could control my eating. I could find time to exercise regularly. I could find low-fat foods that I like to eat.

6. List the things that tempt you to overeat and not exercise.

7. How can you withstand these temptations?

Preparer

1. What do you specifically want to accomplish? (For directions on goal setting, see Chapter 2.)

2. What type of actions will accomplish this goal?

3. Suppose you did change your body composition. How would your life be different?

   Physically: _____

   Socially: _____

   Emotionally: _____

4. Refer back to Chapter 6. Which of the Barrier Busters on page 155 would help you control body fat?

5. Refer back to Chapter 3. What can you do to help yourself adopt a lifestyle that includes physical activity?

6. What is the first step you need to take to accomplish your goal(s) stated in item 1?

7. What makes you think you can accomplish this first step? What makes you think you can accomplish your goal?

8. Complete the following statement:

   I am going to take my first step on _____.
   date within 30 days

Action Taker

1. What are you currently doing to improve your body composition?

2. Are your body composition goals specifically and clearly stated?

3. Are you keeping track of your progress?

   If yes, how? (for example, weighing once a month, keeping a weight-loss journal, measuring changes in inches, experiencing better endurance and/or fitness, having easier breathing)

   If no, would it help motivate you to keep a record of your progress?

4. Are you receiving support or rewards for your effort?

If yes, what kind?

If no, why not? And can you change this?

5. Do you think you will continue? Why?

6. If you were to stop, what do you think would be your major reason for stopping?

7. Is there a way to prevent this (item 6)?

8. How would you get yourself started again if you did stop?

Maintainer

1. How long have you maintained your body composition?

2. What are the top two reasons that make you want to continue?

3. Have you been tempted to stop?

4. If you have relapsed, list the reasons why you think you did and what you did to get back on track.

5. Write down a few things you can do to prevent relapse in the future.

6. Are you happy with your current body composition, or do you wish to continue to improve?

7. What kind of support do you get for your efforts? (for example, these may be some type of self-reward, internal reward, or external reward)

8. How have you changed or how have you changed the environment around you to accommodate a healthier lifestyle? (*Example:* I don't shop when I'm hungry. I take a lunch rather than eat out.)

9. Is there anything else you need to promote your continued maintenance? (for example, information, support, time management)

10. If you listed something in item 9, can you think of a way to attain it or can you think of someone who can help you with it?

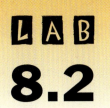

Calculating Daily Caloric Expenditure

Part 1

To estimate the total number of calories you expend per day read and complete the following lab.

Directions

Estimate the average number of hours you spend on each of the following categories and put this figure in the space provided. Remember there are only 24 hours in each day, so your total number of hours should not exceed 24. Write your body weight in kilograms under the weight column (1 lb = 0.4536 kg). For each category multiply hours per day by the calorie per kilogram factor times your body weight. This figure is the number of calories you expended for that particular category of activity. Add the total number of calories expended across the nine categories. This figure equals the total number of calories you expend in one day.

Category 1	Sleeping, resting in bed
Category 2	Sitting, eating, listening, writing
Category 3	Light activity while standing: washing, shaving, combing hair, cooking

Category 4	Slow walking, driving, dressing, showering
Category 5	Light manual work: floor sweeping, window washing, driving a truck, painting, waiting on tables, nursing chores, electrical work, walking at moderate pace
Category 6	Leisure activities and sports in a recreational environment: baseball, golf, volleyball, bowling
Category 7	Manual work at moderate pace: carpentry, construction, snow shoveling, loading and unloading goods
Category 8	Leisure and sports activities of heavy intensity, but not competitive: bicycling, dancing, skiing, swimming, tennis, brisk walking, light jogging
Category 9	Intense manual work, high-intensity sports: lumber cutting, jogging and running, racquetball, cross-country skiing, mountain biking

Category	Average hr/day		Calorie/kg/hr		Body Wt (kg)		Calorie/Category
1	_____	×	1.04	×	_____	=	_____
2	_____	×	1.52	×	_____	=	_____
3	_____	×	2.28	×	_____	=	_____
4	_____	×	2.76	×	_____	=	_____
5	_____	×	3.36	×	_____	=	_____
6	_____	×	4.80	×	_____	=	_____
7	_____	×	5.64	×	_____	=	_____
8	_____	×	6.00	×	_____	=	_____
9	_____	×	8.00	×	_____	=	_____
Total:	24 hours					Total _____ (24-hr energy expenditure)	

Source: Information in part 1 is from C. Bouchard et al. A method to assess energy expenditure in children and adults. *American Journal of Clinical Nutrition* 37:461–467, 1983.

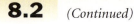

Part 2

To complete this lab you will need to refer to the daily caloric intake you calculated in Lab 6.2. This number was gathered from the nutrition analysis you performed as part of Chapter 6. Part 1 of this lab, which you just completed, shows your total daily energy expenditure. With these two figures and Lab 6.2, you are ready to determine if you are in a positive or negative weight balance. To do so, merely plug your values into the formula below. Remember, the labs you used to determine these figures are only as good as the information you used to calculate them. The weight balance is equal to the daily caloric intake minus the daily energy expenditure. Now determine your own weight balance:

$$\underline{\hspace{2cm}} - \underline{\hspace{2cm}} = \underline{\hspace{2cm}}$$

   daily caloric   daily energy   weight balance
      intake   expenditure

Example

2,380 calories – 2,500 calories = –120 calories
  (Lab 6.2)   (Lab 8.2)

This example individual is expending more calories than consuming because he has a –120 calorie deficit. This means he is consuming 120 fewer calories than he is expending, which may mean he is losing weight.

If your total is negative, you are in a negative energy balance; if it is positive you are in a positive balance, or gaining weight. If your total is around 0, your weight is staying approximately the same and your intake and expenditure is balanced. These calculations are only rough estimates and may include large discrepancies. No one understands your body weight better than you, so be your own guide to weight control.

CHAPTER 9

Preventing Cardiovascular Disease

Objectives

1. Understand the trend of the prevalence of cardiovascular disease.

2. Describe the heart and its diseases.

3. Demonstrate an understanding of the process of arteriosclerosis.

4. Be able to describe the different forms of cardiovascular disease.

5. Know the heart attack warning signs.

6. Demonstrate a clear understanding of the different risk factors and how they can be reduced.

7. Comprehend the processes required to prevent, reverse, diagnose, and treat cardiovascular diseases.

Terms

- Cardiovascular disease
- Arteriosclerosis
- Atherosclerosis
- Ischemia
- Angina pectoris
- Myocardial infarction
- Stroke
- Thrombosis
- Aneurysm
- Hypertension

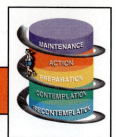

Where Am I?

Precontemplator _____ I am not contemplating finding out about or changing my blood pressure and cholesterol levels.

Contemplator _____ I am considering finding out about and/or changing my blood pressure and cholesterol levels.

Preparer _____ I intend to test and, if necessary, work to change my blood pressure and cholesterol levels.

Action Taker _____ My blood pressure and cholesterol levels have been under control for less than six months.

Maintainer _____ My blood pressure and cholesterol levels have been under control for more than six months.

No single lifestyle is responsible for heart disease. Some of the earlier chapters of this text are designed to help you reduce your risk of heart disease and other diseases caused by such factors as improper nutrition, excessive body weight, and sedentary living. Although this chapter discusses all heart disease risk factors, the Stages of Change Model will focus on achieving healthy blood pressure and blood cholesterol levels.

Choose the statement above that best describes your current behavior. In order to be in the action or maintainer groups, you must know your current levels of blood pressure and blood cholesterol; your blood pressure should be below 140/90 mmHg, and your total blood cholesterol should be below 200 milliliters per kilogram.

One of the last things young adults worry about is dying of **cardiovascular disease** (CVD). It's easy not to be concerned about something that won't happen for fifty years, if it happens at all. Yet, as the number one cause of death, CVD begins early in life and builds up for many years before it becomes critical. The best way to avoid the disease is to start early by adopting a healthy lifestyle.

The word *cardiovascular* can be broken down into "cardio," which means heart, and "vascular," which means vessels. Cardiovascular diseases include more than twenty different diseases that affect the heart and vessels of the body, with the more common forms being coronary heart disease, stroke, and hypertension. The good news is that most forms of CVD share one common characteristic: they are mainly caused by lifestyle factors that can be altered. These modifiable risk factors include diet,

stress, high blood cholesterol, smoking, and sedentary living. This chapter will help you determine your own heart disease risk factors and assist you in modifying your lifestyle to reduce your chances of having heart disease later in life.

CARDIOVASCULAR DISEASES: PAST AND PRESENT TRENDS

In 1953, William Enos, Robert Holmes, and James Beyer conducted a study on the corpses of American soldiers who were killed in combat during the Korean War.[1] Autopsy findings revealed that 77 percent of the 300 soldiers examined showed advanced levels of blood vessel blockage, and many of these had such severe artery blockage that their arteries had narrowed by 50 percent. The shocking part of the study was that the average age of the men was twenty-two years. How could so much blockage occur in men so young? This disturbing news began a scientific inquiry that has produced much of what we know today about the heart and its diseases.

Right now, more than 115 million Americans are living with some form of cardiovascular disease, which affects both men and women and costs society over $135 billion dollars each year in medical expenses.[2] However, not all the reports on heart disease are grim.

The prevalence of heart disease is much lower now than it was from 1920 to 1950, when a large portion of the American work force relocated to cities and towns to work in urban environments. During this transition period, cars became popular, diets changed, and tobacco use increased. But since the 1950s the occurrence of heart disease has dropped 50 percent, with further decreases occurring today. This reduction in mortality has been hailed as one of the greatest public health accomplishments in our century. Men and women of all races have experienced reductions in heart disease occurrence.[3]

Experts have determined that the decline in heart disease is primarily related to changes in lifestyle. As increased health awareness has prompted many Americans to reevaluate their level of health risk and adopt healthier lifestyles, heart disease has declined accordingly. Fewer people smoke, more are aware of the dangers of elevated levels of cholesterol and blood pressure and have taken steps to reduce them, and many people now make exercise part of their daily lives.[4–6]

In addition to people taking action to reduce their risk factors, improvements in medical interventions such as specialized hospital trauma units, coronary care facilities, and advanced treatment of heart disease also contribute to the overall decline in cases of heart disease.

However, despite tremendous reductions in the prevalence of heart disease, it remains the number one cause of death. (See Figure 9.1.) It kills five times the number of people who die of lung or breast cancer and is responsible for almost half of all deaths.[7]

HOW CVD DEVELOPS

The heart is composed of a cardiac muscle fiber that is unlike any other muscle in the body. It beats continuously from about the fifth week after conception until death. In one year it contracts 42 million times and ejects 700,000 gallons of blood. Its primary function is to provide constant blood and nutrients to the cells and remove waste products by circulating blood via the arteries to all parts of the body. At rest, the average heart beats seventy to eighty times a minute, while a heart that is fit beats only thirty to forty times a minute. Such inefficiency puts sedentary and overweight individuals at increased risk.

Because the cardiovascular system has such a critical responsibility in supplying the body with life-sustaining blood, malfunction of the heart or the vessels that carry blood to the heart can result in either death or serious injury to the heart muscle. **Arteriosclerosis** includes any

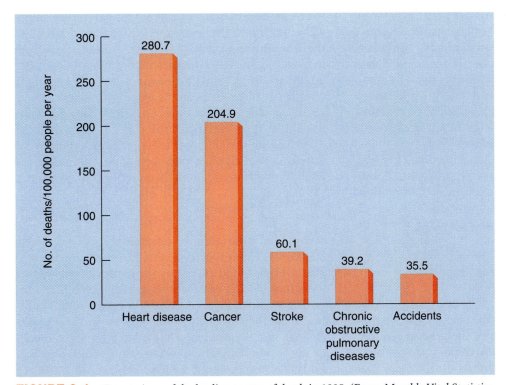

FIGURE 9.1 Comparison of the leading causes of death in 1995. (From *Monthly Vital Statistics Report* 45(11): Supplement 2, June 12, 1997.)

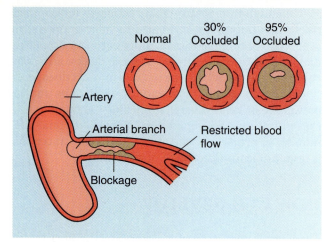

FIGURE 9.2 Atherosclerosis occurs in stages. Plaque deposits in a normal "clean" artery can partially block the flow of blood. As the size of the blockage increases, blood supply decreases until tissues downstream from the block fail to receive adequate blood and are damaged.

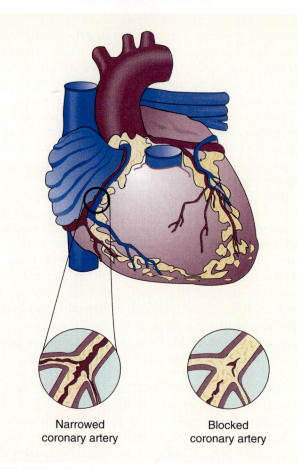

FIGURE 9.3 Narrowed or blocked arteries in the heart result in a heart attack.

arterial disease that leads to thickening and hardening of the arteries. One specific form of arteriosclerosis is **atherosclerosis.** It is characterized by the accumulation of plaque (a lipid-like substance) in the inner layer of large elastic arteries, such as the coronary arteries of the heart or femoral arteries in the upper leg. The middle layer of arteries is composed of smooth muscle that contracts or expands, allowing the artery to constrict or dilate. The buildup of plaque in this layer of muscle causes the vessel to narrow. (See Figure 9.2.)

Atherosclerosis is responsible for 85 percent of all cardiovascular deaths.[8] The plaque deposits can range from small streaks to large lesions that can cause thromboses (blood clots), bleeding, and hardening of the arteries. It is not clear why the plaque is deposited. Some believe the buildup is due to vessel injury caused by abrasion as blood travels through the artery while under pressure caused by high blood pressure. Other factors that may come into play are high blood cholesterol, viruses, toxins, and cigarette smoking.[9,10]

Some researchers believe that certain bad cholesterols can injure the vessel walls and cause the smooth muscle to grow and attract other cholesterols. Regardless of the actual injury mechanism, the process is widespread throughout the population and appears to begin early in life, perhaps as early as childhood.[11–13] (See Figure 9.3.)

TYPES OF CVD

When atherosclerosis forms in the arteries that supply the heart, continued narrowing of the arteries reduces the amount of blood supply and **ischemia** (lack of oxygen) results. During rest or calm periods of the day, the blood being supplied through a narrow artery to the heart is limited, but sufficient to meet the demands of the heart. However, periods of emotional stress or physical activity push the heart's demands for oxygen beyond the amount supplied by the narrow arteries. The resulting oxygen starvation causes severe chest pain called **angina pectoris.** Individuals who suffer from angina are required to take medications quickly to relieve the ischemia and pain. As the emotional stress subsides or the individual stops exercising, the pain usually goes away. This type of partially blocked artery can often be detected by participating in a maximum endurance test while a physician monitors the heart's electrical activity.

Heart Attack

Myocardial infarction, or heart attack, is caused by a blocked coronary artery. The artery may become blocked by a blood clot or by the gradual narrowing of the artery, which eventually closes completely. The portion of the heart that is deprived of oxygen dies. The location of the obstruction determines the amount of damage and the severity. New treatments are quite effective at reducing the severity of the attack and preventing death; however, the time between the onset of a heart attack and initiation of treatment is critical. The sooner the treatment the better.

To help identify a heart attack when it occurs, the American Heart Association has produced a list of heart attack warning signs that indicate when immediate medical attention should be sought (see the box above).

Stroke

Stroke is another form of cardiovascular disease that affects the vessels that supply blood to the brain. The cerebral artery supplies most of the nutrients for the brain. Atherosclerosis, which narrows the arteries of the heart, also narrows other arteries in the body including those found in the brain. The most common cause of stroke is a **thrombosis,** or blood clot, which forms in the arteries of the brain. When this occurs all of the brain tissue being supplied by the blocked artery is starved for oxygen. Some strokes are caused by an **aneurysm** or weakened section of an artery that expands like a balloon until it finally bursts. This hemorrhaging causes severe damage to the brain. One-third of all stroke victims die, one-third are permanently disabled and must live in special-care centers, and one-third are able to gradually return to an acceptable quality of life.

The actual causes of strokes are not clearly understood, but several risk factors have been identified, the most prominent of which is **hypertension,** or high blood pressure. Stroke warning signs include sudden weakness or numbness on one side of the face, arm, or leg, temporary loss of speech or vision, unexplained dizziness, or headaches.

For years doctors have been treating heart attacks with thrombolytic medicines, or "clot busters." The medicine rapidly dissolves the blood clots that have blocked arteries and restores blood flow. Now doctors are using the drugs to dissolve blood clots in the brain. If the blood flow is restored quickly, brain damage is limited. As you might guess, the sooner a stroke patient gets a drug, the less damage is likely to occur. The drug must be given within three to six hours after the signs of a stroke start. After about six hours, the brain damage is permanent.

Hypertension

Aside from being a major risk factor in stroke and heart disease, hypertension itself is considered a disease. It is a condition in which blood pressure is chronically elevated. Hypertension is the most common type of vascular disease, affecting 25 percent of the population of the United States. The cause is sometimes related to problems in other body organs, such as the kidneys or liver; however, physicians are unable to find a cause for almost 90 percent of cases of hypertension. Several factors have been linked to the occurrence of hypertension, including age, African American heritage, obesity, heredity, sodium sensitivity, lack of exercise, and excessive alcohol consumption.

RISK FACTORS FOR CVD

The primary risk factors for heart disease include sedentary living, smoking, secondhand smoke, chronic stress, obesity, and high cholesterol. Other factors that play a lesser role in causing heart disease include age, heredity, race, and gender. These four factors are nonmodifiable risks, or risks that cannot be altered by lifestyle changes. All other risk factors can be changed, and by knowing which modifiable risks you possess, you can develop a plan to modify your lifestyle and reduce your risk for experiencing heart disease. Lab 9.2 gives you an opportunity to assess your risk for heart disease. The factors stress, smoking, exercise, diabetes, and obesity are described in other chapters of this book. This chapter outlines the stages of change for high blood pressure and blood cholesterol. Not all cases of CVD can be attributed to one of these factors, but each of these factors has been shown to be associated with an increased risk of CVD.[14]

Because the major forms of cardiovascular disease share many of the same risk factors, the elimination of one risk factor can potentially lower the risk of several cardiovascular diseases.[15] Cigarette smoking, for example, increases a person's risk of heart disease, arteriosclerosis, and stroke. When two or more risk factors are reduced, the benefit is even greater.

Figure 9.4 demonstrates how the risk of coronary heart disease increases as the number of major risk factors possessed increases. For example, people with just one risk factor are 1.75 times more likely to suffer from

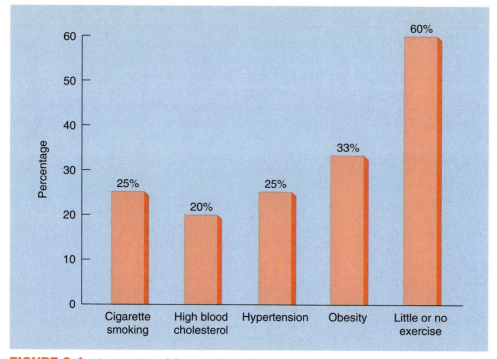

FIGURE 9.4 Comparison of the prevalence of the five major heart disease risk factors. Percentages indicate the percent of the U.S. population who have each risk factor. (Data from B. K. Jacobsen, and D. S. Thelle. Risk factors for coronary heart disease and level of education. *American Journal of Epidemiology* 127:923–932, 1988.)

heart disease than those with no risks, while people with three major risk factors are four times as likely to suffer from the disease.[16]

Now let's take a look at the nonmodifiable risk factors associated with CVD. Then we'll cover the modifiable risk factors, or the ones you can do something about.

Nonmodifiable Risk Factors

In order for a risk factor to be truly nonmodifiable, it must be immune to any attempts made to modify it. Nonmodifiable risk factors include age, heredity, race, and gender.

Age

One out of two deaths after the age of 65 are caused by CVD. As we age, our risk of dying from accidents, infections, and homicide decreases and our risk of CVD increases. Age greater than 65 is associated with 80 percent of all fatal heart attacks.[17] This does not mean that everyone who ages will likely die from heart disease. There is no evidence that increased age causes CVD, only that there is a relationship.

Although many people try to hold back time, it is impossible to change your age. The risk of cardiovascular disease increases as you age, regardless of how old you may look. But older people who exercise regularly, don't smoke, have safe levels of blood pressure and cholesterol, and eat a proper diet decrease their risk of CVD.

Heredity

A family history of heart disease is perhaps the best predictor of heart disease. Individuals who are biologically related to a mother, father, grandparent, brother, or sister who had heart disease before age 65 are considered to have a family history of heart disease. Individuals with a known family history of heart disease often also have a second major risk factor. One study showed that people with a family history of heart disease were more likely to have high blood cholesterol.[18] Having a family history of heart disease does not mean that you cannot reduce your risk of CVD; it simply means that added attention should be paid to the modifiable risk factors that might be present.

Race

Another powerful risk factor is race. African American males an increased risk of stroke and CVD primarily owing to high rates of hypertension. Only 11 percent of the general population is hypertensive; however, 33 percent of African Americans are hypertensive.[19] High rates of hypertension put the African American population at greater risk of stroke and heart diseases. Medical experts believe that the added risk may be due to salt sensitivity, high psychological stress, genetics, or a combination of these factors.

Although African American women do not have the same prevalence of hypertension as men, they have added risk of CVD because of high levels of obesity. The most recent survey by the Centers for Disease Control and Prevention showed that 50 percent of all African American women are overweight as compared to 32 percent of African American men and 33 percent of the general population.[20]

Gender

Women do not have the same risk of CVD as do men. Before menopause, women have some level of protection because of the female hormone estrogen, which their bodies produce naturally. Estrogen tends to keep total blood cholesterol levels lower, which protects against atherosclerosis. Once women reach menopause, they lose the protective effects of estrogen and their risk of CVD increases steadily. By age 65, women have substantially higher rates of CVD, but their risk still does not reach the rate of CVD found among men. Daily adherence to hormone replacement therapy as prescribed by physicians can greatly reduce the increased risk that occurs when natural estrogen is no longer produced.

Modifiable Risk Factors

Reduction of CVD risk begins with identification of risk areas and implementation of successful lifestyle change. Although it is impossible to remove the risk associated with nonmodifiable risk factors, you may be able to reduce your total risk for CVD by changing some current behaviors—in other words, by changing your modifiable risk factors. Each of the following modifiable risk factors can be reduced as we move through the various stages of change.

Sedentary Living

From a public health perspective the greatest reduction in heart disease would be accomplished if more of us became more physically active. In 1991, a national survey on physical activity indicated that 58.1 percent of adults reported irregular or no physical activity, and some studies even show a decrease in the number of adults who exercise regularly.[21] The number of people who get regular exercise has not changed much; however, infrequent exercisers have become regular exercisers.

One of the best predictors of CVD is inactivity. Because sedentary individuals have an increased risk and so many Americans are sedentary, increasing the number of adults who get regular physical activity could result in a large reduction in the number of cases of CVD. The adoption of active lifestyles has the potential to drastically alter the prevalence of heart disease. Cardiovascular disease is associated with low levels of cardiovascular endurance. Researchers have shown that the more fit people are, the less likely they are to suffer from heart disease.

There is considerable debate about the role of fitness and physical activity in the prevention of heart disease. Studies completed on large populations have shown that those individuals who expended at least 2,000 calories of energy per week in physical activity had the greatest reductions in the incidence of heart disease. To expend 2,000 calories per week the average adult would have to walk briskly for 4.77 hours a week or jog for two hours. These calories can be burned in a variety of ways: gardening, hiking, cleaning, mowing the grass, manual labor, and even playing golf (without a cart) are effective ways to expend calories in physical activity. The important conclusion of this research is that doing any type of physical activity can help reduce a person's risk of heart disease. While low-intensity physical activity may not produce much improvement in cardiovascular endurance, there is still a marked reduction in heart disease risk.

In addition to its association with a decrease in cardiovascular disease risk, physical fitness is also related to large decreases in cardiovascular disease death rates. Research conducted at the Institute for Aerobics Research tracked 10,000 adults for eight years to determine the relationship between CVD and fitness. (See Figure 9.5.) The researchers found that moderate and high fitness levels resulted in one-third the amount of heart disease found among individuals who had low levels of fitness. This reduction in risk was found after differences in smoking, cholesterol, blood pressure, age, gender, body fat, and family history of heart disease were considered. There was little difference in risk between the moderate and high levels of fitness. Low- to moderate-intensity activities such as a brisk daily walk are sufficient to produce a level of fitness that can provide substantial reduction in heart disease risk by reducing blood pressure, elevating good cholesterol levels, removing excess body fat, and

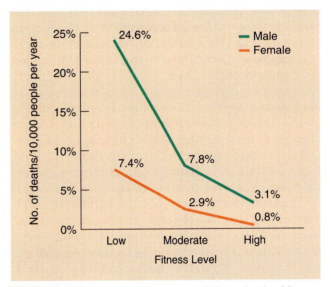

FIGURE 9.5 Relationship between different levels of fitness and death due to cardiovascular disease among men and women. (Adapted from S. N. Blair, H. W. Kohl III, R. S. Paffenbarger, Jr., D. G. Clark, K. H. Cooper, and L. W. Gibbons. Physical fitness and all-cause mortality: A prospective study of healthy men and women. *Journal of the American Medical Association* 262(17): 2395–2401, 1989.)

even assisting in smoking cessation by encouraging a lifestyle of activity and healthy choices.

Cigarette Smoking

Smoking is the number one risk factor associated with death in the United States, causing nearly one out of every five deaths.[22] The general public usually associates cigarette smoking and lung cancer, but smoking is responsible for more deaths caused by cardiovascular disease than deaths due to cancer. Although the association between smoking and heart disease may not be as easy to discern, if a smoker and a nonsmoker have the same blood pressure, the smoker still has at least twice the risk of heart disease. The same relationship holds true for various levels of blood cholesterol. In addition, if a smoker does have a heart attack, he or she is two to four times more likely to die during the attack.[23]

Tobacco users who need a smoke just after awakening are craving the stimulating effects of nicotine. This powerful stimulant increases heart rate and gives smokers an early morning "kick." Nicotine also affects blood lipids by increasing LDL levels and decreasing HDLs, which elevates overall heart disease risk. The carbon monoxide present in tobacco smoke displaces oxygen in the blood and can cause shortness of breath with mild physical exertion. Constriction of blood vessels, reduced oxygen in arterial blood, and higher levels of blood pressure all cause the heart to work harder and can produce cardiac arrhythmias (abnormal heart contractions that can lead to cardiac arrest).

Smoking cessation programs, public health awareness, government intervention, and new smoking laws have all helped to reduce the total number of Americans who are addicted to tobacco. Chapter 14 of this text explores the pros and cons of successful smoking cessation programs. If you are a smoker or are considering smoking or know someone who does smoke, the information in Chapter 14 will help you.

Secondhand Smoke. Environmental tobacco smoke, passive smoking, and secondhand smoke are all terms referring to inhaling other people's tobacco smoke. After years of research and persistent confrontation with the tobacco industry, the National Cancer Institute and the Environmental Protection Agency conclude that there is no longer any doubt that exposure to environmental tobacco smoke is a cause of death and disease among nonsmokers. Nonsmoking spouses are three times more likely to die of a heart attack than spouses of nonsmokers.[24] Children of parents who smoke have a very high incidence of bronchitis, asthma, and other respiratory disorders. For this reason, smoking is now banned on all U.S. domestic flights and some states and municipalities have instituted a "no-smoking" policy in public buildings and restaurants.

Many individuals are unable to quit for themselves, but when they consider the damage they are doing to their family and loved ones, they are sufficiently motivated to break their dependence on tobacco. With the tightening social and legal pressures on the tobacco industry, the gradual decline in the number of smokers is expected to continue.

Chronic Stress

Chronic high levels of stress have been associated with cardiovascular diseases. During the stress response, blood pressure and heart rate increase, there is an increase in the number of fatty acids released into the blood, digestion stops, and muscles tense. If the stress continues, the physiological reactions to the stress will also persist.

To determine the relationship between chronic stress and cardiovascular disease prevalence, several researchers have tested large populations and followed their health status. There appears to be an increase in cardiovascular disease incidence among individuals who are depressed, stressed, or overly anxious. Studies have shown that individuals who experience chronic stress have higher levels of blood cholesterol and blood pressure, which can lead to heart disease.[25]

Chronic stress has been listed as one of the most pressing issues at home and the workplace. Employees experience stress in a variety of settings; this stress, if left unattended, could result in psychosocial difficulties and even disease. Relaxation techniques can ease the tension and anxiety that can influence blood pressure. Regular vigorous exercise has a proven stress-reducing effect that can even help reduce the occurrence of chronic stress. Chapter 11 of this text is devoted solely to the topics of stress, stress reduction, and mental well-being.

Obesity

Another major risk factor for heart disease is excessive body fat. As you have learned, body fat in excess of what is required for healthy living increases heart disease risk. Even when other heart disease risk factors are not present, excessive body fat by itself can raise heart disease risk because of elevated levels of blood cholesterol and blood pressure.

The same lifestyle intervention strategies required to lose excessive body fat are also effective in reducing the risk of heart disease. You can in essence achieve two things at once as you pursue the wellness lifestyle. Regular aerobic physical activity and dietary intervention will help you lose body fat while at the same time reducing your risk of heart disease.

High Cholesterol

The link between cholesterol and heart disease has been fairly well established through long-term studies of high levels of blood cholesterol and the incidence of heart disease. Cholesterol is a substance found only in animal tissues. Like all animals, human beings require cholesterol to build cell membranes and produce hormones responsible for the development of male and female sex characteristics. Cholesterol is also used to help digest fats. Infants and children need cholesterol and related fats for proper development of the nervous system. It is essential that we have some cholesterol for optimal health; however, too much cholesterol can be dangerous.

In order to be transported throughout our bodies, cholesterol, which is fat-soluble, must be made water-soluble. In the liver cholesterol is encased with protein forming a lipoprotein (fat protein). The different types of lipoproteins are classified based on the thickness of the protein shell that surrounds the cholesterol. High-density lipoproteins, or HDLs, have a thick, dense protein wall whereas low-density lipoproteins, LDLs, have thinner walls.

The "Good" Cholesterol

High-density lipoprotein (HDL) cholesterol is commonly termed the "good" cholesterol. Research shows that it takes up cholesterol from the blood and tissues and delivers it back to the liver, where it is converted to bile to be used for digestion or disposed of. Many studies have documented an inverse relationship between HDL and cardiovascular disease. High quantities of HDLs are able to remove cholesterol from artery walls and the bloodstream, causing a reduction in the amount of arterial plaque that in turn lowers the risk of CVD. The higher the level of HDLs the better. Average HDL values are 45 mg/dl for men and 55 mg/dl for women (Table 9.1). HDL levels can be increased with regular, moderate to vigorous aerobic exercise, as well as by weight loss. Being overweight, smoking or chewing tobacco, using steroids, and having some medical conditions, including diabetes, can decrease HDL levels.

The "Bad" Cholesterol

Low-density lipoproteins (LDLs) are the primary transporters of cholesterol. LDLs are considered to be "bad" because they aid in transporting cholesterol to various body cells including vessel walls where LDLs release and deposit cholesterol. As a result, when LDL levels are excessively high, cholesterol begins to accumulate and restrict blood flow, which leads to possible heart disease. The liver has specialized receptor sites that bind LDLs and remove cholesterol from the blood. When LDL levels are elevated, the receptor sites in the liver are all constantly occupied by LDL molecules, allowing the other LDL molecules to roam the body and unload their cholesterol. Table 9.1 displays the risk of cardiovascular disease based on the amount of LDLs found in the blood. Heart attacks are rare with LDL levels below 100 mg/dl of blood. Regular exercise, a diet low in saturated fat, weight loss, and medication if necessary can lower LDL blood levels.

Cardiovascular disease is greatly influenced by levels of HDL, LDL, and total cholesterol. The relationship between cholesterol and heart disease is graded and continuous, meaning that the higher the level of blood cholesterol, the higher the health risk. There are no known risks to having very low blood cholesterol in adulthood.

A seven- to ten-year investigation of 4,000 healthy middle-aged men with high blood cholesterol provided the most convincing argument that cholesterol is directly related to heart disease. Using dietary intervention and medication, high blood cholesterol levels were lowered 25 percent. Not only were lower levels of blood cholesterol associated with 50 percent fewer heart attacks, but the heart attacks that did occur were less severe.[26] The improvements in heart disease risk were related to the decrease in cholesterol by a factor of 1 to 2, meaning that a 1 percent reduction in blood cholesterol caused a 2 percent reduction in heart disease risk. For example, people whose blood cholesterol level drops from 250 to 200 mg/dl (20 percent) lower their heart attack risk by 40 percent. Most experts agree that desirable levels of cholesterol should be below 200 mg/dl, though there are some who believe cholesterol should be less than 180 mg/dl to be ideal.[27]

Where Does Cholesterol Come from?

Cholesterol comes from two sources: the diet and the body. The average American consumes from 500 to 600

TABLE 9.1 ■ Cholesterol Guidelines			
	Desirable	**Borderline High**	**High**
Total Cholesterol	< 200 mg/dl	200–239 mg/dl	≥ 240 mg/dl
LDL Cholesterol	< 130 mg/dl	130–159 mg/dl	≥ 160 mg/dl
HDL Cholesterol	≥ 45 mg/dl	35–44 mg/dl	< 35 mg/dl

Source: Lipid Research Clinics Program. The Lipid Research Clinics coronary primary prevention trial results, II. The relationship of reduction in incidence of coronary heart disease to cholesterol lowering. *Journal of the American Medical Association* 251:365, 1984.

Note: A desirable total cholesterol level may still be associated with heart disease risk if HDL levels are < 35 mg/dl.

milligrams of cholesterol daily in food and naturally produces an additional 1,000 to 2,000 milligrams. The American Heart Association recommends that daily dietary cholesterol be limited to not more than 300 milligrams per day, about half the current amount consumed. Cholesterol produced in the body is mainly manufactured in the liver. Total cholesterol production can vary depending on how much saturated fat and cholesterol is consumed. Americans consume twice the recommended amount of saturated fat. One of the most effective ways to lower elevated levels of blood cholesterol is by reducing dietary cholesterol and saturated fat. Dietary cholesterol is limited to foods that are derived from animal products like meats and dairy products. Plant products contain no cholesterol; however, saturated fat is prevalent in most of the foods we eat, including some plant food.

Most cooking oils are derived from plant sources and do not contain cholesterol. They are also low in saturated fat. When less saturated fat is consumed, the liver slows its production of cholesterol, which keeps total blood cholesterol levels low.

How to Lower Cholesterol

Elevated cholesterol can be reduced by increasing consumption of foods high in soluble fibers like oat and wheat bran, as well as fruits and vegetables. Several studies of oat bran and other sources of bran have found that people who ate diets high in soluble fiber had significantly lower levels of blood cholesterol after six weeks. Increased dietary fiber may cause lower total cholesterol by binding with cholesterol before it is digested, thus reducing the total amount that gets absorbed. Complex carbohydrates that include high quantities of fiber have also been effective in reducing blood cholesterol, simply by the fact that a diet high in complex carbohydrates is automatically low in fat. Adults can expect to see a 5 to 10 percent reduction in blood cholesterol simply by eating two low-fat oat bran muffins a day or by increasing the amount of complex carbohydrates they consume. (For further information, see Chapter 6.)

Exercise and weight loss are also effective ways to produce a favorable level of HDL blood cholesterol. With endurance-type regular physical activity, levels of HDLs increase; LDL and total cholesterol levels drop only slightly. Studies of exercise and cholesterol have produced mixed results because of the confounding effect of weight loss, which usually occurs with exercise programs.[28] Active weight loss also results in decreased cholesterol levels, which is an added reason to achieve and maintain ideal body weight. But it is less clear whether total cholesterol reductions from exercise are due to weight loss or exercise or both. In varying degrees, tobacco use through either smoking or chewing is associated with elevated cholesterol. And we know that psychological stress can cause cholesterol to increase.

Cholesterol reduction through dietary intervention, weight loss, exercise, smoking cessation, and stress reduction requires lifestyle changes. Medical treatment for high blood cholesterol always includes lifestyle intervention. Medications such as Cholestipal and Cholestyramine are usually prescribed after attempts at lowering cholesterol with lifestyle intervention have failed. Cholesterol-lowering medications are most effective when combined with lifestyle changes, but they do have side effects. If your blood cholesterol is high, see your physician.

High Blood Pressure

Blood pressure is the force exerted against vessel walls as blood is pumped by the heart to all areas of the body. The pressure is caused by the resistance the blood encounters as it travels through arteries, arterioles (small arteries), and capillaries. When vessel walls exert too much tension on the flowing blood, a condition called hypertension—high blood pressure—results. For the most part, individuals with hypertension have no symptoms or outward signs of the problem, which is why it is sometimes called the "silent killer." Without any outward manifestations, hypertension often goes unnoticed until years of elevated pressure have had time to damage blood vessels and certain organs.

Blood pressure measures consist of two pressures. A typical blood pressure measure of 120/80 mmHg includes a systolic and diastolic pressure. The first number is the systolic pressure or the pressure in the vessels when the heart is physically pushing blood out into the vessels. The second number, the diastolic pressure, refers to the pressure in the blood vessels when the heart is at rest, between beats.

Any measured blood pressure that has a systolic pressure above 140 mmHg or a diastolic pressure of greater than 90 mmHg is considered elevated. True hypertension is not diagnosed until several blood pressure readings are averaged and the mean is above 140 mmHg systolic or 90 mmHg diastolic. (See Table 9.2.)

TABLE 9.2 ■ Blood Pressure Levels and Risk Classifications		
Category	Systolic mmHg	Diastolic mmHg
Normal	<130	<85
High normal	130–139	85–89
Hypertension		
Stage 1 (mild)	140–159	90–99
Stage 2 (moderate)	160–179	100–109
Stage 3 (severe)	180–209	110–119
Stage 4 (very severe)	≥210	≥120

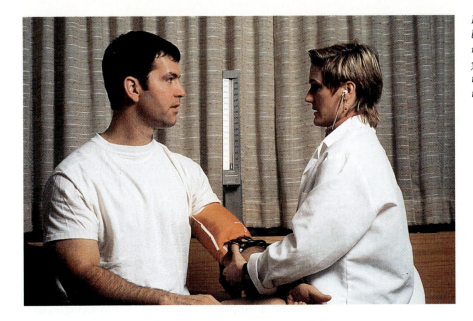

High blood pressure can be a "silent" killer because it quietly causes damage that you may not know of until it's too late. Identify your blood pressure to determine if it is in the healthy range, and monitor it regularly to make sure it stays there.

Why Is High Blood Pressure Dangerous?

You will recall that the vessels of the body can harden or become lined with plaque through a process called arteriosclerosis. The middle lining of arteries is made of smooth muscle that can contract and expand, causing the vessel to constrict or dilate. The blood vessels' ability to adjust their internal diameter provides our bodies with a way to control the flow of blood. Have you ever stood up too fast and become light-headed or dizzy? When you stand suddenly, the pressure of your blood is not sufficient to supply blood to your brain and you feel light-headed. Moments later, the sensation goes away and you feel better. Sufficient blood has been restored to your brain because heart rate has increased and the main arteries of the body have constricted, causing blood pressure to increase.

Prolonged hypertension causes the smooth muscle in arteries to lose their ability to contract and expand, resulting in a hardened or rigid artery. Without flexible arteries, the only way the body can constantly control blood pressure is for the heart to alter the force it exerts on pumped blood. When faced with constant elevated blood pressure, the muscle of the heart is forced to pump harder, causing it to gain extra muscle mass and enlarge. The heart sits in an enclosed sac in the chest, which does not have sufficient room to support an enlarged heart. The enlarged heart is forced to operate in an extremely tight space and fails to pump sufficient amounts of blood because it has become too restricted (constrained).

Smooth muscle damaged by hypertension is more susceptible to the deposition of plaque. When hypertension and high blood cholesterol are present simultaneously, the entire process of atherosclerosis is accelerated, often leading to blocked arteries in the heart (heart attack) or damaged arteries in the brain (stroke). Other organs of the body are also sensitive to elevations in blood pressure. The kidneys, liver, and eyes can all be permanently damaged by the effects of uncontrolled hypertension.

How to Control High Blood Pressure

Like other forms of CVDs, hypertension is primarily caused by lifestyle factors. In the United States and other high-tech societies, increased age is strongly associated with increases in blood pressure. In less advanced countries, blood pressure does not increase with increased age. These countries also do not have the United States' high rates of obesity, sodium intake, inactivity, and alcohol consumption. Thus it appears that age does not have to be associated with hypertension if modifiable risks are reduced. The risk factors associated with hypertension are the same risk factors that are associated with most of the chronic diseases afflicting adults.

Lose Excess Body Weight. If you connected all of the various blood vessels found in the body, the total length would exceed 60,000 miles! Every pound of excess body fat adds many more miles of vessels to the heart's already difficult workload. Excess body fat has been found to cause a two- to sixfold increase in the risk of developing hypertension.[29] Likewise, fat loss can result in decreased systolic and diastolic pressures. Weight control has been identified as the most effective way to control blood pressure. Refer to Chapters 6 and 7 for information on how to effectively lose excess body fat.

Reduce Sodium Intake. A careful eye at the grocery store will reveal a whole new marketing scheme directed at consumers concerned with reducing dietary sodium. Food products proudly announce that they are "reduced

Tips to Help You Reduce Sodium

Here are five tips that have been shown to be effective in helping people reduce sodium intake:

1. Limit the use of foods with visible salt on the surface (pretzels, snack chips, salted nuts).
2. Choose more fruits and vegetables.
3. Instead of using salt when cooking, try herbs, spices, or salt-free seasonings.
4. Read food labels and avoid foods high in sodium.
5. Don't use the salt shaker on processed foods such as lunch meats, soups, and hot dogs. They are already high in sodium.

sodium" or "sodium free" in an effort to increase sales. Americans consume between six and twelve grams of salt a day. Only 40 percent of the weight of salt is sodium, so ten grams of salt supplies about 4.5 grams of sodium. Experts citing large-scale studies agree that Americans consume about two to four times too much sodium and recommend that daily amounts of sodium not exceed 2.5 grams. To put all this in perspective, less than one teaspoon of salt a day is safe for most healthy adults; Americans still consume two to four times this amount. Buying foods that are low in sodium or sodium free is a good idea for everyone.

A reduction of one-half teaspoon of salt a day has been shown to reduce systolic pressures by an average of 5 mmHg and diastolic pressures by 2.5 mmHg. Lifelong habits of salt consumption can be altered with aggressive behavior change and social support. Successful salt reduction programs have resulted in 30 to 50 percent reductions in total salt consumption and reduced blood pressure.[30]

Reducing dietary sodium is no different from making other lifestyle changes. We change in stages and start by viewing sodium reduction as an essential part of wellness.

Limit Alcohol Consumption. There is a strong connection between alcohol consumption and high blood pressure. Regular consumption of three or more drinks a day increases blood pressure, and heavy drinkers have four times the risk of being hypertensive. The amount of alcohol found in one beer, glass of wine, or shot of spirits is approximately the same. Interestingly, some studies have shown reduction in heart disease risk among individuals who drank fewer than two drinks per day. Researchers propose that ethanol, the alcohol found in alcoholic drinks, may reduce the blood's ability to clot and may increase HDL cholesterols when consumed in moderate amounts. The combination of less clotting and improved blood lipids may reduce overall heart disease risk.

Contradictory findings about the dangers and possible benefits of alcohol consumption are understandably confusing. Too much alcohol will increase hypertension, but just a little might reduce overall risk. Although these findings are equivocal, the medical community is united in their opinion on alcohol consumption. There are no circumstances when alcohol consumption should be prescribed as a part of a healthy lifestyle. Any benefit that may arise from moderate consumption is potentially overwhelmed by the societal, personal, and community problems its abuse can cause. It does not make much sense to promote a treatment that might cause more harm than good. Most experts feel that the best advice is not to start drinking, but if you do drink, to do so in moderation.[31]

Get Some Exercise. Physical activity causes arteries to expand and contract as the body's requirement for additional oxygen and nutrients increases during exercise and decreases as the body slows to a resting state. The contracting and expanding of smooth arterial muscle that occurs during exercise is beneficial in reducing elevated levels of blood pressure. Immediately following an exercise session, blood pressure levels for hypertensive individuals are usually 10–20 mmHg lower than before the exercise session began. Even normal levels of blood pressure decrease 8–12 mmHg following exercise. The reduced levels of blood pressure persist from 20 minutes to 2 hours after the exercise session has concluded. It is believed that regular daily physical activity can produce permanent decreases in blood pressure. The research consensus on exercise and blood pressure reveals that a physically active lifestyle can reduce systolic and diastolic pressures by 10 mmHg.[32]

Activity 9.1
Know Your Numbers

The test to measure blood pressure uses an inflatable cuff around your upper arm. The cuff is inflated until circulation is stopped. As the air in the cuff is slowly released, the return of the blood flow can be heard through a stethoscope. The point at which the first sound is heard is called the systolic pressure—the pressure of the blood vessels as the heart beats. The point at which the sound stops is called the diastolic pressure—the pressure between heart beats. A normal adult blood pressure is 120/80 (read 120 over 80).

Identify your average blood pressure by having it read four separate times under usual conditions. You should be able to see a pattern.

Date	BP Reading
_____	_____
_____	_____
_____	_____
_____	_____

The amount of activity required to achieve this reduction is equal to three to five exercise sessions a week for at least 20 minutes. The intensity of the activity should be between 40 and 60 percent of the person's maximum oxygen uptake. Exercise at this same intensity can also result in an improved cholesterol profile, weight loss, and increased cardiovascular endurance. The activity should be aerobic in nature. Resistance training is not considered to be effective in reducing blood pressure; in fact, during actual lifting periods, blood pressure measures have been recorded at 350/250 mmHg and higher. The postexercise pressure reduction experienced with endurance activities is not seen after a session of weight lifting. Resistance training has other benefits and can be included as part of a balanced fitness program.

Treat Hypertension with Medication. With all cases of hypertension, lifestyle interventions will be the first method of treatment. As we have discussed, behavior change including dietary intervention, exercise, smoking cessation, and weight control has been shown to reduce hypertension and can be the long-term solution to keeping it under control. Few if any side effects are associated with the adoption of lifestyle changes, there is no additional cost, and changes can reduce the risk for a wide range of other illnesses not associated with hypertension.

Treatment of hypertension with medication has been shown to reduce cardiovascular disease mortality. Many people prefer to take medication every day rather than alter their lifestyles. Blood pressure medication does not treat the cause of the disease; it only treats the symptoms. Some individuals fail to take their prescribed medication and only one in five adults on hypertensive medication is able to get his or her blood pressure below 140/90 mmHg. Some of the side effects of medication include weakness, leg cramps, stuffy nose, diarrhea, impotence, and skin rash.

Perhaps the greatest blood pressure lowering effects can be seen when successful lifestyle modification and medication are combined. Effective lifestyle changes can reduce the needed dosages of medications and the number of medications that a person must take.

CAN HEART DISEASE BE REVERSED?

Clearly the best way to avoid cardiovascular disease is to prevent its occurrence through a long-term commitment to a life of healthy living. Few individuals have lived their entire lives in accordance with wellness lifestyles. But it is never too late to start. When a patient is hospitalized because of a blocked coronary artery, the atherosclerosis that caused the block is not confined to just that artery in the heart. Atherosclerosis is systemwide, meaning that it affects all arteries of the body. Clearly, it is important to repair the blocked artery, but what about the rest of the body? Is it reasonable to expect a person with

advanced arterial damage to be able to reverse the damage? The answer is yes.

Atherosclerosis will do one of three things: worsen (progress), be somewhat reduced (regress), or not change at all. Progression is characterized by the worsening of the disease, which ultimately results in premature death. A lifestyle that has produced atherosclerosis in the past will continue to do the same if nothing is done to alter the health risks that are present; however, we have seen the many steps one can take to avoid arterial disease or to reduce its severity if one already has it. If advanced levels of arterial disease can be kept from getting any worse, either through lifestyle changes, medication, or both, present quality of life can be maintained.

The intent of this chapter has been to empower the reader with tools and knowledge to prevent the occurrence of heart disease in the first place. The same lifestyles that can prevent heart disease have been shown to be effective in slowing the progress of or even reversing existing heart disease. Weight loss, exercise, diet intervention, stress reduction, smoking cessation, and medications are all effective in preventing and reversing heart disease.

Studies have demonstrated that drug and diet therapy can lower LDLs and raise HDLs and are effective in retarding the progression of artery plaque and promoting plaque regression. Several studies have evaluated medication, diet, and lifestyle intervention in cardiovascular disease patients who were assigned to either a treatment or control group. The treatment group received medication and education and support for lifestyle changes. This group experienced half the amount of progression and three times the amount of regression as the control group. The most interesting aspect of the study revealed that the treatment patients experienced 50 percent fewer cardiovascular events (death, heart attacks, and so forth). Several studies evaluated the effect of lifestyle interventions without the effect of medication. Patients who consumed very low-fat vegetarian diets, exercised, and practiced stress management lost an average of 22 pounds and experienced a 24 percent reduction in total cholesterol, and over 82 percent of all subjects in the treatment group experienced regression of plaques compared to 42 percent of the control group.[33]

Most of the interventions used in these studies were drastic and were used for relatively short periods. Changing a normal American diet to one with less than 10 percent fat would be difficult for most individuals. But in order for behavior changes to have a lasting reversal on CVD, healthy habits must be maintained for life, not just short term. Some individuals have been able to make very low-fat eating a part of their lifestyles.

DIAGNOSING CVD

Regular medical examinations and evaluation of family history of heart disease can help a physician diagnose early stages of heart disease. If heart disease is suspected,

Healthy Food Substitutes

When trying to manage your weight, sometimes slight changes in the foods you eat can make a tremendous difference. Following are some suggestions for making healthy food substitutions.

Fish, Meat, and Poultry

Decrease or avoid these foods:
fatty cuts of beef, lamb, pork, spare ribs, organ meats
regular cold cuts
bacon
sausage
hot dogs
fried fish
chicken fingers

Choose these instead:
fish
poultry without skin
lean cuts of beef, lamb, pork, or veal
shellfish

Milk and Dairy Products

Decrease or avoid these foods:
whole milk, 2% milk, evaporated or condensed milk
cream, half and half, imitation milk products, nondairy creamers, whipped toppings
whole-milk yogurt
whole-milk cottage cheese
all natural cheeses
cream cheeses, sour cream, including low-fat or "lite" products
ice cream
egg yolks

Choose these instead:
skim or 1% milk
buttermilk
nonfat or low-fat yogurt, low-fat cottage cheese
low-fat cheeses
sherbet, sorbet

egg whites, cholesterol-free egg substitutes

Fruits and Vegetables

Decrease or avoid these foods:
vegetables prepared in butter, cream, or other sauces

Choose these instead:
fresh, frozen, canned, or dried fruits or vegetables

Breads and Cereals

Decrease or avoid these foods:
commercial baked goods: pies, cakes, doughnuts, croissants, pastries, muffins, biscuits
high-fat crackers and cookies
egg noodles
breads in which eggs are a major ingredient

Choose these instead:
homemade baked goods using unsaturated oils sparingly
angel food cake, low-fat crackers and cookies
rice and pasta
whole-grain breads and cereals (oatmeal, whole wheat, rye, bran, multigrain)

Fats and Oils

Decrease or avoid these foods:
chocolate
butter, coconut oil, palm kernel oil, lard, bacon fat
dressings made with egg yolks
coconut

Choose these instead:
baking cocoa
unsaturated vegetable oils: corn, olive, canola, safflower, sesame, soybean, sunflower
margarine or shortenings made from one of the above unsaturated oils
diet margarine
mayonnaise, salad dressings made with unsaturated oils
low-fat dressings
seeds and nuts

---

a number of tests can confirm or disprove a physician's suspicions.

One of the most common screening tests requires the individual to jog on a treadmill. After a few minutes of jogging at a certain speed, the speed is increased little by little until the person cannot continue. Because the treadmill requires maximum cardiovascular output, the heart is forced to work at its maximum effectiveness. Each time the heart contracts and relaxes, a small electrical current is conducted through the body. This electrical activity is monitored with small sensors taped to the chest and is used to produce a printout called an electrocardiogram (ECG). A cardiologist reads the ECG print-

out and looks for specific signs or deviations that may indicate abnormalities in the heart. Because the test makes the person exercise at maximum level, if any problems are present, they will likely surface when the heart is working at its peak of performance. An electrocardiogram may also be taken when the patient is lying down, although signs of heart problems are not always present at rest.

A more sensitive test to detect heart damage is the thallium test. Radioactive thallium is injected into the bloodstream during the last minute of a treadmill test. As the thallium circulates through the vessels of the heart, a three-dimensional picture of the heart is produced by sensors that detect radioactivity. From this picture, physicians are able to see the exact location of the arteries and determine the status of any that are currently blocked. Another diagnostic tool uses sound waves to produce three-dimensional images of the heart called echocardiographs. This test gives doctors the ability to measure heart size and heart wall thickness and to determine if heart valves are functioning properly.

Each of these diagnostic tools is effective in determining the presence of atherosclerosis in the vessels of the heart. Vessels that have enough blockage to reduce the heart's function will require medical treatment and lifestyle changes.

TREATING CVD

Several medications can be used to lower blood pressure and blood cholesterol, control abnormal heart rhythms, and relieve angina pain. Anticlotting drugs called clot-busters have been shown to be effective in reducing the seriousness of heart attacks by dissolving clots that may be blocking arteries. These are only effective if used in the early stages of the heart attack, which is why people who think they may be having a heart attack should seek immediate medical attention.

Invasive treatment for heart disease primarily involves two procedures: balloon angioplasty (technically called percutaneous transluminal coronary angioplasty or PTCA) and heart bypass surgery. PTCA involves inserting a balloon-tipped catheter into the blocked artery. When the tip of the catheter is positioned in the blockage, the balloon is inflated, causing the blockage to be smashed and the plaque to be cracked. Once the catheter is removed, the blocked area is wider and blood flow is restored.

Coronary artery bypass surgery shunts blood around blocked areas in a coronary artery by rerouting blood through a surgically attached vessel. Part of the patient's own leg vein is removed and reattached to the heart in a position that bypasses the blockage. One end of the vein is sewn into the aorta and the other sewn into an artery below the blockage. This allows blood to flow despite a blockage.

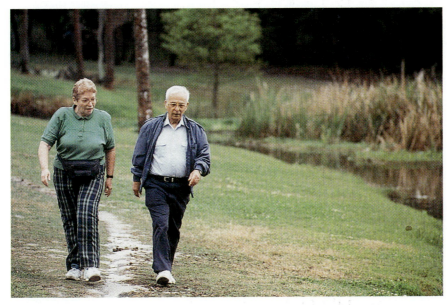

At all stages of life, establishing and maintaining a regular exercise routine is one of the most important steps you can take to prevent heart disease. It's also an important recuperative step for those living with heart disease.

An increasingly common treatment is heart transplant. In this procedure the defective heart of a patient is removed and replaced with a heart taken from a cadaver donor. Tissues are matched by blood type, and the donor heart is usually flown to a hospital where it is prepared for implant. Approximately 65 percent of heart transplant patients are alive after five years.

In most cases, major heart disease causes a greatly decreased quality of life and reduced life span. The only way to avoid the disease is through consistent lifestyle change that reduces those risk factors that are known to cause the disease.

SUMMARY

Even though cardiovascular disease is the leading cause of death for half of all Americans, very few young adults experience the disease. For many, the disease is something you get when you are older. Heart disease is the most preventable of all the major causes of death, but prevention must begin early in life to be effective. College age students are ideally positioned to prevent this disease. Making good choices about the use of tobacco, exercise, and dietary habits can all help in prevention. Even if you do get the disease, treatments are available, but they too will require you to adopt healthy behaviors. So why wait? If you start reducing your risk now, chances are you will never have to experience the disease.

SUGGESTED READING

American Heart Association. *Heart and stroke facts.* Dallas, TX: 1995.

Editors of Consumer Guide. *Cholesterol: Your guide for a healthy heart.* Lincolnwood, IL: Publications International, 1994.

Fischman, J. Type A on trial. *Psychology Today,* February 1987.

Hamann, B. *Disease: Identification, prevention, and control.* St. Louis: Mosby, 1994.

Lorig, K., D. Laurent, H. Holman, V. Gonzalez, D. Sobel, and M. Minior. *Living a healthy life with chronic conditions.* Palo Alto, CA: Bull Publishing, 1994.

What Can I Do?

At the beginning of this chapter, you determined your stage of readiness to change with regard to preventing cardiovascular disease. Now take out a sheet of paper and complete the corresponding section of this lab: precontemplator, contemplator, preparer, action taker, or maintainer.

Precontemplator

1. Precontemplators have many reasons for not checking blood pressure and blood cholesterol or reducing elevated levels. Below are listed several reasons why people are resistant to change. From the list, check those items that best describe your reasons for not wanting to change.

   _____ I'm too lazy.

   _____ I don't have a regular doctor.

   _____ Nobody in my family has had high blood pressure or high cholesterol, so I don't think I need to worry.

   _____ A family member died of heart disease, and I feel I am unable to do anything about my risk.

   _____ I don't have enough self-control to alter my diet.

   _____ I love too many foods that are high in saturated fat and cholesterol.

   _____ I still do not know what my cholesterol and blood pressure are.

   _____ I'm not worried about heart disease because I'm young.

   _____ Other reasons _____

2. List the main barrier why you do not actively try to reduce your elevated levels of blood pressure and/or cholesterol.

   Example: I just don't care about CVD.

3. List three benefits of having a lower heart disease risk. Refer to material in this chapter for ideas.

4. Do your answers in item 3 outweigh your answers in item 1?

5. Think of a relative or acquaintance who has heart disease. How would his or her life be different if he or she did not have the disease?

6. If you could re-live the past, what could you tell this person that might have helped him or her avoid cardiovascular disease?

7. Is any of that advice applicable to you today?

Contemplator

1. In the left column below, write the high-fat and high-sodium foods you consume regularly. Using the list shown in the box on page 224 or your own ideas, list foods you could use as substitutes to your current diet. You may not like all substitutes so rather than write in a substitute food write "reduce" or "eliminate" in the substitutes column.

   Current High-Fat Foods   *Substitutes*

   _____   _____

   _____   _____

   _____   _____

   _____   _____

   _____   _____

   _____   _____

   _____   _____

   _____   _____

   _____   _____

   _____   _____

2. Why do you think about reducing your risk of CVD?

3. What actually prevents you from doing anything to reduce your risk?

4. Make a list of your reasons for being for and against reducing your risk.

5. Can you think of anyone who can help you reduce your risk? Ask them to do so.

Preparer

1. Write a long-term goal regarding your high level of cholesterol or blood pressure. (*Examples:* I will lower my blood pressure 10 mmHg during the next six months. I will lower my blood cholesterol to less than 200 mg/dl in the next six months.)

2. With this goal in mind, make a specific plan of attack to help you overcome your barriers and change your behavior. Remember, you can't do everything at once. Pick one aspect of your behavior and develop a plan to change it. Review the chapter for the various methods to reduce blood pressure and cholesterol as you develop your plan. For example: If your goal was to lower your level of blood cholesterol to below 200, then you might form the following plan:

    a. Identify foods in your diet that are high in fat and cholesterol.

    b. Make a detailed plan on reducing the amount of fat and cholesterol in your diet. (See Chapter 6 for help.)

    c. Make a detailed plan to begin an exercise program. (See Chapter 3.)

    d. Set goals and deadlines to accomplish these details.

3. What friends or family members can help you attain your goal?

4. Complete the following statement:

    I am going to take my first step on _____ .
    date within 30 days

Action Taker

1. What things are you currently doing to lower your risk of heart disease?

2. What success are you having? Is your blood pressure or cholesterol lower because of them? If they are not working, try to explain why not.

3. Are your goals specifically and clearly stated? What is your long-term risk reduction goal?

4. What can you do differently to increase your success?

5. After reviewing the chapter, list some other strategies that can be used to lower your risk.

6. What is the biggest temptation for you?

7. Is there a way to prevent this (item 6)?

8. It is easy to get discouraged when change does not happen quickly. Whom can you talk to to get ideas, encouragement, or support?

9. How is your life different now that you have been working on lowering your risk of CVD?

10. How might your future be affected by the changes you are making today?

Maintainer

Congratulations, you are doing great. If you are a maintainer, either you have reduced your blood pressure and/or blood cholesterol or you never had a risk to begin with. If you have lowered your risk, complete the next section. If you never had high risk, go to the section entitled, "I'm risk free."

I Lowered My Risk!

1. List three of the successes you have had in your attempts to lower your heart disease risk (for example: I avoid eating greasy fast foods and I have lost weight).

2. If you stop taking blood pressure medication or you stop living a low-risk lifestyle, don't get discouraged. Quickly start over again. If you have relapsed in the past, list the reasons why you did and what you did to get back on track.

3. Write down a few things you can do to prevent relapse in the future.

4. What advice do you have for individuals who are struggling to become maintainers?

I'm Risk Free!

1. Blood pressure and blood cholesterol increase with age. What can you do now to keep your risk low?

2. You may have a poor diet and still have low levels of blood pressure and cholesterol. Besides high blood pressure and cholesterol, what other health risks might you have because of your diet?

L A B 9.2

Assessing Heart Disease Risk

Using this simple worksheet, you can calculate your heart disease risk score. Circle one number by each risk factor that applies to you. Total your score, and use the table at the end of the assessment to determine your risk classification. You will need your systolic blood pressure (the higher pressure when the heart beats) and blood cholesterol measurements to take this test. If you have not been measured, we highly recommend you see your doctor or local public health department very soon.

Heredity

Do you have a father or brother who had heart disease before age 55 or a mother or sister with heart disease before age 65?

No	0
Yes, but just one individual in family	3
Yes, with more than one individual	4

Age/Gender

Are you a male 45 years of age or older or a female 55 years of age or older?

No	0
Yes	4

Cigarette Smoking

Never have smoked or quit more than 15 years ago	0
Ex-smoker (quit less than 15 years ago)	1
Smoke 1–20 cigarettes a day	2
Smoke 21–40 cigarettes a day	3
Smoke 41 or more cigarettes a day	4

Blood Pressure

Your systolic blood pressure is

< 120 mmHg	0
121–129 mmHg	1
130–139 mmHg	2
140–149 mmHg	3
> 149 mmHg	4

Blood Cholesterol

Your serum cholesterol is

< 200 mg/dl	0
200–219 mg/dl	1
220–239 mg/dl	2
240–259 mg/dl	3
> 259 mg/dl	4

Inactivity

How often do you usually engage in physical exercise that moderately or strongly increases your breathing and heart rate, and makes you sweat, for at least a total of 30 minutes a day such as in brisk walking, cycling, swimming, jogging, or manual labor?

5 or more times a week	0
3 or 4 times a week	1
2 times a week	2
1 time a week	3
None	4

Source: Based on information from the Framingham Heart Study, *Circulation* 83:356–362,1991, and the MRFIT research project, *Archives of Internal Medicine* 152:56–64, 1992.

Obesity

How would you rate your body weight?

Close to ideal	0
About 10 to 20 pounds overweight	1
About 21 to 50 pounds overweight	2
About 51 to 100 pounds overweight	3
More than 100 pounds overweight	4

Stress

How would you describe the stress you experience?

Low or moderate levels of stress	0
High stress, but am able to cope with it	1
High stress, and often feel unable to cope	2
Very high stress, but trying to cope with it	3
Very high stress, and unable to cope with it	4

Diabetes

Have you been diagnosed with diabetes by a doctor?

No	0
Yes	4

Your Heart Disease Risk Classification

Total your points here: _____

Now use the scale below to determine your CVD risk classification.

Classification	Total Points
Very low risk	Fewer than 5
Low risk	6–10
Moderately high risk	11–15
High risk	16–20
Very high risk	More than 20

All of the above risk factors except heredity, age, and gender are modifiable. That means if you scored high, chances are you can do something about it.

CHAPTER 10

Cancer and Other Common Threats to Wellness

Terms

- Cancer
- Tumors
- Benign
- Malignant
- Metastasize
- Oncogenes
- Carcinogens
- Carcinomas
- Sarcomas
- Lymphomas
- Leukemia
- Mammogram
- Malignant melanomas
- Biopsy
- Radiation therapy
- Chemotherapy
- Immunotherapy
- Noninfectious
- Diabetes mellitus
- Type I diabetes
- Type II diabetes
- Hypoglycemia
- Tension headaches
- Psychological headaches
- Secondary headaches
- Migraine headaches
- Allergens
- Hives
- Anaphylactic shock

Objectives

1. Define cancer and discuss the theories regarding how cancer develops.

2. Learn the major risk factors and causes for the most common forms of cancer.

3. Learn how some cancers can be prevented.

4. Adopt lifestyles that prevent cancer.

5. Understand the roles of diet and exercise in cancer prevention.

6. Discuss cancer detection and treatment, including radiation, chemotherapy, and immunotherapy.

7. Learn about headaches, asthma, allergies, and diabetes.

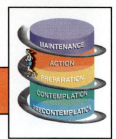

Where Am I?

Precontemplator _____ I do not practice cancer-prevention strategies, and I do not intend to start.

Contemplator _____ I often think about reducing my cancer risk, but I just haven't done anything about it yet.

Preparer _____ Not only do I think about reducing my cancer risk, but I'm planning to do something about it within the next thirty days.

Action Taker _____ I am actively reducing my cancer risk but have done so for less than six months.

Maintainer _____ I practice regular cancer-prevention activities and have done so for at least six months.

Healthy cancer prevention strategies include regular breast self-exams for women and a regular mammogram for women over 50. Other lifestyle choices that may help prevent cancer include using safeguards to protect against sun exposure, avoiding tobacco and secondhand smoke, consuming a healthy diet, limiting or avoiding alcohol consumption, and exercising regularly. Read the statements above, which describe cancer-prevention practices, and determine which stage best fits your current cancer-prevention attitudes.

Some diseases are not affected by the way we live our lives. Down syndrome, for example, is an inherited condition caused by a gene defect. You cannot develop Down syndrome by having a poor diet or not exercising; it is entirely inherited. Unlike Down syndrome, most of the common diseases of our time are only slightly related to genetics. Experts estimate that 76 percent of all disease is determined by lifestyle, suggesting that when you look at the big picture, genetics play less of a role in the disease process than we previously thought.[1]

Individuals can choose where and how to live. Some people live reckless, high-risk lives, whereas others follow more conservative paths in hopes of avoiding disease and death as long as possible. This chapter has been included to convince readers that cancer can be postponed or even avoided through adoption of a wellness lifestyle and that chronic conditions such as diabetes or headaches don't have to lower quality of life even though they may be part of daily living. Those who understand these conditions are often better able to deal with illnesses if and when they do occur.

CANCER: THE BIG C

During his successful acting career, John Wayne used to call cancer "The Big C." In 1979, he died after a long struggle with lung cancer. Even today it seems everyone is talking about cancer. Researchers are constantly finding new ways to treat, detect, prevent, and survive cancer, and the media are quick to report any cancer-related news. Almost everyone has a relative or knows someone who is suffering from some form of the disease. It seems that cancer is everywhere; perhaps "The Big C" *is* big when it comes to death and disease.

Recent statistics from the U.S. Department of Health and Human Services reveal that cancer is the number two cause of death in this country and that one out of every three people will eventually have some form of the disease. Cancer is responsible for one out of every five deaths.[2] Overall, with the exception of lung cancer, which is on the rise, the numbers of cases of cancer are either remaining the same or declining slightly. Many individuals who were heavy smokers during the seventies and eighties are now developing lung cancer. At one time, 54 percent of the population smoked; now the prevalence of lung cancer is a direct reflection of the days when smoking was popular. Today, even though fewer people smoke (26 percent of the U.S. population), it will take several years for the lung cancer rate to reflect this change.

Although there are many types of cancers, lung, colorectal, and breast cancer account for over half of all cancer cases. Figure 10.1 demonstrates the cancer rate for the various types of cancer for men and women.

Because of improved treatments and early detection, the average survival time for cancer victims is increasing. Of those who developed cancer in 1990, half were still alive in 1995. However, the prospect of surviving cancer is not the same for all people. White patients have a 50 percent survival rate, while African Americans have a 37 percent survival rate. The difference is partly explained by socioeconomic factors such as access to health care early

in the disease or access to state-of-the-art technology if the disease has progressed. Future reductions in cancer incidence and increases in cancer survival rates will depend primarily on the prevention and early diagnosis of cancer.

What Is Cancer?

Cancer is not one disease, but a group of over 100 different diseases, each of which is characterized by the uncontrolled growth and spread of abnormal cells. Normally the cells that make up the body reproduce and divide in an orderly manner, so that old or injured cells are replaced with new ones. Several factors in the environment or within the cell itself can cause a new cell to undergo an abnormal change that makes it different from the parent cells. A single mutated cell will divide into two and then four and eight and so on, eventually forming clusters of abnormal cells called **tumors.** Unlike normal cells, which divide, grow, and replace old cells in an orderly fashion, abnormal cells grow and reproduce randomly. This uncontrolled growth is the common characteristic of all cancers.

A tumor that grows inside a confined space and does not spread usually does not pose a threat to life. These

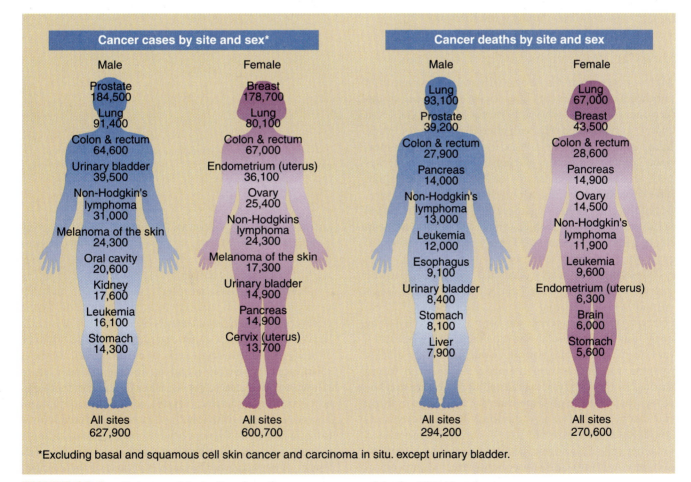

FIGURE 10.1   Estimates of the leading sites of new cancer cases and deaths, 1998. (American Cancer Society, *Cancer facts and figures—1998*, p. 9. Reprinted by permission of the American Cancer Society, Inc.)

tumors are said to be **benign** and include many common growths like freckles and moles. If a benign tumor continues to enlarge in a crowded space, other neighboring organs may get squeezed so much that they stop functioning normally. This is the only circumstance in which a benign tumor may be life threatening and is the reason why benign tumors are often removed.

The abnormal cells of a cancerous, or **malignant,** tumor, however, are dangerous and can become fatal quickly if not recognized and treated early. These cells can cause problems either by invading tissues in the surrounding area or by spreading throughout the body like seeds in the wind. Wherever the abnormal cells land, they start other abnormal growths. Cancer cells can be transported by the bloodstream or through the lymphatic system of vessels that transport a liquid called lymph. The purpose of the lymphatic system is to drain infectious, toxic, and other waste materials from the body. Once cancer cells enter the lymphatic system, they rapidly spread to other areas. (See Figure 10.2.) The term **metastasize** refers to the spreading of cancerous cells. Once new cancer growths start appearing at other locations of the body, organ damage and dysfunction soon result, and it is possible to have two or more malignant tumors growing at the same time in different areas of the body. The only way to tell if a cancer cell is benign or malignant is to examine it under a microscope.

How Cancer Develops

All forms of cancer display growth and reproduction of abnormal cells. Scientists have focused on trying to determine how and why apparently normal cells can change and produce cells with altered genetic properties. Many experts believe that cancer results from a spontaneous error that occurs during cell reproduction. Genetic errors may be caused by cells that are older or that have been subjected to extreme stress or injury. It is believed that the genetic sequence of the normal parent cell is broken or changed, which affects the genetic makeup of any cells that are created. The altered cells continue to reproduce as they form tumors.

Research that was conducted on cancer-causing viruses has led scientists to believe that all chromosomes contain a few genes that may be cancer causing.[3] These genes, termed **oncogenes,** are found in all cells of the body, but are almost always dormant. Once activated they begin to grow and reproduce uncontrollably, quickly forming tumors. Although oncogenes may be found throughout the body, it is believed that they are activated by the influence of some external agent or condition such as age, stress, toxins, radiation, viruses, or even sunshine. Researchers are not sure if oncogenes are passed on genetically or if normal genes are somehow altered by certain conditions and subsequently turned into oncogenes. New knowledge about genetics and cancer is being discovered every day as researchers study cancer-related problems. The governments of the United States

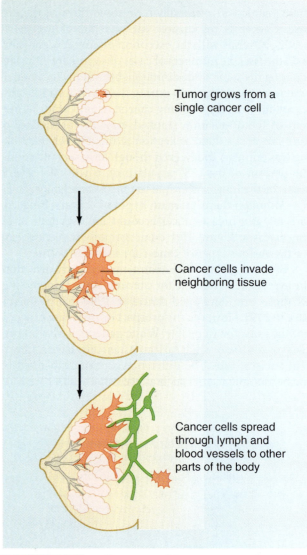

FIGURE 10.2   Illustration of the progression of a malignant breast tumor.

- Tumor grows from a single cancer cell
- Cancer cells invade neighboring tissue
- Cancer cells spread through lymph and blood vessels to other parts of the body

and several European countries currently support several large research projects to answer gene-related cancer questions in an attempt to find effective methods of preventing and treating cancer.

Perhaps the most accepted cancer theory states that normal genes can be altered and made cancerous by the effects of certain external agents or substances that enter the cell and cause the genetic sequencing of the cell to be altered. Cancer-causing agents, or **carcinogens,** are those substances or environmental agents that are believed or known to be related to cancer. They include tar from cigarette smoke, radiation, nitrates, certain hormones and hormone drugs, ultraviolet light, asbestos, some medications, alcohol, and many other substances, including a variety of chemicals that surround us every day. The length of exposure or the larger the dose of the carcinogen tends to determine the extent of the damage.

The most frustrating aspect of carcinogens is the difficulty researchers have in proving that a substance can absolutely cause cancer. For decades the tobacco industry has been able to evade legal and government actions because of the lack of absolute, clinical proof that smoking causes cancer. It is not ethical to randomly designate a few individuals to become long-term smokers and then track them for several years to see whether they develop cancer. Researchers can only develop circumstantial evidence of the possible cancer-causing effects of a substance. But this evidence has grown to the extent that experts feel confident in stating that tobacco smoke does cause cancer and it appears that the courts agree. The Liggett Group, the smallest of the big four tobacco companies, recently agreed to a settlement to repay state Medicaid money spent treating sick smokers. This settlement has acted as a catalyst that has brought every major tobacco manufacturer into the largest lawsuit in history. The details of the settlement are still being worked out, but one thing is certain, for the first time ever, the tobacco industry has been forced to rethink its pursuit of corporate profits at the expense of human suffering.

Causes of Cancer

Because so little is known about cancer and its causes, the general public is quick to suggest that many substances are probably cancer causing even though there may be little hard evidence to support these claims. Scientists all over the world are working to unravel the reasons why some substances are related to cancers, but until more information is obtained, the only prudent thing to do is to avoid suspected agents or factors as much as possible. In the future, researchers may be able to state that certain substances are proven causes of cancer, much as they have already done with tobacco and tobacco products.

Heredity

The offices of the National Institutes of Health are currently involved in a gene identification program called the Human Genome Project. Its main goal is to map the entire human gene sequence, which involves the identification of each gene sequence for each of the twenty-three chromosomes. Using this information, cancer researchers have identified several abnormal gene sequences that are related to some forms of cancer. Every cell in the body contains the entire genetic sequence, including any inherited gene abnormalities. But just because a person has a known defective sequence does not mean he or she will develop cancer. At this time, the number of cancer cases largely caused by genetics is thought to be very small. The complex interaction among genetics, environment, and lifestyle makes the identification of inherited cancers extremely difficult.

Family histories of cancer suggest a genetic link, but this may not mean the cancer was genetic. If a grandmother, mother, and sisters all suffer from breast cancer, it is reasonable to assume that they inherited a high risk for the disease. However, this phenomenon might also be explained by lifestyle or environment. Perhaps all members of the family lived in the same area and were all exposed to the same carcinogen. Possibly they all had comparable diets or shared other known cancer risk factors. The difficult task of teasing out the genetic influence on cancers keeps everyone wondering what the real causes are. Cancers of the breast, stomach, colon, prostate, uterus, ovaries, and lungs appear to run in families more than some other kinds of cancer.

Race

Race is another genetic factor related to cancer. The highest rates of cancer are found among black males. As can be seen in Figure 10.3, black males have twice the death rate of cancer as all other races and genders, with the exception of white males who have a third less deaths. The races with the lowest cancer death rates are Native Americans and Native Alaskans. Even though race is genetic and is related to cancer, it is not a cause of cancer. The differences in cancer death rates between Asian men and African American men, for example, are most likely due to differences in education, access to quality medical care, diet, or other social and cultural differences.

Gender

Gender is also an important inherited factor that can increase risk of certain cancers. Many are surprised to learn that breast cancer also occurs in men, but these cases are rare when compared to the fact that one out of eight women will have breast cancer in her lifetime.[4] Gender-specific organs such as the prostate, uterus, ovaries, and testes are common cancer sites. It is of course impossible for men to get uterine cancer or for women to get prostate cancer. Gender is inherited and these cancers are gender-specific. Although gender plays a role in certain cancers, other factors are perhaps of greater importance.

Environment

The world in which we live is perhaps the biggest cause of cancer. We work, sleep, and play in an environment filled with known and unknown carcinogens. Occupational hazards include exposure to carcinogens that are commonly found at worksites. (See Table 10.1.) These include asbestos, a fiberlike substance formerly used in ceiling and floor tiles, insulation, and other construction materials.

When tiny asbestos fibers are inhaled, they damage the lungs and require new cells to replace old damaged cells. Repeated exposure increases the risk of an abnormal cell being produced. Other occupational risks include coal dust, which is often inhaled by miners and mining employees. Painting and auto repair specialists are exposed to inhalants and solvents known to be related to lung cancer. Farmers who repeatedly work with herbicides and pesticides are known to suffer from in-

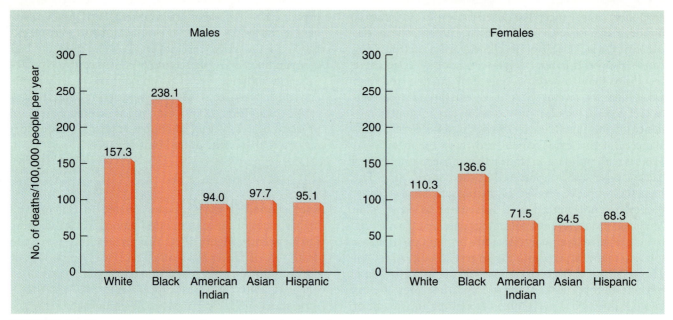

FIGURE 10.3   Cancer death rates by race and gender. (Data from U.S. Department of Health and Human Services, *Health United States, 1994.* Public Health Service, Centers for Disease Control and Prevention, National Center for Health Statistics. DHHS Publication No. (PHS)95–1232. Hyattsville, MD, May 1995.)

creased rates of various cancers. Environmental carcinogens can also be found in public water supplies, especially in private wells where regular testing in not required. There is also a possibility of increased cancer risk for those living in homes that have measurable amounts of radon—a naturally occurring radioactive substance—in the soil or surrounding bedrock.

Food Additives

Whenever a new food additive is proposed, the Food and Drug Administration requires extensive animal and human testing before the additive is permitted in foods. Any additive that demonstrates possible health dangers does not get FDA approval. Too often, fear of food additives is fueled by unsubstantiated stories of cancer vic-

tims who claim that their cancer was caused by a specific additive found in the foods they ate.

The food and beverage industries have adopted saccharin as an artificial sweetener that can be used to replace high-calorie sweeteners. Many scientists labeled saccharin a carcinogen, only to be outvoiced by the American Diabetic Association, which saw saccharin as a vital and important breakthrough for people with diabetes. They believed that any cancer-causing effects that might be associated with saccharin were outweighed by the risks associated with not maintaining proper blood sugar levels. The FDA gave its approval for saccharin, but with the condition that all products containing the additive carry a warning label similar to the one found on cigarettes. Other artificial sweeteners such as NutraSweet and Equal have been developed and marketed aggres-

TABLE 10.1 ■ Carcinogens and Occupations		
Occupation	**Suspected Carcinogen**	**Type of Cancer**
Automobile mechanic	Petroleum products	Larynx, lung, nasal passages, scrotum, skin
Carpenter	Wood dusts	Nasal passages, sinus cavity
Dyer	Benzene and other aromatics	Bladder, leukemia
Farmer	Ultraviolet rays of the sun	Skin
Miner	Arsenic, asbestos, coal, iron oxide, uranium	Liver, lung, skin; lung; bladder, larynx, lung, scrotum, skin; larynx, lung; bone, lung, skin
Painter	Benzene	Leukemia
Rubber worker	Vinyl chloride	Liver
Textile worker	Cadmium	Kidney, lung, prostate

sively and can now be found in many food products. Sugar substitutes, preservatives, coloring agents, and artificial flavors are used extensively in processed foods. The limited studies on these additives have been unable to demonstrate any consistent evidence that they are related to or can cause cancer. At the present time, there are no known dangers in consuming these substances, but this may change as researchers evaluate long-term data on the use of additives. There is, however, some evidence that links nitrates with esophageal and stomach cancer. Nitrates are used to smoke or cure meats like bacon, sausage, and other dried meats.

Cigarette Smoke

If you smoke, or if you live and work in a smoke-filled environment, you will have a greater risk of cancer. Cigarette smoke is the largest known cause of cancer and the most preventable. People who smoke two or more packs a day are fifteen to twenty times more likely to die of cancer than are nonsmokers. Cigarette smoke causes most cases of lung cancer and is clearly related to cancer of the throat, mouth, esophagus, pancreas, and bladder. Pipe smokers or users of chewing tobacco have an increased risk of cancers of the mouth and throat. Breathing secondhand smoke can cause a threefold increase in lung cancers.[5]

A study of cigarette smoke and pregnant women compared pregnant women who smoked, who lived or worked in a smoky environment, and who were not exposed to any smoke at all. When their children were born, a small sample of the babies' hair was taken and analyzed for smoke-related chemicals. Babies born to mothers who smoked had the highest amount of chemical residues in their hair, but amazingly, the mothers who were nonsmokers but were exposed to secondhand tobacco smoke also gave birth to babies whose hair had high amounts of the same chemicals. This study demonstrated that environmental smoke has a permeating effect on unborn babies.[6] The dangers imposed on these infants are not clearly known, but it would be prudent for expectant mothers to not smoke or live in a smoke-filled environment.

Radiation

The word *radiation* is generally associated with the emission of subatomic particles. Exposure to this type of radiation does cause cancer, but unless you live or work around materials that are radioactive, the risk of exposure to this cancer-causing substance is extremely rare.

Another form of radiation, ultraviolet light from the sun, is a much greater cause of cancer. Sunlight is responsible for 600,000 cases of skin cancer every year. Lifeguards, sailors, construction workers, farmers, or anyone else who spends considerable time outside is at risk of getting skin cancer. Most skin cancer is easily treated by burning or surgically removing the abnormal

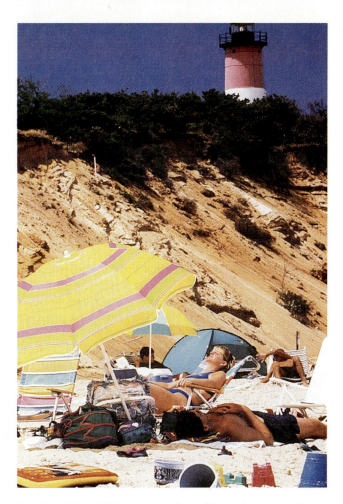

Despite evidence of the negative effects of the sun's rays, people continue to place themselves at risk for skin cancer while searching for "the perfect tan."

cells. However, 4 to 5 percent of all skin cancers are serious enough to be potentially fatal.

Viruses

It's easy to catch a cold, but can you "catch" cancer? Researchers have known for some time that viruses can cause tumors in animals, but only recently have they shown a connection between viruses and cancer in humans. Leukemia, lymphomas, and cancers of the liver and cervix can be caused by viruses. The human immunodeficiency virus (HIV) can lead to certain types of cancers and the herpes virus can cause leukemia. Most likely the presence of a virus will not cause cancer unless the immune system is also compromised.

TYPES AND FORMS OF CANCER

Oncologists (physicians who specialize in the study and treatment of cancer) can determine the type and severity of most cancers using laboratory results. Cancers that receive a high rating have spread further and are more difficult to cure. Cancers are also classified according to the type of body tissue they have affected.

Carcinomas are found in the epithelial tissues (tissues that line body surfaces or cavities) and account for most forms of cancer. They include cancers that affect the breast, skin, lung, intestines, pancreas, mouth, and other similar tissues. Malignant carcinomas spread to adjacent tissues and eventually enter the lymphatic and/or blood vessels as they spread throughout the body.

Sarcomas are forms of cancer that occur in muscle and bone, and in connective tissue that is found in the mesodermal, or middle, layers of the body. They are less common, and spread through the blood during early stages of the disease.

Lymphomas are cancers that form in the lymphatic system. When this type of cancer spreads, it travels quickly throughout the body as it metastasizes to other lymph nodes and vessels. Hodgkin's disease is one type of lymphoma.

Leukemia occurs in the blood-forming parts of the body, including the marrow of long bones and the spleen. Leukemia is characterized by an abnormal increase in the number of white blood cells.

Of the four types of cancers, carcinomas are the most common and are responsible for most cancer deaths. To help you better understand and prevent these cancers, we will discuss a few of the most common types.

Lung Cancer

Because smoking is related to more than 75 percent of all lung cancer cases, avoidance of tobacco products will eliminate most of the risk of lung cancer. Chemicals in the smoke irritate the cells of the lungs and cause many of them to die. The rapid replacement of destroyed cells eventually produces a cancerous cell that starts to metastasize. Smokers who quit often experience some tissue restoration and may even see improvements in their cancer prognosis if they quit as soon as cancer has been detected. The risk of developing lung cancer drops almost to the same level as that of nonsmokers after ten years of tobacco-free living, even though the lungs may still be damaged.

Risk factors for lung cancer include smoking for twenty or more years, exposure to industrial substances such as asbestos and coal dust, passive smoke, and radiation. Symptoms of lung cancer include a persistent cough, blood in the sputum, recurring bronchitis or pneumonia, and chest pain. If the cancer is localized, surgery is performed to remove the tumor; spreading tumors are treated with surgery, chemotherapy, and radiation therapy. Lung cancer stands out from other forms of cancer because of the low survival rates seen five years after the cancer is diagnosed. Only 13 percent of lung cancer patients live longer than five years after cancer is identified. It is deadly, painful, and almost entirely preventable. (See Chapter 14 for information on quitting.[7])

Breast Cancer

Over the past sixty years, there has been a slow and steady increase in breast cancer among American women. By the early 1990s one out of eight women could expect to contract breast cancer sometime during her lifetime. In 1994, more than 182,000 American women were diagnosed with breast cancer.

Warning signs of breast cancer include changes in the breast such as a lump, thickening, swelling, dimpling, skin irritation, distortion, nipple discharge, pain, or tenderness. Risk factors for breast cancer include age greater than 50 years and family history of breast cancer, especially in a grandmother, mother, or sister. Other risk factors include sedentary lifestyle, never having had children, not breast feeding, and having a first child after the age of 30. Some studies that evaluated the relationship between alcohol and breast cancer found that women who drank as few as three drinks a week were 30 percent more likely to have breast cancer than women who seldom or never drank.[8]

Even though studies have not been able to find an association between dietary fat and breast cancer, women

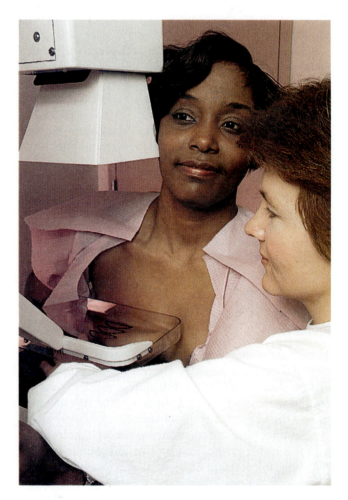

Mammograms, in conjunction with self-exams and medical examinations by a doctor, improve a woman's chances of early detection, one of the most successful weapons in fighting breast cancer.

who are overweight and carry excessive body fat may be at increased risk. The link between estrogen and breast cancer has been clearly established.[9] The more estrogen in a woman's body over her lifetime, the greater her risk of developing breast cancer. Early menarche, late menopause, and obesity can increase exposure to estrogen and all have been linked to breast cancer. Women who have undergone hysterectomies or who are postmenopausal and taking hormone replacement therapy need to know that an extensive review of hormone treatment studies has failed to demonstrate a conclusive association between hormone replacement therapy and breast cancer.

The best defense against breast cancer is early detection. To detect changes or lumps that could indicate breast cancer, all women should perform monthly breast self-exams and have a professional breast exam every three years between the ages of 20 and 40, and yearly after that. Figure 10.4 shows the correct method for doing breast self-exams (BSE).

The best tool for detecting breast cancer is the **mammogram,** an x-ray exam of the breast. Mammography can detect tumors that might not be detected by manual examination for another two or three years. Women over the age of 50 should have a yearly mammogram. Some physicians recommend a baseline mammogram for women between the ages of 35 and 49. Women should discuss mammography with their physicians, who will assess individual risk factors and recommend early mammograms if necessary.[10] Research on women 50 years or older has shown that clinical breast examination and mammography can reduce breast cancer mortality by one-third.

Increased awareness, better diagnostic tools, and improved treatments have caused the five-year breast cancer survival rate to increase from 78 percent in 1940 to 92 percent today. If the cancer has not spread, the survival rate is 100 percent. Breast cancer treatment includes lumpectomy (removal of the lump), radical mastectomy (complete removal of the breast and surrounding tissue), chemotherapy, and radiation therapy.

Skin Cancer

Caught early, skin cancer is not life threatening. The most common types of skin cancers affect the squamous and basal layers of the skin and usually do not spread. However, 3 to 5 percent of skin cancers are **malignant melanomas,** which spread quickly and are much more dangerous. The overall risk of getting melanoma is about one in 120, but the risk goes up with each of the following factors: red or blond hair, freckling on the upper back, family history of melanomas, three or more severe sunburns as a teenager, and two or three years of outdoor work during the summer.

Changes in a wart or mole or a sore that does not heal may signal skin cancer. Avoiding excessive exposure to the sun and other artificial sources of ultraviolet light is the best method of preventing skin cancer.

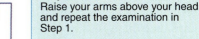

How to Examine Your Breasts

Do you know that 95% of breast cancers are discovered first by women themselves? And that the earlier the breast cancer is detected, the better the chance for a complete cure? Of course, most lumps or changes are not cancer. But you can safeguard your health by making a habit of examining your breasts once a month – a day or two after your period or, if you're no longer menstruating, on any given day. And if you notice anything changed or unusual – a lump, thickening, or discharge – contact your doctor right away.

How to Look for Changes

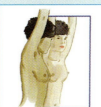

Step 1
Sit or stand in front of a mirror with your arms at your side. Turning slowly from side to side, check your breasts for
• changes in size or shape
• puckering or dimpling of the skin
• changes in size or position of one nipple compared to the other

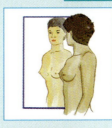

Step 2
Raise your arms above your head and repeat the examination in Step 1.

Step 3
Gently press each nipple with your fingertips to see if there is any discharge.

How to Feel for Changes

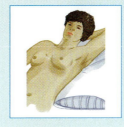

Step 1
Lie down and put a pillow or folded bath towel under your left shoulder. Then place your left hand under your head. (From now on you will be feeling for a lump or thickening in your breasts.)

Step 2
Imagine that your breast is divided into quarters.

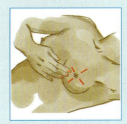

Step 3
With the fingers of your right hand held together, press firmly but gently, using small circular motions to feel the inner, upper quarter of your left breast. Start at your breastbone and work toward the nipple. Also examine the area around the nipple. Now do the same for the lower, inner portion of your breast.

Step 4
Next, bring your arm to your side and feel under your left armpit for swelling.

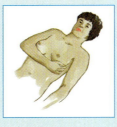

Step 5
With your arm still down, feel the upper, outer part of your breast, starting with your nipple and working outwards. Examine the lower, outer quarter in the same way.

Step 6
Now place the pillow under your right shoulder and repeat all the steps using your left hand to examine your right breast.

FIGURE 10.4 Steps to use when learning to do breast self-exams.

Indoor sunlamps or tanning lights are dangerous because they emit ultraviolet radiation, which after one-half hour of exposure is equal to a full day of outdoor sunlight.

It is possible to spend many hours outside in the sun and still not significantly increase your risk of skin cancer. Skin cancer prevention requires careful planning and application of a few basic principles: avoid sunburn by using effective sunblock lotions and creams [those with a Sun Protection Factor (SPF) of at least 15], wear a hat, and wear a long-sleeved shirt and long pants if possible. And remember, there is no such thing as a healthy tan.

Colon and Rectal Cancer

More than 55,000 Americans died of cancer of the colon and rectum during 1992, the last year for which actual figures are available. It is the third most common type of cancer for both men and women, affecting some 156,000 people yearly. There is strong evidence that lifestyle is the biggest factor in determining who develops this cancer, because diets high in fat and low in fiber as well as a sedentary lifestyle are all strongly related to colon cancer. Men develop it more often than women and adults older than fifty have the greatest risk. Blood in the stool, bleeding from the rectum, and changes in bowel habits are serious warning signs. Colon and rectal cancers tend to spread slowly, which greatly increases the survival rate after surgical treatment. Part of an annual physical exam includes a digital rectal examination.

Prostate Cancer

One in eleven men will suffer from prostate cancer, which is more common than either lung or colon cancers. It is also the second most deadly cancer for men, killing an estimated 32,000 men a year. Risk factors include age greater than 45, family history, a high-fat diet, multiple sexual partners, and a history of sexually transmitted diseases (STDs). Race also seems to play a role. African Americans are more susceptible to this cancer than are males of other races and should start regular screening at age 45. The signs and symptoms of prostate cancer are vague and nonspecific and include pain or difficulty when urinating, pain in the lower back or pelvis, and blood in the urine. In those men whose prostate cancers are still localized, the survival rate is 88 percent. For this reason, digital rectal exams and prostate-specific antigen tests should be conducted every year after age 50.

Other Forms of Cancer

Women should get a regular Pap test to identify cervical and uterine cancers. The Pap test requires that cells be taken from the cervix and surrounding areas and examined for abnormal cell activity. The test works well for cervical cancers, but is less effective in detecting uterine cancers. Risk factors for both types of cancer include early age of first intercourse, multiple sex partners, cigarette smoking, and exposure to sexually transmitted diseases. Unusual bleeding, including bleeding after menopause, or unusual discharge is a warning sign that something might be wrong.

Testicular cancer is one of the few cancers that affect men between the ages of 15 and 34. No exact cause is known. Testicular self-examination is the best way to detect unusual lumps or nodules on either testicle. To examine each testicle, place the index and middle fingers of both hands under the testicle and the thumbs on top. Gently roll the testicle between the thumbs and fingers, feeling for small lumps. If you locate a suspicious lump or thickening, seek medical attention right away.

PREVENTING CANCER

The Diet Connection

You have already read about the significant role diet can take in promoting wellness. The link between diet and cancer has been widely researched. Colorectal, stomach, breast, esophageal, and uterine cancers have all been linked to diets high in fat.[11,12] The average intake of dietary fat accounts for 38 percent of total daily calories, but should be less than 30 percent. You've heard it before, but we'll say it again: the average American eats too much fat. Reductions in dietary fat will lower the incidence of cancer.[13]

Dietary fiber may help prevent colon cancer. Fiber is needed in our diets because it reduces foods' *transit time,* the time it takes for consumed foods to pass through the digestive tract. When the passage of food through the large intestine is slowed because of lack of sufficient water or fiber, constipation occurs and transit time of undigested food increases. A diet high in fiber introduces nondigestible fiber (roughage) into the colon. The fiber retains water, helping fecal matter pass through the colon more quickly. Fecal material may contain cancer-causing substances that continually make contact with the wall of the large intestine. The longer it takes fecal matter to pass through the colon, the greater the exposure to the carcinogens.

One of the differences between white and whole-wheat bread is the substantial amount of fiber found in whole-wheat bread. Natural foods such as fruits, vegetables, whole grains, and cereals also contain large amounts of fiber and should be the mainstay of a healthy diet.

In addition to dietary fiber, fruits and vegetables also contain large amounts of vitamins A, C, and E, which have been classified as antioxidants. Some researchers believe that antioxidants may prevent gene damage inflicted by free radicals, which may be a direct cause of cancer (the vitamin section of Chapter 6 has more information on antioxidants). Overall cancer risk may be reduced by eating a diet that is low in fat and high in fiber, and that contains ample antioxidants. As you may have

Dietary Guidelines to Reduce Cancer Risk

The American Cancer Society has provided several dietary guidelines that can significantly reduce your risk of cancer. Some researchers estimate that 40 to 50 percent of all cancers are related to diet. Put in perspective, one out of three people will get some form of cancer and approximately half of all cancers can be avoided by eating a proper diet.[a]

Maintain desirable weight. Sensible eating habits and regular exercise will help you avoid excessive weight gain. Being 40 percent overweight significantly increases your risk for colon, breast, gallbladder, prostate, ovarian, and uterine cancer.

Eat a varied diet. A varied diet consumed in moderate quantities seems to lower the risk of getting cancer.

Include a variety of vegetables and fruits in your daily diet. Five servings daily of fruits and vegetables may help reduce your chances of getting lung, prostate, bladder, esophageal, and stomach cancer.

Include cruciferous vegetables in your diet. Cruciferous vegetables include cabbage, broccoli, Brussels sprouts, cauliflower, and kohlrabi. These seem to prevent the development of certain cancers because of their high antioxidant content.

Eat more high-fiber foods such as whole-wheat cereals, bread, and pasta. Diets high in fiber may reduce the risk of colon cancer. Legumes such as pinto beans, black beans, chickpeas, lentils, and kidney beans are other low-fat sources of fiber.

Reduce total fat intake. A high-fat diet has been associated with several cancers. Choose leaner cuts of beef, pork, and lamb. Substitute chicken, turkey, fish, and shellfish for some of the red meat in your diet. Eat reduced-fat, low-fat, and fat-free dairy products, salad dressings, and snacks and eat these in moderation.

Limit animal foods charred by grilling or broiling. Mutagens formed from high-temperature charring of muscle protein have been linked to a variety of cancers in animals.

If you drink alcohol, do so in moderation. The heavy use of alcohol is associated with increased rates of mouth, larynx, throat, esophageal, and liver cancers. When alcohol use is combined with cigarette smoking, risk of these cancers may increase even more.

[a]American Cancer Society, *1996 Guidelines on Diet, Nutrition, and Cancer Prevention.*

---

noted, experts recommend the same diet for reducing the risk of cardiovascular disease.

Exercise and Cancer

A number of studies have evaluated the relationship between exercise and cancer. Regular, moderate to vigorous physical activity seems to significantly reduce the risk of several cancers, especially colon cancer. The effects of exercise on cancer were first studied in small animals by injecting them with cancer-causing chemicals and assigning them to either an exercise or sedentary group. Most animal studies have found that exercise tends to retard cancer growth, though the reasons for

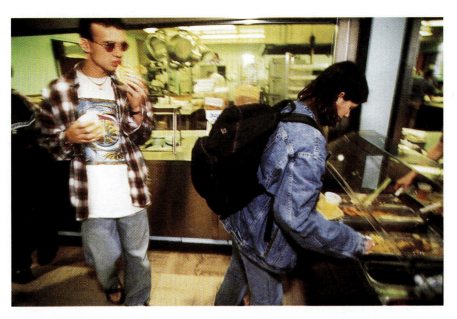

The dietary choices you make go a long way in helping your efforts for preventing cancer.

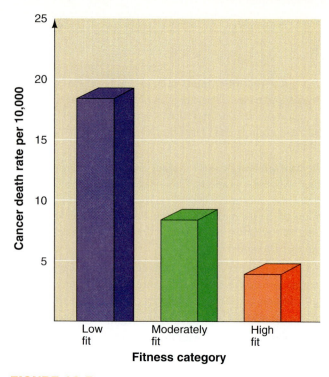

FIGURE 10.5   The rate of death due to cancer is significantly lower with elevated levels of fitness. (Data from S. N. Blair, H. W. Kohl III, R. S. Paffenbarger, Jr., D. G. Clark, K. H. Cooper, and L. W. Gibbons. Physical fitness and all cause mortality: A prospective study of healthy men and women. *Journal of the American Medical Association* 262:2395–2401, 1989.)

this slowed growth are not clearly understood. Some believe that exercise enhances immunity, which helps to destroy abnormal cancer cells.[14,15]

Studies involving human subjects have provided the most compelling evidence that exercise can protect against cancer. In 1989, a long-term study of cardiovascular fitness and cancer mortality evaluated over 13,000 people. The results of the study indicate that cancer death rates for poorly fit subjects are substantially higher than death rates for subjects who had average or good fitness levels. (See Figure 10.5.) For men, poor fitness was associated with three to five times more cancer when compared to men who had average or good fitness levels respectively, and women who had good fitness had only one-sixteenth the risk of cancer death.[16,17]

Although genetics can affect a person's fitness, it is generally impossible to attain fitness without participating in regular physical activity. Regular physical activity can cause a reduction in body fat. Studies that controlled for differences in body fat have been able to demonstrate that individuals whose lifestyles include regular physical activity have lowered rates of cancer.

One study found that active women have less cancer of the breast and reproductive organs. In the study, Dr. Leslie Bernstein at the University of Southern California Norris Cancer Center reported that one to three hours of exercise a week over a woman's reproductive lifetime (between the teens and about age 40) can bring a 20 to 30 percent reduction in the risk of breast cancer. Exercise that averaged four or more hours per week resulted in a 60 percent reduction. The research also pointed out that breast cancer risk was reduced even for those who didn't start exercising until their 20s or 30s.[18]

Cancers of the breast and reproductive organs are also less common among women who were athletes in college than among nonathletes. Women who were former college athletes demonstrated a significantly lower incidence of cancers of the breast, uterus, and cervix. As a whole, women who were former athletes were leaner, had a later age of menarche (probably because of being physically active children), and were younger when they reached menopause than were women who were not athletes in college.[19]

In general, women who exercise regularly from childhood through adulthood tend to reach menarche later and menopause earlier than those who are less physically active. Exercise shortens the organs' exposure to estrogen, which reduces the risk of cancer. Not every woman needs to be a college athlete in order to get some protection against certain cancers; regular, moderate to vigorous aerobic exercise will provide comparable levels of protection.[20,21]

The strongest evidence supporting exercise as a cancer deterrent comes from research that evaluated colon cancer and physical activity. This research indicates that sedentary individuals have 30 to 100 percent greater risk of colon cancer than those who are active. It is believed that exercise stimulates muscle movement of the large intestine, which forces fecal material to move through the intestine more quickly. As discussed earlier, the longer it takes fecal matter to pass through the colon, the greater the exposure to carcinogens. It is also interesting to note that exercisers are constipated less often than their sedentary counterparts, which is likely associated with the short digestion time.[22]

Decreased rates of colon cancer among the physically active may also be related to eating a high-fiber, low-fat diet. The wellness lifestyle includes a variety of health promoting activities that collectively and individually can reduce cancer risk. People who exercise regularly also tend to participate in other health-promoting activities such as eating a sensible diet.

DETECTING CANCER

Because one in three Americans will develop cancer, there has been much fear and anxiety about the disease.[23] New diagnostic and treatment methods are being discovered all the time. With these advances, the chances of surviving cancer have never been better. A diagnosis of the disease is no longer a death sentence and many cancer survivors go on to lead long, productive lives.

It is important to remember that the earlier the cancer is detected the better the chances of survival. Most

TABLE 10.2 ■ Summary of American Cancer Society Recommendations for the Early Detection of Cancer in Asymptomatic People

Site	Recommendation
Cancer-related Checkup	A cancer-related checkup is recommended every 3 years for people aged 20–40 and every year for people age 40 and older. This exam should include health counseling and depending on a person's age, might include examinations for cancers of the thyroid, oral cavity, skin, lymph nodes, testes, and ovaries, as well as for some nonmalignant diseases.
Breast	Women 40 and older should have an annual mammogram, an annual clinical breast exam (CBE) performed by a health care professional, and should perform monthly breast self-examination. The CBE should be conducted close to the scheduled mammogram. Women ages 20–39 should have a clinical breast exam performed by a health care professional every three years and should perform monthly breast self-examinations.
Colon & Rectum	Men and women aged 50 or older should follow *one* of the examination schedules below: • A fecal occult blood test every year and a flexible sigmoidoscopy every five years. • A colonoscopy every 10 years. • A double-contrast barium enema every five to 10 years. • A digital rectal exam should be done at the same time as sigmoidoscopy, colonoscopy, or double-contrast barium enema. People who are at moderate or high risk for colorectal cancer should talk with a doctor about a different testing schedule.
Prostate	The ACS recommends that both the prostate-specific antigen (PSA) blood test and the digital rectal examination be offered annually, beginning at age 50, to men who have a life expectancy of at least 10 years and to younger men who are at high risk. Men in high risk groups, such as those with a strong familial predisposition (e.g., two or more affected first-degree relatives), or African Americans may begin at a younger age (e.g., 45 years).
Uterus	**Cervix:** All women who are or have been sexually active or who are 18 and older should have an annual Pap test and pelvic examination. After three or more consecutive satisfactory examinations with normal findings, the Pap test may be performed less frequently. Discuss the matter with your physician. **Endometrium:** Women at high risk for cancer of the uterus should have sample of endometrial tissue examined when menopause begins.

Source: American Cancer Society, *Cancer facts and figures—1998, p. 31.* Reprinted by permission of the American Cancer Society, Inc.

---

cancers are discovered when people seek medical attention after they realize that their bodies are not functioning properly. If you have a cancer warning sign or feel that something is not right, contact your health care provider. If you think you may have something wrong, seek medical help quickly rather than delaying. Early diagnosis may mean the difference between life and death. See Table 10.2.

Physicians who suspect cancer have a variety of diagnostic tools, among them specialized computers and high-tech imaging machines to take three-dimensional pictures of the suspected cancer area. Such diagnostic tools make it possible to view internal organs and structures without having to do exploratory surgery. Two of the most common diagnostic tools are magnetic resonance imagery (MRI) and computer axial tomography (a CAT scan). In addition to imaging, a sample of the suspected cancer tissue (**biopsy**) can be taken using a small needle or other instrument and analyzed for the presence of cancer cells. With the results of three-dimensional pictures and biopsies, physicians are able to suggest a best course of treatment.

TREATING CANCER

Localized cancers that give no evidence of spreading are typically treated by surgically removing the cancerous cells. Surgery is the oldest and most widely used approach to cancer treatment. Today **radiation therapy** is often used in conjunction with surgery to destroy any remaining cancer cells. Radiation is helpful in treating cancers that are difficult to remove surgically or that have not responded well to drug or immune treatments.

The sun feels good on my skin.

The sun feels just as warm on your skin when you wear clothing and/or sunscreen.

I feel healthy when I have a good tan.

There is no such thing as a healthy tan.

I look better when I have a tan.

You might think you look better now, but later in life when you have many wrinkles and leathery skin you may regret your sunbaked years.

Mammograms hurt.

Mammograms may be slightly uncomfortable but are not supposed to hurt. If you feel pain, tell the medical staff.

I'm young and I'm not worried about cancer.

Cancer prevention should begin early and last a lifetime. Starting young will pay off later in life.

I don't have time to prepare high-fiber foods.

Try frozen vegetables, whole-grain cereals, and breads.

Fruits and vegetables are expensive and I don't like to cook.

Most fast foods are more expensive than high-fiber foods. Fast-food restaurants now offer many high-fiber alternatives.

I like foods high in fat.

Don't eliminate all high-fat foods from your diet. Start slowly by eliminating one high-fat food or replacing it with a low-fat or fat-free substitute.

If a known cancer has spread, other treatment options may be used to kill spreading cancer cells. **Chemotherapy** uses powerful drugs or hormones to kill cancer cells, which usually reproduce rapidly if left untreated. Another powerful cancer treatment is **immunotherapy,** which stimulates the body's own immune system to attack cancer cells. This rapidly evolving approach requires that the cancer patient receive injections of antibodies or vaccines grown from the patient's own tumor cells. These injections stimulate the immune system to attack all cells that are foreign to the body.

Most cancer treatments affect not just cancer cells, but also healthy cells that may be in the surrounding area or have similar characteristics. The damage done to healthy cells is minimal when compared to the damage cancer cells can do if left untreated.

For those who experience the pain and sorrow associated with cancer, there is hope and support available from both medical and nonmedical groups. Cancer support groups, cancer information workshops, and even discussion groups on the information highway are available in most communities and on any computer linked to the Internet. For most people, there is life after cancer. Each year the chances of surviving cancer increase; today there are at least 8 million cancer survivors in the United States living happy, productive lives.

OTHER HEALTH IMPEDIMENTS TO WELLNESS

In addition to cancer, certain chronic diseases can reduce quality of life and even cause death. Like cancer, these diseases are **noninfectious,** meaning that they cannot be passed to another individual through casual contact. True wellness involves prevention and treatment of any disease that can hamper quality of life and health. We will discuss just a few here: diabetes, headaches/migraines, allergies, and asthma.

Diabetes

Diabetes mellitus is a common metabolic disease that occurs either because the pancreas fails to produce sufficient insulin or because the insulin being produced is not being used efficiently. Insulin is a hormone that makes blood glucose available to cells for use and storage. Without sufficient insulin, glucose accumulates to such a level that the kidneys cannot process it and it spills over into the urine where it is excreted.

Each year 30,000 Americans die from the disease and 300,000 more die from complications stemming from it. As a result, it is the seventh leading cause of death. There are an estimated 10 million people with diabetes in the United States and approximately 4 million are unaware that they have the disease. Those with the disease have twice the risk of heart disease and stroke and account for one-third of all cases of kidney failure. Diabetes is also the number one cause of blindness.[24]

Type I diabetes, or insulin-dependent diabetes, results from the destruction of insulin-producing cells in the pancreas. Under these conditions, no insulin is produced. Type I diabetes usually strikes in childhood or adolescence, but can develop at any time before age 35. It typically comes about suddenly, the result of the body's own immune system destroying the insulin-producing cells. It is believed to be linked to a viral infection. There are no known risk factors. Treatment for this type of diabetes consists primarily of insulin replacement therapy through regular daily injections. Because too much or too little insulin causes side effects that can range from weakness to death, people with diabetes must monitor their blood sugar levels and make regular adjustments in exercise and diet.

Over 90 percent of diabetes cases are **type II diabetes,** which results from a combination of changes in insulin sensitivity and insulin production. Its occurrence is gradual, with most cases striking adults over age 35 who are overweight. Researchers have identified several risk factors for type II diabetes, which include having a family history of the disease, being overweight, and being sedentary. Heredity also seems to play a role. Native Americans, African Americans, and Hispanics have a higher risk than Caucasians. People with type II diabetes may not need daily insulin injections, but they do need to take steps to maintain normal blood glucose levels. Regular exercise, normal body weight, and consistent dietary intervention and control are usually sufficient to control the condition.

Diabetes and Diet

The American Diabetes Association suggests that those with type II diabetes consume 60 percent of their calories from complex carbohydrates. This means eating lots of cereals, grains, beans, pasta, vegetables, and fruits. It is also important to reduce consumption of sugars, either by avoiding them or by using sugar substitutes. Although these dietary guidelines were developed for people with diabetes, they may help prevent diabetes from occurring among those who do not have the disease, especially those who are at above-average risk for it.

Diabetes and Exercise

People with either type I or type II diabetes may participate in any form of exercise if they are careful to monitor blood glucose levels. If not performed as prescribed, however, exercise may be harmful.[25, 26] During exercise, blood glucose levels tend to fluctuate; the major problem for a person with diabetes is the occurrence of **hypoglycemia** or low blood sugar. Blood flow increases during exercise, which mobilizes the insulin injected earlier in the day. Large increases in insulin cause the cells to take large amounts of glucose from the bloodstream, leaving very little glucose for later use. This condition can result in unconsciousness, due to inadequate glucose to the brain. To prevent this, a person with diabetes should always carry a small amount of candy or other sweet food that can be consumed if low blood sugar occurs. To ensure that a proper exercise regimen is followed, people with diabetes should consult with a health care provider.

Headaches

Headaches are a common noninfectious condition. They occur at all ages and across all races. Not all headaches are the same. Some are caused by stress, whereas others are related to physiological changes in the body. Most headaches involve a mild throbbing, but 20 percent of Americans experience severe headaches of such excruciating pain that they can cause dizziness, nausea, and even temporary visual impairment.

Common headaches or **tension headaches** are caused by muscle tension, usually because of sustained contraction of the muscles of the neck and head. Muscles can contract without conscious control, and these involuntary contractions can occur during periods of stress, boredom, fatigue, and physical labor, or because of poor posture. The resulting tension can produce the dull, throbbing headache with which many people are familiar. These headaches are easily treated with mild pain relievers, sleep, relaxation, and stress reduction. (See Chapter 11 for stress reduction techniques.) Frequent tension headaches are best treated by eliminating their cause. This usually involves reducing stress, managing time effectively, and participating regularly in leisure or recreational activities.

Psychological headaches feel just like tension headaches, but are psychological rather than physical in nature. They are caused by anxiety, depression, mental stress, and emotional disturbances. Because no muscle or physical tension is involved with these headaches, treatment consists of social and psychological therapies designed to relieve depression and emotional stress. When psychological balance has been restored, the headaches usually subside.

Secondary headaches happen as a side effect of some other underlying condition. For example, the common cold often causes blockage of the sinuses; sinus pressure often increases and causes secondary headaches. In addition, flu, fasting, hypertension, excessive heat, allergies, bodily pain or injury, and poor eyesight can lead to headaches. As you might guess, treatment for secondary headaches addresses the underlying cause, not the headache itself, although common medications taken for headaches may also relieve some of the problems of underlying illnesses.

All arteries in the body have the ability to contract and expand as demands for blood change throughout the day. **Migraine headaches** are caused by rapid constriction and subsequent dilation of blood vessels in the brain. So far, researchers have been unable to determine why the blood vessels react this way. These vessel changes are accompanied by the release of various chemicals that seep through the vessel walls and inflame brain tissues. The pain associated with migraines is usually limited to one side of the brain, but can last from minutes to days. The pain can be excruciating and may worsen with time. Migraines can become so severe that a sufferer can experience temporary visual impairment and hypersensitivity to light. Migraine sufferers are often unable to continue daily work and home activities. Because relaxation and rest are only partially effective in reducing the pain, powerful painkillers are usually prescribed. While painkillers have been only moderately effective, in recent years many new treatments show promise in alleviating the pain. People who suffer from migraines may want to consult with a physician about these treatments.

Allergies

For some people with allergies, springtime and summer can be difficult times of the year when winds carry virtually invisible particles of pollen and mold through the air. When inhaled, these cause the sneezing and wheezing of an allergic reaction. An allergic response can also be triggered by insect bites, drugs, synthetic materials, animal dander, and various foods. Some people are so allergic that they suffer all year.

Allergies and the allergic response are caused by a person's own immune system. Under normal conditions, any foreign microorganism that enters the body is quickly identified, attacked, and eliminated by the immune system. Viruses that cause colds or flu and bacteria that cause infection are quickly destroyed by a properly functioning immune system. However, in some people, exposure to certain allergy-causing substances (**allergens**) initiates an overly aggressive immune response that vigorously attacks and eliminates the foreign substance. The immune system goes too far in its attempt to remove the foreign substance. Those who have such overly protective immune responses are said to be hypersensitive towards the substances that cause allergic reactions.

Part of the immune response involves the production of histamines, which dilate blood vessels, increase mucus secretions, and can cause swelling and other allergy-related symptoms. A running nose and watery eyes are classic signs of excess histamine production. Other symptoms include sneezing, nasal congestion, and itching of the ears, nose, and throat. Sometimes allergic responses result in skin discoloration and rashes called **hives.** A severe allergic reaction can cause blood pressure to drop drastically and restrict respiration so severely that death can result. This type of allergic response is called **anaphylactic shock.** It is rare and requires immediate medical attention.

Researchers have determined that the tendency to be allergic is inherited. Those who live in rural, agricultural areas are more exposed to common allergens and suffer from allergies more frequently. Urban residents do not have the same exposure and typically do not demonstrate high allergy rates. A health history, a detailed list of symptoms, and an allergy skin test are the most common medical methods used to detect allergies. During an allergy skin test, small amounts of known allergens are either scratched or injected into the skin and signs of redness or swelling are monitored.

Once allergens have been identified, the best treatment is to avoid the offending substances. Because this is not always possible, several medical therapies have been developed. Medications are commonly used either to reduce the immune response or to reduce the symptoms associated with allergies. Allergy "shots" that contain minute amounts of allergens can sometimes desensitize an allergy sufferer. This process may take several years.

Asthma

Asthma is a chronic disease of the lung airways and is characterized by a spasm of the muscles surrounding the airways and by inflammation of the airways. The spasms cause constriction and inflammation of the airway linings, which swell and secrete extra mucus, further blocking air passages. Most asthma attacks begin when an allergen or an irritant such as exercise, smoking, cold air, pollutants, stress, or infection initiates a spasm in the bronchial tubes. Treatment for asthma includes the use of prescription inhalers, which are used to spray a small dose of a muscle relaxant, bronchodilator, or anti-inflammatory medication into the lungs. New medications use a combination of approaches to cause airways to reopen.

Over the last ten years, the number of Americans with asthma increased by over one-third and the number of asthma-related deaths doubled. Worldwide, there has been a consistent increase in asthma cases and deaths, although the medical community is unable to determine why the increases are occurring. Most severely affected are adults over 65, children, and African Americans living in inner-city communities.

There appears to be an increase in the number of children and adults who experience exercise-related asthma attacks. Increased respiration that results from heavy exercise can cause bronchial constriction and labored breathing. Exercise-induced asthma, however, can be controlled effectively. During the 1984 Olympics, seventy athletes suffered from exercise-induced asthma. Of

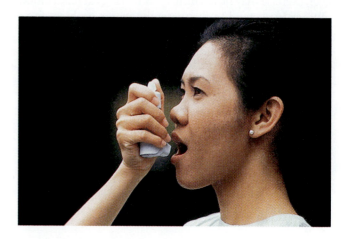

Health officials have noted a marked increase in recent years in the number of people developing asthma. Although precautions and care need to be followed, asthma does not have to interfere with your fitness needs.

these athletes, forty competed well enough to earn medals.

An effective way to prevent exercise-induced asthma is to inhale a dose of prescribed asthma medication fifteen to thirty minutes before beginning an exercise session. If you have chronic asthma and want to exercise regularly, keep an inhaler with you at all times so that at the earliest signs of chest tightening or breathing difficulty, you can quickly treat the problem before it worsens. Work closely with your physician to determine the exercise regimen and medications that are best for you.

SUMMARY

Cancer is the second leading cause of death in the United States. Like heart disease, it is caused by several factors, the most important of which may be lifestyle. Of the various forms of cancer, lung cancer is the most common and the most preventable. Tobacco use is the primary cause of this disease. Other forms of cancer may not be as easily prevented, but many can be detected early enough to increase one's chances of a complete recovery. A wellness lifestyle uses diet and exercise to reduce the risk of many cancers. It also employs the use of early detection practices such as breast or testicular self-examination.

Other common ailments such as diabetes, headaches, allergies, and asthma may not be completely preventable, but they are treatable. Knowing how to recognize these conditions and how to treat them can add significantly to a person's quality of life.

SUGGESTED READING

Blum, A., ed. *The cigarette underworld—A front line report on the war against your lungs.* New York: Lyle Stuart, 1985.

Fiore, N. A. *The road back to health: Coping with the emotional side of cancer.* New York: Bantam Books, 1985.

Prescott, D. M., and A. S. Flexer. *Cancer—The misguided cell,* 3rd ed. New York: Charles Scribner's Sons, 1986.

Simone, C. B. *Cancer and nutrition.* New York: McGraw-Hill, 1983.

Behavioral Lab 10.1

What Can I Do?

The following labs are designed to help you make cancer prevention behaviors a part of your everyday life. At the beginning of this chapter, you determined your stage of readiness to change with regard to cancer prevention. Now take out a sheet of paper and complete the corresponding section of this lab: precontemplator, contemplator, preparer, action taker, or maintainer.

Precontemplator

1. Listed below are the main reasons why you may not be motivated to practice cancer-prevention behaviors. Write down those that apply to you.

   The sun feels good on my skin.

   I feel healthy when I have a good tan.

   I look better when I have a tan.

   Mammograms hurt.

   I don't like vegetables.

   I don't like to exercise.

   I'm addicted to tobacco.

   I like to drink alcohol.

   Breast and skin cancers do not affect young adults, so I'm not worried about them.

2. Practicing cancer prevention behaviors might make your life better. Which of the following benefits appeal to you?

   You'll prevent most forms of cancer.

   As you age, your skin will look and feel better.

   Regular exercise will help you feel and look better.

   You'll be constipated less.

   Your teeth will not have tobacco stains.

   You'll save money by not drinking, smoking, or tanning.

   You might live longer and have a higher quality of life.

   You will likely lose excess body fat.

3. Do your answers in items 2 and 3 outweigh your answers in item 1?

4. In your opinion, which of the reasons you listed in item 1 is the hardest for you to overcome? Why?

5. If you were going to make one change to prevent yourself from getting cancer, what would it be?

Contemplator

1. List any activities you are currently thinking about doing to avoid or prevent cancer.

2. What would be the benefit to you if you adopted a low-cancer-risk lifestyle?

3. List any disadvantages to your prevention activities. (For example: it's not cool to wear a hat to protect against the sun.)

4. Based on what you listed in items 2 and 3, do the benefits outweigh the disadvantages? If they don't, you might want to review the chapter.

5. Identify and list the barriers that prevent you from doing cancer-prevention behaviors.

6. What do you think you could do to overcome the barriers you listed in item 5?

Preparer

1. Write a long-term goal regarding cancer prevention. *Examples:* I will consume at least five fruits and vegetables each day. I will perform monthly breast self-exams. I will stop smoking. I will get a baseline mammogram this month (if between 40 and 49 years of age).

2. Now break your goal into at least three short-term goals that you can complete in the next six weeks.

3. With your main and short-term goals in mind, make a specific plan of action to help you overcome your barriers and change your behavior. Remember, you can't do everything at once. Pick one small aspect of your behavior and work on it.

Example: If my goal were to do monthly breast self-exams (BSE), I would use the following plan: (1) Follow the information in the chapter to learn how to do BSE. (2) Set a date each month to do it. (3) Do this month's exam today.

4. Look at the action plan you created in item 3. What makes you think you can accomplish your first step?

5. Complete the following sentence:

I am going to take my first step on _____ .

date within 30 days

Action Taker

1. List the things you are currently doing to lower your risk of cancer.

2. Are any of these working? *Example:* Is your diet low in fat and high in fiber? Has tobacco use stopped? If so, is anything different in your life? If they are not working, why not?

3. After reviewing the chapter, what else can you do to lower your cancer risk?

4. What is your long-term risk-reduction goal?

5. Are you receiving support for your efforts? (For example: parents support your actions, friends do it too, you are saving money, you feel your health has improved.)

   If yes, what kind?

   If no, why not and what can you do to increase your supports?

6. Do you think you will continue? Why?

7. If you were to stop, what do you think would be your major reason for stopping?

8. Is there a way to prevent this (item 7)?

9. How would you get yourself started again if you did stop?

Maintainer

Congratulations, you are doing great.

1. List three benefits you have experienced as you lowered your cancer risk. (For example: I no longer spend money on cigarettes. I feel better eating a low-fat diet.)

2. How have you changed or how have you changed the environment around you to accommodate a healthier lifestyle? (*Examples:* I don't go to smoky places any more. I eat more salads.)

3. Are there any situations or events that tempt you to give up your current lifestyle? What are they?

4. If you have relapsed, list the reasons why you did and what you did to get back on track.

5. Write down a few things you can do to avoid temptations in the future.

6. The risk of cancer increases with age. What can you do now and in the future to keep your risk low? (See Table 10.2 for recommendations to lower cancer risk as age increases.)

7. Is there anything else you need (information? support? time management?) to continue your healthy lifestyle?

8. If yes, can you think of a way to attain it or can you think of someone who can help you with it?

CHAPTER 11

Understanding and Managing Stress

Terms

- Stress
- Stressor
- Strain
- Distress
- Eustress
- Stress response
- Homeostasis
- Arousal
- Inverted "U" Hypothesis
- Fight-or-flight response
- General adaptation syndrome (G.A.S.)
- Adaptive energy reserve
- Perception
- Cognitive intervention strategies
- Reframing
- Imagery
- Progressive relaxation
- Autogenic training
- Meditation
- Biofeedback
- Hypostress

Objectives

1. Know that stress can be both positive and negative, and provide examples of both kinds in your life.

2. Understand the multifaceted nature of stress and define it accordingly.

3. Explain the basic tenets of biological (physiological), psychological, and social stress theory.

4. List the personality traits most associated with a stressful lifestyle and those of "hardy" individuals.

5. Explain how arousal, performance, and stress are related.

6. Recognize symptoms of, and responses to, stress in yourself and others.

7. Select and practice one or more coping and stress reduction strategies.

Stages of Change

Where Am I?

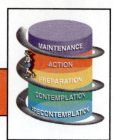

Precontemplator _____ I have not attempted to manage the stress in my daily life and I do not intend to in the next six months.

Contemplator _____ I have not attempted to manage the stress in my daily life but I intend to in the next six months.

Preparer _____ I have not attempted to manage the stress in my daily life but I intend to in the next thirty days.

Action Taker _____ I have been managing the stress in my daily life for less than six months.

Maintainer _____ I have been managing the stress in my daily life for more than six months.*

Stress management includes regular relaxation, physical activity, talking with others, and making time for social activities. To place yourself in the action taker or maintainer category, you must be practicing this definition of stress management. If you are able to sustain some stress management behaviors but not meet the whole goal yet, your efforts should still be applauded. For example, you may have successfully incorporated ten-minute relaxation breaks into your day, but haven't yet made exercise a regular part of your life. It is important to feel good about each of your healthy lifestyle behaviors and use this positive attitude to build confidence; then try to take another small step toward managing your stress.

Stress can bring out our best performance or make us faint of heart. It is one of the great contradictions of life. Living involves stress—only death is stress free. In a broader definition than most people give it, stress provides the stimulation we need to grow and prosper. Too much stress, however, can make us irritable, anxious, and ill. Seven out of ten respondents told the U.S. News/ Bozell survey that they feel stress at some point during a typical weekday—30 percent say they experience a lot of stress; 40 percent say they feel some stress. Forty-three percent of all adults suffer noticeable physical and emotional symptoms from burnout. Somewhere between 75 percent and 90 percent of all visits to the doctor's office stem from stress. By one account, the country loses $7,500 per worker per year to stress, through either absenteeism, decreases in productivity, or workers' compensation benefits.[1]

Too much or too little stress can hurt us, but the "right" amount of stress enables us to be healthy, motivated, and productive. The challenge is to find the balance, the magical amount that lies between boredom and panic, between nonproductivity and workaholism, and between not caring and worrying yourself sick. Healthy coping strategies can help you maintain this balance during the many changes, challenges, and surprises that lie in your future.

WHAT IS STRESS?

If you were to mention "stress" in a roomful of friends, chances are everyone would nod as if to say, "Oh yes, I know what stress is." But when asked to define it, most people hesitate. Eventually your friends might suggest

---

Source: Personal communication with Dr. Joseph L. Fava, Associate Professor (Research), Cancer Prevention Research Center of the University of Rhode Island.

252

that stress is pressure to do something within a specific time frame; pressure to perform; emotional tension; physical and mental strain; a nervous reaction; an inability to cope. It can be all these things and more, which is precisely why stress researchers have been grappling with the problem of how to define it for years. Stress can be both cause and effect.

Because of its complex nature and the ensuing necessity to study it with a variety of approaches, stress is defined in different ways by different researchers. Nonetheless, a starting point is needed, so here are three ways that the term *stress* is commonly used.[2]

1. **Stress** is something external to the person (an event, person, or environmental condition) that causes mental and/or physical tension and arousal. For example, stress is the angry customer waiting to chew your head off, or stress is waiting for the starting gun to go off before the race. The term **stressor** is frequently used in place of stress in this definition. Stressors can be physical, such as hot, humid weather; emotional, such as a death in the family; mental, such as an exam; or social, such as a blind date.

    Research on stressors started with inquiry into the nature of combat and natural disaster trauma. The focus then turned to major life changes and events, including marriage, divorce, and employment changes, and more recently to some common chronic types of stressors like occupational, marital, and financial difficulties. Researchers are also interested in the smaller, chronically irritating stressors (hassles) such as busy traffic and deadlines. Environmental characteristics under study include noise, overcrowding, and pollution.

2. Stress is the internal state of a person. Sometimes the term **strain** is used in place of stress in this definition. This refers to both the physiological and emotional states of a person. When a demand is placed on the body, the body reacts by rising to a higher level of arousal so that it is prepared either to defend itself against something harmful or to perform at a level needed to meet the challenge. Comments reflecting this meaning of stress are, "When you scare me like that, I can feel my heart pounding and my skin crawl," or, "Right before I go on stage, I feel an adrenaline rush."

    Emotional responses, such as anger and joy, also constitute your internal state. Stress of this nature may cause you to say, "I am emotionally drained," or "The idea of parachuting is both frightening and exhilarating." There is an interesting "chicken or egg" debate among experts as to whether you react first emotionally or cognitively to a stressor. In other words, do you get frightened (emotion) and then decide (cognition) to run, or do you decide you need to run and then get scared? The answer is probably both, and the details, while fascinating, are beyond the scope of this book. What is impor-

tant to recognize, from a practical standpoint, is that emotional, cognitive, and physical responses to stress can be successfully managed with practice.

3. Stress arises from a transaction between a person and the environment. Stress in this case is a combination of the stressor and the way the stressor is perceived or interpreted by the individual.[3] If a person believes that a situation will result in loss, harm, threat, or challenge, the individual will experience stress.[4] For example, students who are unable to enroll in a course will experience stress if they believe that this will harm their academic progress. The same stress will not be experienced if the course is an elective and can be easily replaced. The environmental condition (a closed-out course) does not create stress by itself. The situation and the person's appraisal of the situation work together to create the stress.

    Some experts believe that less emphasis should be placed on personal appraisal and more on the resources available to the individual to meet the challenge. In other words, if you have a lot of resources available, you will experience less stress. For example, if your car breaks down and you have the money to fix it and a friend to pick you up and take you to campus or a job, you will experience less stress than if you can't afford to fix the car and know that without transportation you will lose your job. Of course, whether or not you believe you have resources available may also be subjective. Consider the difference between two people lost in the woods—one, trained in survival, sees resources for shelter and food; the other does not.

Stress and Physical Wellness

When astronauts began spending time in space, losses in their bone and muscle tissue were discovered. This loss was attributed to a lack of weight-bearing activity—too little physical stress—in the gravity-free environment. Today's space shuttle is equipped with foot straps and a pull cord to be used like a rowing machine (no seat is required since the astronaut can float just above the floor). Pushing off the shuttle floor and against the resistance of the pull cord allows the astronauts to exercise their legs, arms, and backs. This push–pull physical stress helps them maintain their muscle tissue and bone density.

Some professional athletes, such as football linemen, trade a career of excessive physical stress for fame, fortune, and the pursuit of excellence. As a result many live with chronic pain. But it's not just the professionals—weekend athletes or weekend project doers can also find themselves in pain from blisters, shinsplints, or a sore back if they overexert themselves. Carpal tunnel syndrome (irritation of the nerves in the wrist), which develops from highly repetitive tasks like keyboarding, is another example of the way excessive chronic physical stress can result in disability.

So whether in space or on earth, too little physical stress can lead to physical weakness and too much can be injurious. The right amount is what keeps the body strong and healthy. (See Chapter 2 for a detailed discussion of physical fitness.)

Stress and Social and Emotional Wellness

Human beings are social creatures by nature. A lack of social interaction can be as harmful as negative social relationships. It starts in infancy; babies whose basic physical needs are met but who are left alone rather than cuddled and caressed show poorer weight gains and delayed neurological development. Recent studies have found that a mother's caresses seem to help moderate production of a hormone that affects the body's reaction to stress. Abnormal levels of this hormone have been linked to changes in a part of the brain involved with learning and memory. Children, like the institutionalized Romanian orphans, who are deprived of such attention show wide fluctuations in the levels of this hormone, and those with the greatest peaks and valleys scored lowest on tests of mental and motor ability.[5] As the individual grows older, a lack of social interaction can manifest itself as loneliness, isolation, and doubts of self-worth. Such feelings may affect both a person's physical and mental health.[6,7] This is a special concern for the elderly. Being surrounded by friends and family (good relationships) may help you live a longer, healthier life. Interestingly, married people live longer than their unmarried, divorced, or widowed counterparts.[8] It may be that marriage supplies life-giving social support or that people somehow better equipped to live a long life tend to get and stay married. There is also some evidence that it isn't marriage per se, but companionship and social support that make the difference. Mothers who have the support of a companion during labor and delivery experience fewer childbirth complications and less postpartum depression.[9] It appears that appropriate social and emotional support can be stress buffering and therefore health promoting.

Unfortunately the reverse is true: emotional and social distress can have a negative impact on health. Abusive, degrading, or highly demanding relationships can create excessive interpersonal tension. When trying situations are teamed with a lack of social support and dwindling financial resources, coping is even more difficult. Common social and emotional stressors include employment conditions, financial status, racial acceptance, and balancing the obligations of home and work responsibilities.

People who live alone or who receive very little social contact often suffer quietly. So too can those in poor and abusive relationships. Social and emotional stress balances are achieved by developing positive relationships and having at least one other person you can depend on, someone who will always listen to you. Improving coping skills, establishing new contacts, getting out of abusive situations, and learning how to relax may help.

Stress and Spiritual Wellness

Spiritual stress may include ethical and moral decision making, feelings of guilt, and the acceptance or rejection of religious beliefs. Too little spiritual stress may result in a failure to resolve issues such as death and the meaning of one's life. At the other extreme, too much spiritual stress can manifest itself in spiritual coercion (such as cults) or in the kind of overwhelming guilt that results in suicide. It is important to work through difficult spiritual issues and develop a philosophy of life. The latter can guide you when difficult decisions and issues arise. Finding a spiritual balance provides comfort, joy, and a sense of purpose.

Stress and Mental Wellness

Too little stress can result in the underdevelopment of mental capabilities. Those who are bored or unmotivated (perhaps because life appears hopeless) fail to progress and may even regress, while those who are intellectually stimulated and challenged tend to thrive. Good parenting and good educational opportunities are essential to the mental development and well-being of children. Children who are encouraged to read at home tend to do better in school, and their linguistic development may have long-reaching health effects. A recent series of studies called the Nuns Studies[10] (because many nuns have volunteered their brains for study upon their deaths) discovered that those nuns who demonstrated more complex linguistic patterns early in life were less likely to develop Alzheimer's disease when they grew older. While this link is not completely understood, perhaps the more developed the brain, the greater the protection against disease.

But of course, too much stress is bad. Mental challenges that exceed a person's capabilities and coping abilities cause distress. Too much mental stress hinders development and interferes with motivation. Burnout, the result of chronic stress, can be seen in children and young adults who are pushed too hard to excel in school or extracurricular activities, and in adults who are expected to do too much or too difficult work. Stress is often the result of demanding tasks, few resources, and limited decision-making control.

To maintain a healthy mental outlook, challenge your brain, but at the same time, try to avoid long periods of mental stress. Seek out both challenging mental activities (for example, problem solving) and relaxing activities (for example, listening to music).

The Stress Continuum

The bases are loaded . . .

The deadline is now . . .

A bump is heard in the night . . .

Stress in the Work Environment

Creates Stress	What's at Stake	Relieves Stress
• Inadequate space, lack of privacy, unsafe or poorly fitting equipment, too hot or cold an environment	Physical Wellness	• Adequate space, privacy, control over noise and temperature, ergonomically correct equipment, health insurance
• Not enough work time, frequent interruptions, work assignments are too hard or too easy, micro-managing boss, little or no on-the-job training or professional development	Mental Wellness	• Decision-making power, budgetary and personnel control, tools needed to do the job, challenging but doable assignments, control over the work schedule, job training/professional development
• Target of prejudice or pressures concerning gender, race, religion, socioeconomic background, an overly competitive environment	Social Wellness	• A supportive and mutually respectful work environment, opportunities for advancement
• Threat of being laid off, passed over for promotion, promoted to a level that exceeds one's present competence/ability	Emotional Wellness	• Stable job, recognition for quality work and achievement, supportive employer and coworkers, self-improvement workshops
• Work that does not fit one's moral, ethical, or spiritual values, such as being a non-drinker who serves drinks at a restaurant, a pro-lifer who works for a company that manufactures birth control products	Spiritual Wellness	• Work is meaningful, work is compatible with personal values and beliefs, opportunity to change company policies

A baby is being born . . .

A wedding is being planned . . .

What do all of these things have in common? *Stress!*

Notice that some of these events are considered positive, but others have a negative connotation. The stress continuum ranges from bad stress (house burned down) to good stress (getting married). Hans Selye, who pioneered stress research and is considered the first person to isolate stress as a separate field of study, called bad stress **distress** and good stress **eustress**.[11] A bad haircut, being stuck in traffic, a death in the family, a tornado, an athletic event, a big date, and meeting a movie star are all stressors but the first four evoke distress and the last three eustress. An individual's frame of reference also plays a role in determining the positiveness of the situation. For example, tornado damage is usually devastating but an individual who loses a failing but well-insured business may actually feel some relief. As another example, public speaking pumps some people up, while others would rather "die" than talk in front of a group. Clearly one person's distress can be another person's eustress.

Regardless of whether you are experiencing good or bad stress, the physical **stress response,** the physical reaction to a stimulus (stressor), is similar. For example, both the anticipation of an oral exam and an exchange of wedding vows can cause sweaty palms, a racing heartbeat, and a flood of adrenaline. The stress response also occurs regardless of whether the stressor is real or imagined. The monster under the bed can be very stressful!

Unfortunately we do not have direct control over most stressors. For example, you cannot prevent most deaths, traffic jams, or exams (at least not if you want a college degree!). Life is full of potential distress. What you do have control over is how you perceive and react to situations. You can decide whether an exam is a terrifying experience designed to demonstrate your ignorance or an opportunity to show what you have learned. One of our favorite stories illustrates this point.

> A student received a grade of 27 percent on his first exam. The teacher told him he had to buckle down and study harder. On the next exam the student received a grade of 54 percent. In exasperation the teacher asked the student if he had studied. He responded excitedly, "Yes I did, and look at this, I did twice as well!"

This student will no doubt live a long, healthy, well-balanced life. Being able to see the "high side" is called "reframing" and will be discussed in more detail under the coping strategies in this chapter.

Although eustress can cause the same physiological responses as distress, it is not linked to stress-related disease. It is not as chronic in nature. This means that following the stressor, a person returns to **homeostasis** (a stable internal environment) more quickly, thereby conserving energy and other bodily resources. You can usually act on eustress—you can jump for joy or scream in triumph. And although reframing can turn the negative into a positive, its effect is usually one of neutralizing negative stress rather than causing high levels of eustress. Eustress is less common, not harmful, and possibly health enhancing.

Stress and Performance

Arousal is a form of stimulation, of stress, that affects performance. If you are excited, pumped up, and ready to go, you will perform better than if you are not particularly aroused. On the other hand, too much arousal can cause a decrease in performance quality. This is often the case when an athletic team that has played extremely well all season makes senseless errors in the beginning of a playoff game. As overexcited players settle into the game, they calm down a little (decrease their arousal levels), and their performance improves. Another classic case of over-arousal, often stereotypically portrayed on television, is the very excited father-to-be who on hearing that his wife is in labor, rushes around trying to find the car keys and suitcase and then jumps in the car, leaving his wife behind.

Can you think of times when excitement or nerves overaroused you and affected your performance? Do you remember when you were "lulled into complacency" and your underarousal affected your performance?

The Yerkes–Dodson Law, known as the **Inverted "U" Hypothesis,** describes the relationship between arousal, stress, and performance. (See Figure 11.1.) Low arousal and excessive arousal result in low performance. The top of the inverted "U" represents the amount of arousal that results in the best performance. The actual amount depends on several factors. A greater amount of arousal is needed for what are referred to as "simple tasks" such as strength, speed, and muscular endurance activities than for "complex tasks" such as accuracy, agility, and balancing activities. The reason for this is not totally understood, but is believed to have something to do with how information is processed in the brain. (In relationship to tasks, the words *simple* and *complex* refer to the number of parts or components that make up a response or skill; they do not describe the difficulty of the task.[12]) Simple skills like weight lifting require more arousal than complex skills like serving a tennis ball. Getting pumped the right amount is the secret.

In rare cases people have experienced incredible adrenaline rushes that have allowed them to perform fantastic feats of strength such as lifting up a car that has fallen on a friend or family member. These are cases where very high arousal levels led to all-time peak performances. However, it is also possible to be overaroused for a strength move, lose technique, be a less efficient lifter, or apply more force to a situation than is helpful. Finding optimal arousal levels for different activities is one of the goals of stress management.

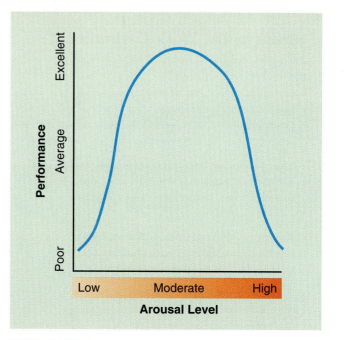

FIGURE 11.1   The Inverted "U" Hypothesis. Increased arousal improves performance only to a point, after which further increases in arousal degrade performance. (Reprinted by permission from Schmidt, R. A. *Motor learning and performance: From principles to practice,* Champaign, IL: Human Kinetics, 1991, p. 26 (Figure 2.5).)

THEORIES ABOUT STRESS

The concept of stress is so broad that researchers and scholars have approached it from a variety of perspectives. Physiologists study the body's physical reactions to stress such as elevated heart rate, increased hormone production, and higher rates of illness, whereas psychologists examine mental and emotional stress through issues such as perception and personality. A third focus comes from human engineers and sociologists who concentrate on how environmental conditions and societal pressures influence stress.[13] Rice compares this multidirectional research approach to the ancient eastern parable of the three blind men who investigate an elephant. Each man's report on what the elephant "looks like" is dramatically different because each comes in contact with a different part of the elephant (trunk, ears, legs, etc.). It is not until the three men put together all of their information that the "whole truth" of the elephant is known. It may be a long time before we see the whole stress picture, but in the meantime it is certainly worthwhile to examine the wealth of available information. The following overview of some of the prominent stress theories is useful for understanding how to interpret the work of different researchers and the stress-management strategies that have grown out of their work.

Stress and the Physical Response

Walter Cannon, a noted Harvard physiologist, contributed the idea of *homeostasis*, defining it as the tendency of organisms to maintain a stable internal environment.[14] He noticed that initial or low-level environmental stressors could be withstood, and the organism would adapt and "bounce back," quickly restoring homeostasis, but that high-intensity or continued physical stressors resulted in a disturbance of homeostasis that, if prolonged, could lead to a breakdown of biological systems.[15] Cannon also provided insight into the body's emergency **fight-or-flight response,** which is explained in more detail on page 258.

Influenced by Cannon, Hans Selye also concentrated on the body's physical responses to stress. He called these reactions the *stress response.* (Today the stress response is considered both physical and psychological.) While still a student, Selye was struck by the similarity of certain symptoms experienced by the ill. Regardless of the nature of the illness, a set of common physiological responses (for example, elevated heart rate and body temperature) that were not necessarily linked to the illness occurred alongside symptoms specific to the illness. In 1942 Selye was again intrigued when British physician Thomas B. Curling reported acute gastrointestinal ulcers in patients who suffered extensive skin burns. That the ulcers could not be directly caused by the burns led Selye to believe they were the result of stress experienced during and after the burn incident. Upon further research, Selye defined stress as "the nonspecific response of the body to any demand made upon it."[16] Specific responses are those that are linked to a specific illness such as blistering skin in reaction to a burn. Nonspecific responses are those that occur without a specific link to the illness. The nonspecific response, therefore, refers to the stereotypical reaction of the body regardless of the specific nature of the stressor. In Hans Selye's own words:[17]

> The businessman who is under constant pressure from his clients and employees alike, the air-traffic controller who knows that a moment of distraction may mean death to hundreds of people, the athlete who desperately wants to win a race, and the husband who helplessly watches his wife slowly and painfully dying from cancer, all suffer from stress. The problems they face are totally different, but medical research has shown that in many respects the body responds in a stereotyped manner, with identical biochemical changes, essentially meant to cope with any type of increased demand upon the human machinery. The stress-producing factors—technically called stressors—are different, yet they all elicit essentially the same biological stress response.

But if we all react with the same response, why, when subjected to chronic stress, does one person get ulcers while

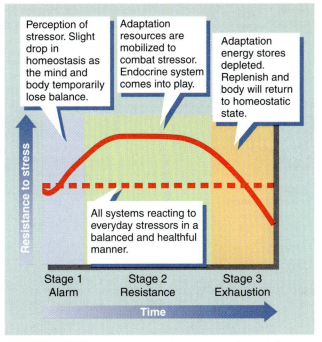

FIGURE 11.2 The General Adaptation Syndrome. If stress is chronic, the body follows a pattern of alarm, resistance, and finally exhaustion. If stress is resolved and rest obtained, homeostasis is reestablished.

another suffers from migraine headaches? Selye argues that in times of chronic stress our bodies respond much like a chain giving out at the weakest link. The most vulnerable parts of our body give out and manifest stress symptoms and diseases. Other scientists argue that there are individual differences in how people respond to stress and that even the type of stress can make a difference in the response.[18] For example, potentially ego-damaging situations such as academic failure may produce different stress responses from potentially physically painful situations, such as having a root canal.

General Adaptation Syndrome

Selye identified a three-stage stress response to explain how the body responds to sudden stress, chronic stress, and excessive stress resulting in physical collapse. Selye's description of this stress response, which he named the **general adaptation syndrome (G.A.S.),** has three stages: alarm, resistance, and exhaustion.[19] (See Figure 11.2.)

The Alarm Response.   The alarm response is the immediate response to a stressor. Your equilibrium is disturbed and you automatically react. You know these symptoms well—just think how you feel when a pop quiz is announced, when you are presented with an award and asked to say something, when you discover a bee in your car while you're driving, or when you think someone is

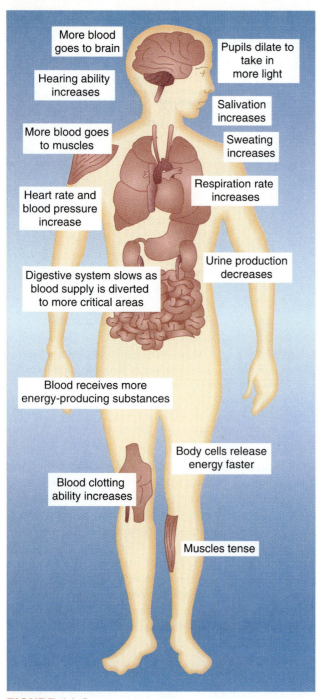

FIGURE 11.3 Physiological changes that occur during an alarm reaction.

Image labels:
More blood goes to brain
Hearing ability increases
More blood goes to muscles
Heart rate and blood pressure increase
Digestive system slows as blood supply is diverted to more critical areas
Blood receives more energy-producing substances
Blood clotting ability increases
Pupils dilate to take in more light
Salivation increases
Sweating increases
Respiration rate increases
Urine production decreases
Body cells release energy faster
Muscles tense

muscles tense in readiness. Even the goosebumps that appear are important; they are the result of the constriction of blood vessels in the skin—a response that minimizes blood loss if you are wounded. Body hair standing on end is also part of this response. It doesn't help *you* a lot, but this same physical response is important to other members of the animal kingdom. For example, a bristling cat looks larger and therefore more threatening! See Figure 11.3 for a more complete list of physical reactions initiated by the sympathetic branch of your autonomic nervous system.

When you are physically threatened and you respond by either fleeing or fighting, your body has the opportunity to use the energy and relieve the tension created by the nervous system to meet the situation. This allows your body to return to a state of homeostasis. If, however, no physical action occurs, as is more true of the stress response today, the body has no way of using up the energy and hormones marshalled to meet the challenge. Our fight-or-flight reaction allows us to face life-threatening situations, something that was more common in primitive societies. Now that most stressful situations are usually psychological and not life threatening, such as deadlines, tests, and financial decisions, the repeated triggering of the alarm response results in a bottling up of energy and emotion that may ultimately lead to stress-related disease. Occasional fight-or-flight responses are, however, normal and healthy, even in modern society. When another driver suddenly veers into your lane, you may be heart-poundingly frightened, but your quick response may save your life.

The Resistance Stage. When stress becomes chronic, the body begins to view it as a normal condition and adjusts to establish a new level of homeostasis. This new level might be compared to an arm-wrestling match, where two evenly matched opponents expend a lot of energy resisting one another and yet their hands remain in a neutral position. The effort of maintaining that position is exhausting and cannot be sustained indefinitely.

In the case of a sudden, high-intensity stressor, the alarm response occurs and then dissipates, followed by a resistance phase in which the adaptive energy remains elevated. As an example, imagine that you have just discovered a project deadline is two days away instead of seven. Instant panic! As the initial panic subsides, you find the energy to redouble your effort and get the project done. Assuming the stressor is eliminated (you finish the project) and rest and relaxation are obtained (you get some downtime), your body will return to its original level of homeostasis. But suppose that after meeting this deadline, you also have an exam and a major paper due and your boss asks you to work overtime at your part-time job. This kind of continued stress leads to exhaustion. If allowed to continue, chronically fatiguing stress may diminish the body's ability to resist illness, which can open the door to serious problems such as chronic high blood pressure, cancer, or cardiorespiratory disease.[20] Paradox-

breaking into your home. Your nervous system goes to work, in particular the autonomic nervous system, which can act rapidly and without conscious thought.

The autonomic system is broken down into two branches: the sympathetic and parasympathetic. The sympathetic nervous system controls the many quick adaptations needed to either stand and fight or run away (flight) from a perceived threat. Your senses sharpen, you become more alert, epinephrine (adrenaline) pours into your bloodstream, your heart starts pounding, and your

ically, the more pressed we are for time, the more important it is to make time for rest and relaxation.

The Exhaustion Stage.

When stress is very intense or lasts too long it can literally wear you out. The length of time an individual can maintain the resistance phase depends on individual coping ability and the nature and intensity of the stressor(s). When the body can no longer resist, it slumps into exhaustion. This is not the kind of exhaustion you feel at the end of a busy day; this kind of exhaustion is more serious. The inability to work, physical collapse, and even death can result. In Japan, where the work hours are long and demands very high, there has been an increase in the number of deaths attributed to exhaustion.

It is easy to understand how high-profile people like basketball coach Mike Krzyzewski and the President of Harvard, Neil Rudenstine, have suffered stress-related exhaustion and had to take leaves from their jobs. It is also evident that some occupations are chronically stressful; certainly air-traffic controllers, inner-city police, and emergency-room personnel fall into this category. What may be less obvious is the high stress felt by people like secretaries and blue-collar workers. Job stress mounts when demands are high and the employee has little or no control over job-related decisions. For example, blue-collar workers can lose their jobs because of decisions made by upper management, and good waiters and waitresses can lose tips when the cook does a bad job. When you can take control and resolve problems, you can reduce stress, but when someone else has the control, and especially when the behavior of the controller is erratic, such as the case of an inconsistent supervisor, stress soars. Three more stress recipes are (1) high demands and not enough time, (2) frustrated idealism, and (3) financial difficulties.

Interestingly, this type of exhaustion can occur even when a person is eating a nutritious diet and getting enough sleep. Selye concluded that something less obvious but critical to health is depleted during the resistance phase. He refers to this something as the **adaptive energy reserve**—a stockpile of energy available for adapting to difficult situations. Each time you use some of it, according to Selye, you deplete your reserves, which cannot be replaced. Regular energy levels return to normal with rest, but the adaptive energy reserve does not. If Selye is right, how would you like to spend your reserve? On big important issues? Or on everyday irritants? Selye's idea of a depleting adaptive energy store is now controversial (others believing that with adequate rest and restoration of resources a person can fully recover), but the idea of only sweating the big things remains appealing and will no doubt improve the quality of your life and the lives of those around you!

Selye's theory helps explain the physiological phenomena of stress, but it does not address psychosocial issues, cognitive processes, or the selection, use, and effectiveness of coping strategies. Today there is evidence that the stress response is not as nonspecific as Selye suggested. Different physical stress patterns have been discovered between individuals and in response to different kinds of stressors.

Psychological Aspects of Stress

J. W. Mason challenged Selye's biologically based theory by suggesting that the physiological system is sensitive to, and influenced by, emotional input.[21] As an example, in one study Selye provoked the physiological alarm reaction by subjecting people to extreme temperatures, but Mason showed that a gradual change of temperature (which minimized the emotional impact of the temperature change) did not elicit the alarm reaction even when the same extreme temperatures were reached. At about the same time, Lazarus[22] suggested that the nature and severity of a stress disorder is tied to the interaction between environmental demands, the quality of the individual's emotional response, and the coping process selected. A worst-case scenario would be high environmental demands (final exams), an extreme emotional response (panic or depression), and a poor or incorrect coping strategy (binge drinking).

To understand the different positions taken by physiological and psychological theorists regarding stress, take the example of shivering. A biologist would explain shivering as a natural biological reaction that occurs when a cold environment disrupts homeostasis. Shivering acts to restore body temperature by using muscle movement to generate heat. A psychologist or cognitist would argue that the physical reaction of shivering only occurs when the brain believes the body is cold. If, in your mind, you aren't cold, theoretically you won't shiver. Following this logic, you should be able to walk across hot coals without getting burns, assuming that you really believe they won't burn. This example appears to place these theories in opposition, when in truth both biological and psychological responses complement one another.

One of the most prominent psychological theories of stress is Richard Lazarus's cognitive transactional model of stress. In this model, stress is described as a relationship between demands and the power to deal with them without suffering unreasonable and destructive costs.[23,24] The demands are determined by an individual's perception rather than by an absolute value. This means that the demands of the same situation may be considered very high by one person and low by another. The same person may even perceive the demands as different at different times. For example, think how much harder it is to deal with things or to accurately appraise a situation when you are tired or emotional. How different is your reaction to an "out of order" sign on the copy machine when you have plenty of time to turn in a paper and when it is due within the hour? As we have discussed, the ability to deal with stress also varies according to things like available resources, one's emotional state, and coping strategies.

Chronic stress may have cognitive side effects such as emotional outbursts, anger displacement, distorted perception, and a lessening ability to plan rationally and make decisions. Recognizing the real source of these problems is important for understanding yourself and others during stressful times. Here is an example of chronic stress and cognitive side effects:

> Jim is an intelligent, easygoing guy with lots of friends. This semester his mother was diagnosed with cancer (stressor). He and his mother have decided that he should stay in school and visit on the weekends (resistance stage). Having trouble concentrating, Jim's grades have gotten very low and he may be endangering his chances for medical school (added stressor). He tries to make a study plan, but can't figure out where to start (difficulty planning). Thirsty, he goes to a soda machine and discovers it is out of his selection. Jim starts kicking and swearing at the machine (emotional outburst, anger displacement). Frustrated, he decides to go visit some friends. When he gets there, they are studying and turn down his offer to go to the student union for a break. Grumbling, he walks away thinking they don't want to hang around with a "dummy" like himself (distorted perception). Unsure whether to go back to studying or head to the union, he sits down on a bench and stares into space.

Someone who wasn't aware of Jim's situation might think that he was vandalizing the soda machine "just for kicks" and was too lazy to make good grades. Recognizing stress's role in behavior does not excuse harmful behavior, but it does enhance our understanding of ourselves (and others) and opens the door for clearer communication.

Can you think of a time or times when someone yelled at you when you knew that person was really mad at something or someone else? Can you identify a time or times when you became angry or upset with someone else when in fact you were really upset by something or someone else?

Perception's Influence on Stress

Three students trying to register for courses are standing in a long line. One mutters about the time being wasted and lambastes the school for an inefficient process. Another is chatting excitedly with a friend—they haven't seen each other all summer. The third spends the time in line trying to figure out how to make the courses for a double major fit together. If these three people were polled on how stressful the registration process was, we'd probably get three very different answers. Different things stress different people differently. It is important to recognize how our **perception,** the way we interpret and frame things, can create stress, not only for ourselves but also for others. Later in this chapter you will see how **cognitive intervention strategies** can be applied when problems of a perceptual origin have been identified.

Perceptual differences can easily lead to miscommunication—one of the greatest sources of interpersonal tension. Checking for understanding by asking others what they think you said is a quick way to see if you have communicated clearly. Restating someone else's words can verify whether you heard and understood them correctly. A mother who told her young daughter to "throw the empty cup in the sink" realized her mistake a moment later when the cup splintered into pieces.

Miscommunication often occurs when people work from different frames of reference. Deborah Tannen, a sociolinguist and author of the book *You Just Don't Understand,* reveals some fascinating gender differences in the area of communication. For example, a woman complaining about something may be looking for empathy and mutual understanding, and she is likely to receive that from another woman. However, a man hearing the same complaint may feel the need to help the woman by fixing the problem. Attempting to do this, the well-intentioned man will then wonder why his perfectly good suggestions are met with such disinterest.

Differing cultural backgrounds can create funny or disastrous mishaps. For example, in the United States wedding gifts are traditionally wrapped in white paper. In Japan, white paper represents death. We also expect a gift we are giving to be opened right away so we can see the receiver's expression—one of pleasure, we hope. The Japanese open their gifts in private so that if they don't like the gift the giver need not be embarrassed and the receiver does not have to pretend to like it. In Italy, the American OK sign made with your fingers is considered an obscene gesture. An effort to study other cultures and a willingness to admit ignorance and accept advice can eliminate many awkward and stressful situations. Recent debates concerning standardized test language in the SAT, GMAT, and so on also highlight the differences between ethnic cultures within the United States. Interacting with people of diverse backgrounds is one way to broaden your frame of reference and become aware of the assumptions you make based on your own background. A willingness to learn can help you turn potentially awkward situations into enlightening ones.

Can you think of examples of how two different perceptions or frames of references coming together on a college/university campus can result in tension? Here is an example to start you thinking:

> *Professor's perception:* Students need to understand the theoretical basis for a field of study in order to intelligently turn theory into practice in a changing world.
>
> *Student's perception:* Theoretical information is nice but it isn't relevant. What I need from this course are the practical skills needed in order to get and hold a job.

In summary, people often react differently to the same situation because of their differing perceptions of the event and their frame of reference. The actual stressor does not dictate a response; the perception of the demand of the stressor and the ability to meet the demand determine the response. It can then be argued that one's outlook on life, and one's perception of life's events, can lead toward or away from stress-related disease.

Personality and Stress

Psychologists are interested in the relationship between personality and stress. Research has been done to determine if one type of personality handles stress better than another and/or if one type is more susceptible to stress-related disease. Four major types of personalities have been identified. Type A personalities are considered hard driving, ambitious, competitive, high-strung, and high achieving. Not very long ago, it was believed that Type A personalities were high-risk candidates for cardiovascular disease. However, additional research has revealed that only those who exhibit chronic hostility and anger have a higher risk.[25,26] Control is a major factor in managing stress and Type A people are often in a position to control important job and lifestyle decisions, which may help them control their stress levels. Thus, for very driven individuals, others' well-meaning suggestions that they slow down may actually cause them to become more stressed.

Type B personalities are relaxed and easygoing—the opposite of Type A—but they too can experience stress, particularly if they are passive aggressive. Type C, a blend of A and B without the aggressive hostility that a Type A can exhibit, is the most stress-resistant type of personality. Type Es are the "please everyone" type of folk. These people may suffer from the feeling that they haven't accomplished enough, or that their efforts are inadequate. They may also experience guilt for not doing something or not including someone. Stress runs high for them when plans don't run smoothly.

Researcher Suzanne Kobasa has studied stress and personality and identified characteristics of what she calls "hardy" personalities.[27] A hardy person is one who accepts new developments as exciting challenges, is committed to work, has a sense of control and responsibility both on the job and in community or outside activities, and looks upon change as a normal part of life, not a stressor. It may be that children who are raised in a positive environment that encourages problem solving of problems difficult enough to be challenging but not so hard as to promote frustration and hopelessness will develop hardy personalities.

It is difficult for adults to change their personalities. Being aware of your personality traits, however, can help you select coping strategies and also avoid some of the things that are most likely to increase your stress. For example, a very athletically competitive person in need of relaxation will not get it by entering an athletic contest. This is just competitive stress wrapped in a new package. However, this same individual may be bored or irritable sitting on a sunny beach, perceiving it as a waste of time. Something active but noncompetitive like snorkeling might be the solution. To find out whether you have a type A personality take the quiz in Activity 11.1.

Activity 11.1
What's Your Personality Type?

Answer yes or no to the following statements:

1. I hate to wait for anyone or anything.
2. I often interrupt others when they are speaking.
3. I am usually rushed. There's never enough time in the day.
4. I feel guilty when I have nothing to do or when I play.
5. I get impatient when others perform tasks that I can do faster.
6. I eat faster than most of my friends.
7. I feel stretched to my limits at the end of the day.
8. I think about other things during conversations.
9. When driving, I get irritated at drivers who cut me off or drive too slowly. I frequently blow my horn and try to pass them.
10. I react with gestures, raised voice, and increased heart rate when someone does something incompetent, messy, inconsiderate, or unfair or after an irritating encounter.
11. I think cashiers will shortchange me if they can.
12. I feel my anger is justified. I feel an urge to punish people—plot to get back at them.
13. I frequently feel irritated when I stand in line or drive.
14. I like to have the last word in an argument.
15. In a checkout express line, if the person in front of me has more items than the limit, I get frustrated.
16. If a see a nonhandicapped person park in a handicapped driver's space, I feel anger inside.
17. When I am angry, I keep things bottled-up inside, pout, and sulk.

Scoring:

Statements 1 through 8 demonstrate Type A behavior. If you said yes to three or more of these statements, you probably fall into the Type A behavior category. Statements 9 through 17 demonstrate angry/hostile/cynical/hot reactor behavior. Even one yes response to any of these statements is too many. Have a friend or loved one who knows you also check the statements for you. Was there a change in any of the responses?

From G. Robbins, D. Powers, and S. Burgess. *The wellness way of life*, 3rd ed. Madison, WI: Brown & Benchmark, 1997, Table 7.3 ("Quiz to Identify Your Type A/Hostile, Hot Reactor Behavior"), p. 151. Reproduced with permission of The McGraw-Hill Companies.

If you are interested in taking a more comprehensive personality inventory, speak with someone with a background in psychology. There are a number of different ways to assess personality. In this text we are most concerned with a discussion of hostility, since this has been found to be a predictor for stress-related illness.

Some scientists also suggest that certain people have a genetic predisposition for stress-related illness.[28] Their research focuses on linking genetic makeup to physical characteristics that lower the person's general ability to resist stress. This does not mean that a person will definitely fall victim to stress, but that there is a higher risk.

Social Aspects of Stress

Social stress theorists study how stress results from the relationship between the individual and society. Issues of tension include compliance with social norms and laws, opportunities for education and work, financial gain, family growth, political voice, power, and status. Stress may be the result of a conflict between a desire for something and the inability to obtain it. For example, you may want to go to college, but the congressional statutes that have made it more difficult for you to get the financial aid you need may make this seem like an impossible goal.

Life change theory explains stress in terms of the changes in our lives that require adaptive energy. A relationship has been found between the number and intensity of negative life changes you experience and the risk of disease.

More recently A. D. Kanner and colleagues[29] have challenged the life-change theory, suggesting that daily *hassles* and small, irritating problems are more significant to health risk than major stressors. The effects of hassles may be cumulative, and their nagging appearance may be the day-to-day manifestations of larger issues. People are more apt to resolve the big life changes and let the smaller problems continue to irritate. Whenever possible, eliminate the daily hassles in your life. Begin by thinking of some hassles in your life and brainstorm ways to eliminate one or more of them. When brainstorming, put down all your ideas (or ideas of the group) no matter how ridiculous they sound. Stopping to judge each one may limit creativity. You can eliminate the far-fetched ideas later. Here is an example:

Hassle: No convenient parking on campus.

Solutions: Park far away and enjoy the walk.
           Ride a bike, the bus, or car pool.
           Arrive early before all the spaces are taken.
           Move closer to campus and walk.

Environmental-ecological theory, also considered a social theory, examines the stress caused by our surroundings. Loud noises, crowding, poor air quality, bright or dim lighting, and chemical hazards are examples of the kinds of things that can cause discomfort, poor health, tension—and stress. Something as simple as a poorly adjusted chair can be a factor in repetitive stress syndrome, headaches, and backaches. With more women in the workforce, changes are being made to address their special needs. As an illustration, women who want to breastfeed have had to pump their milk in a bathroom stall during their coffee breaks. Now many employers are adding nearby daycare and lactation centers to allow women to better combine work and family obligations. Can you think of any environmental factors that stress you?

The Interdisciplinary Approach to Stress Management

Stress researchers and other professionals have learned a great deal about stress in the past sixty years, and now, as they grapple with how to put together their knowledge, more and more interdisciplinary research is being initiated. Psychoneuroimmunology, the study of the effects of the psyche on the neurological and immunological systems, is one such area. Researchers try to answer questions like "Can positive or negative thinking raise or lower the body's immunity to disease?"

Another example of an interdisciplinary approach is Gary Swartz's biopsychosocial model for health and illness. According to this model, medical diagnoses and treatments should consider the matrix of biological, psychological, and social factors represented in a patient's history and current condition.[30]

TECHNIQUES FOR MANAGING STRESS

The Stress Survival Kit

Managing stress is paramount in this high-pressure, high-tech, low-touch society. The simplest things can gang up on you . . . like trying to hook up a new modem or choose a long-distance carrier. Ironically, we tend to handle traumatic events better than small problems. When something major happens, people often stop everything else and attend to the problem. This allows them to make a plan and bring resolution to the problem. During traumatic times, friends and family usually come rushing to your side with loving support. So while traumas are intensely stressful for a short period of time, over the long haul the ongoing daily hassles may take more of a toll. There should be five rules in everyone's "stress survival kit":

1. *Identify the stressors in your life.* Since stress is tied in with perception, personality, environmental conditions, demands, and available resources, only an individualized assessment will work well. Identify your stressors by looking for stress symptoms or by keeping a journal that includes not only how you spend your time, but also how you feel about what you do. Sometimes just the act of putting things down on paper provides relief.

   If you experience any of the following, try to figure out what triggers them.

   Clenching your jaw

   Making fists

Backache

Tension headache

Neck and shoulder tension

Irritability

Depression

Anxiety

Excitability

Jumpiness

Getting hot and flushed

Reaching for relief through alcohol or drugs

2. *Take control.* Where and when it is possible, minimize distress by taking control. Preplanning is one way to do this. If you know that you can't make big decisions late in the afternoon, set aside time in the morning for them. If you hate traffic, establish a schedule that will allow you to avoid it. Anticipate problems and put in place some contingency plans. Not everything can be controlled, but eliminating foreseeable problems leaves you the time and energy to deal with the unexpected.

Sometimes it is possible to increase the amount of control you have. If, for example, you see a problem, think of some possible solutions before approaching the person in authority. People are much more interested in listening to ideas on how to fix things than to someone simply voicing a complaint. You may be rewarded with additional authority and more decision-making power. Taking the initiative may provide you with control.

Put yourself in charge of the problem. One frustrated employee, unable to get the equipment she needed, finally asked to be in charge of equipment disbursement. It took her less time to develop an efficient way to handle equipment assignments than it had previously taken to search for the equipment she needed.

3. *Accept your limitations.* When you cannot control a situation or simply don't have the time to handle everything, accept that you can't do it all. The "I shoulds" are killers. You can only do so much, and kicking yourself for things you should have done will not improve the future. Decide what is important and set priorities. This means focusing on the really important items and delegating or letting others go. A working parent, for example, may need to accept that the house won't be spotless in exchange for quality time to spend with the children.

4. *Change your attitude toward stressors you can't change.* If you can't change it, try to understand it or put it in its best light. Sometimes you can't avoid distress, in which case, confront it, cope, give yourself positive reinforcement when you cope well, and move on.

5. *Use stress-management strategies to reduce or escape distress.* A number of stress intervention strategies have been developed and research on their effectiveness is mixed. Like all behavior change strategies, they take time and effort. The stress intervention programs that seem to be the most effective are those that (1) are offered over a period of weeks or months; (2) include ongoing training and assessment; and (3) follow up and provide for discussion on the effectiveness of the techniques in the individual's life.

Like stress theories, different intervention strategies approach the problem in different ways. A cognitive intervention strategy uses mental tactics to reduce psychological stress, whereas a relaxation strategy aims to release muscular tension. Because of the nature of stress, use of a variety of strategies is often most effective. The rest of this chapter presents stress-management techniques. This information is meant as a guide to what is available with the hope that it will stimulate you to do additional reading for in-depth information and to use the additional sources of clinics, other courses, and mental health professionals when necessary. If you feel that you suffer from a serious stress disorder, you should seek professional guidance and training without delay.

Applying Cognitive Interventions

If thoughts and emotions can influence the stress response, then "thinking" interventions ought to be able to alleviate distress. If we can think ourselves into distress, then we ought to be able to think ourselves out. This is the basis behind cognitive interventions. In order to intervene, however, you must first recognize how you are "thinking" yourself into distress. Here are three examples:

1. *Problem:* Negative self-talk.

   Examples: I just can't do it. I'm no good. I am such an idiot to have made that mistake.

   Intervention: Positive self-talk. As soon as you realize you are doing negative talk, you say "stop" and convert your thoughts to positive talk. Positive talk can enhance self-esteem and act like a form of goal setting. To accomplish something, you must believe in yourself. Be your own cheerleader. Keep telling yourself positive thoughts like, "I can do this," "Just ten more," and "It's worthwhile." This will help keep negative thoughts and fears from generating unproductive tension and doubt.

2. *Problem:* Personalizing a situation instead of recognizing that not everything is about you.

   Example: I am a lousy salesperson because this customer is unhappy and yelling at me.

   Intervention: Only worry about the things you actually have control over. If the customer is unhappy with a product over which you had no control, his anger is really directed at the company, not you personally. Remembering this can help you deal with the customer calmly and objectively.

In stressful situations, try to identify the "real" reasons for things. Look beyond the obvious, look for clues. For example, an angry customer at 5:30 P.M. may be coming off a bad day on the job, be hungry, and be in a hurry—none of which is under your control.

3. *Problem:* Filtering other people's actions through your frame of reference and then passing judgment.

Example: A car has gone off the road and smashed into a tree in someone's front yard. A member of an anti-drunk-driving group who sees the accident gets angry at the thought of another irresponsible drunk. A physician passing by pulls over, suspecting that the driver might have had a seizure or heart attack at the wheel. A parent of a teenager points out the danger of flirting with a passenger instead of concentrating on the road. A pet lover wonders if the person lost control while trying to miss an animal in the road.

Intervention: Look for clues before making conclusions. Try to see events from other people's perspectives.

Public relations professionals are sometimes called "spin doctors." Their job is to interpret and present events and news in such a manner that you believe their version, their "spin" of what happened and what it means. For example, following a political debate, spin doctors are hard at work convincing you that the candidate they represent came out the winner. They want you to look at things from their point of view, so they "reframe" the event, putting the facts in the best possible light. You can use a similar **reframing** technique to control stress. When faced with a stressful situation, you have the opportunity to put your own spin on it. Try it while reacting to the statements below:

> "The boss wants to talk to you right now."
>
> "Professor M. wants to see you about your paper."
>
> "Your doctor's office called and asked you to call back today."
>
> "The IRS is on the line."

For many people these statements would cause alarm, anxiety, and worry. But maybe the boss wants to promote you, the professor wants permission to keep a copy of your excellent paper, the doctor's office wants to remind you of an appointment, and the IRS wants to tell you that you overpaid your last tax bill.

The point is, you can choose to look at events from a positive direction or a negative one. Sometimes sheer optimism can change the situation for the better. Enthusiasm can also go a long way in getting others to support you. Some remarkable people have such positive energy and tremendous coping abilities that they emerge from tragic circumstances with a plan that touches all those around them. Television host John Walsh is such a person. After mourning the terrible murder of his young son, Adam, John committed his life to getting criminals off the streets. Today he hosts the very successful *America's Most Wanted* television show.

Think of something that has been bothering you and then reframe it.

Be aware that there is a difference between reframing and rationalizing. During rationalizations the truth of the situation may be lost. For example, a professor can rationalize that students don't seek out extra help because they are lazy, when the truth may be that the professor is intimidating. Rationalization, denial, and fantasy are usually considered poor stress-management techniques, but there is also evidence that these processes can be valuable during the initial stages of trauma since they allow the person time to cope without being hit by the enormity of the situation.

Imagery

Our imagination is a powerful tool. We know that an overactive imagination in the dark can conjure up all kinds of horrors, and we also know that positive images can help us diminish fears and achieve our goals. **Imagery** as a cognitive stress-management technique involves the use of visualization to imagine yourself in, and successfully handling, stressful situations. Olympic athletes often mentally rehearse their skills right before an event. They picture themselves performing their event perfectly. Research indicates that mental and physical practice together are better than just physical practice. Being able to "see" yourself do something helps you do it. One of the best times to do mental imagery is when you are totally relaxed.

One way to relax is to imagine a favorite hideaway or vacation retreat. When performing mental imagery, try to use all of your senses. For example:

> The sand is warm on the soles of my feet and I can feel the light breeze blowing through my hair. The cry of wild birds is distant but clear coming across the ocean waves. As I wade in the cool water's edge, I can smell the salt air mixed with the scent of wood burning from a nearby campfire.

When you are feeling relaxed, focus on an activity you are having trouble with and try to picture a positive outcome. The activity does not have to be a sport skill; it could be rehearsing a conversation, successfully mingling at a party, giving a presentation, or boarding an aircraft without feeling afraid. Focus on performing well at whatever it is you have chosen. It takes practice to keep negative thoughts and scenarios from creeping into your mind. If your mind takes off in a negative direction, refocus and try again. If you are an external imager, you will be looking at someone (in your mind) doing the activity. You may even be looking at yourself perform much as you would if you were reviewing a videotape. If you are an internal imager, you will not see a separate image performing the task; instead you will "feel" (in your mind) yourself doing it. Both work well.

Asking for Help

The "hardy" do it. To recognize that you need help and then get social support by asking is crucial. Sadly most people are too busy keeping their own lives together to notice when others need help. Yet when asked for help, these same busy individuals are often happy to make room in their schedules for you. Numerous hotlines and professional services are also waiting to help.

Learning to be more assertive can help at those times when you feel unsure of yourself and can assist in overcoming feelings of unworthiness. Assertive training programs are available on college campuses, through evening adult education classes, and at the YMCA. You may want to put together a list of people and organizations you can call on for help and keep their phone numbers handy.

Solving Problems Creatively

The tree limb that can bend in the wind survives. Or as Tao tradition suggests—move like water . . . do not try to push through the immovable rock; instead seek the path of least resistance around the rock. In time the jagged immovable rock will be changed (smoothed) by the water. In the nineties we are challenged to think "outside of the paradigm," to find solutions that are unorthodox but, like the water, allow progress in what otherwise seems like an impossible situation.

Two men lived in the same apartment building. One would get up in the morning and take a long, hot shower. The second would get up a half hour later and get nothing but cold water. The second man politely knocked on the first man's door and asked if he could take a shorter shower. The first man refused, saying he needed to steam his sinuses. Rather than argue, the second man went home, set his alarm clock for an hour earlier, woke up, turned on the shower, and went back to bed. The "immovable rock" was soon at the door offering a compromise. If you have what looks like an impossible problem, brainstorm with your friends and see whether you can come up with a creative solution.

Working on Communication Skills

Being an effective communicator prevents misunderstandings and facilitates positive interactions. Learning how to speak comfortably to a group of people (or to a person of authority) will make many of life's experiences easier, including serving on committees, interviewing for a job, presenting an idea to clients, or meeting your potential in-laws.

Managing Your Time

Stress? Excuse me, I don't have time to talk about stress. A chapter on stress in the nineties is not complete without talking about time or the perceived lack thereof. Time, for many, has become the number one most desired commodity. People are trading in high salaries and fast-track lifestyles for more time. Others just dream about having it. The superwomen and supermen of the world are trying to manage the time demands of work, families, and in many cases education or retraining. Developing good time-management skills will give you more time, as long as you avoid the trap of filling that new time with more work and added pressures. Here is an overview of some time management tactics.

1. Prioritize. Make lists of things to do and decide which are the most important.
2. Make a daily plan. Take fifteen minutes in the evening to outline your goals for the next day. You might even try ordering the goals. Then be sure to stick to your plan.
3. Keep a journal to find out where your time is going. See Lab 11.3.
4. Set aside "closed door" or personal work time.
5. Handle paper once. Make a decision the first time.
6. Break large projects into smaller units that you can tackle during smaller time blocks.
7. Limit interruptions when possible. Let your answering machine get the phone. Shut your door or go to the library to study.
8. Do the most difficult task first. This stops you from doing a lot of little things that can be done quickly later on and leaves you fresh to tackle larger or more complicated projects.
9. Delegate. This means to get someone else to do what you don't have time for. Once you delegate, be sure not to oversupervise.
10. Beware of perfectionism. Being obsessive about perfection will backfire—you don't have time for it!
11. Learn to say no.

If you are having time management problems, you might want to focus on one of these skills for a behavior change.

Learning to Relax

As discussed earlier, the Inverted "U" Hypothesis describes the relationship between arousal and performance. When arousal is too high, performance declines. When performance declines, people get frustrated and their anxiety creates more tension, which in turn makes performance even worse. A vicious cycle is set up. Relaxation techniques allow you to break the cycle and reduce your arousal level. Whether you are trying to sink a $50,000 putt or get a passing grade on a paper, the right level of arousal is important. When you find yourself getting "too wound up," a little relaxation may be what you need. Relaxation techniques include progressive relaxation, autogenic training, transcendental meditation, and biofeedback. Each of these techniques takes months

Progressive Relaxation

Get in a comfortable position and relax. Now clench your right fist, tighter and tighter, studying the tension as you do so. Keep it clenched and notice the tension in your fist, hand, and forearm. Now relax. Feel the looseness in your right hand, and notice the contrast with the tension. Repeat this procedure with your right fist again, always noticing as you relax that this is the opposite of tension—relax and feel the difference. Repeat the entire procedure with your left fist, then both fists at once.

Now bend your elbows and tense your biceps. Tense them as hard as you can and observe the feeling of tautness. Relax, straighten out your arms. Let the relaxation develop and feel that difference. Repeat this, and all succeeding procedures at least once.

Turning attention to your head, wrinkle your forehead as tight as you can. Now relax and smooth it out. Let yourself imagine your entire forehead and scalp becoming smooth and at rest. Now frown and notice the strain spreading throughout your forehead. Let go. Allow your brow to become smooth again. Close your eyes now, squint them tighter. Look for the tension. Relax your eyes. Let them remain closed gently and comfortably. Now clench your jaw, bite hard, notice the tension throughout your jaw. Relax your jaw. When the jaw is relaxed, your lips will be slightly parted. Let yourself really appreciate the contrast between tension and relaxation. Now press your tongue against the roof of your mouth. Feel the ache in the back of your mouth. Relax. Press your lips now, purse them into an "O." Relax your lips. Notice that your forehead, scalp, eyes, jaw, tongue, and lips are all relaxed.

Press your head back as far as it can comfortably go and observe the tension in your neck. Roll it to the right and feel the changing locus of stress, roll it to the left. Straighten your head and bring it forward, press your chin against your chest. Feel the tension in your throat, the back of your neck. Relax, allowing your head to return to a comfortable

position. Let the relaxation deepen. Now shrug your shoulders. Keep the tension as you hunch your head down between your shoulders. Relax your shoulders. Drop them back and feel the relaxation spreading through your neck, throat, and shoulders, pure relaxation, deeper and deeper.

Give your entire body a chance to relax. Feel the comfort and the heaviness. Now breathe in and fill your lungs completely. Hold your breath. Notice the tension. Now exhale, let your chest become loose, let the air hiss out. Continue relaxing, letting your breath come freely and gently. Repeat this several times, noticing the tension draining from your body as you exhale. Next, tighten your stomach and hold. Note the tension, then relax. Now place your hand on your stomach. Breathe deeply into your stomach, pushing your hand up. Hold, and relax. Feel the contrast of relaxation as the air rushes out. Now arch your back, without straining. Keep the rest of your body as relaxed as possible. Focus on the tension in your lower back. Now relax, deeper and deeper.

Tighten your buttocks and thighs. Flex your thighs by pressing down your heels as hard as you can. Relax and feel the difference. Now curl your toes downward, making your calves tense. Study the tension. Relax. Now bend your toes toward your face, creating tension in your shins. Relax again.

Feel the heaviness throughout your lower body as the relaxation deepens. Relax your feet, ankles, calves, shins, knees, thighs, and buttocks. Now let the relaxation spread to your stomach, lower back, and chest. Let go more and more. Experience the relaxation deepening in your shoulders, arms, and hands. Deeper and deeper. Notice the feeling of looseness and relaxation in your neck, jaws, and all your facial muscles.

David, M., Eshelman, E. R., and McKay, M. *The relaxation and stress reduction workbook,* 4th ed., 1955, pp. 36–37. Reprinted by permission of New Harbinger Publications, Oakland, CA; www.newharbinger.com.

to master, but once learned, can elicit relaxation in a matter of minutes.

Progressive Relaxation

Believing that a person cannot be nervous or tense in any body part where muscles are relaxed, Edmond Jacobson developed a technique for **progressive relaxation** of the muscles. He surmised that a technique that systematically relaxes your skeletal muscles will also relax nearby organs and involuntary muscles. Jacobson's program consists of alternately tensing and relaxing muscles in a predetermined order. Creating tension helps you recognize tension in a muscle and consciously learn to let it go.

To begin progressive relaxation, take up a comfortable position lying on your back on the floor with your knees straight or bent but not crossed and your arms by your side. (You may also sit relaxed in a comfortable chair.) Next spend a few minutes clearing your mind and concentrating on deep breathing. Proper breathing for relaxation is to draw the air in, let it fill your abdomen, and then let tension release as you breathe out. Once you are comfortable and focused you can begin tensing and relaxing your muscles. See the box above for an example of a progressive relaxation routine. Jacobson's full training procedure takes months, with whole sessions dedicated to relaxing a single muscle group. However, it is possible to achieve significant relaxation benefits in less time. A session should begin with muscle tensing, but most of the session should be devoted to achieving full relaxation. In the beginning it may take a while to achieve muscle relaxation, but with practice (usually several months), you will be able to elicit the relaxation response quickly and counteract stress-induced tension. Progressive relaxation, a physiological technique, is often combined with mental imagery, a cognitive technique.

Autogenic Training

Something that is autogenic is, according to Webster, "produced independently of external influence or aid" and "originating within or derived from sources within the same individual."[31] **Autogenic training** in relaxation terms requires individuals to imagine conditions such as warmth and heaviness in their muscles, thereby inducing relaxation. The feeling of warmth is generated from within the person, not by an external warming of the room. A variety of mental images may be used to further relax the person, such as glowing warm like the sun and sinking into the deepest, downiest cloud. To relax a tense muscle, a person might picture the aching muscle as red and then try to mentally change the color to a cool blue, or imagine the tension as a liquid and let it run out like water. The technique involved is very similar to Jacobson's progressive relaxation technique and often begins with a muscle-tensing and -relaxing exercise.

Autogenic training, developed by German physician Johannes H. Schultz, is made up of a series of six psychophysiologic exercises that take about four months to learn. Many professionals have developed programs and commercial tapes for autogenic training, often in combination with progressive relaxation.

Meditation

Meditation is a form of relaxation and concentration that allows you to free yourself from the bombardment of conscious thought (immediate situation) and achieve a more objective perspective. Transcendental meditation (TM), a religious/mystical technique with historical roots in India, uses breathing, visualization, and muscular relaxation techniques. Deep mental concentration is achieved through repetition of the mantra, one word or a simple sound that is repeated over and over. The mantra helps you to free your mind of other thoughts. In the beginning it may be difficult to keep thoughts from interfering, flitting into your consciousness, but with practice a deep relaxed state of concentration is possible. It is believed that TM allows you to move past subtler levels of thought and experience the source of a thought. Most Eastern forms of meditation are taught sitting with the eyes closed but TM may also be practiced standing. For more information on medi-

tation, look to local college courses and courses taught by professionals at community centers and elsewhere. Be sure the trainer is well educated in the technique he or she is teaching.

Biofeedback

It was once believed that the autonomic nervous system was totally automatic and that we had no control over it. **Biofeedback** techniques teach you how to exert voluntary control over certain functions of the autonomic nervous system. If, for example, your heart starts racing at the thought of something you find frightening, you can use this technique to bring your heart rate down and reduce your anxiety. The term *biofeedback* means that one of your biological responses is monitored with an instrument that provides information, "feedback," to you. A number of instruments are used to monitor different physiological responses. You may have performed biofeedback using a skin temperature instrument. A number of companies have produced the "stress card" or "stress dot," which starts out black but turns red, green, yellow, or blue depending on your skin temperature. Mood rings work on the same principle. The idea is that when you are aroused (stressed, tense, anxious) blood is pumped to the vital organs and away from the skin, making the skin cool or clammy. The goal becomes to warm your hands and make the dot, card, or ring change colors. (As with all instruments there is room for error—a person may be mentally relaxed but feel chilled in a room and hence have cold hands. Poor circulation may also be caused by age and disease, and the instrument used may reflect physiological stress, but not psychological stress.)

Physicians use a number of common instruments to monitor physiological responses, including an EKG or pulse monitor for heart rate, EEG for brain waves, and computer-generated visual representation of respiration rate and blood pressure. After a period of training, the person may no longer need the feedback from the instrument to induce relaxation or stimulation. Progressive relaxation, meditation, and autogenic training are all used in combination with biofeedback.

Laughter

It is impossible to laugh and stay tense for very long. Laughter diffuses physical tension and triggers a relaxation response. Humor is a wonderful way to work yourself out of feeling stress in a difficult situation. It won't necessarily change the situation, but it can change your response to it. Comedians are very good at looking at things from a different perspective and making us laugh at ourselves. Although we can't all be standup comics, we can learn how to produce humor and take life a little less seriously. For example, next time you are standing in a line at the book store, try saying something like, "Gee, I

My stress level is tied to other people's actions. I can't change things myself.

Take on projects in which you will have control over decisions and the quality of the final product. When possible, turn down jobs in which you will not have any control. Negotiate for control and resources before taking on a job.

Example: If you are in charge of ordering team shirts, only do so after everyone has given you money so that you don't waste energy hounding people later when you are "out" the money.

- Change your attitude rather that trying to change others.
- Use humor to gain a new perspective on the situation.
- Write down your frustrations on a piece of paper and throw it away.

I don't have time to figure out how to lower my stress.

Learn time-management techniques first. Reexamine your priorities.

It's just my nature. I like being busy and living on the edge.

- No problem if this is true. But keep track of how many times you say, "I wish I had time to. . . ." Determine whether you would like to be busy doing other things.
- Check your health. Do you suffer from headaches, tension, or other conditions that might be stress-related?

The thrill outweighs the risks.

- Make sure you understand exactly what the risks are.
- Look around. Are your thrills hurting anyone you love?

I am not a hardy person.

- Practice stress-management techniques.
- Preplan events to eliminate as many stressors as possible.
- Know your limits and work within them, and perhaps work to extend them little by little.

Change sounds hard and I don't have any friends to help me.

- Call a hotline or support service.
- Talk to a minister, priest, or rabbi.
- Meet people through church or community service or by joining a leisure activity such as a bowling league or cooking class.
- Make one change at a time. And remember, you *can* do it.

---

hope we get out of here before the authors have written a new edition" or "At the rate this line is moving, these will all be history books." No doubt others will come back with their quips and before you know it, you'll be checking out with a smile on your face.

Seeking a Balanced Level of Stress

Too little stress is called **hypostress.** For those who are always distressed, it is hard to believe that there are many people who suffer hypostress. These individuals are bored, lonely, and often isolated. To combat this, seek out stimulation. How much "stress" do you like? Do you watch horror movies, read suspense novels, ride rollercoasters, take on job challenges that you aren't quite sure how to accomplish, or agree to go on a blind date? Some people crave even more tension and excitement. These thrill seekers bungee jump, white water raft, and parachute. It is unhealthy, however, when the thrill becomes more important than anything else or the risks become too high. Drug and alcohol abuse, driving recklessly, and playing Russian roulette are examples of very destructive thrill-seeking behaviors.

Taking Care of Yourself

Eat right, get enough sleep, exercise, limit or avoid alcohol and caffeine intake, and avoid tobacco and drugs. Don't always rush around—take timeouts and vacations. Be patient with yourself and others. Take time to develop good relationships. In short, live a wellness lifestyle. Suffice it to say that taking care of yourself is an excellent antistress strategy.

SUMMARY

Stress is a multifaceted phenomenon. It has been studied from psychological, biological, and social perspectives, all of which provide us with part of the "picture" of stress. Stress-management techniques vary according to the nature of the stress.

There are many kinds of stressors, both good (eustress) and bad (distress). Stressors can be beyond our control or preventable. Often the stressor does not itself cause stress; rather, our perception of the stressor is the problem. The intensity and duration of distress, the resources available, and our coping abilities all determine the impact of the stress. Being aware of how our perceptions can shape events and affect others can also help to reduce or prevent stressful situations.

Sources of stress vary a great deal from person to person, as do personality, hardiness, and perception. An effective stress program must be tailored to the individual, and as with any behavior change program, both short- and long-term goals should be established. When stress, anxiety, and depression are too high, professional help is needed. On the other hand, sometimes just a little help is needed to get through a tough period and friends, families, and community resources can make the difference.

Challenge is good for personal and professional growth. The important thing is to prevent challenge from becoming chronic distress. Letting off steam through exercise, eating right, getting plenty of sleep, and maintaining a sense of humor can all help you keep a healthy perspective.

SUGGESTED READING

American Heart Association, Greater Long Beach Chapter. Stress—bona fide A.H.A. risk factor. *Heart Lines* 41: 1, February 1984.

Cotrell, R. R. *Stress management.* Guilford, CT: The Dushkin Publishing Group, 1992.

Crews, D., and D. Landers. A meta-analytic review of aerobic fitness and reactivity to psychosocial stressors. *Medicine and Science in Sports and Exercise* 19: 5114–5120, 1987.

DeLongis, A., J. C. Coyne, G. Dakof, S. Folkman, and R. S. Lazarus. Relationships of daily hassles, uplifts, and major life events to health status. *Health Psychology* 1: 119–136, 1982.

Hobfoll, S. E. *Stress, social support and women.* Washington, D.C.: Hemisphere Publishing, 1986.

International Society of Sport Psychology. *Physical Activity and Psychological Benefits: Position Statement* 20: 179, 1992.

Morse, D. R., and M. L. Furst. *Stress for success.* New York: Van Nostrand Reinhold, 1979.

Selye, H. *The stress of life,* 2nd ed. New York: McGraw Hill, 1976.

Stanford, S. C., and P. Salmon, eds. and J. A. Gray, consultant ed. *Stress: From synapse to syndrome.* San Diego: Academic Press, 1993.

5. Take the activity you selected in item 4 and decide what you need to do to start doing that activity or behavior. Decide on a first step.

6. What makes you believe you can accomplish your goal? *Or* What makes you believe you can accomplish this first step?

7. If your first step doesn't work, then what will you do?

8. Complete the following statement:

   I am going to take my first step on _____ .
   date within 30 days

Action Taker

1. What are you currently doing to balance the amount of stress in your life?

2. Are you keeping track of your progress?

   If yes, how?

   > Journal
   >
   > Discussions with a professional
   >
   > Stress tests (physical or psychological)

   If no, would it help motivate you to keep track?

3. Are you receiving support or rewards for your effort?

   If yes, what kind?

   If no, why not? And can you change this?

4. Do you think you will continue? Why or why not?

5. If you were to stop, what do you think would be your major reason or temptation for stopping?

6. What strategies can you use to prevent the temptations or situations listed in item 5 from making you stop your new behavior? In other words, how can you prepare yourself against temptation?

   Examples

   Set aside a specific time of day for ten minutes of progressive relaxation and make it clear to others that you do not want to be disturbed.

   Have a friend help you identify beginning signs of stress or stress triggers.

   Ask for time to think before committing to something that might overload your schedule.

7. How would you get yourself started again if you did stop?

8. Are your stress-management goals specifically and clearly stated? (See Chapter 2.)

9. Do you have confidence in your ability to continue your new behavior?

   If yes, what kinds of things are you doing that are building your confidence?

   If no, what kinds of things lower your confidence? How can you change or change the environment around you to eliminate or neutralize the effect of these things?

Maintainer

1. For how long have you maintained your stress-management program?

2. What are the top two reasons that make you want to continue?

3. Have you been tempted to stop? If so, what tempted you?

4. How did you convince yourself to continue?

5. Can you prevent such temptation? If so, how?

6. Do you have confidence in your ability to continue your new behavior?

   If yes, what kinds of things are you doing that are building your confidence?

   If no, what kinds of things lower your confidence? How can you change or change the environment around you to eliminate or neutralize the effect of these things?

7. Are you at a level of stress you are happy with or do you wish to continue to improve?

8. If you would like to improve, how are you keeping track of your improvement?

   > Tests
   >
   > Journaling
   >
   > Other

9. What kind of support do you get for your efforts?

   > Self-rewards, internal
   >
   > External rewards

10. How have you changed or how have you changed the environment around you to accommodate a healthier lifestyle?

11. Is there anything else you need to promote your continued maintenance? Information? Support? Time management?

12. If you listed something in the previous statement, can you think of a way to attain it or can you think of someone who can help you with it?

The Distress-Eustress Continuum

Stressors can affect us mentally, emotionally, spiritually, physically, and socially. Here are some examples of stressors for each of the categories. Use the following scale to rank each stressor (or perhaps seven to ten from each category) and then compare your answers with others in the class and discuss your differences. Remember: something that is eustress for you can be distress for someone else.

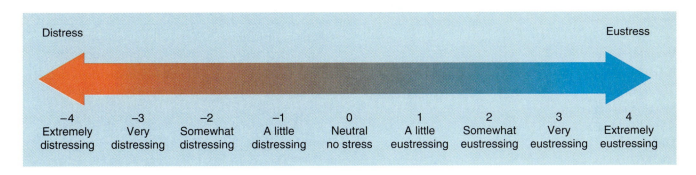

Distress								Eustress
−4	−3	−2	−1	0	1	2	3	4
Extremely distressing	Very distressing	Somewhat distressing	A little distressing	Neutral no stress	A little eustressing	Somewhat eustressing	Very eustressing	Extremely eustressing

Physical Stressors

Exercise/physical activity

Dancing

Sex

Pregnancy

Massage

Loud noise

Temperature extremes

Bright lights

Injury

Illness

Headaches

Prescriptive drugs

Recreational drugs

Sleep deprivation

Jetlag

Sunburn

Emotional Stressors

Marriage

Birth of a child

Graduation

New job

Major purchase (car, jewelry, house)

Dating

End of a semester

Interview

Loan payments

Helping a friend in crisis

Confrontation to resolve a problem

Meeting a celebrity

Asking for help

Seeing a horror movie

Watching a violent news story

Reading a romance novel

Arguing or fighting with a friend or member of your family

Disagreement with an authority figure (boss, police officer, professor, parent)

Illness of parent, friend, self

Failing a course or being reprimanded by the boss

Injury to self or others

Unfair treatment of self or others

Victim of crime (robbery, assault, rape)

Not being able to spend the holidays with family

No date

Loss of loved one

Loss of a pet

Loss of a job

Car problems

Mental/Intellectual Stressors

Doing well on an exam

Recognition for scholarly achievement

Solving a puzzle

Finding a unique solution that encompasses everyone's needs

People wanting your advice or help

Being a major player in decision making

Building or creating something

Job interviewing

Being in charge of a project

Meeting an expert in your field

Learning new computer software

Mental fatigue or boredom

Frustration, which can lead to burnout

Being responsible for and making big decisions when you are working with inadequate information or funds, and a lack of control over the situation

Studying, especially with time restraints

Working on financial papers (income tax, budgets)

Not being recognized for achievements or hard work

Social Stressors

Being part of a group

Finding an outfit for a special occasion

Being the center of attention (and wanting to be, or handling it well)

Running for office

Isolation—no friends, no relationships

Supporting an unpopular cause

Trying to "fit in"

Meeting other people's expectations (parents, boss, friends)

Peer pressure

Spiritual Stressors

Giving to or helping others in need

Supporting the spiritual community

Playing a role in a service (reader, greeter, choir member)

Ethical, moral, and religious decisions

Medical decisions tied to your spiritual belief system

Religious decisions

Guilt

Name _____ **Section** _____ **Date** _____

How Do I Spend My Time?

Do you often wish you had more time? Wonder where it goes? Does a lack of time add stress to your life? This lab will help you focus on the types of things that eat up your time and cause stress. Awareness is the big first step toward managing time and taming stress.

Keep a timed journal as follows:

In a notebook that is easy to carry with you, record what you are doing every 15, 30, or 60 minutes. Add to this how you are feeling mentally, emotionally, and physically. If you have used a stress reduction strategy, make a note of it and its effectiveness. Maintain this journal for three days. Here is an entry example:

	Activity	*Comments*
7:00 A.M.	Got out of bed. Drank some coffee. Watched cartoons.	Tired, four hours sleep. Dread exam. Knot in stomach. Cartoons funny, laughed, relaxed a little.

Review your journal.

1. Identify three to five activities that ate up big amounts of your time. Add up the time spent in each of these activities over three days. Then try to write down some ways to eliminate or cut back the time needed for these activities.

2. Identify the amount of time you spend relaxed or happily engaged in activities. How much of the time are you engaged in stressful activities? Would the activities that are stressful be less so if you had more time for them?

3. Identify stress symptoms like headaches, stomach upset, burnout, and feeling overwhelmed. Do you see a relationship between these and where, how, or with whom you spent your time?

4. Identify stress and time management strategies that worked for you. Identify times when you wished you had used a management strategy.

5. If you were to make one change in how you spend your time what would it be? Do you think you could successfully make this change? Maybe you should give it a try!

CHAPTER 12

Creating and Maintaining Healthy Relationships

Objectives

1. Be able to describe and define healthy relationships.

2. Understand why healthy relationships are an important part of total wellness.

3. Understand and describe the three phases of social maturity.

4. Learn how to be a good friend and why it is important to have good friends.

5. Discuss the pros and cons of marriage.

6. Describe the characteristics of healthy marriages and families.

7. Identify the physical and social disadvantages of loneliness.

8. Determine your healthy relationship stage of change and complete the appropriate laboratory exercises.

Terms

- Intimate relationship
- Selfishness
- Learned tolerance
- Selflessness
- Safety net
- Infatuation
- Traditional family
- Blended family
- Family violence
- Loneliness

Where Am I?

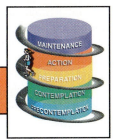

Precontemplator _____ I am currently not participating in a healthy relationship, and I do not want to begin one.

Contemplator _____ I am considering developing a healthy relationship or improving a relationship in which I am involved, but I have not done so yet.

Preparer _____ I am currently intending to develop a healthy relationship or improve a relationship in which I am involved within the next month.

Action Taker _____ My close relationship is sometimes healthy and supportive, but I need to do more to strengthen it.

Maintainer _____ I currently have a close, healthy relationship, and I want to maintain it.

ealthy relationships are those based on love, trust, kindness, good communication, acceptance, and intimacy. With this in mind, think about the types of relationships you have with other people. Most of us are involved in many different kinds—relationships with parents, siblings, friends, boyfriend, girlfriend, or spouse. In staging yourself, first think of a type of relationship that is important to you. Then think about that relationship in terms of the definition of a _healthy_ relationship. Choose the statement above that you think best describes your relationship in this category. You may want to circle the relationship for which you are staging yourself:

Relationship:

friend family member spouse boyfriend/girlfriend

other _____ .

Many people feel that a high quality of life and true happiness are perhaps most easily achieved when the physical aspects of wellness (healthy body weight, proper nutrition, and fitness) are combined with the intangible benefits found in participating in healthy relationships. However, many people with disabilities or other chronic conditions adapt wellness guidelines to their own situations and maintain mutually supportive relationships. They, too, live happy, healthy, and productive lives.

An individual can possess an appropriate level of fitness, maintain proper nutrition and body weight, and demonstrate other physical attributes of wellness and still be at a considerable disadvantage without the powerful emotional, mental, and social benefits that come from healthy relationships. These benefits are not easily measured and do not receive as much attention as do other aspects of wellness, but they are just as important and are vital to achieving wellness. People who fail to maintain healthy relationships often suffer from social isolation, depression, loneliness, and low self-esteem. All human beings have the need for intimacy, the need to be loved, and the need to give love, but all too often we neglect or fail to succeed in forming enduring, joyful relationships.[1]

Healthy relationships are not exclusive to the union formed between couples, but also include the attachments formed in short- and long-term friendships. Healthy relationships exist when there is close, personal communication between individuals. This closeness involves emotional, spiritual, or physical intimacy—sometimes all three.

Too often we associate intimacy with physical intimacy or sexuality, even though physical intimacy is only one type of intimacy found in healthy relationships. A true **intimate relationship** is one that has a high degree of closeness in the form of a friendship, relationship, or association. For example, it is possible for two people to have an intimate intellectual association if they share and discuss personal and deep intellectual ideas. Healthy social interactions are built on a foundation of love, trust, kindness, respect, communication, and many other forms of intimacy.

Human sexuality can mold and bind relationships in such a way that individuals can experience mature feelings of love, kindness, selflessness, and complete trust. On the other hand, improper use of physical intimacy can completely destroy a relationship by introducing distrust, heartache, and, in some cases, physical disease. We will discuss human sexuality in detail in Chapter 13. The purpose of this chapter is to encourage individuals to enhance the quality of life and achieve optimal health and wellness by developing healthy relationships.

FROM SELFISHNESS TO WELLNESS: THREE STAGES OF SOCIAL MATURITY

Despite cultural, ethnic, and demographic differences, almost everyone in a healthy relationship has passed through three common phases of social maturity: selfishness, learned tolerance, and selflessness. At birth, newborns are completely helpless and dependent; they rely upon others to do everything for them. As infants develop, they learn to get what they want by crying, and later, they find that pointing and yelling become effective methods of communicating needs. Most of a child's early years are filled with getting what he or she wants and needs. The ability to think about other people's wants and needs is a learned characteristic that requires many years to acquire. **Selfishness** and being self-centered characterize the first phase of social maturation. (See Figure 12.1.)

As babies grow out of infancy and into childhood, they learn tolerance; they may not consider others' opinions or feelings and they may still be selfish, but they learn that they cannot always have what they want. This second stage, **learned tolerance,** is often demonstrated by adolescents. Many teenagers learn to accept the rules and guidelines that have been placed on them even though they may not understand the reasons for the rules. They tolerate the situation, although they may not like it, and they accept that they are not going to get everything they want.

The transition from selfishness to learned tolerance is typically long, difficult, and painful. In most cases, it takes years to change. Some people never mature beyond the selfishness stage. These individuals find it hard to be happy because their happiness depends on getting what they want. These individuals often have difficulty sustaining relationships because they lack the ability to show true, caring, selfless compassion. It is impossible to have a healthy relationship when one or both individuals are selfish.

The third and final stage of social maturity is described by the word **selflessness.** One of the defining characteristics of healthy relationships is the ability to put someone else first. This does not mean that a person must give in to every need and want of the companion; it merely suggests that healthy relationships are "give and take" in nature rather than "take and take." When individuals learn and practice the value of selflessness and compassion, they have reached the highest level of social maturity and are able to experience true happiness, love, empathy, and joy. This level of maturity allows an individual to form and maintain healthy relationships; as those relationships prosper, one's quality of life and physical and mental well-being may increase.

THE LINK BETWEEN HEALTHY RELATIONSHIPS AND WELLNESS

A comprehensive review of the research on health and quality relationships reveals that social support is a key factor in protecting health. For example, sharing life experiences and having someone to depend on may be one of the most powerful ways to manage stress.[2,3] People who have rich resources of family and friends tend to have a buffer against stress-related illness and premature death.

Some researchers have coined the term **safety net** to describe the effect that a network of close personal relationships can have on supporting a person who is suffering from life's major stresses. When life gets more diffi-

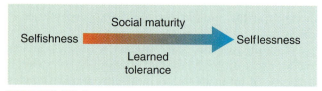

FIGURE 12.1 The continuum of social maturity. As individuals learn to be accepting and loving, they gradually become selfless.

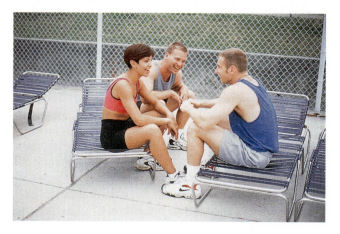

Social relationships provide individuals with a sense of strength and support that can serve as a buffer against illness.

cult because of a significant negative life event, the safety net is there to provide unfailing support and comfort. This support provides the person with faith and hope, which has the physical effect of maintaining a person's level of immunity.[4] Thus, people without a safety net may be more prone to a variety of diseases. Given the large body of research supporting the health benefits of social support, it is clear that caring relationships are an important ingredient for wellness.

TYPES OF HEALTHY RELATIONSHIPS

Healthy relationships take a variety of forms: close friendships, dating, marriage, family, or even an association with a pet. Casual friends play a role in our social wellness and quality of life, but they do not supply the same level of commitment and loyalty that is found in long-term relationships.

Close Friendships

Family relationships sustain individuals during the early stages of life, but as they grow older children spend more time with friends and less time with family. Most long-term friendships are formed during adolescence. Most people feel fortunate if they have one or two very close friends throughout their lifetime. Long-term friends can be a source of happiness, they can be a shoulder to lean on in times of sorrow and disappointment, and they can be trusted. True friendships provide value and a sense of self-worth to both parties. In the best and worst of times, friends are understanding because their love is unconditional. Best of all, true friends are always there when they are needed and are willing to accept personal faults and weaknesses without being critical or judgmental. It is not easy to make lasting friendships because like any long-term relationship, they require an investment of trust, acceptance, support, and intimacy.

Men and women develop and maintain friendships in slightly different ways. Women who are friends value the closeness and intimacy that comes from talking and listening to each other. Communication between women is emotionally expressive and supportive. They tend to talk about large issues and simple day-to-day events, and each friend gives and receives validation, support, and love. The time spent together, the sharing of emotions, joys, and concerns, all help to further develop a close emotional attachment. Women want to share their personal selves with someone who understands and relates to them, and they want to understand the personal lives of others. Such sharing of deep insights requires communication that is expressive and tactile. This is one reason why women communicate with both verbal and nonverbal feedback such as a warm hug or holding a hand.

Strong friendships are also formed by doing things together. In fact, the act of doing something may be the reason why some friendships even exist. Male friends are more prone to skip the talking and go do something together. Activities such as watching and participating in sports, working on weekend projects, and fixing things are examples of how some friendships among men are sustained without the intimate personal communications seen in typical friendships among women. Even during difficult times, male friends are more likely simply to pat each other on the back or shoulder rather than hug. By doing things together, all friends can gradually learn about each others' personal lives, strengths, and weaknesses. Even joking around about a problem is common among good friends because there is an unspoken code of acceptance that lets everyone know that they are trusted.

Underlying all strong friendships is a foundation of absolute trust and support. Confidence in others to be dependable and follow through with promises and commitments is an essential requirement of close friendships. When you know that a friend will keep private information private, that good friendship becomes a real asset. Trustworthy friends provide us with valuable opportunities to talk about private problems and concerns without worry that outsiders are learning information that could be personally damaging. Trust puts meaning to the words, "I care about you." The support that comes from trustworthy friends sustains us during difficult times and provides us with a valuable resource when a need arises.

To develop trust in a friend it is necessary to take on a little risk. Early in a friendship, trust is tested when personal or intimate bits of information are shared. As confidentiality is maintained, trust increases, and the risk of exposing personal information decreases. Gradually, complete trust is developed and each individual's level of commitment to the relationship grows.

The following are some simple suggestions for nurturing a good friendship:

- Be appreciative of the things your friends do for you and express this to them.
- Be willing to share your most personal thoughts and ideas. By confiding in a friend, you show him or her the level of your trust.
- Be willing to share material things. True friends are part of your "family" and often are closer than related family members.
- Accept your friend's mistakes and shortcomings. Everyone is going to mess up sometime, so don't let this ruin your friendship. Accept your friend for who he or she is and don't let faults ruin a good thing.
- Spend time together. Friendships can only develop when substantial time and energy are committed to the relationship.

Dating

Dating is any social occasion shared by two individuals. These might be lovers, friends, or total strangers, and the

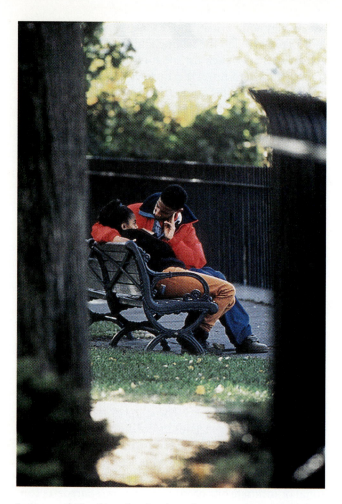

Intimate relationships often involve at least some degree of physical or social attraction.

How to Say No to Sex

Intimate relationships require communication, commitment, love, kindness, and selflessness. Sex, too, is important, but it should not be the only basis for a relationship. Here are some ways to say no to sex:

1. If saying no to sex ends a relationship, then so be it; it wasn't a very good relationship to begin with.
2. If you believe sex is proper only in marriage, be true to your beliefs. Tell your partner how you feel and let him or her know early on, so that you can avoid awkward situations.
3. Be aware of your sexual signals. Frequent touching, sexual advances, and suggestive comments may be sending signals to your partner that you are inviting sex. You may not even be aware of the messages you send. Don't invite what you don't want.
4. Determine early on a date not to put yourself in situations where it will be difficult to say no. Avoid settings like late-night dates when you are alone, sleeping together, or excessive alcohol consumption. In these settings, personal inhibitions often are quickly forgotten and desire is easily aroused.
5. True love requires communication and respect. If you are being pressured to have sex, tell your partner to stop. A partner who says, "You'd do it if you love me," can be told, "If you love me, you'll stop."
6. Date as a group. You are not as likely to be pressured to have sex when there are others nearby.

event might be a dance, sporting event, dinner, or walk in the park. Variations of dating include group dating, single dating, steady dating, and blind dating. Dating is a time to meet new friends, lovers, and potential mates; it is often one of the more difficult times in life because interacting with others can be confusing, awkward, stimulating, challenging, depressing, rewarding, and terrifying.

Dating can be an emotional roller coaster. One day you can flip over someone and the next day you can be devastated. When a relationship runs into problems or is unhealthy, it can leave emotional scars that take years to heal. One study found that problems in dating relationships were the most frequent complaints voiced by undergraduates using a college counseling center.[5] When having trouble dating, the best place to turn is to friends, family, or counselors in whom you can trust and confide and from whom you can get valuable advice.

Physical attraction is often the main reason why young people date. Sexual attraction is the primary reason a couple comes together in a dating situation. Physical attraction initially draws people together, but after the first infatuation fades, a reevaluation of the relationship needs to take place. If the relationship is based largely on physical attraction, it will likely fail. Commit-

ted, healthy relationships take time to develop and cannot be based solely on sex. If you find that you really care about the other person and not just about his or her body, you are developing a strong relationship, and sex will be an important aspect of that relationship. Dating is a time to learn to communicate, listen, trust, love, and have fun. Successful dating can contribute to a high quality of life and happiness. When dating, a couple should strive to learn more about each other. They should share interests, feelings, and opinions and strive to develop all of the characteristics found in successful long-term friendships. Because dating often leads to the more committed institutions of marriage and families, it should be used as a barometer of married life. If a couple has frequent problems while dating, it is highly unlikely that the relationship will be any different after marriage.

Marriage

As couples become more committed to each other, their relationship often turns from one based on **infatuation** (initial physical attraction) to a relationship founded on principles of trust, sharing, and commitment. The institution of marriage is a natural, traditional course of action for many committed couples as their level of commitment increases.

In all cultures, there are specific advantages and disadvantages to being married. The vast majority of Americans (90 percent) will marry sometime in their lives.[6] From a practical standpoint, married couples can share resources by pooling their personal belongings and finances and thus are often better off financially. Substantial legal protection supports marriage, including making health and life insurance available for spouses and in some cases providing retirement incomes for spouses who are widowed. Taxation, employee benefits, and even automobile insurance all favor married individuals. Married couples enjoy a high level of social acceptance and within the bonds of a faithful marriage, it is impossible to become infected with a sexually transmitted disease, assuming that both partners were disease free at the time of the marriage. Children especially benefit from having two parents who provide role models, support, and unconditional love.

Good marriages help people live happy and healthy lives. Studies have found that married men and women live longer than those who are unmarried. Married men are also less prone to alcoholism, accidents, and illness. Divorced, widowed, and single people are more likely to die of heart disease and to have weaker immune systems.[7] Differences in health between married and unmarried individuals may be partly due to the fact that, statistically, single individuals tend to drink more alcohol, smoke more, exercise less, and have poorer diets than married people. Marriage can also provide lifelong emotional support above and beyond the support provided by close friends.[8]

Happily married couples seem to demonstrate several qualities of good health. In general they experience less illness and disease and recover more quickly when they do become ill. In one study, men who married added almost ten years to their life span.[9] Interestingly, couples who are unhappily married do not experience any added health benefits and actually die earlier.

From a health and wellness perspective, living in a poor marriage may be worse than being divorced.[10] Unhappy marriages typically involve conflict, contention, poor communication, and stress. The body reacts to conflict with changes in the immune system, elevated blood pressure, hormone changes, and the general stress responses we have discussed in Chapter 11. These changes, plus the emotional effects of hostility, distrust, and blame, combine to increase the risk of illness. Hurtful words, demeaning remarks, and selfishness can damage self-esteem and accelerate a downward health trend. It appears that marriage in and of itself does not translate into physical and emotional health, but rather the quality of the relationship determines whether or not a couple will experience improved length and quality of life.

A couple may want to think twice about taking the important step into marriage if the following conditions exist in the relationship.

- You are constantly arguing or quarreling.
- You are pregnant and feel pressured to marry.
- Your partner wants you to change the way you are: dress differently, change jobs, or stop doing something that you feel enhances your life.
- You think about your partner and say to yourself, "After we're married she (or he) will change or the problem will go away." Be willing to tolerate flaws, but don't expect the other person to change after marriage.
- If friends and family have serious misgivings about your relationship, at least listen to their concerns. Good friends and close relatives may be able to give you an unbiased appraisal of your relationship.
- You are both still young (under age twenty).

Recognizing Unrealistic Expectations

All too often, couples struggle because partners fail to meet each other's expectations. It is not realistic to think that a partner will always look attractive, act perfectly, or be willing to agree with every opinion. Successful relations require a give-and-take arrangement in which one partner doesn't expect perfection from the other. Happiness requires the willingness to live with and accept personal flaws and weaknesses.

Arguing

Living in a close relationship with a partner reveals the full range of emotions, opinions, and problems that beset all of us. The differences of opinion and arguments common to almost all committed couples can actually be good for a marriage because each person learns to listen and understand another's point of view. Long-term studies of married adults reveal that couples who learn to fight fairly and effectively have a 50 percent lower divorce rate. Fighting fairly or arguing in a nondestructive manner reduces the likelihood of physical violence, teaches children how to handle disagreement as adults, and helps couples stay together longer.[11]

Managing Money

One of the main stumbling blocks of marriage is money. The amount of money a couple has is not as important as how it is spent. Who decides how much money is spent? Who determines the wants and needs of the family? Who pays the bills? Each of these questions must be resolved within the relationship. A spouse who stays home to tend children or maintain the home is a working spouse. This person may not get paid at the end of the month, but he or she may work harder than the

Working on relationships takes more time than I have to give.

Building strong relationships does require you to invest time and energy. Instead of trying to have many friends, try to focus the time you do have on a few people whose company you especially enjoy. Look at your schedule, and save some time for visiting and doing things with these friends. Review the list on how to be a good friend on page 279.

I can't seem to find someone I want to date.

Think about how you currently meet people, for example, in classes, at parties, or at bars. Are there other places you could go or other activities you could participate in to meet a new group of people who share your interests? Perhaps you could join a club on campus, participate in intramural sports, join a volunteer organization, or attend a church near campus. New outlets mean opportunities to meet new people.

The relationship I'm thinking of is too far gone to bother repairing it now.

Refer back to Table 12.1 to assess how you and your friend, relative, or partner resolve disagreements. Share the suggestions for nondestructive approaches with the other person and ask that you both agree to work on improving the way you handle disagreement. If your relationship is in trouble because of problems managing money or differences in goals, you may want to see a professional counselor for help. Remember that being able to work through problems will make your relationship stronger.

that make parenting especially difficult. For example, most single-parent families experience greater financial difficulties than do traditional families. Being a single parent is perhaps one of the most challenging and difficult tasks a person can face. Because of the added financial burdens of supporting a family on only one income, many single parents are forced to work long hours or at low wages. Many divorced or single parents never anticipated being the only provider for a family. At the end of a long work day, single parents must return home and take on the role of homemaker, tending to children, cleaning the home, and trying to spend time together. The burden carried by single parents is heavy, which may be one reason why 80 percent of previously divorced single parents remarry.

Family Violence

Contrary to popular belief, family violence is not an occasional incident that occurs in a select group of broken homes. It occurs increasingly across all segments of society: rich and poor, Caucasian, Asian, and African American, and in rural communities and urban communities. **Family violence** includes spouse-battering, sexual abuse and marital rape, and child abuse and neglect. It also encompasses violence between brothers and sisters, violence against elderly relatives, and all forms of psychological abuse. Regardless of who commits the violent act, the goal is to demonstrate power dominance.

When a violent event occurs, it is typically preceded by a cycle of events and circumstances that are often predictable and repeated. The first stage of the cycle includes a period of time when the individuals avoid each other in an effort to avoid provoking each other. This is followed by a time when grievances are not expressed, but are

internalized and begin to accumulate. As grievances accrue, emotions take over and eventually erupt into violence. After the parties involved are physically and emotionally removed from each other for a while, a spirit of conciliation and remorse often brings the conflict to a temporary truce. In many families this cycle is ongoing and is often accepted as a normal part of the relationship. The remorse and conciliation on the part of the abusing partner tend to lessen the impact of the violence on the battered or abused partner and provide a false sense of hope for the future of the relationship. This is why so many abused women leave their husbands temporarily—for example, to stay in a battered women's center—but then decide to return to the abusive relationship.

If you know someone who is in a violent relationship, help by encouraging him or her to see a counselor, seek out a battered women's center, or call the local police.

ENDING RELATIONSHIPS AND FACING DIVORCE

It would be ideal if all relationships were healthy, but in reality, not all relationships are and some may even be detrimental to wellness and physical health. Making a relationship last requires high levels of commitment and hard work by both parties throughout the life of the relationship. It has been said that if a couple considers separation as an alternative, they will most likely separate. Just the consideration of ending a relationship is a sign that the relationship may be in trouble.

Breakdowns in relationships begin when couples fail to communicate effectively with each other. Often, communication breakdowns are very subtle and go unnoticed until emotional confrontation brings them to attention. Either partner may stop listening or cease to be emotionally present. Feelings of being unwanted, ignored, or unappreciated are damaging to individual self-esteem and cause individuals to want to seek validation elsewhere. Unresolved conflicts can escalate and generate problems in a couple's sexual relationship, which can lead to even deeper emotional trauma. Couples who previously spent much time together may find that they have grown apart and spend more time with others or by themselves. Unless balanced with regular communication and joint activities, dramatic changes in the amount of time a couple spends together may signal problems in the relationship.

Any relationship that involves physical, sexual, or emotional abuse signals a need for the abused partner to seek professional counseling. Abuse of any kind is demeaning, hurtful, immoral, and punishable by law, and should never be tolerated in a relationship. The cycle of abuse must be broken or it will likely be passed on to the children and other future generations. Counseling can often help, but if the abuser is unwilling to make changes, it is best to end the relationship.

Terminating a dating relationship or a marriage is a very painful and difficult experience. When families are broken up by divorce, children may experience emotional scars that may never heal. Couples who go through divorce often require years to recover fully from the emotional trauma of being overwhelmed with feelings of despair, disappointment, loneliness, and anger. The decision to divorce is often a difficult one to make, yet there are times when it is the correct thing to do.

Each year at least one million marriages will end in divorce.[16] Reasons for divorce may include unmet expectations, unacceptable differences in sexual behavior, career failure, or financial difficulties. Divorce is only one of many possible solutions to the problems that beset many marriages. There are numerous professional, religious, and social organizations that can assist couples in successfully overcoming marital difficulties. Marriage counselors have experience in solving marital problems, and their advice may be helpful in resolving conflicts and strengthening the bonds of marriage.

The difficulties found in marriage are indeed challenging, but the rewards are high. The joy and happiness found in living in a relationship in which both partners are faithful, honest, and caring can instill the feelings of belonging and love that are the basis of social and spiritual wellness.

LIVING SINGLE

Despite the advantages of marriage, many individuals choose not to marry. The number of single adults has been increasing over the past few decades. Currently, just over 37 percent of the U.S. population is single at any given time. This group includes young men and women who have yet to marry, divorced adults who may or may not have children, widows and widowers, homosexual partners who cannot legally marry, and other adults who simply choose to be single rather than marry.[17] There are several reasons for the increase in the number of single adults, with the most obvious being the high level of divorce. In addition, Americans are getting married later, and thus are among the ranks of "adult singles" for a longer period of time than in the past. In general, women live longer than men, which accounts for a large number of elderly single women.[18] Surveys of single adults show that most singles would prefer to be married, but have not yet had the right opportunity.[19]

Intimate, healthy relationships can be maintained by single adults. Singles still date, enjoy active social lives, and have close friendships with both sexes. Close friendships can provide social and emotional support for single as well as married adults. Many single adults are also parents who devote much of their lives to raising and caring for children.[20] Recent reports from the Department of Health and Human Services indicate that more than 30 percent of all children are born to single mothers. Many of these women will keep their babies and raise them alone, at least for a while.

LONELINESS

Nearly everyone will be single at some point in his or her adult life. Single life can be a great deal of fun for some and a time of independence, but it can be difficult for those who do not like being alone. Whether married or single, true **loneliness** occurs when current social relationships fall short of ideal, or when the social network surrounding a person becomes deficient in quality or quantity. Loneliness directly affects a person's self-esteem and sense of self-worth, and when self-esteem is lowered, depression, anxiety, or physical illness can set in

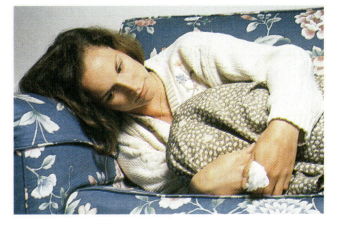

Loneliness can be common among people unable to maintain close relationships or pursue social interests. For some, it is easy to lose perspective and fall into periods of depression.

———— I will ask someone out for a date this week.

———— I will spend more time with my best friends doing things they want to do.

———— I will help someone this week.

———— This week I will attend a social gathering (club, dance, party, church) where I might meet new friends.

———— Today I will make a list of my acquaintances and decide which ones I would like to be closer to.

———— I will show my partner I love him or her by doing an act of kindness or compassion.

———— I will spend one hour each day with someone in my family.

———— Other ————————————————————————

3. Based on what you answered in item 1, list five steps you can take to develop or improve this relationship.

4. What first step are you ready to take toward your goal?

5. Complete the following statement:

I'm going to take my first step on ————————————.
date within 30 days

Action Taker*

1. What are the benefits of your close relationship?

2. Below is a list of areas in which different types of relationships need strengthening. Write down those that apply to you.

———— Our expectations of the relationship are not being met.

———— We fight too much.

———— We have different goals in life.

———— We disagree about how to spend and handle money.

———— We don't apologize and take responsibility for our mistakes.

———— We are not satisfied with our sexual relationship.

———— We don't seem to have many common interests.

———— We don't communicate very well.

———— We have difficulty deciding who is responsible for things that have to be done.

———— We don't spend much time together.

———— The relationship struggles because one or both parties is being selfish.

———— We aren't willing to accept each other's shortcomings.

———— Other reasons ————————————————————

3. Based on your comments above, list four steps you can take to help strengthen your relationship. Here are some examples:

Read and follow the steps found in Table 12.1.

Talk and listen to each other's concerns.

4. It's always easy to point fingers and assign blame, but it's good to consider your own behavior first. Read through the questions below to help you determine what you could work on.

———— Do you promise to do things and then forget?

———— Do you try to "top" stories told by others?

———— Do you exclude others from your group of friends?

———— Do you tell friends what is wrong with them?

———— Must you always be the center of attention?

———— Do you ask others to do trivial tasks for you?

———— Do you drop in unannounced and then stay?

———— Do you tell secrets?

———— Are you rarely in a good mood?

———— Do you rarely comment on the good in others?*

If you checked any of these statements above you can see where you might need to improve. Look at them often to remind yourself how you need to

---

*List adapted from M. M. Klein. You can learn the fine art of friendship. *USA Today*, May 28, 1983, p. 4D. Copyright 1983, *USA Today*. Reprinted with permission. As cited in Brian Williams and Sharon Knight. *Healthy for Life*. Pacific Grove, CA: Brooks/ Cole, 1985, p. 8.4.

change. Then have your friend or partner do the same.

Maintainer

1. Maintainers enjoy many of the benefits of healthy relationships. List five benefits you are experiencing from your relationship.

2. Which of these benefits is the most important to you?

3. In your own words, state why your relationship is important to you.

4. Does your spouse, friend, or partner know why this relationship is important to you? If not, tell him or her what you stated above. You'll make his or her day.

5. What can you do now to liven up a healthy relationship that might need a boost in the future?

6. Healthy relationships require full confidence and trust between individuals. Long-term success requires continued efforts to maintain the relationship. Following is a list of things you can do to keep your relationship healthy and avoid relapse.

In the next week, which of these would you be willing to do?

_____ Be spontaneous in some way. For example, surprise a friend with tickets to an event, give flowers to your partner or friend, or ask your spouse for a date.

_____ Tell your friend or spouse that you love him or her.

_____ Set individual and family goals with your spouse.

_____ Go out on a regular date, without children or other people.

_____ Meet your friend for an afternoon treat at the local café.

_____ Make a list of all of your friend or partner's qualities that you really like and appreciate.

_____ Tell your friend or partner that you recognize and appreciate these qualities.

_____ Other ideas _____

_____

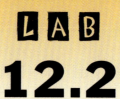

L A B

12.2

How Healthy Is Your Relationship?

Read each question. Determine how frequently you could answer yes for each one and write down the appropriate number in the space provided.

0—never, 1—rarely, 2—sometimes,
3—often, 4—almost always, 5—always

If a particular question does not apply, just skip it and go on to the next one. Complete it first by yourself, then suggest that you and your partner answer the questions together.

Feelings of Warmth

_____ **1.** Do you feel a warm glow when you see or think about your partner?

_____ **2.** Do you have tender feelings when you're together?

_____ **3.** Do you miss your partner when you're apart?

Expressions of Affection

_____ **1.** Do you use terms of endearment with your partner?

_____ **2.** Do you express affections in your normal tone of voice?

_____ **3.** Do you show affection through physical contact—touching, holding hands, and so on?

Caring

_____ **1.** Are you concerned about your partner's welfare, pleasure, or pain?

_____ **2.** Do you try to show your partner that you care?

_____ **3.** Do you avoid saying or doing things that will hurt your partner?

Acceptance and Tolerance

_____ **1.** Do you accept differences of opinion, tastes, and style?

_____ **2.** Do you accept your partner in totality, as someone with weak points as well as strong points?

_____ **3.** Do you avoid being judgmental or punishing your partner for his or her mistakes?

Empathy and Sensitivity

_____ **1.** When your partner is feeling down, do you find you can share some of that feeling?

_____ **2.** Are you able to sense that your partner is feeling bad without being told?

_____ **3.** Are you able to determine and respect your partner's sensitive areas?

Understanding

_____ **1.** Do you find that you can understand why your partner may be upset?

_____ **2.** Can you see things through your partner's eyes even though you might disagree?

_____ **3.** Can you tell what your partner is upset about when he or she complains?

Companionship

_____ **1.** Do you enjoy doing exciting things with your partner?

_____ **2.** Do you like your partner's company when doing routine things?

_____ **3.** Do you enjoy just having your partner around when you're not doing anything in particular?

Intimacy

_____ **1.** Do you share your private thoughts and wishes?

_____ **2.** Do you feel free to tell your partner things that you wouldn't tell anybody else?

_____ **3.** Do you like your partner to confide in you?

Friendliness

_____ **1.** Do you feel an interest in your partner as a person?

_____ **2.** Do you like to know what your partner is thinking or how he or she is doing?

_____ **3.** Do you like to solicit your partner's opinions about your problems?

Pleasing

_____ **1.** Do you try to think of things the two of you can do that will make your partner happy?

_____ **2.** Do you try to make yourself more attractive for your partner?

_____ **3.** Do you say or do things that please your partner?

Support

_____ **1.** Do you try to bolster your partner when he or she is discouraged?

_____ **2.** Do you help out when your partner is feeling overwhelmed?

_____ **3.** Do you encourage your partner when he or she wants to engage in a new venture?

Closeness

_____ **1.** Do you feel emotionally close to your partner?

_____ **2.** Do you have a feeling of closeness to your partner even when you're apart?

_____ **3.** Do you enjoy being physically close to your partner?

This survey can be helpful in identifying the ways in which you and your partner show each other affection and caring. Although there are no absolute scores for rating your relationship, the questionnaire can be useful as a guide for evaluating the present status of your relationship and determining possible areas of improvement. Questions marked with 0, 1, or 2 may indicate areas that need attention. Talking about your responses may provide new insights into your relationship.

Preventing Sexually Transmitted Diseases

Objectives

1. Explain what sexually transmitted diseases (STDs) are and what causes them.

2. Recognize the signs and symptoms of the most common STDs and know when to seek medical attention.

3. Identify risky sexual behavior and its potential consequences.

4. Assess personal risk of disease using demographic and personal choice factors.

5. Identify the steps you can take to diminish or eliminate your risk of contracting (or passing on) a sexually transmitted disease.

6. Recognize the role that relationship skills, especially communication skills, play in STD management and safe sex.

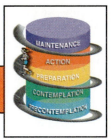

Precontemplator _____ I never, or almost never, use a condom when having vaginal or anal sex, and in the next six months I do *not* intend to start always using one.

Contemplator _____ I never, or almost never use a condom when having vaginal or anal sex, but I intend to start in the next six months to always use one.

Preparer _____ I never, almost never, or sometimes use a condom when having vaginal or anal sex, but I intend to start in the next 30 days to always use one.

Action Taker _____ I always use a condom when having vaginal or anal sex, and I have been doing this for less than six months.

Maintainer _____ I always use a condom when having vaginal or anal sex, and I have been doing this for more than six months.

In this chapter safer sex is defined as all the actions needed to help prevent the transmission of STDs or an unwanted pregnancy. We use the term "safer sex," rather than "safe sex," because no precautions are 100 percent foolproof. Abstinence is the only sure way to prevent sexual transmission of a disease and pregnancy.

Use of a latex condom will provide for safer sex. In some cases, partners must take additional steps to protect against STDs. For example, a condom may not sufficiently protect someone from contracting herpes from a partner with open sores. Specific prevention needs are discussed with each of the STDs within the chapter. Al-

ways being as safe as possible is the goal. The problem with STDs is that a single unprotected sex act can result in disease; therefore, it is important that you aim for full protection each and every time you have sex.

The set of behavior-staging questions above assumes sexual activity and refers only to the use of a latex condom to provide safer sex. If you have been practicing abstinence for less than six months consider yourself an action taker, for more than six months consider yourself a maintainer. If you wish to work on a different safer sex behavior (for example, communication, abstinence, or not sharing needles) substitute your desired behavior for condom use and stage yourself accordingly.

Let's assume a flood has occurred and the health authorities who have not had time to test the water warn you that your tap water may not be safe to drink. If you are really thirsty will you drink it anyway? Hand a glass to a close friend or lover? Give the water to a baby? Suppose the authorities haven't said anything, but you have heard that it is dangerous to drink tap water following a flood. Will you call and ask the authorities? Will you have the water tested before drinking it? Or imagine that your friend finds out the water isn't safe and doesn't tell you. How will you feel toward your friend if you do get sick or someone you care about gets sick? Will you be angry at your friend even if you don't become ill?

Parents, some school programs, and the media have warned the public that unprotected sex can be hazardous to health, and can cause serious illness or even death—yet millions of people continue to have unprotected intercourse and contract sexually transmitted diseases. Substituting sex for the water in the preceding example, how would you answer the questions? Would you check first to make sure sex is safe? Would you take the risk of putting an unborn child at risk? Would you be less cautious about sex than you would be about drinking water? And if so, why? The "why?" makes a big difference, because the "why?" leads a person either toward or away from participating in safer sexual activity.

How we perceive our life roles affects our sexual behavior. At one end of the spectrum are people who view sex as a sacred part of marriage and a means of procreation. At the other end are people who are comfortable with multiple partners and casual sexual activity. Examine your sexual activities in light of your values and beliefs. How much of an influence have your parents or friends had on shaping your views of appropriate sexual behavior? How do gender issues influence your sexual behavior? If you are sexually active and considering behavior change, think about not only your sexual lifestyle and sexual behaviors, but also those of the person(s) with whom you are intimate. STDs are preventable; you can lower or eliminate your risk through personal actions.

When people are trying to make a decision about a behavior, they weigh the pros and cons, and if the behavior will result in more perceived benefits than drawbacks, they usually choose it. Notice the word, *perceived*. Perceptions shape our actions, making it extremely important that our perceptions are well founded. When perceptions are distorted or based on faulty information, it is easy to make mistakes. For example, a common myth or perception held by teenagers is that "you can't get pregnant the first time." One youth went as far as to say that you can't get a girl pregnant early in the morning because the sperm are asleep at that time! People who believe that they are invincible to disease are more apt to select riskier sexual actions.

People who are afraid to talk about STDs and protection are also more apt to take unnecessary risks. Others may refuse to believe that such a "nice" person as their partner could possibly have a disease. It is also possible that some people see life as so hopeless that they do not care if they contract a disease and may even purposely put themselves and others at risk. Many people under the influence of drugs and alcohol take risks that they would not otherwise take.

Perhaps most startling is that some people who have been educated about the risks of sexual activity and disease and agree they should be careful, still don't take any precautions. Even more frightening are people who are willing to put others at risk rather than communicate with and protect them. Individuals have the right to put their life, their ability to have children, and their physical comfort on the line, but do they have the right to make that decision for someone else? Already the legal system is grappling with the problem of whether a person is guilty of murder for intentionally infecting a person with HIV. Sadly, most of the people who become infected are the infected person's friends, spouses, lovers, and newborn children. STDs, like drugs, seem most often to hurt those we love.

Taking care of someone may mean abstaining from, postponing, or talking about sex, using a condom, or getting a medical test. If you have a disease and choose to be sexually active, it is critical that you be honest with your partner and protect him or her from contracting it.

If you think you may have infected someone, respect your partner's right to know and encourage him or her to get tested right away. Early treatments can minimize the spread of some diseases and cure others. If you aren't comfortable talking about sex, STDs, and protection with a partner, then you aren't fully ready for sex. When you really care about someone, your desire to see him or her happy, safe, and protected is as natural and strong as your desire to be intimate.

This chapter is not about whether you should abstain from or engage in sexual activity. Rather, it is about behaviors that increase or decrease the risk of contracting a sexually transmitted disease. **Abstinence** (no sexual activity) or a disease-free **monogamous relationship** (sex with one partner) eliminates the risk of contracting an STD through sexual activity. Unfortunately, even this does not completely eliminate risk of an STD since a few of them can be contracted through nonsexual means. For example, HIV infection can be the result of needle sharing or blood-to-blood contact at the scene of an accident. And although a yeast infection can be passed back and forth between sexual partners, it can also be caused nonsexually by things that upset the vaginal environment, such as a course of antibiotics or a hormonal shift. Therefore, eliminating all STD risk from your life may involve changes in both sexual and nonsexual behaviors.

Overviews of the major diseases are included, but the focus is on changing risky sexual behavior to safer behavior. Although sexual risk has traditionally been discussed in an "all or none" manner—safe sex or unsafe sex, period—any behavior change that results in less risk is worthwhile. Smoking fewer cigarettes reduces your risk of lung cancer. Walking around the block reduces your risk of cardiorespiratory disease. And any step of precaution reduces your risk of getting or transmitting a sexually transmitted disease. Whenever you decrease your risk, you increase your odds of staying healthy. If you were about to have an operation, would you rather hear that you had a 75 percent chance of survival or a 50 percent chance? Even one small step toward safer sex is significant. Successful behavior change is often accomplished through a series of small steps. However, always remember that anything less than safe sex is unnecessarily risky.

WHAT ARE STDs?

Sexually transmitted diseases (STDs) are diseases that are passed from one person to the next through sexual contact. As of 1989 STDs had infected an estimated 12 million people in the United States, 86 percent of whom were between the ages of 15 and 29.[1] More than fifty organisms and syndromes are recognized as being involved in sexually transmitted diseases.[2] Most are caused by bacteria or viruses. **Bacteria** are microscopic organisms that can live inside the human body. Some bacteria are health-promoting, whereas others act as pathogens (disease-causing agents). STDs caused by bacteria can usually be treated and cured, especially when treatment is started early. Syphilis and gonorrhea are examples of bacterial STDs. **Viruses** are submicroscopic organisms made up of complex proteins that can grow and multiply inside living cells and cause infectious diseases. While treatable, viral STDs are not curable, and therefore can recur or progress. Viral STDs include HIV, herpes simplex, hepatitis B, and human papillomavirus (HPV). These are often called the "4 Hs." Viral STDs can be transmitted through both sexual and nonsexual means. For example, HIV and hepatitis B can be transmitted through needle sharing. They are called sexually transmitted diseases because they can be transmitted through sexual contact although not exclusively. Fungal and parasitic agents can also be transmitted sexually.

After being infected with an STD, people may remain **asymptomatic** (free of symptoms) for extended periods ranging from days to several months. During this period, however, people can transmit the infection to others. Symptoms related to bacterial or viral STDs often dissipate and recur. Because of long periods in which an infection may not produce symptoms, public health officials and other medical experts recommend that people at risk for STDs regularly seek an **STD risk assessment,** including a physical examination and laboratory tests to detect infections that may be asymptomatic. When symptoms do occur, they typically include one or more of the following: burning or pain during urination or defecation, itching or burning around the genitals, mucus discharge or bleeding from the genitals, ulceration or blistering, rashes on the body, and flu-like symptoms. STD infections can also lead to a variety of other illnesses, including pelvic inflammatory disease (PID), cancer, and death.

The rest of this chapter is designed to help you (1) recognize your own risk both by demographics and by personal choice, (2) identify what risky behaviors are, (3) provide information on STDs, and (4) identify some steps you can take to diminish your risk of disease.

HONEST COMMUNICATION ABOUT STDs

Trust is one of the essential ingredients of a mature, intimate relationship. You can relax when you are with someone you trust because you know that you are safe, that that person will look out for you, just as you will look out for him or her. The question is, when can you trust someone? In order to protect yourself from STDs, you either have to take precautions "just in case" or determine whether or not your partner has a communicable disease. Unless you can verify beyond any doubt that your partner is disease free, the risks are high, especially now that AIDS is at an epidemic level. The fact that many STDs do not manifest symptoms makes it even more difficult. Your partner may not even be aware that he or she has an infection. Here are several steps you can take toward establishing a trusting and caring sexual relationship.

1. Talk to one another even if it feels awkward or uncomfortable at first. Discuss your sexual history and any concerns you might have. If one of you has an infection, telling the other person allows you

both to come to terms with it and decide on a plan. Trust your partner to be understanding and to appreciate your honesty.

2. Have a medical checkup before initiating a sexual relationship. "I'll show you mine, if you show me yours," now refers to medical health histories!

3. Look for outward signs of disease—such as genital warts or sores—on yourself and on your partner. Sex in the dark leaves you in the dark. If you see anything suspicious, consult a doctor before having sex.

4. Finally, remember you are the one making the decision about your own health. If you have any reservations, it may be best to postpone sex until you are more comfortable.

The better the communication and the longer the monogamous relationship, the better your chances are for avoiding an STD. Trust is rarely a part of casual sex or of sex initiated under the influence of drugs or alcohol.

Some individuals may fear losing a partner or losing a partner's trust by raising the issue of disease. These decisions are compounded when the partner is helping support the family and a breakup of the relationship would put the other partner and any children in financial difficulty. In these situations consideration must also be given to the importance of being a healthy parent. Children are being orphaned by the AIDS epidemic. If you fear losing a partner's trust or support by raising the issue of sexually transmitted disease, talk with a counselor who can help you weigh the benefits and risks.

As awareness of the risk for contracting HIV and other STDs grows, more people recognize the importance of regular medical checkups and honest communication with partners. By approaching the subject in an "up front" manner, much of the awkwardness and tension can be avoided. It is difficult to ask for this information; it is much easier when someone volunteers it. If you are sexually active, or considering it, help your partner by starting the conversation.

DEMOGRAPHICS, PERSONAL CHOICE, AND RISK

Demography is the statistical study of the human population. Sexual orientation, gender, and socioeconomic class are the demographic factors most often associated with STDs. Much demographic risk can be eliminated through personal choices. For example, a person living in a town in which 90 percent of the people are infected has very high demographic risk, but that same individual can drop personal risk to zero by choosing to be abstinent. Demographic information is valuable for studying a disease and for knowing where to target educational materials.

Unprotected sexually active heterosexual women and homosexual men are at an increased risk (demographi-

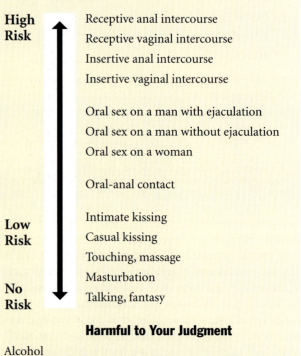

The Spectrum of Risk

Cognitive Corner

Sexual behaviors have different levels of risk for different STDs. *Using condoms lowers the risk of transmitting STDs by anal, oral, or vaginal intercourse.*

The following chart depicts risk assuming no protection is used for these behaviors.

High Risk
Receptive anal intercourse
Receptive vaginal intercourse
Insertive anal intercourse
Insertive vaginal intercourse

Oral sex on a man with ejaculation
Oral sex on a man without ejaculation
Oral sex on a woman

Oral-anal contact

Low Risk
Intimate kissing
Casual kissing
Touching, massage
Masturbation
No Risk
Talking, fantasy

Harmful to Your Judgment

Alcohol
Amphetamines (speed, crystal meth, Ecstasy)
Amyl Nitrite (poppers)
Marijuana
Cocaine, Crack
LSD

cally speaking) because they are sexually receptive, meaning that when the male partner introduces infection, it is deposited inside his partner's body. This increases the disease's chance of survival. Women are also at greater risk than men because they tend to be less symptomatic, providing the disease a longer period of growth without treatment. The structure of a woman's reproductive organs also makes her more susceptible; disease can easily travel up the uterus and into the fallopian tubes and ultimately into the pelvic cavity. Hormonal changes due to menstruation may also provide the disease with a desirable environment for growth. Finally, women are considered higher risk because they can become pregnant and pass the disease to the fetus *in utero* or during childbirth. Homosexual women have the least risk of contracting an STD since neither partner is sexually receptive. This does not mean that they are totally risk free as they can still pass some sexually transmitted diseases through oral-genital contact or other mutual contact of internal body fluids.

Individuals' sexual behavior and the characteristics of their social group interact to increase or diminish risk. A promiscuous person having sex exclusively with disease-free individuals will remain healthy, while a person in a monogamous relationship practicing unsafe sex with an infected person is likely to become infected. Urban areas are often statistically cited as high risk. However, risk is high anyplace that there is a pocket of disease. For example, a rural town may have a low overall incidence, but there can be a group of infected individuals who are at high risk as they pass the diseases back and forth within the group. Similarly, there can be pockets of very little disease in areas of high incidence. Urban areas, it is believed, have overall high incidence because of dense populations and high numbers of socioeconomically disadvantaged individuals. Again, it is important to note that being poor does not mean a person will become infected; it means that there are more infected people who are poor. In the past, many studies in the United States pointed to race as a risk factor; it may be, however, that STD infections are less race dependent and more class dependent. Studies from other countries (where race is more uniform in their populations) have noted socioeconomic class as the significant risk factor, meaning more cases of disease have been found in socioeconomically depressed populations. It is hypothesized that individuals living in despairing situations, not sure whether they will survive conditions of violence, crime, and hunger, are less concerned with contracting disease. It may also be that this population is the least educated about the risk and prevention of STDs.

Sexuality is a lifelong dynamic process. It encompasses gender roles, gender orientation, our relationship with ourselves and with others, feelings, dreams and fantasies, attitudes, values and beliefs, sexual behaviors, and reproductive decisions. There is a sense of an ebb and flow of importance in these issues as you progress through life. Sexual behavior change is related to all of these things and must be thought of in the context of your life.

STDs

Some of the most common STDs are discussed in this section. Prevention material that can be applied to all of the diseases is presented in the next section. When there are specific additional prevention tips for a particular STD, they are included with the disease. Otherwise the "prevention" category will not be listed individually. The key to prevention is stopping transmission. For this reason, pay special attention to how each of the following diseases is transmitted.

HIV and AIDS

Names: HIV infection, acquired immune deficiency syndrome

Cause: The human immunodeficiency virus (**HIV**). HIV can damage the immune system, the body's defensive system made up of a variety of blood cells that work together to defend the body against infection and disease. HIV can damage and destroy a number of different cells, making it difficult for the immune system to recognize and defend against infection. One of the cells most closely watched by clinicians is the T-cell. The number of T-cells in your body is an indication of the health of your immune system. Doctors use blood tests to monitor the number of T-cells of HIV positive individuals. As the AIDS virus kills T-cells, the immune system is weakened. This allows "opportunistic" infections like PCP (pneumocystis carinii pneumonia), tuberculosis, or a skin cancer known as Kaposi's sarcoma to enter the body and take hold. A healthy immune system can usually fight these diseases off, but in someone weakened by HIV, they are often fatal.

Cases: Over one million cumulative cases of AIDS have been identified or are suspected in more than 165 countries, and it was estimated as of 1993 that more than ten million people worldwide were infected with HIV.[3]

Transmission: HIV can be transmitted whenever the internal fluids of one individual come in contact with the internal fluids of someone carrying the virus. (See Figure 13.1.) HIV is found in blood, semen, vaginal fluids, and breast milk. During unprotected sex, HIV can enter the body through tiny breaks in the tissue lining the vagina, anus, penis, rectum, and mouth. HIV can also enter the body through cuts or sores in the skin. Sharing

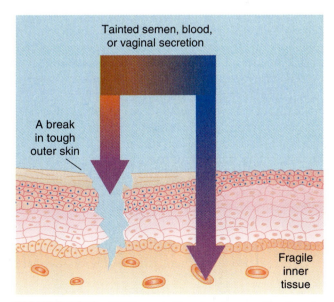

FIGURE 13.1 HIV is carried in tainted semen, blood, vaginal secretions, and breast milk. HIV can enter the body through the fragile tissue of the vagina, penis, anus, and mouth.

needles or equipment ("works") with an infected individual can also result in transmission. Tiny amounts of blood remain in the needle and are then injected directly into the next person's bloodstream. This includes needles used for tattooing, body piercing, and injecting vitamins, as well as those used for shooting drugs including anabolic steroids.

An HIV positive woman has a one in four chance of passing the virus on to her child before or during birth. She can also pass it on while breast-feeding. A woman who has HIV and is pregnant can receive medical treatments with AZT during pregnancy and labor, which may reduce the risk of infecting the baby to about one in twelve. If a woman is thinking of getting pregnant and has at any time (even years ago) engaged in a behavior that may have brought her in contact with HIV, she should seek counseling and testing so that she can make an informed decision about becoming pregnant.

AIDS was first discovered in the United States in 1978. Risky behaviors in the United States prior to this date may have resulted in transmission of other STDs but probably not HIV.

In 1985 stringent tests for donated blood were established. In the United States, all blood is thoroughly screened and the risk of receiving HIV through a blood transfusion is now very small. In the case of elective surgery, however, you may want to consider donating some of your own blood well ahead of time. This will also limit your risk of receiving other bloodborne diseases. Sex with someone who received transfusions prior to 1985 may put you at risk. You will not get AIDS from giving blood because hospitals and blood banks use sterile equipment and discard it immediately.

Small amounts of HIV have been detected in saliva, but not enough to cause infection. Casual or social kissing is considered safe. Since 1986 the Centers for Disease Control and Prevention has recommended couples not kiss deeply if one of them has the AIDS virus, mostly because of the risk of infection from bleeding gums or open sores in the mouth. The CDC has reported one case of infection through kissing (1997) and emphasizes that both partners had gum disease, which allowed the virus to be passed through the blood, not the saliva.

There are a lot of misconceptions about how HIV can be transmitted. HIV is a fragile virus that cannot live long outside the body. This means you can't get it by shaking hands, hugging, or touching things an infected person has touched. Nor is it airborne or foodborne, so you can't "catch" it like a cold or flu from coughs or sneezes or from eating something. Here are some more ways you *won't* become infected:[4]

- You won't get HIV through everyday contact with infected people at school, work, home, or anywhere else.

- You won't get HIV from clothes, drinking fountains, phones, or toilet seats. It isn't passed on by things like forks, cups, or other objects that someone who is infected with the virus has used.

Activity 13.2
Am I at Risk for HIV?

There is evidence that HIV, the virus that causes AIDS, has been in the United States at least since 1978. If you have engaged in any of the following behaviors since that time, you may be at increased risk for infection. If you answer yes to any of the following, speak with a trained counselor about getting HIV tested. Early detection is important.

_____ I have had unprotected sex with a partner who has had sex with other partners.

_____ I have shared needles or syringes to inject drugs or steroids or had unprotected sex with someone who has.

_____ I have had blood transfusions between 1978 (the date AIDS was discovered) and March 1985 (the date blood screening for HIV began) or had unprotected sex with someone who has.

_____ I have had unprotected sex with a prostitute or multiple partners.

_____ I have had unprotected sex with someone whose medical and sexual history I do not know.

_____ I have had or have a sexually transmitted disease (STD).

Am I taking precautions to prevent HIV infection?
A yes answer indicates prevention, a no answer means you are engaging in risky behavior—something you may wish to change.

_____ I abstain from sexual activity or have a monogamous relationship with a disease-free individual.

_____ When having vaginal or anal sex, my partner and I always use a latex condom. (This assumes that there is a risk of infection from one or both partners and that pregnancy is not a goal.)

_____ When (if) giving oral sex I always use a moisture barrier such as a condom, a dental dam, a cut-open and flattened condom, or household plastic wrap.

_____ I never re-use injection needles or syringes or frequent a place (such as a disreputable tattoo parlor) that might.

- You won't get HIV from eating food prepared by an infected person.

- You won't get HIV from a mosquito bite. HIV does not live in a mosquito, and it is not transmitted through a mosquito's bite like other germs, such as the ones that cause malaria. You won't get it from bedbugs, lice, flies, or other insects, either.

- You won't get HIV from contact with sweat, saliva, or tears.
- You won't get HIV from a simple kiss.

Symptoms: HIV may remain dormant for years, in which case individuals may feel very healthy, may show no symptoms, and may not even realize that they are HIV positive. During this time, however, a person can infect others. When the virus becomes active, symptoms begin to develop, often slowly at first and gradually worsening. At first a person may develop swollen lymph glands, or experience fever, night sweats, skin rashes, diarrhea, sores, weight loss, and tiredness. (This stage is sometimes called **AIDS-related complex or ARC.**) In full-blown AIDS the person's immune system is very weak, allowing other opportunistic infections to spread uninhibited.

Diagnosis: Three to six months following infection, the body will have produced sufficient HIV antibodies to be detected by a blood test. The antibodies, which are not capable of eradicating HIV, may be the only sign of infection. T-cell counts are also monitored to follow the course of the disease and its effect on the immune system.

Treatment: There are no successful cures or vaccines for AIDS at this time. There are, however, a number of antiretroviral therapies available to help manage HIV. The Food and Drug Administration (FDA) has approved eleven drugs through an accelerated approval process. This has made these drugs available more quickly, but at the same time long-term effectiveness and safety of these drugs is as yet unknown. Drug therapies require strict adherence and close management. They are also costly, as much as $10,000 a year. In many cases antiretroviral therapies have succeeded in slowing down the virus and helping AIDS patients live longer. There is also evidence that some drugs slow down the progression to illness in asymptomatic people. This means that people who are HIV infected but not showing symptoms may be able to follow a treatment plan and stay healthier longer, a very good reason for getting tested early.

Hepatitis B

Name: hep B

Cause: The hepatitis B virus.

Cases: Although an effective genetically engineered vaccine for **hepatitis B** was introduced in 1986, the number of new cases has remained the same. (Not everyone receives the vaccination.) The proportion of hepatitis B cases attributed to sexual contact between men has declined in recent years, while the proportion attributed to heterosexual contact and injection drug use has increased.

Transmission: It is estimated that up to half of all hepatitis B infections are sexually transmitted. Multiple sex partners and high-risk sex practices, especially receptive anal intercourse, place both gay men and heterosexual women at increased risk for hepatitis B transmission. Hepatitis B may also be transmitted to a fetus during pregnancy or to a child at birth, and from one person to another by using contaminated injection materials.

Symptoms: Because this disease affects the liver, the skin and whites of eyes may turn yellow (a condition called jaundice). Other symptoms include fever, nausea, and abdominal pain. People infected with hepatitis B may develop cirrhosis, carcinomas, and chronic active hepatitis. This disease can, in a small percentage of people, become chronic and, for some, be fatal.

Diagnosis: Hepatitis B is diagnosed using a blood test.

Treatment: The best "treatment" for hepatitis B is prevention in the form of a vaccine. Alcohol should be avoided as this aggravates the condition. Although there are no curative treatments at this time, hepatitis B will usually resolve itself spontaneously, but the damage it causes may be permanent. Health workers, teachers, and people who travel to less developed countries are all encouraged to get vaccinated.

Gonorrhea

Names: The clap, the drip, a dose

Cause: A bacterium called *Neisseria gonorrhoea,* usually found in white blood cells.

Cases: **Gonorrhea** is one of the most commonly reported diseases in the United States, with approximately 700,000 cases reported each year to the CDC.[5]

Transmission: Gonorrhea is transmitted through direct contact of mucus membranes during vaginal, anal, or oral sexual contact. Babies can be infected during birth. It is possible to contract gonorrhea repeatedly; having been infected does not ensure immunity against future exposures. Condoms will block transmission from the vagina or penis, but the disease can still be spread from the mouth or anus.

Women are particularly susceptible to this disease. It is believed that 90 percent of women will become infected after a single episode of vaginal intercourse with an infected partner. Men have a 33 percent chance of contracting the disease during a single act of vaginal intercourse with an infected partner.[6]

Symptoms: Up to 80 percent of infected women will not have symptoms and between 10 and 30 percent of infected men will have either minor or no symptoms.[7] When symptoms do appear, they do so from two to ten days after exposure. Both men and women may experience pain and/or burning during urination, and a yellowish white or yellowish green discharge. Women may mistake this discharge for a normal ovulation discharge. Gonorrhea can affect the rectum, throat, tonsils, and eyes, the urethra in men and the reproductive organs in women.

In women it most commonly affects the genital tract, specifically the cervix, and is the most common cause (approximately 30 to 60 percent) of **pelvic inflammatory disease**. Fifteen percent of women with gonorrheal infections of the cervix will develop PID.[8] These women may experience lower abdominal pain, cramping, abnormal vaginal bleeding, and fever. Scar tissue in the fallopian tubes can also affect fertility.

Pelvic inflammatory disease (PID) occurs when infectious bacteria escape into the pelvic cavity. More than one type of bacteria may be involved, and because the bacteria have access to all the reproductive organs, the infection can cause extensive damage.

Consider these facts about PID:

- There are about 1 million cases of PID per year in the United States, of which about 150,000 result in surgical procedures.[9]

- One out of four women with PID has serious complications including infertility, ectopic pregnancy, or chronic pelvic pain.[10]

- Infected women are six times more likely to have an ectopic pregnancy and four times more likely to develop chronic pelvic pain.[11] Ectopic pregnancies occur outside the fallopian tube (in the pelvic cavity)—a life-threatening condition.

- Twenty percent of women with a single episode of severe PID may become infertile due to tubal damage.[12] Tubal infertility becomes even more likely with repeat episodes of PID because of the increased likelihood of fallopian tube scarring.

- PID most often occurs in women who have gonorrheal or chlamydial infections. Together, these infections are responsible for 30 to 60 percent of PID infections.

- Younger women are at more risk, partly because as a group they tend to use less protection, but also because they are more prone to gonorrhea and chlamydia. An adolescent woman has a one in eight chance of PID, as compared to a one in eighty chance for a woman over age 25.[13]

- Douching frequently can increase a woman's risk of developing PID three- to fourfold as compared to women who douche only once a month.

- IUDs may increase the risk of PID.

There are some things that *reduce* the risk of PID. Oral contraceptives decrease the risk of PID 70 percent and barrier methods (like a condom) decrease risk by 60 percent. Delaying sexual intercourse (beyond the adolescent years), protecting against and being screened for vaginal infections, and having fewer sex partners will all decrease risk.

Symptoms of PID may include fever, fatigue, severe lower abdominal pain, lower abdominal tenderness, enlargement of the fallopian tubes, and vaginal discharge. PID is treated with multiple antibiotics, and in severe cases, hospitalization and IV antibiotics may be required. Medical costs of managing PID and its complications are estimated to be between 3.5 and 5 billion dollars.[14,15]

In men, gonorrhea most commonly infects the urethra. Men may notice swollen lymph glands in the groin along with penile discharge. Damage to the penis can make urination difficult and erection impossible. The epididymis (part of the scrotum) may become infected and scar tissue may block the flow of semen from the testicle.

Babies' eyes can be infected when they come in contact with the bacteria in the birth canal during birth. This infection can lead to blindness if not treated with antimicrobial eyedrops. Men and women can also get eye infections from contact with infected secretions carried by the hand to the eyes.

If gonorrhea spreads to the bloodstream of either gender, it can cause gonococcal arthritis of the joints, damage heart valves, and affect the spinal cord or the brain.

Diagnosis: A lab technique called the gram-stain using fluid from the penile discharge is highly accurate in diagnosing gonorrhea in men. Women are encouraged to have a culture of the cervical discharge done to determine infection. In both cases, fluids are obtained by a simple swab technique.

Treatment: Gonorrhea is treated through oral antibiotics, such as penicillin. Abstinence should be maintained

STDs—Race and Ethnicity

When we examine STD statistics by race/ethnicity, we continue to see very wide discrepancies among racial/ethnic groups. For example, gonorrhea rates among black adolescents (15–19 years of age) are more than twenty-six times greater than the rate among white adolescents. The rate of P&S syphilis among blacks is nearly sixty times that in whites; P&S syphilis among Hispanics is about four times that in whites. Congenital syphilis has decreased nationally in recent years. However, in 1995, of the 1,534 reported cases with known race/ethnicity of the mother, blacks and Hispanics accounted for 91 percent of all reported cases, while accounting for only 21 percent of the female population. Although there are no known biologic reasons to explain why racial or ethnic factors alone should alter STD risk, race and ethnicity in the United States serve as risk markers that correlate with other more fundamental determinants of health status such as socioeconomic status, access to quality health care, and health-care-seeking behavior. Reporting biases may also play a role in race differentials.

Division of STD Prevention. *Sexually transmitted disease surveillance, 1995.* U.S. Department of Health and Human Services, Public Health Service. Atlanta: Centers for Disease Control and Prevention, September 1996.

until the clinician confirms the cure. Notification and treatment of partners is essential to stopping the spread of gonorrhea, whether they have symptoms or not.

Although penicillin historically has been the most widely used treatment to cure gonorrhea, strains resistant to penicillin have developed in recent years. Therefore, suspected gonorrhea cases are now treated with other medicines, even though these are often many times more expensive than penicillin.

Syphilis

Names: syph, pox, bad blood, blues, the imitator

Cause: A bacterium called *Treponema pallidum.*

Cases: The number of cases of **syphilis** in the United States averaged about 70,000 a year until 1988, when a 33 percent increase occurred, mostly among heterosexuals.[16] This increase was believed to be due to an increase in sex for drugs, especially in crack houses. Although much of the increase was among heterosexuals, this disease has also been a problem among homosexuals. With this increase the incidence of syphilis shot over 100,000, hitting its high in 1990 at 135,000. Since then, the number of reported cases has steadily declined. By 1995, the number of cases reported to the Centers for Disease Control[17] for all stages of syphilis was down to 68,953. Of these, only 16,500 were cases of primary and secondary (P&S) syphilis, the fewest cases reported since 1960.[18] Cases of congenital syphilis have likewise declined.

Although the U.S. syphilis rate is at its lowest level in many years, this disease remains an important problem in certain geographical areas, particularly among African Americans. In addition, syphilis, a genital ulcerative disease, facilitates the transmission of HIV infection, and may be particularly important in contributing to HIV transmission in those parts of the country, such as the South, where rates of both infections are high. Untreated early syphilis during pregnancy results in perinatal death in up to 40 percent of cases, and, if acquired in the previous four years, may lead to infection of the fetus in over 70 percent of cases. For syphilis, as for other STDs, differential reporting of cases from public and private sectors may magnify the differences in reported rates by race/ethnicity.[19]

Transmission: Syphilis can be transmitted from one person to another through direct contact with the sores of someone who is infected, or through contact with mucus membranes during kissing, vaginal or anal intercourse, or oral-genital contact. Bodily fluid contact between persons through a break or opening in the skin or mucus membrane can also result in infection. An infected mother can pass the disease to her fetus through the placenta. It is possible to contract syphilis repeatedly.

Symptoms: Syphilis passes through four stages if it is not treated and cured. The stages are as follows:

Primary stage: Ten to ninety days (average of twenty-one days) after exposure, a small painless open sore, or chancre, develops at the entry site of the infection. The chancre can be as small as the top of a pin or as large as a dime. It can appear anywhere intimate contact occurs: on the genitals, in the mouth, vagina, cervix, or rectum, on the fingertips, lips, tongue, or breast, but usually on the shaft of the penis or around the vaginal opening. Depending on where the chancre is located, it may not be noticed at all. The chancre disappears without treatment after about three to six weeks. This does not mean the infection is cured.

Secondary stage: Two to twelve weeks after the appearance of the chancre, a nonitchy pinkish to brown rash may cover the whole body or appear in a few places like the face, hands, or feet, or around the genitals. Symptoms at this time may include a low-grade fever, headache, malaise, swollen lymph nodes, white patches on the mucus membranes of the mouth and throat, patches of hair loss, and open sores around the genitals and mouth. Clear fluid from these sores is full of bacteria and may be easily passed to another person by any physical contact—sexual or nonsexual. At this stage the infected individual is highly contagious. Lesions tend to heal with or without treatment in several weeks or months, but may recur for as many as two to three years after the initial infection.

Latent stage: (This stage is not always listed separately. Sometimes it is considered part of the tertiary stage.) The infecting bacteria continue to multiply but the individual appears to be healthy. The individual is usually not contagious during this time, except when a mother passes the disease through pregnancy or in the event that open moist sores reappear. This stage may last for one to forty years.

Tertiary stage: People with untreated latent syphilis risk progression to tertiary disease. In this stage the syphilis infection that has continued to multiply attacks the brain, heart, and other organs, and can be fatal. Any part of the body is susceptible to attack. Victims may experience facial tremors, slurred speech, impaired vision or headaches, deafness, convulsions, heart disease, paralysis, memory loss, depression, insanity, and death. This stage may appear in as little as two or three years or as long as forty years after the initial infection.

Diagnosis: During the first stage, the disease is identified by examining tissue from the chancre under a microscope. In the second stage a blood test looking for antibodies is used for diagnosis. The blood test may miss syphilis in the first six weeks since it takes that long for antibodies to develop.

Treatment: Antibiotics (usually penicillin) provide an effective treatment. Sexual abstinence is required until a clinician confirms the cure; otherwise, partners may pass the disease back and forth.

Chlamydia

Names: The silent STD (male nongonococcal urethritis)

Cause: A bacterium called *Chlamydia trachomatis*.

Cases: **Chlamydia** is the most widespread bacterial STD in the United States today, infecting three to five million people each year.[20] It has reached epidemic proportions, and is thought to infect about 20 percent of all college students.[21] Approximately 30,000 newborns born to infected mothers are also affected each year.[22] Chlamydia frequently occurs along with gonorrheal infections. In STD clinics in Washington, D.C., and Baltimore, 20 percent of men with infections of the urethra from gonorrhea also had chlamydial infection, and 40 percent of women treated for gonorrhea also had chlamydial infections of the cervix.[23] Chlamydia may also cause PID (see page 300) in as many as half a million women.[24]

Transmission: Chlamydia is transmitted through direct contact of mucus membranes during vaginal and anal sexual activity. Whether chlamydia can be transmitted orally is as yet unclear. It may be accidentally transmitted from the genitals to the eyes by the fingers. Mothers can transmit chlamydia to their babies during childbirth. Chlamydia can be contracted repeatedly; prior infection does not ensure immunity against future exposures.

Symptoms: Chlamydia is known as the silent STD because its early symptoms are so mild. In fact, up to 50 percent of women and 25 percent of men do not experience any early symptoms.[25] This is one of the things that makes this disease so dangerous. If chlamydia is not diagnosed, severe damage to the reproductive organs can quietly occur. When symptoms do occur in women they include vaginal discharge (most common), spotting between periods, abdominal pain, sometimes with fever and nausea, burning on urination, and painful inflammation of the fallopian tubes. Ultimately the disease can affect the cervix, uterus, fallopian tubes, ovaries, urethra, Bartholin's glands, eyes, mouth, and rectum. It can lead to PID, premature birth, ectopic pregnancy, and sterility. Together, chlamydia and gonorrhea cause sterility in 150,000 women each year.[26]

Symptoms in men include burning on urination, testicular pain, and a watery, white penile discharge. This discharge may only occur in the morning and can disappear spontaneously. Disappearance of the symptoms does not mean that the infection is gone. Chlamydia is the leading cause of urinary tract infection in men and is also responsible for half of the 500,000 cases of epididymitis (inflammation of the testicles) that are seen annually in the United States.[27] Ten to 30 percent of men with this condition may become permanently sterile.[28] Chlamydia can affect the urethra, testicles, rectum, mouth, or eyes. Rectal chlamydia in both men and women is most commonly caused by anal intercourse and is characterized by itching, watery discharge from the rectum, cramping, and diarrhea. Eye infections result from contact with infected secretions usually transmitted by the fingers and hands.

Four to 10 percent of all pregnant women have chlamydia, and unless they receive treatment, more than half of their babies will be born with eye infections, and 10 percent of their babies will develop a potentially fatal form of pneumonia. Ear infections may also occur.

Diagnosis: Chlamydia is very similar to gonorrhea, and one disease can be mistaken for the other. After ruling out gonorrhea, doctors can diagnose chlamydia using several tests, including microscopically examining a culture of tissue taken from the infected area. Since chlamydia mimics gonorrhea's symptoms and the diseases often occur together, physicians will frequently treat for both when one is found. Accurate and affordable diagnostic tests have only recently become widely available. Public health efforts to screen for chlamydia to diagnose asymptomatic cases have proven effective.

Treatment: When diagnosed, infections can be cured by taking tetracycline or other antibiotics. Notification and treatment of partners is essential to stopping the spread of chlamydia, whether the partners have symptoms or not. Both partners must be treated and cured before resuming intercourse; otherwise, one partner will reinfect the other.

Herpes

Names: Herpes I, type 1 (HSV-1): cold sores, cankers, fever blisters
Herpes II, type 2 (HSV-2): genital herpes

Cause: **Herpes** is caused by two forms of the herpes simplex virus (HSV). HSV-1 tends to stay above the waist, causing minor health problems like cold sores. HSV-1 infections may occur on the mouth, lips, or skin, and may be spread to the genitals. HSV-2 tends to occur below the waist and is usually known as genital herpes. HSV-2 may cause infections of the genitals or the anus. It can also infect the mouth, spread by the hands or by oral-genital contact.

Cases: Some experts argue that the number of herpes-infected individuals is difficult to estimate since many are symptom free. As many as one in four people may be carriers of the virus. Each year about half a million new cases of genital herpes are reported in the United States.[29] Women are four times more likely to get the disease from men than men are to get it from women.[30]

Transmission: Genital herpes is usually contracted through sexual contact with someone who has an outbreak of genital sores. It is less common, but transmission can also occur when the carrier does not have sores or other symptoms. When lesions are present, the infected person should abstain from sex because of the increased risk of infecting a partner.

Symptoms: Herpes is an ulcerative disease that causes painful blisters on the genitals, mouth, anus, and other mucus membranes, and sometimes on the skin of other areas of the body. Over a period of days the blisters crust over and heal without leaving scars. Other symptoms include a burning sensation when urinating, vaginal discharge, pain in the legs or genitals, fever, swollen lymph nodes, malaise, and abdominal pressure. If herpes is spread to the eyes, a serious infection can occur.

Men and women infected with the herpes virus are often asymptomatic for long periods. Women can have a longer asymptomatic period and a more severe initial manifestation of disease than men, and women can transmit the virus during pregnancy and childbirth. Infected babies may develop blindness or brain damage, or even die. Delivery by Caesarean section may prevent infection if a mother has genital herpes.

Herpes symptoms may appear as soon as two days or as late as thirty days after initial exposure. There is no cure for herpes, but the virus may remain dormant for long periods of time. The virus travels up the sensory nerve and settles in the ganglia near the spinal cord. For unknown reasons (although emotional triggers may be responsible in some cases) the virus will periodically travel back down the nerve and start multiplying near the skin again. These recurrent episodes are common, but the number of recurrences and time between episodes vary dramatically between individuals. Generally the outbreaks are less severe over time. Some people will feel a tingling sensation just before a reoccurrence. Some reoccurrences are asymptomatic, meaning a person can be infectious without being aware of it.

Diagnosis: A diagnosis is usually made through visual examination of the sores (lesions).

Treatment: The drug Acyclover helps heal the sores and alleviate pain, but it is not a cure. It may also help reduce the number and severity of occurrences.

Human Papillomavirus (HPV)

Names: HPV, genital warts. Also rectal, cervical, or venereal warts, and condyloma acuminatum.

Cause: Over sixty different forms of the **human papillomavirus,** 15 percent of which cause genital warts.

Cases: Currently about 40 million people in the United States are infected with the virus and one million new cases of genital warts are reported each year.[31] Some types of HPV cause genital infection, and a small number produce benign genital warts, which are nonulcerated and frequently recur. Only a small percentage of HPV cases have visible warts.

Certain types of HPV are linked to precancerous lesions or cancer of the cervix, vulva, penis, anus, and throat. A person with warts will not necessarily get cancer, but the warts do increase the risk; therefore, regular checkups are recommended. Warts are generally removed so that they can't turn into precancerous tissue. It is also very possible to have HPV, not have visible warts, and be unaware of an infection.

Warts may appear on the tip or shaft of the penis or around the anus in men, or around the vulva, in the vagina, on the cervix, or around the anus in women. The warts are often cauliflower-like in their appearance and do not go away on their own. They may also appear in the mouth or throat of either sex.

Transmission: The highly contagious HPV enters the skin through microscopic tears and abrasions that occur during sexual activity. In women the cervix is the most common site of infection since it has a very thin skin layer. HPV DNA has been found in semen, but whether this is a means of transmission remains unclear. About two-thirds of people who have sexual contact with an infected person will go on to develop this common STD.[32] HPV can be transmitted to the larynx of babies during childbirth. It is possible to contract HPV repeatedly; having the virus once does not ensure immunity against future exposures.

Symptoms: Genital warts can be larger than a dime or so small that they can only be seen with magnification. They can be white, flesh colored, brownish, or pink, and they can look like miniature cauliflowers or be completely flat. Genital warts are sometimes associated with itching or local soreness, but most often produce no symptoms. The tongue or larynx is involved in rare cases in both sexes. The incubation period varies widely; it can range from three weeks to many months, or even years.

Without treatment, warts may spontaneously clear up, stay the same, or multiply and spread, increasing the chances of infecting others or becoming cancerous. Warmth, moisture, pregnancy, and vaginal infections encourage rapid growth and spreading. Twenty percent of women with warts have vaginal infections, which makes the virus harder to treat.

Diagnosis: In addition to visual identification of warts, diagnosis includes a Pap smear to detect HPV infection and precancerous tissue. The new Virapap test screens for five types of HPV that have been linked to cancer risk. A colposcopy, a procedure that uses a small lighted magnifying scope to view the woman's internal organs, may also be performed to detect flat cervical warts.

Treatment: Although there is no cure for HPV, treatment can help manage genital warts. After successful treatment the virus usually becomes latent or dormant. But since recurrences are possible throughout a person's lifetime, it is recommended that individuals with a history of HPV see a physician regularly.

The exact treatment depends on the location of the warts. External warts can be treated with an acidic solution applied by a physician directly to the infected area. Freezing (cryotherapy) individual warts with liquid nitrogen can be used for both external and cervical warts. For persistent external genital warts and cervical warts, more potent treatments such as electrocautery and laser therapy may be used. Electrocautery, the burning off of warts under local anesthesia, has largely been replaced by laser therapy, which involves vaporizing warts with a laser beam. Vaginal and rectal warts can be treated by inserting a strong chemical in a cream base (often 5 percent Fouracil Cream) at bedtime for several nights. This causes the vaginal or anal lining to slough off, destroying the infected skin. All of these treatments help manage warts and prevent cancerous lesions from developing; they do not eradicate the HPV infection.

Trichomoniasis

Name: trich (pronounced "trick")

Cause: A parasite called *trichomonas vaginalis,* which is a protozoan that thrives in warm, moist places.

Cases: Trichomoniasis is one of the most common protozoan infections in the United States, with an estimated three million annual cases.[33]

Transmission: Although this STD is occasionally transmitted nonsexually (through wet towels, bathing suits, and so forth), the primary mode of infection is sexual. It is highly contagious and it is possible to contract trichomoniasis repeatedly; having been infected once does not ensure immunity against future exposures. Men and women are equally vulnerable to this parasite and asymptomatic men represent a common pathway for reinfection of women.

Symptoms: Both men and women with the disease may be asymptomatic for extended periods. When symptomatic, women experience mild to severe vaginitis, including intense itching, burning, vaginal or vulvular redness, a heavy frothy white, yellow, or green-grey foul-smelling vaginal discharge, frequent and/or painful urination, discomfort during intercourse, and abdominal pain. Men are usually asymptomatic, but when symptoms do occur they consist of a pus-like or watery penile drip, and pain upon urination. Men may also experience painful swelling of the penis and/or epididymitis.

Diagnosis: A diagnosis is determined through microscopic examination of vaginal and penile secretions.

Treatment: The oral antibiotic metronidazole (common brand name Flagyl) is 90 percent effective in curing the disease. Failure is most often attributed to a lack of testing and treatment of one partner (usually the man). The untreated partner, if infected, will reinfect the healthy partner. Sexual activity should be suspended until the infection has been eliminated. Vinegar and water douches may help alleviate symptoms.

Candidiasis

Names: yeast infection, vaginitis (type of), candida

Cause: An overgrowth of fungus that is normally present in the vagina as well as on the skin and in the mouth and digestive tract.

Cases: Vulvovaginal **candidiasis** is one of the most common infections of the female genital tract. About 75 percent of women at some time in their lives experience the discomfort of a vaginal yeast infection.[34] Most of these cases are easily treated but a small percentage of people develop chronic or recurrent episodes.

Transmission: Yeast infections can occur without any sexual contact or may be passed to a partner through oral or genital intercourse. An infection occurs when there is an overgrowth of the naturally occurring fungus. This can be the result of additional fungus being introduced through sexual contact. Other precipitating factors can be pregnancy, use of oral contraceptives, diabetes mellitus, systemic diseases requiring the use of antibiotics or corticosteroids, or HIV infection, but usually the infection occurs without any of these underlying medical problems. Reinfection may be caused by sexual contact with an infected partner, introduction through the gastrointestinal tract, or an infection that during treatment becomes temporarily suppressed and later reemerges. Nursing women can develop a monilial infection of the breast as a secondary complication of vaginal candidiasis or from a fungal infection in the infant (thrush or a candidal diaper rash).

Symptoms: Women may experience intense itching, and/or a thick cottage-cheesy discharge smelling of yeast. Symptoms often worsen just before menstruation. Men may experience burning or itching during urination. Oral contact can result in a throat infection called thrush. Infants can also get a thrush infection.

Diagnosis: Microscopic examination of vaginal and penile discharges as well as a visual examination of the vagina looking for white patches on the walls or on the vulva. A throat culture is taken to diagnose thrush.

Treatment: A variety of treatments may be used to treat candidiasis, the most common of which are vaginal creams and suppositories. These may be over-the-counter products or prescribed medicines. Symptoms usually abate in a few days, but treatment should be continued until all of the prescribed or over-the-counter medication is used. This helps prevent recurrence.

Plain yogurt with live lactobacillus cultures can be inserted into the vagina or smoothed onto irritated areas. Relief may also be obtained by taking saltwater baths and/or douching with a mild vinegar and water douche every day for one to two weeks beginning at the onset of symptoms. If infection persists or reoccurs frequently see a physician.

Prevention: Use condoms and latex squares (a barrier for oral sex) or remain abstinent when the infection is

BARRIER Busters

Using a condom or other protection method kills the romance.

- Familiarity with condoms and other protection and birth control devices will enhance your willingness to use them. The same is true for your partner. Practice with your choice of protection before you need to use it.
- Protection is more romantic than itching, blisters, oozing lesions, and the risk of a fatal disease. Being infected and putting someone else at risk dampens romance even further.
- Consider safer sex an expression of concern and love.
- Practice increases the speed and efficiency with which a condom can be put on—this makes it less of an intrusion.
- Be creative and make using protection "fun" or "sexy." Help each other with whatever form you choose.

Asking a partner about STDs and safer sex can interfere with relationship trust by questioning a partner's honesty or forthrightness.

- Minimize this problem by offering information about yourself first. Then your partner may feel freer to disclose information to you.
- Discuss issues of safer sex and disease prevention prior to intimate moments. This minimizes emotional reactions.
- Agree to exchange mutual medical information.
- If a relationship cannot bear this type of discussion, con-

sider whether you would be better off out of the relationship.
- Involve a professional counselor who can mediate the discussion.

I don't always know when I'm going to have sex.

- Carry protection with you and keep a supply available at home.
- Be wary of casual sex with a partner of unknown history. Consider not having sex under these circumstances.
- Consider abstinence or a monogamous relationship.
- Say no to sex if you aren't prepared.

Condom use is inconvenient.

- It is far more inconvenient to have an STD and have to take precautions to prevent from spreading it to someone you care about.
- Keep supplies in a convenient location(s) and practice with products ahead of time so that they can be used comfortably and in a way that enhances rather than interrupts the mood.

I am sexually active, but I'm not at risk.

- This is true only if sexual activity occurs exclusively with another disease-free individual. This assumes that you also don't share IV drug needles.
- Unless you have always abstained from risky behaviors, the only way you can be sure you are disease free is through several medical examinations (over a period of time so that

diseases have time to manifest themselves).
- A sexual partner may in good faith tell you that she or he is not infected, but because some diseases, especially HIV, take time to show up on medical tests, that individual may be infected and not know it yet. People who are infected but asymptomatic may also believe they are healthy and therefore not seek early medical testing.

HIV is a homosexual disease.

- Check the Center for Disease Control's statistics. HIV in the United States is spreading most quickly through contaminated needle use. Both heterosexual and homosexual individuals are at risk.
- Read the stories of Mary Fisher (wife and mother infected by her husband), Arthur Ashe and Ryan White (infected through blood transfusions), and Magic Johnson (infected through sexual relations with a woman).
- Borrow the free video on AIDS available at movie rental stores.

I want to get pregnant but I have an STD.

- Consult a physician.

  Treatment may be able to clear up the disease.

  Learn about how your infection could affect a baby and then make informed decisions.

  New procedures are available whereby a physician can place sperm directly into a woman's uterus or fallopian tubes, thereby eliminating risk to a partner.

present. Change from high-dose estrogen oral contraceptives to low-dose or to a different form of birth control after consulting with your physician. Wipe from front to back after urinating or defecating. Wear cotton, rather than nylon, underwear to allow the area to breathe.

Because these infections like warm, damp environments, it helps to remove your bathing suit immediately after swimming and regularly wash any clothing, especially bathing suits, pantyhose, underpants, etc., that come in contact with the vulva.

Pubic Lice

Names: crabs, crab lice, cooties

Cause: Parasite (insect) that breeds primarily in the pubic hair. This is a different parasite than those that cause body and head lice. It gets its name from its appearance; it has a short, crablike body and three pairs of large legs.

Cases: Common.

Transmission: **Pubic lice** are transmitted through sexual contact or contact with infected clothing, sheets, towels, or toilet seats. The pubic louse attaches itself to the skin around the genitals and lays eggs (nits) on a pubic hair shaft. It can also migrate and be transmitted to the chest, scalp, underarm, and facial hair. It is possible to contract this disease repeatedly; having been infected once does not ensure immunity against future exposures.

Symptoms: Intense itching in pubic hairs, around the anus, in the armpits, and occasionally in the beard and mustache. Bites can cause a rash or small blue spots. Brown specks may also be seen in underwear.

Diagnosis: Examination by a clinician to identify lice and eggs attached to hairs.

Treatment: Topical creams, lotions, and medicated shampoos will kill the lice. Lice must also be eradicated from clothing and bed linen. This can be done by washing them in hot soapy water and drying them in a hot dryer. Sexual partners should be treated simultaneously.

Prevention: Bathing and changing underclothing every day. Regular inspection of pubic hair and partners' pubic hair.

RELATIONSHIP BETWEEN HIV AND OTHER STDs

Researchers have identified a complex relationship between HIV and other STDs that results in a synergistic interaction—that is, the presence of both HIV and another STD has an effect that neither one would have alone. Of the major STDs, syphilis, chlamydia, gonorrhea, genital herpes, trichomoniasis, genital warts, and hepatitis B have been investigated for their impact on HIV. Researchers have discovered that the presence of these STDs, both ulcerative and nonulcerative, increases the risk of HIV transmission. Ulcerative STDs like syphilis and genital herpes appear to promote HIV transmission by causing inflammation and lesions of the genital tract, which provide an accessible place of entry for HIV. Increased risk of HIV transmission can also be attributed to nonulcerative STDs such as chlamydia, gonorrhea, and trichomoniasis, which weaken the body's defenses against disease. However, research related to the relationship between nonulcerative STDs and HIV has been limited.

It appears that the suppressive effects of HIV on the immune system worsen the symptoms of other STDs and decrease the healing effects of STD therapies. For example, genital herpes ulcers normally heal within two to three weeks, but persist much longer in people with HIV. Similarly, syphilis treatments sometimes fail or the disease develops more severely in people with HIV.

AVOIDING STDs: FACTS ABOUT PREVENTION

While there are over fifty different infecting organisms, the ways to protect yourself are relatively simple and few. Abstinence and exclusive sex with a disease-free individual are the safest methods. The next safest is use of a latex condom in combination with a spermicide. The spermicide alone is not sufficient but it adds some effectiveness. Lamb and natural skin condoms are effective for birth control, but are too porous to stop many STDs, including the AIDS virus. Be careful adding lubricants, because the wrong lubricants can damage a condom. Avoid oil-based products like petroleum jelly and Vaseline. Instead, use water-soluble products available at your drug store. Finally, put the condom on properly. (See Figure 13.2.) A latex female condom was

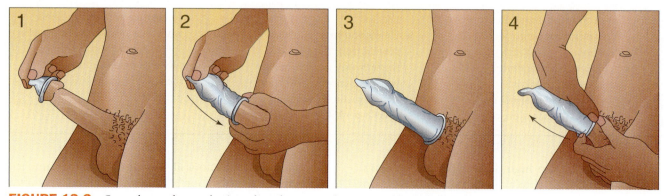

FIGURE 13.2   Grasp the condom at the tip and gently squeeze the air out of it. Leaving about one half inch of room at the tip, roll the condom on. Following ejaculation, hold on to the rim of the condom and withdraw the penis.

approved for sale in the United States by the Food and Drug Administration in 1993 with a warning that it had been found to be less effective. It is also often more expensive but it has two advantages. First, it covers more area on the female body, and second, it can be put in place ahead of time as opposed to a condom, which requires an erect penis. If you want to use this method of protection, discuss the pros and cons more fully with your health care provider.

Earlier in the chapter, two ideas were introduced: (1) that a person's STD risk is based on a combination of demographics and personal choice and (2) that while the goal is maximum disease prevention and daily practice of safer sex, it is better to take any step of precaution rather than none because it will reduce risk. For example, use of a condom every single time you have sex is optimum. However, use of a condom 50 percent of the time is better than never. You are still running a 50:50 chance of getting something but you are also half as risky as before. Similarly, if you get a little information from your partner, that is better than none and it may lead to more discussion as your relationship develops. As you consider the choices below, remember that taking even one small step is better than standing still. Here are some additional steps of prevention:

- Get to know your partner. Discuss your sexual histories and talk about concerns and precautions ahead of time.

- Abstain from sexual intercourse. Use other ways of expressing intimacy such as hugging, kissing, masturbation, or giving massages.

- Avoid sexual activity during an infectious outbreak (warts, lesions, discharge, and so on) or abstain during treatment.

- Look at your own and your partner's genitals. Watch for signs of infection. If you see any, delay having sex and ask a physician how to treat the disease and how to protect one another from infection or reinfection.

- Use a latex condom during any kind of sex. A dental dam (barrier for oral sex) can be created by cutting a regular condom.

- If you have multiple partners, get tested regularly.

- If you think you might have become infected, see a doctor. Early treatments are more effective and can prevent unnecessary damage to your body.

- Avoid high-risk situations like sex with multiple partners, sex with prostitutes, mixing alcohol and drugs with sex, and trading sex for drugs.

- Have a mutually monogamous relationship (both of you having sex only with each other).

- Live a wellness lifestyle. Eating balanced meals, sleeping well, being active, and moderating your stress can all help keep your immune system healthy and your body resistant to disease.

SUMMARY

STDs are uncomfortable and sometimes deadly diseases, only some of which are curable, and all of which are preventable. As long as individuals engage in unprotected sexual activity with infected partners, STD incidence will continue to increase, in some cases to epidemic levels. Although scientists are struggling to find better treatments, the best way to stop the spread of STDs is through responsible low-risk behavior.

Changing sexual behaviors is a most difficult task. For those who are sexually active, the benefits of spontaneous, unplanned, no-hassle sex must be weighed against the risks of pregnancy, infection, and even death. As long as perceived benefits outweigh perceived risk, a person will not change. Young people are especially susceptible to risky sexual behavior because many of them do not believe that the risk is "real," or they doubt that their relationship can handle an honest and open discussion of STDs. Decisions are also influenced when sex is mixed with drugs and alcohol, or for some, by the appeal of "no-attachment" casual sex.

The important thing to remember if you are sexually active is that you can control the amount of risk you take. The decision is yours. Abstinence, a monogamous relationship, or protected sex provides you with the lowest risk. Unprotected sex, sexual activity with multiple partners, or sex with a member of a high-risk group dramatically increases your risk. If you choose to be sexually active and you plan ahead, you can enjoy both the passionate moment and good health.

SUGGESTED READING

Centers for Disease Control. *Division of STD/HIV Prevention annual report, 1989.* Atlanta, GA: U.S. Department of Health and Human Services, 1990.

Centers for Disease Control. 1985 STD treatment guidelines. *Mortality and Morbidity Weekly Report Supplement,* September 1985.

Chlamydia: cloak and dagger, *Harvard Medical School Health Letter* 13(12):7, 1988.

Holmes, K. K., P.-A. Mardh, P. F. Sparling, P. J. Wiesner, W. Cates Jr., S. M. Lemon, and W. E. Stamm, eds. *Sexually transmitted diseases,* 2nd ed. New York: McGraw-Hill, 1990.

Larson, D. E., ed. *The Mayo Clinic family health book.* New York: William Morrow, 1990.

Shilts, R. *And the band played on: Politics, people and the AIDS epidemic.* New York: St. Martin's Press, 1987.

U.S. Department of Health and Human Services. *Healthy people 2000: National health promotion and disease prevention objectives.* DHHS Publication No. (PHS) 91-50213. Washington, D.C.: U.S. Government Printing Office, 1990.

U.S. Department of Health and Human Services. *Medicine for the public: Sexually transmitted diseases.* Public Health Service, National Institutes of Health Publication No. 93-3057, April 1993.

RESOURCES

CDC National AIDS HOTLINES
    1-800-342-AIDS (2437)—English
    1-800-344-SIDA (7432)—Spanish
    1-800-AIDS-TTY (243-7889)-TTY-service

CDC National STD Hotline
    1-800-227-8922

National Herpes Hotline (American Social Health Association)
    1-919-361-8488

Behavioral Lab 13.1

What Can I Do?

The following stage-based worksheets are for those individuals who are presently sexually active or considering becoming active. Safer sex in these worksheets will refer to behaviors that limit the transmission and potential infection of STDs. Someone who practices sexual abstinence could be considered either a precontemplator or a maintainer. In this text, the latter is assumed, which means a precontemplator is one who practices risky sexual activity whereas a maintainer practices either abstinence or safer sex.

Precontemplator

1. Even though you haven't considered changing your behavior, has your behavior ever worried you? If so, in what way? What were the circumstances?

   Examples

   I was worried about getting a disease when I found out one of my previous partners had one.

   I've worried a little more about sleeping with a prostitute because he or she might have AIDS.

   I've worried about getting pregnant or getting someone else pregnant.

   I sometimes worry about infecting someone else.

2. Think about what you gain from risky sex that you lose with safer sex. Refer to the barriers in the Barrier Busters feature for ideas.

3. Have you ever caught yourself rationalizing or downplaying the risks of unsafe sex? If yes, why do you think you do this?

   Examples

   I'm healthy, I won't catch it.

   The media make it sound worse than it is.

4. If you knew for sure that the next time you had unsafe sex, you would get AIDS, would you act any differently?

   What if it was herpes, syphilis, chlamydia, or another STD?

   What if you knew there was a 50 percent chance of getting it? 25 percent chance? 10 percent chance? What chance is acceptable to you?

5. Does reading about or seeing pictures of STDs upset you?

6. How do you feel about the idea that you may have already had intimate contact with someone infected with an STD?

7. How do you feel about someone passing a disease to you without telling you? Or you passing on a disease to someone you care about?

8. Have you or one of your friends been infected in the past? How does this make you feel?

9. Do you know if you are disease free right now? If your answer is yes, how do you know? If your answer is no, what are the implications of not knowing?

10. Do you think that society and the people around you support the idea of safer sex? How do their beliefs influence you?

11. Looking at your answers in items 3 to 10, do they outweigh your answer for item 1?

12. If you wanted to practice safer sex, what is the first thing you would do?

Contemplator

1. What behavior change are you thinking about making?

2. What changes will this action (item 1) bring about that are important to you? (Why are they important?)

3. Is there something you'd like to know more about before making this change?

Examples

What questions should I ask my partner?

How do I select and use a condom?

How do I say no without offending my significant other?

4. What conditions do you need in order to consider making this change? Try to finish this statement:

I would consider changing if . . .

5. How can you overcome or accomplish the items listed above? If you don't know how, can you think of someone who could help you come up with some ideas?

Preparer

1. What do you specifically want to accomplish? (For directions on goal setting see Chapter 2.)

2. What type of activities will accomplish this goal?

Examples

Talk with partner.

Purchase a product.

3. Experiment with some of the ideas you listed in item 2.

Examples

Role play what you would say to a partner.

Buy or look at products in the store or ask a friend if he or she has products you can look at.

4. Based on items 1, 2, and 3, select one activity you would like to incorporate into your lifestyle.

5. Take the activity you selected in item 4 and decide what you need to do to start doing that activity or behavior.

6. What kinds of things do you think might stop you from taking this first step or accomplishing your overall goal?

7. What strategies can you use to prevent the temptations or situations listed in item 6 from stopping you from adopting your new behavior? In other words, how can you prepare yourself against temptation?

8. What makes you believe you can accomplish your goal? *Or* What makes you believe you can accomplish this first step?

9. If your first step doesn't work, then what will you do?

10. Complete the following statement:

I am going to take my first step on _____.
date within 30 days

Action Taker

1. What STD prevention or safer sex practices are you currently doing?

2. How long have you sustained this behavior or what percentage of the time have you succeeded in using it?

3. If you are still inconsistent with your behavior, what do you think is causing this?

4. Can you think of ways to control the factors you listed in item 3, or do you know anyone who can help you find solutions?

5. Are you receiving support or rewards for your effort?

If yes, what kind and from whom?

If no, why not? And can you change this?

6. Do you have confidence in your ability to continue your new behavior?

If yes, what kinds of things are you doing that are building your confidence?

If no, what kinds of things lower your confidence? How can you change or change the environment around you to eliminate or neutralize the effect of these things?

7. If you were to stop or slip up, what do you think would be the major reason for doing this?

8. Is there a way to prevent this (item 7)? Are there actions you can take to minimize the temptations of less-safe sex?

9. How would you get yourself started again if you did stop?

10. Are you clear about what it is you are doing and why? Can you state your action in the form of a clear and specific goal?

If you are still somewhat uncertain about whether you are taking the right action, can you formulate some questions you'd like to have answered? To find the answers to these questions where can you look or whom can you talk to?

11. How have you or your environment changed to accommodate and support this new behavior?

Maintainer

1. How long have you practiced safer sex (or abstinence)?

2. What are the top two reasons that make you want to continue this behavior?

3. Have you been tempted to stop practicing safer sex? If so, what tempted you?

4. How did you convince yourself to continue?

5. How can you prevent such temptation or a relapse in the future?

6. How confident are you that you will continue to practice safer sex? What kinds of things increase your confidence? Decrease your confidence? How can you optimize the former and diminish the latter?

7. Do you feel as though you have support for your action? If yes, from whom (significant other, spiritual leader, and so on)? How does this support or lack thereof make you feel?

8. Is there anything you need (information? support?) to promote your continued maintenance?

9. If you listed something in item 8, can you think of a way to attain it or can you think of someone who can help you with it?

10. How have you changed or how have you changed the environment around you to accommodate this healthier lifestyle?

LAB
13.2

Safer Sex Scenarios

A number of dilemmas are presented here in the form of hypothetical scenarios. The names of colors are used in place of people's names. Read each of the scenarios, explain the dilemma(s) and discuss possible plans of action. A number of issues are involved in each of these scenarios, including the risk of STD infection, moral beliefs, drug dependency, and family relationships. It is unrealistic to propose preventions and treatments of STDs outside the context of relationships. Keep this in mind as you search for ways to deal with each situation.

1. Blue comes back to her dorm room and is met in the hallway by her roommate Yellow. Yellow explains that her boyfriend is spending the night and asks Blue if she can find another place to sleep. Blue knows that Yellow's boyfriend has slept with a mutual friend who has chlamydia.

2. Red is HIV positive. He has been dating Purple and feels that it is time to reveal his HIV status. He is afraid that by telling Purple, he will lose what he needs most, Purple's love and support.

3. Brown is watching TV with a groups of friends when, after a few beers, her date Orange invites her into his bedroom.

4. Gray suspects that his sexual partner Tan is involved with illegal IV drugs. Meanwhile Tan thinks she has an STD but is worried about treating it because then White might find out about it.

5. Violet is single, pregnant, and no longer seeing the baby's father. She has a good relationship going with Green, who has Herpes II. What are the risks to the fetus? To her?

6. Silver has discovered that the initiation into a group he has always wanted to belong to is sex with a member of the club or "scoring" with a certain number of people.

7. Gold suspects her partner Bronze of cheating on her. In addition to the emotional pain, she is concerned that he may expose himself, and ultimately her, to disease. Currently they don't use any barrier protection because he has had a vasectomy.

8. Black is concerned about getting his partner Blue pregnant or exposing himself to disease. He wants to use a condom but is afraid Blue will consider it an intrusion and less romantic.

9. Red and Yellow have been dating for several months. Red has been dropping hints about having sex but Yellow would like to wait until after marriage. Yellow would also like Red to take a test for HIV before they sleep together. Yellow is afraid to tell Red, in case Red gets upset and breaks off the relationship.

10. Pink and Blue want to get married and have children. Blue has gonorrhea and has been exposed to HIV. Pink is disease free.

CHAPTER 14

Understanding and Avoiding Substance Abuse

Terms

- Substance abuse
- Addiction
- Physical dependence
- Psychological dependence
- Psychoactive
- Depressant
- Blood alcohol content
- Smokeless tobacco
- Secondhand smoke
- Marijuana
- Stimulants
- Cocaine
- Amphetamines
- Methamphetamine
- Caffeine
- Hallucinogens
- Opiates and narcotics
- Inhalants
- Designer drugs

Objectives

1. Recognize the problems created by substance abuse and be able to discuss the impact at both a personal and societal level.

2. Understand some of the reasons why people abuse substances.

3. Be able to define and give examples of abuse and addiction.

4. Know the effects and risks of alcohol, tobacco, and drug abuse.

5. Know how and where to obtain help for yourself or for someone else.

6. Take a critical look at the picture being presented to you by advertisers and pressuring peers concerning the use of certain substances.

7. Identify an abusive behavior you would like to alter or a proactive stance you would like to adopt to help fight substance abuse in your community.

Where Am I?

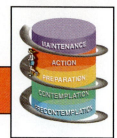

SUBSTANCE ABUSE

Alcohol

Please check one of the following that best describes your alcohol use. In each statement *three drinks* applies to women; *four drinks* applies to men.

Precontemplator _____ I have no intention in the next six months to stop typically drinking three/four or more drinks one or more times a week.

Contemplator _____ I plan to stop typically drinking three/four or more drinks one or more times a week in the next six months.

Preparer _____ I plan to stop typically drinking three/four or more drinks one or more times a week in the next thirty days.

Action Taker _____ I stopped typically drinking three/four or more drinks one or more times a week less than six months ago.

Maintainer _____ I stopped typically drinking three/four or more drinks one or more times a week more than six months ago. *Or*

_____ I have never typically drunk three/four or more drinks one or more times a week.

Tobacco

Select the statement that best answers the following question: Have you quit smoking or using other tobacco products?

Precontemplator _____ No, and I do not intend to quit in the next six months.

Contemplator _____ No, but I intend to quit in the next six months.

Preparer _____ No, but I intend to quit in the next thirty days.

Action Taker _____ Yes, I quit less than six months ago.

Maintainer _____ Yes, I quit more than six months ago. *Or* I was never a smoker or tobacco user.

Drugs

Please check one of the following that best describes your drug use:

Precontemplator _____ I do not intend to stay off drugs completely in the next six months.

Contemplator _____ I am thinking about staying off drugs completely in the next six months.

Source: alcohol: Modified with permission of Jeff Migneault. *tobacco:* From J. Prochaska and M. Goldstein. Process of smoking cessation: Implications for clinicians. *Clinics and Chest Medicine.* 12(4):727–734, December 1991. Reprinted with permission of W. B. Saunders Company. *drugs:* Tsoh, J. Motivation and stages of change among drug addicts in drug abuse treatment programs. Thesis. University of Rhode Island, Kingston, 1993. Modified with permission of the author.

Preparer	_____	I intend to stay off drugs completely in the next thirty days.
Action Taker	_____	I have stayed off drugs completely for less than six months.
Maintainer	_____	I have stayed off drugs completely for more than six months.
Other	_____	I have never used drugs.

ABUSE PREVENTION

Precontemplator	_____	I have no intention of being active in ways that help prevent or reduce substance abuse in my community.
Contemplator	_____	I plan to be active in at least one way that will help reduce or prevent substance abuse in my community in the next six months.
Preparer	_____	I plan to be active in at least one way that will help reduce or prevent substance abuse in my community in the next thirty days.
Action Taker	_____	I have been active in one or more ways that help reduce or prevent substance abuse in my community, but have been active for less than six months.
Maintainer	_____	I have been active in one or more ways that help reduce or prevent substance abuse in my community for more than six months.

Substance abuse can take many forms. Each instance of abuse has to be handled within the context of the specific substance and the individual's personality and contributing environment. In some cases, a person can stop an abusive habit without any professional treatment; in other cases, years of rehabilitation and therapy are required. With the understanding that substance abuse covers a wide spectrum of behaviors, the behavior change information in this chapter is offered as a tool for focusing awareness and beginning a change process that will likely require additional resources. As with other lifestyle behaviors, any change that you can sustain is worthwhile, even though the end goal is to stop abusing substances altogether. The behavior change staging information in this chapter and the Barrier Busters have been organized into four areas: alcohol, tobacco, drug abuse and drug abuse prevention. Abuse prevention is any activity—at either the personal or community level—that helps prevent someone from becoming a substance abuser or helps stop continued abuse by someone already abusing.

The behavior change lab at the end of the chapter is organized into two headings: substance abuse and abuse prevention. If the substance abuse section of Lab 14.1 is too generalized, adjust it to better fit the behavior you are trying to change. Now, to begin, select the behavior change area(s) that is (are) important to you and stage yourself using the appropriate set(s) of questions in the Where Am I? section on this and the previous page.

In the United States today, substance abuse represents a societal menace. The problem takes many forms: It may be an elderly person addicted to prescription drugs, an athlete taking anabolic steroids, a truck driver using speed to stay awake, a baby born addicted to heroin, a teenager smoking a cigarette or pot to be cool, a college student who has three drinks and then drives, a parent who overdrinks and then abuses a child, or a crack addict who will do anything to get money for another hit. The price we are paying in health care, rehabilitation, law enforcement, lost productivity, and most important, personal loss and tragedy, is beyond calculation.

The substances themselves are not inherently good or bad, it is how they are used. Many abused substances have beneficial effects when used medicinally. For some cancer victims, marijuana reduces nausea during chemotherapy. Cocaine is used as a topical anesthetic, and for some, modest alcohol intake may help prevent heart disease. It is only when these substances are exploited that they become a problem.

Different cultures define what responsible or acceptable use is according to their values and traditions. For example, in some cultures wine is an acceptable beverage for teenagers. By contrast, the consumption of alcohol is completely unacceptable among people who practice the Islamic religion.[1] Different standards may also exist within a culture, depending on the circumstances. In the United States, for example, it is socially acceptable to drink excessively at a bachelor party, but not at a fund raiser. Social mores may also set different standards of acceptability for men and women. For example, society is more accepting of a man chewing tobacco than a woman.

WHAT IS SUBSTANCE ABUSE?

Cultural differences aside, **substance abuse** can be defined as use of a substance even though the substance is harmful to the user or to the people around the user. Thus, even if you are a moderate drinker, you are an alcohol abuser when you drink and drive. And if you normally drink one or two cups of coffee a day, but you use caffeine pills to stay up all night, you are a caffeine abuser. Prescription drugs can be abused by giving them to a friend, using too many, or using too few. The latter is often done by the poor and the elderly in an effort to reduce the cost of their medical care.[2] You can abuse a substance without being addicted to it. With cocaine, the abuser may not even have a chance to become addicted since the first hit can be lethal. As Figure 14.1 indicates, substance abuse contributes directly to thousands of deaths in the United States each year, with the leading substances being tobacco, alcohol, and crack cocaine.

WHAT IS ADDICTION?

Addiction is an advanced form of abuse, which includes a physical or psychological dependence. **Physical dependence** is characterized by tolerance to the drug and withdrawal symptoms if the level of drug in the body drops. As the body becomes accustomed to a substance, it desensitizes itself to the effect of the drug. This forces the user to take a higher dose to achieve the same result. When the blood concentration of a substance drops, the shock to the system results in withdrawal symptoms such as the shakes, nausea, and convulsions. If withdrawal is severe enough, death can occur.

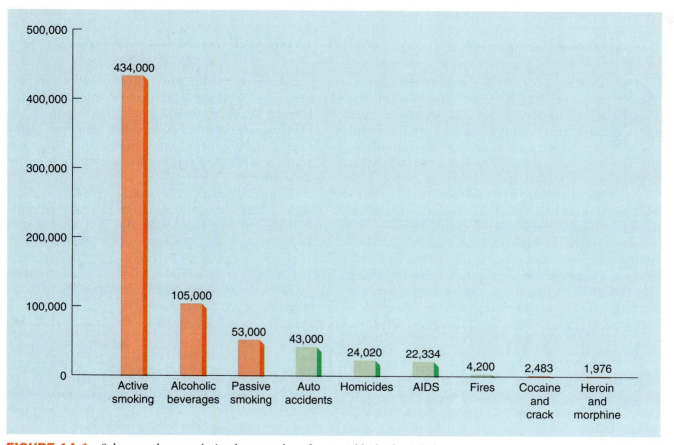

FIGURE 14.1 Substance abuse results in a large number of preventable deaths and plays a major role in accidents and crime. (Data from *The chemical people newsletter*, Summer 1993.)

Psychological dependence includes an intense craving or compulsive desire for the mood-altering effects (such as euphoria) that the **psychoactive** ingredient in certain substances provides. A person can be psychologically dependent without being physically dependent. Some experts, however, argue that because brain chemicals are altered (a physical phenomenon) during psychological dependence, there is no such thing as purely psychological dependence.

Addictions, particularly drug addictions, affect all aspects of wellness. Addictive substances can cloud mental judgment, interfere with or contradict spiritual beliefs, cause negative emotions like guilt and anxiety, and result in poor physical health.

WHY DO PEOPLE ABUSE SUBSTANCES?

People abuse substances for many reasons. There are biological explanations such as genetic predisposition and prenatal drug exposure; psychological ones, including peer, family, and religious influences as well as personality traits; and social factors such as socioeconomic background and present living conditions. Recent research evidence suggests that certain brain chemical deficiencies in some people predispose them to addiction. This genetic condition may help explain why addictions like alcoholism tend to run in families.[3,4] Exposure to drugs in utero may also make a person more susceptible to drug dependency.

The research on whether or not there is an addictive personality is somewhat inconclusive. People who have low self-esteem, suffer from depression, or have a tendency to take high risks may be more prone to addiction. Children of abusers are more likely to abuse substances than other children.

Curiosity about and experimentation with substances often initiate the tragic trip toward abuse and addiction. Casual users become abusers as the desired pleasurable effect requires more and more of the abused substance. What may have started as a daring act of rebellion, or as an effort to act mature and be independent, can end with the user a slave to a chemical. It is ironic that people think they can be independent by becoming dependent.

Also ironic is that the people who begin using a drug to gain acceptance in a social group often find themselves in a spiral of increasing isolation. Addicts will shoot up or drink by themselves, and to get money for a habit they will steal from their parents, employers, and friends. Sadly the drug, not the company they are keeping, becomes their focus of attention.

For others, drugs offer an escape from reality. The problem is that reality keeps coming back, and too often the solution seems to be an intensification of drug use. The person may lose all sense of reality or the ability to cope with reality. This is why drug rehabilitation includes facing the underlying issues that led to drug abuse in the first place. Failure to deal with these issues leads to relapse.

The decision concerning which substance to abuse is often dependent on what is available and what is being used by people around the individual, or at least what is perceived to be socially acceptable. Peer pressure and, in the case of alcohol and tobacco, advertising pressure may encourage a person to try a substance. Many young people also claim to experiment with drugs to combat boredom.

Finally, a person may seek out a substance for its specific effect. For example, someone who is tired or depressed may turn to something for a lift. This can be anything from a caffeinated drink to snorting cocaine. On the other hand, someone who feels tense or wired or who can't fall asleep may rely on a **depressant** like a sleeping pill, "downers," or an alcoholic drink. Other people want mood-altering drugs in order to experience increased sensations and a rush of euphoria.

WHAT ARE THE COSTS TO SOCIETY?

It is difficult to ascertain all the costs to society that the abuse of alcohol, tobacco, and other drugs exact. Certainly many lives are lost—100,000 annually to alcohol, 419,000 to tobacco, and many more to drug-related illness, overdose, and crime. Forty percent of traffic fatalities[5] and an estimated 47 to 65 percent of all drownings are alcohol related.[6] Alcohol is also typically found in the offender, victim, or both in about half of all homicides and serious assaults.[7]

The cost to society is twofold: first there are the expenses of trying to prevent abuse from starting, stop ongoing abuse, and provide treatment for abusers. Second there are the dollars lost through a lack of productivity. Expenditures include prevention education, treatment programs, health care, traffic accidents, and law enforcement. Work productivity is lost when the quality of an employee's work is erratic, drug-related accidents occur, absenteeism from work increases, and premature deaths occur. Alcohol, tobacco, and other drugs are at the root of many of this country's most serious problems: violence, injuries, disease, rape, child and spousal abuse, AIDS, teen pregnancy, school dropouts, car crashes, escalating health care costs, low work productivity, and homelessness.[8] Babies born with drug-related problems need costly medical care, special education programs, and in some cases lifetime institutional care. Substance abuse can put a drain on personal and family finances, escalate child and spousal abuse, and tear families apart. In 1993 drug-related costs were estimated at $200 billion. Approximately $90.4 billion in health care costs alone could be saved if alcohol and other drug problems were stopped before they were started.[9]

On campus, half of college students who were victims of campus crimes said they had been drinking or using other drugs when they were victimized.[10] Furthermore, it is estimated that alcohol use is implicated in one- to two-thirds of sexual assault and acquaintance or date rape cases among teens and college students.[11] Before you make drinking alcohol a regular college habit, consider the research evidence that students with GPAs of D or F drink three times as much as those who earn A's.[12]

SUBSTANCE ABUSE AND BEHAVIOR CHANGE

Behavior change for substance abuse can include the decisions to: (1) start abusing a substance; (2) stop abusing a substance; and (3) help an abuser or potential abuser.

We will discuss the decision-making process that leads to abuse of a substance, first by providing information on the most commonly abused substances, and then by illustrating some of the situations that can lead to abuse. If you are trying to quit an abusive habit, this chapter offers some motivating reasons for stopping, strategies on how to stop, and where to go for help and support.

Many people are not abusers but hesitate to take actions to help or stop others. In fact, in some cases people inadvertently add to the problem. For these reasons the information and behavior change materials in this chapter go beyond the abuser to address the involvement of others in the prevention (and halting) of substance abuse. Are you a precontemplator, someone who doesn't believe that society's drug problem is your problem? A contemplator thinking about helping? A preparer ready to help but not sure how? Or are you an action taker? Actions can be as simple as being a designated driver, volunteering for a hotline, coaching a youth sport, peer counseling, or just being there when someone needs to talk. If you aren't a substance abuser, consider working through a behavior change lab on abuse prevention.

THE USE AND ABUSE OF ALCOHOL

Alcohol is part of the cultural tapestry of peoples all over the world. We picture the French romantically sipping a fine wine, the Germans festively raising a robust beer, and Russians saluting friendship with a shot of vodka. For many, alcohol is intertwined with a good portion of what is good in life: it is the champagne toast at a best friend's wedding, the red wine sipped at communion, the drink that seals the business deal, a beer after the game, a round "on me" to celebrate a new job. Unfortunately for some it is also a hangover with blackouts, throwing up on a date, drinking up the grocery money, waking up in bed with a stranger and maybe a sexually transmitted

Activity 14.1
Helping or Hurting?

Because of the widespread use of alcohol and other drugs among the college age group, it is likely that you will be faced with issues of abuse—as a friend or relative of an abuser, as a victim of alcohol- or drug-related crime, or perhaps as someone struggling with a personal abuse problem. There is a strong temptation to look the other way, deny that a problem even exists, or even help make excuses for someone with a problem.

Someone who helps a person cover up for a drinking or drug problem (consciously or unconsciously) is called an *enabler*. People often enable substance abusers without realizing the full impact of their actions. Have you ever enabled someone to abuse alcohol or other drugs or has someone else ever enabled you? Here are a few questions to help you think about this:

- Have you ever excused someone's behavior by blaming it on the alcohol or drug? Or have you ever said, "Oh, I didn't mean it. I was drunk at the time." Or, "Please don't judge me by my behavior last night. I was high."
- Have you purchased alcohol for someone underage or asked someone to purchase alcohol for you? Have you ever borrowed or lent money to purchase drugs or alcohol?
- Have you covered for someone or asked someone to cover for you after a drinking or drug episode?

Can you think of other ways that you or someone else might purposely or accidentally act as a substance abuse enabler?

disease, or taking one last drink before driving a best friend through a telephone pole. There are many innocent victims of alcohol. Babies are born mentally retarded and disfigured, people are killed by drunk drivers, children of alcoholics suffer abuse, and one way or another, all of us pay for the violence, crime, and disease related to alcohol.

Is Alcohol a Drug?

Alcohol is a drug—but because it is legal, many people dismiss this fact. Anyone who abuses alcohol is a drug abuser. Alcohol is a mood-altering drug that can become both physically and psychologically addicting. The psychoactive ingredient in all fermented and distilled liquors is ethyl alcohol (ethanol), a colorless liquid with a sharp burning taste that functions as a depressant on the central nervous system (CNS). In particular, ethyl alcohol modifies the brain's control functions of motor coordination, reaction time, information processing, and inhibition. Ethyl alcohol should not be confused with other alcohols such as rubbing or wood alcohol, which are poisonous if consumed. As is done in common usage, the word *alcohol* in this chapter will refer to ethyl alcohol and beverages made with it.

Alcohol is usually diluted with water or another liquid to make an alcoholic beverage. The measure of how much alcohol is in a drink is known as the *proof*. The proof is twice the percentage of alcohol contained in the beverage. Pure alcohol is 200 proof. A beverage that is twelve proof like beer is 6 percent alcohol.

How the Body Metabolizes Alcohol

When you consume alcohol, it is absorbed into the bloodstream. The amount of alcohol in your blood is referred to as your **blood alcohol content** (BAC). When you consume alcohol faster than your body can metabolize it, your BAC rises. Alcohol-laden blood circulates to the brain, where its influence on brain function is related to the BAC. The higher the BAC, the greater the effect.

When you drink alcohol, a small amount is absorbed into the blood through the membranes in the mouth and about 20 percent of it is absorbed out of the stomach. Food in the stomach slows down the rate of absorption by slowing down the rate alcohol moves into the intestines. About 75 percent of the alcohol you consume passes from the small intestine into the bloodstream. The carbon dioxide (bubbles) in carbonated beverages like champagne or a rum and cola cause the stomach contents to move more quickly into the intestines, which means that these beverages are absorbed faster into the bloodstream. A regrettable choice would be several rum and colas in a small amount of time on an empty stomach.

Alcohol-laden blood circulates through the liver every four minutes. The liver extracts the alcohol and converts it into various chemical substances, finally breaking it down into carbon dioxide and water. This process requires about three hours for every ounce of alcohol consumed. The liver does not take rush orders, so drinking coffee has no effect and won't sober a person up. Excessive alcohol has to wait its turn. The liver of a heavy drinker works very hard and, as a result, becomes prone to disease.

A small percentage of alcohol, between 2 and 10 percent, is not metabolized; instead, it is excreted through the urine, breath, and sweat. This is the basis for using urine and breath tests to determine alcohol concentrations. In most states individuals are considered legally intoxicated if they have a BAC of .08 or higher. In a few states the minimum value BAC is .10.

The quantity and type of enzymes with which we are genetically endowed play a role in our ability to metabolize alcohol. Women, for example, metabolize alcohol more poorly than men because they produce lower amounts of alcohol dehydrogenase, a stomach enzyme that breaks down alcohol before it reaches the bloodstream.[13] This means that women experience higher BACs over a shorter time and have an increased vulnerability to liver damage.[14] Genetic differences in alcohol metabolizing enzymes have also been found in certain minority groups. The flushing reaction that occurs most commonly among people of Asian ancestry involves a reddening of the face and neck and can be accompanied by headaches, nausea, and other symptoms. For some, even small amounts of alcohol (one drink) can cause illness.[15] For this reason, the flushing reaction appears to deter excessive alcohol use, but some people with the trait continue to consume alcohol.[16] In contrast, a liver enzyme found in the Japanese has been associated with a faster rate of elimination of alcohol from the body compared with whites.[17] While much more research is needed, evidence like this suggests that certain minority groups possess genetic traits that predispose them to, or help protect them from, becoming alcoholic.

Some people are naturally more tolerant of alcohol than others, but this tolerance does not necessarily protect them from disease. An acquired tolerance develops when a person drinks over a period of time. As tolerance is acquired, individuals must drink more alcohol to obtain the same effect. Alcoholics can lose this acquired tolerance if their liver is damaged because this condition diminishes their ability to metabolize alcohol. (Therefore either an increase or decrease in tolerance can be a warning sign for alcoholism.)

Body size also influences BAC. A larger body and corresponding larger volume of blood dilute the alcohol more than is possible in a smaller body. On average,

---

TABLE 14.1 ■ Effects of Increasing Blood Alcohol Content

BAC	Effect
.03–.05	social euphoric effect
.05–.10	(legally drunk = .08 or .10) impaired coordination, especially fine motor, exaggerates things, slow reaction time
.10–.15	unsteady, loss of peripheral vision
.15–.30	drunken stagger, slurred speech, pain perception dulled
> .30	stupor or unconsciousness, alcohol poisoning, death possible at or above .35
.40–.60	drinker is comatose and in danger of dying from respiratory failure

Source: Information from Mothers Against Drunk Driving and PRIDE.

women are smaller than men and are therefore apt to become more intoxicated after drinking the same amount of alcohol. Body fat plays a role in BAC as well. Alcohol, which is water soluble, does not concentrate in fatty tissues, which are not water soluble. Therefore people with a higher percentage of fat will experience higher concentrations of alcohol in their blood and other nonfat tissues. The average healthy woman has a higher percentage of fat than her male counterpart and so again will therefore become more intoxicated after drinking the same amount of alcohol.

Choices That Affect Blood Alcohol Content

Fortunately there are three ways that you can control your BAC. First, you are the one who decides what you are going to drink. Selecting beverages that are nonalcoholic or low in alcoholic content allows you to avoid the pitfalls of intoxication. Drinking a nonalcoholic beverage first to quench your thirst will also help you limit your alcoholic intake and prevent a rapid spike in BAC. Second, food in your stomach helps slow down the absorption rate of alcohol. It all must be absorbed eventually, but you will be able to avert a surge of alcohol into your bloodstream. Finally, the rate at which you drink makes a difference. The average male can metabolize about one drink an hour. If the rate of consumption exceeds this, blood alcohol concentrations will rise. For this reason, binge drinking is very dangerous; it sharply increases the BAC, putting the drinker at risk for alcohol poisoning—a life-threatening condition that requires emergency medical attention.

When Is It Abuse? Addiction?

Abuse occurs when people drink excessive alcohol and then proceed to do things that are unsafe—such as driving a car, piloting a plane or a boat, or using heavy machinery. Other unsafe activities include mixing alcohol with prescription drugs, over-the-counter medications, or illegal drugs. Abuse leads to addiction when consumption continues even when individuals are aware that they have a problem and that the alcohol is going to make the problem worse. As discussed earlier, addiction includes physical and/or psychological dependence. Alcoholics are usually both psychologically and physically addicted.

Although many people picture a pathetic drunken individual when they hear the word *alcoholic,* addictive drinking follows a variety of patterns. Some people drink large amounts daily, some "party hearty" on the weekend, and others have long, dry periods between episodes of binge drinking. Behind all of these is heavy consumption, often with the intent to become intoxicated.

Alcoholism often has been attributed to weak character or lack of will power. Some people say, "If alcoholics would just try harder, they could clean up their act and stay off the booze." In 1956 the AMA declared alcoholism

a disease. Since then there has been evidence of a gene that may predispose people to alcoholism. That doesn't mean that people with this gene will become alcoholics, but rather that they are more susceptible to alcoholism. Personality research has not revealed a complete profile for alcoholism, but it has identified some characteristics of addictive personalities—those people who may easily become addicted to a variety of things. Treatment must get to the underlying reasons for drinking, or one addictive habit may be replaced with another.

Two-thirds of the population drink, but only a small percentage, about 10 percent, drink half (50 percent) of all the alcohol consumed in the United States.[18] White men and women are the most likely to drink, followed by Hispanics and then African Americans. Men drink larger quantities, drink more frequently, and report more drinking-related problems than women.[19] Among women, the highest rate of drinking is found in single women (unmarried, separated, or divorced). Women with a history of sexual abuse are twice as likely to be problem drinkers than those without. Children of alcoholic parents are more likely to become alcoholics themselves, and these children are more likely to marry alcoholics, have an eating disorder, or become involved with drugs.

What Are the Short-Term Effects?

Alcohol use depresses the brain center that controls a person's inhibitions. As a result, the person is more likely to engage in risky behavior. The risk may be as harmless as getting up the nerve to ask someone out on a date or as dangerous as committing suicide. Brain function slows, which means that reaction time decreases, alertness is dulled, and motor coordination is impaired. All of these make it very dangerous to drive or to participate in activities like sports, in which quick, coordinated movements are important. Although alcohol commercials on television often picture their product alongside fast-paced sporting events, the combination can be hazardous. Sports—for example, driving a skimobile, skiing, or surfing—don't mix with alcohol.

Judgment and the ability to reason are also affected by alcohol consumption. Poor decisions may lead to accidents, to sex with a stranger or sex without protection, or simply to saying or doing something that you will regret the next day. Alcohol may intensify emotions. You can probably think of someone who becomes very excited, talkative, the life of the party while drinking, and you can probably also think of someone who becomes angry and irritable, or very depressed and tearful. Alcohol's effect can also be different at different times for the same person. One of the worst short-term effects is the hangover. For some people the headache and queasy stomach hit right away; others have a pounding head and watch the room spin the next morning.

In social situations people often drink for the feelings of euphoria or relaxation it creates. Tension and worrying

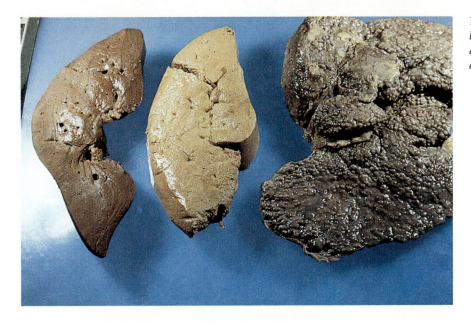

Years of alcohol abuse can turn a healthy liver (far left) into a diseased liver—jaundiced (center) and cirrhotic (far right) livers are shown.

may, at least for a short time, be relieved. A group of people with diverse backgrounds, perhaps strangers to each other, may find themselves comfortably swapping stories after a drink. Care must be taken, however, for these positive short-term effects can be overshadowed by other negative short- and long-term effects.

What Are the Long-Term Effects?

Psychological effects of alcohol abuse include alcoholic paranoia, delusions, and memory gaps. Physical effects of alcohol abuse include cirrhosis of the liver; heart disease; pancreatic inflammation, vomiting, stomach pain, nausea, digestive problems; ulcers and gastritis (stomach lining irritation); brain cell damage; depressed immune system; cancer of the mouth, throat, stomach, intestine, and pancreas; delirium tremens (muscular shakes/convulsions); malnutrition; nerve damage; menstrual irregularities; deep sleep interference; impotence; decreased vaginal lubrication; interference with body temperature regulation; increased risk of osteoporosis; increased risk of kidney disease; fetal alcohol syndrome, mental retardation, and developmental delays; and miscarriage.

One of the most common alcohol-related diseases is cirrhosis of the liver. Alcohol slows down the liver's metabolism of fats, allowing fat to accumulate in the liver cells. Eventually the cells burst and are replaced with fibrous scar tissue that impedes blood flow, ultimately causing liver failure and death. Early signs of liver trouble are jaundice (yellow skin) and fluid in the stomach or lower extremities. As we have noted, women are more susceptible to liver disease because less alcohol is metabolized in the stomach, which means more of it reaches the liver. Heavy alcohol use is also linked to heart disease and some cancers. Malnutrition and its deleterious effects to the heart and body are also common among alcoholics who concentrate their efforts on getting their next drink rather than on consuming nutritious foods.

Alcohol and Pregnancy

When a pregnant woman drinks, her unborn child drinks. Alcohol crosses the placenta and can interrupt normal fetal development. The child may suffer severe physical deformity, behavioral problems, clumsiness, stunted growth, or mental retardation. Each year 4,000 to 12,000 babies are born with the physical signs and intellectual disabilities associated with *fetal alcohol syndrome* (FAS), and thousands more experience the somewhat lesser disabilities of fetal alcohol effect.[20] FAS children may have broader, flatter faces, heart defects, and a wide variety of physical and mental deficiencies. Alcohol during the first trimester is usually the most hazardous, as this is the time during which the central nervous system and many of the organs are developing. *Fetal alcohol effect* (FAE) refers to a more subtle condition in which children may experience memory and judgment problems and a reduced ability to learn from experience. Although this may be caused by alcohol, it often goes undiagnosed and the child is simply considered a slow learner. The amount of damage alcohol causes is not necessarily related to the volume drunk during pregnancy. One woman can drink very little and give birth to a severely affected child, whereas another may drink more and give birth to a normal child. Because there is no way to predict the scope of alcohol's effect on a pregnancy, the only safe thing a woman can do is to abstain from alcohol during pregnancy.

Because many women do not know that they are pregnant for the first one to three months, the critical developmental time for the fetus, someone trying to get pregnant should also avoid alcohol. Women who breastfeed also need to be aware that breast milk can pass alcohol on to the baby. If you are considering drinking alcohol while you are pregnant, think of the risks to your unborn child and the added difficulties of raising a mentally retarded child. For more insight, read the book, *The Broken Cord* by Michael Dorris, a heart-wrenching (and heartwarming) story of life with an FAS child.

Where Is Treatment Available?

Treatment starts with the individual, who must recognize the problem of alcoholism and want to do something about it. However, there is good evidence that concern, confrontation, and help from friends, family, colleagues, and employers have a positive and significant cumulative impact. Concerned individuals should not wait for the problem drinker to bottom out or ask for help.

Twenty-five percent of alcoholics successfully stop or reduce their drinking on their own, meaning without a formal treatment program, but not necessarily without support from friends. Others need the help of a more formal treatment program. Alcoholics Anonymous (AA) was started in the 1930s by two desperate alcoholics, Robert Smith, a surgeon, and William Wilson, a stockbroker. AA has now grown to over 800,000 members in the United States and over 2 million members worldwide. AA teaches members a twelve-step program that includes an admission that they cannot control their use of alcohol and must therefore place their lives in God's hands. New members are given a sponsor who is always

there for them, and a twenty-four-hour hotline. Today there are also secular organizations, like Rational Recovery and Secular Organizations for Sobriety (SOS). These are similar to AA but do not have the same spiritual tone.

Al-Ateen is specifically for young drinkers, youthful friends of drinkers, and children of alcoholics. Al-Anon is an organization for friends and families of alcoholics. At meetings they can learn about the disease of alcoholism and what they can do to help themselves and the alcoholic.

Almost 1.9 million Americans age twelve and older entered a treatment program in 1992, with people ages eighteen to thirty-four significantly more likely to seek treatment than those older or younger.[21] Treatment usually includes three stages: detoxification, medical treatment, and discussion and planning for long-term behavior change. Because alcohol causes a physical dependency, withdrawal can be physically painful. Common symptoms are sweating, weakness, and delirium tremens (trembling or convulsions).

A variety of treatment programs are available. To find one in your area, look in the phone book or call one of the resource phone numbers at the end of this chapter. Colleges and universities offer free, confidential services to students, either on campus or through a referral to a nearby treatment center. Employers may have an employee-assistance program, or can offer a referral. For younger people, there are school-based programs. Those who need to check themselves into a facility should investigate inpatient hospital programs as well as privately run centers. And as previously mentioned, there are a number of support groups like AA and SOS. A treatment program that works will not only address the physical addiction, but will also deal with psychological issues behind the drinking, such as stress, self-esteem, or psychiatric problems.

THE USE AND ABUSE OF TOBACCO

Tobacco products represent a major economic, political, and social force in the United States. Since colonial days, tobacco has been one of America's largest exports; today it is the seventh largest cash crop. Big tobacco producers and distributors are influential people, and as such, they have a powerful influence on Congress. The small family tobacco farms are also an economic factor in tobacco states. The strength and leverage of the tobacco companies and their lobbyists are evident in the time and effort it has taken to change public opinion and pass antitobacco legislation.

Public opinions and attitudes concerning tobacco have changed dramatically over the years. In the 1940s and '50s movie stars like Mae West, Clark Gable, and Humphrey Bogart glamorized smoking. Even Fred Astaire tapped out a number on the big screen with a cigarette clenched between his teeth. By the 1960s about half of all Americans were smokers. Then, in 1964, when the Surgeon General's office published its first report on the dangers of tobacco use, the era of carefree smoking ended. Tobacco's glamour began to fade. Bogart and the unstoppable John Wayne eventually died of lung cancer. Researchers found increasing evidence relating tobacco use to heart disease, respiratory disease, and numerous cancers. Then with the news that even secondhand smoke could cause illness, parents began to think twice about smoking around their children and nonsmokers started to lobby for clean air in the workplace.

Antitobacco legislation has been successful in increasing public awareness of the dangers of tobacco use, limiting how and where tobacco advertisements can appear, and restricting where people can smoke. Health risk warnings appear on all cigarette packages and advertisements. Government buildings are, by law, off-limits for smoking, and many private companies have followed suit. About 80 percent of states have laws banning smoking in public-sector workplaces and 30 percent have similar legislation for the private sector. Congress banned smoking on all domestic flights under six hours. Now, confronted by a changing public opinion, some shopping malls, restaurants, and bars have become completely smoke free. Recognizing consumer preferences, most hotels offer nonsmoking rooms and some car rental companies offer smoke free cars.

In 1995 the Surgeon General labeled nicotine an addictive drug, and in 1997 the FDA took the same action. If the FDA's decision survives legal action brought by the tobacco interests, nicotine will remain a controlled substance under more restrictive government regulations than before. Tobacco companies have also been feeling pressure from class action and law suits and those brought by states. States argue that tobacco companies have known about the risks of their products, have not been forthcoming with the public, and should now pay for the high costs of health care resulting from tobacco-related illnesses. The White House has targeted tobacco companies for advertising campaigns allegedly aimed at children. In 1996 President Clinton supported the FDA regulation that included banning vending machines in places where minors have access, banning advertisements within 1,000 feet of schools, allowing only black-and-white outdoor advertisements, requiring age verifi-

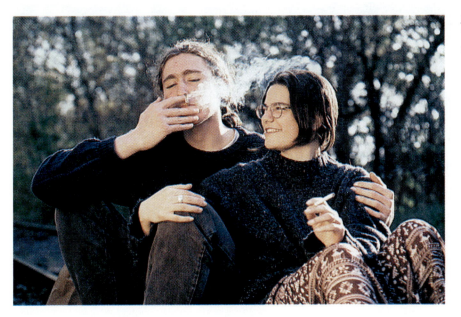

Mistakenly, smoking continues to be seen as "cool" by many young people, who often think they won't become addicted.

cation for all over-the-counter sales, and more. Despite all the pressure and restrictions, tobacco companies service over 48 million American smokers, and the number of teenagers starting to smoke is on the rise.

Today about one-third of adults[22] and one-third of adolescents smoke.[23] The overall number of adult smokers declined 40 percent between 1965 and 1990 and then leveled off between 1990 and 1994.[24] Unfortunately smoking among young people is on the rise, and the largest increase is happening among the youngest smokers. The average age for starting to smoke cigarettes is thirteen, for smokeless tobacco an appalling age ten. The University of Michigan's Monitoring the Future Project reported a 30 percent increase in smoking among eighth graders between 1991 and 1994.[25] Children who grow up around smoke are more likely to become smokers themselves. And according to the U.S. Department of Health and Human Services, white adolescents (20 percent) are more apt to smoke frequently than African American (5 percent) and Hispanic (10 percent) students.[26] Education is also a predictor of who smokes. Adults with less than a twelfth-grade education are twice as likely to be smokers than college graduates, and school dropouts are three times more likely to smoke. This does not mean, however, that tobacco is absent from college campuses. In 1993 one in seven college students was a daily smoker.

Another trend is the increased use of smokeless tobacco, particularly among young men. Snuff, once an older man's product, is now more popular with teenage boys. The Centers for Disease Control and Prevention's 1995 Youth Risk Behavior Survey reported that about 20 percent of male high school students used **smokeless tobacco.**[27] A small percentage of girls also use it to curb their appetites. About 6 percent of men and 1 percent of women eighteen years and older use snuff or chewing tobacco nationwide.[28] Smokeless tobacco is being aggressively marketed with an image of athleticism and machismo; sales have increased 40 percent since 1970. Studies indicate that 20 to 50 percent of college-level athletes (varsity and intramural athletes) use it, along with about 34 percent of the major league baseball players.[29, 30]

Why Do People Smoke?

Tobacco-related illnesses are completely preventable. If you don't smoke, chew tobacco, or put up with secondhand smoke, you drop your risk to zero. Why is it, then, that tobacco-related illness remains so prevalent in the United States? A number of reasons were given at the beginning of the chapter, such as seductive advertising, rebellion, and emulation of a role model. Additional reasons, more specific to tobacco use, are discussed in Activity 14.2.

In addition, many new smokers underestimate the strength of a nicotine addiction or overestimate their ability to control it. They may think that they are invincible, too smart, or too healthy to succumb to an addiction. For many, however, quitting is very difficult. Ninety percent of new smokers are children or teenagers. Almost all first use of tobacco occurs before high school graduation.[31] In other words, people who don't start smoking in high school (or earlier) usually don't start at all. If you are already a smoker, this information is not personally helpful; however, if as a community we can stop young people from starting, we can have a huge impact.

What's in a Tobacco Product?

The *psychoactive* (mood-altering) drug in tobacco is an alkaloid poison called *nicotine*. In low doses, nicotine

---

Activity 14.2 Why Do You Smoke?

Identify the reason(s) you smoke, then consider the intervention ideas in parentheses.

———— I enjoy the stimulation and the lift of energy I get when I smoke. (substitute exercise, nutritious foods, rest)

———— I enjoy handling the cigarette and playing with it in my hand. (substitute doodling, manipulating clay, or marbles)

———— Smoking helps me relax; it's pleasurable. (substitute talking to a friend, exercise, a hobby, or relaxation techniques, for example, meditation or massage)

———— I tend to smoke when I'm uncomfortable or stressed. (It's a crutch.) (confront your feelings, learn and use coping strategies, use humor, lean on a friend)

———— I crave smoking. I have a psychologically and/or physical need to smoke. (quit cold turkey, use a nicotine patch or gum to cut down slowly)

———— I smoke out of habit. I just automatically light up. (change your habits to gain awareness; for example, store your cigarettes in a different pocket)

———— I smoke to depress my appetite and control my weight. (moderate exercise before a meal can help suppress appetite, frequent small meals prevent dips in blood sugar that increase appetite; see Chapters 6 to 8)

acts as a stimulant, increasing heart rate, blood pressure, alertness, the ability to concentrate, and the speed at which information is processed. At higher doses, it acts as a sedative, reducing aggression and alleviating stress. These sound like pretty good reasons to smoke; the problem is, they come at a very high price.

A marine biologist put some of life's risks in perspective. He asked his audience to imagine a beautiful sunny day with people playing happily in the ocean surf. Suddenly a shrill cry of "shark" is issued. A stampede of panicked swimmers hit the beach, run to their cars, roll up the windows, and light up their cigarettes. He then added with a smile that in fifty-three years (1916–1969) there have been thirty-two attacks resulting in thirteen deaths by great white sharks, while fifty people die *each hour* from smoking-related illnesses. The sharks, he declared, are a much better risk!

How the Body Processes Nicotine, Tar, and Carbon Dioxide

Nicotine enters the bloodstream either through the lungs (cigarettes, cigars, pipes), through the membranes of the mouth (chewing tobacco or moist snuff), or through the membranes of the nose (dry snuff). Once in the bloodstream, it takes only a few seconds for nicotine to reach the brain. Users will smoke or use snuff at regular intervals in order to maintain a level of nicotine in their blood that produces a good feeling. The actual amount of nicotine required to induce this feeling varies among individuals. In one research study the amount of nicotine in the cigarettes was varied (raised or lowered) without the subjects' knowledge. The subjects unconsciously changed the number of cigarettes they smoked in order to achieve their desired level of nicotine. If the nicotine level drops, withdrawal symptoms occur, including a strong nicotine craving. This nicotine dependency is one of the main reasons quitting is so difficult.

Cigarette smoke contains tar, which is made up of over 4,000 chemicals, including forty-three known to cause cancer.[32] The dark sticky residue of tar and other substances coats clothing, hair, and furniture, giving them that characteristic smoker's odor. Tar also settles in your air passages. Smokers cough more but are less effective because the tar interferes with the cilia, hairlike structures that normally sweep foreign particles out of the lungs and bronchial tubes. With chronic bombardment the lung tissue beneath the cilia becomes susceptible, cells are altered, and the door is opened to cancer and/or chronic obstructive pulmonary disease (COPD).

Other chemicals found in cigarette smoke include cyanide, benzene, formaldehyde, methanol (wood alcohol), acetylene (the fuel used in torches), and ammonia.[33] Carbon monoxide, an odorless, colorless gas, is a by-product of burning tobacco (or gasoline). When carbon monoxide is inhaled into the lungs, it preempts oxygen, readily combining with hemoglobin. As a result poorly oxygenated blood is circulated out to the body. Low levels of carbon monoxide cause shortness of breath; higher levels can result in death by asphyxiation. (This is why people die when they inhale car fumes in an enclosed space.)

What Are the Short-Term Effects of Tobacco Use?

Everything on and around a smoker smells like smoke. Although this may not bother the smoker, it bothers other people and may drive away potential friends and turn off potential employers and clients. Snuff and chewing tobacco cause bad breath, stained teeth, tooth decay, gum disease, increased blood cholesterol, and dulled senses of taste and smell. Nonsmokers have been known to compare kissing a smoker to kissing an ashtray; needless to say, this could have an effect on your social life. Cigarette ash often burns holes in clothing and furniture, an added expense, and increases risk of injury or death by fire. Smoking is also detrimental to sports performance because it cuts down endurance. Other short-term effects of smoking include a loss of appetite that may result in unwanted weight loss, fatigue, hoarseness, stomach pains, insomnia, diarrhea, and impaired visual acuity, especially at night. When a person stops smoking, these symptoms usually disappear.

In small doses nicotine can make you ill; in high doses it is a poison. When a person first starts smoking, the effects of nicotine and other chemicals sometimes make him or her sick. Symptoms may include nausea, dizziness, clammy skin, light-headedness, rapid pulse, confusion, and vomiting. (This is the body's way of trying to tell us something.) As tolerance to nicotine develops, short-term sickness disappears, but long-term illnesses quietly begin.

What Are the Long-Term Effects of Tobacco Use?

Every year an estimated 419,000 U.S. smokers "quit" by dying of tobacco-related illnesses such as cardiovascular diseases, cancers, and respiratory diseases.[34]

Tobacco-related health problems in adults include lung, oral, larynx, esophageal, pancreatic, bladder, cervical, and uterine cancers; coronary heart disease; peripheral arterial disease; chronic obstructive pulmonary (lung) disease; emphysema; peptic ulcers; and miscarriages. Health problems in the infants and children of smokers include low birth weight, sudden infant death syndrome (SIDS), asthma, and respiratory infections.

Cardiovascular Diseases

The majority of tobacco-related deaths are the result of cardiovascular diseases, particularly coronary heart disease (CHD). This is why smoking is considered one of the primary risk factors for coronary heart disease. (Can you name the others?) Most people associate cancer with smoking and are unaware of the enormous impact smoking has on the circulatory system. Nearly one-fifth of deaths from cardiovascular diseases are attributable to smoking.[35] Smokers double their risk of heart disease[36] and significantly increase their risk for strokes. Tobacco substances affect the cardiovascular system by (1) causing a shortage of oxygen, (2) promoting atherosclerosis, and (3) forcing the heart to work harder than normal. Oxygen shortages occur when carbon monoxide interferes with normal oxygen-hemoglobin loading in the lungs and when arteries become too narrow to circulate oxygenated blood adequately. The mechanism is unknown, but somehow tobacco substances encourage atherosclerosis. One reason may be that the ratio of high-density lipoprotein (HDL) cholesterol to low-density lipoprotein (LDL) cholesterol is lower in cigarette smokers than nonsmokers.[37]

Pulmonary heart disease—damage to the right side of the heart—occurs when the arteries feeding the lungs are affected and the heart must push harder to force blood into these vessels. Smoking is also linked to an increased incidence of aortic aneurysm, a dangerous condition in which the aorta, the main artery taking blood to the body, becomes weakened and bulges. Finally, when a peripheral artery such as one supplying oxygen to the leg narrows or becomes blocked, leg cramping, numbness, and even gangrene can occur. Smoking is not the only cause for arterial disease but it is a major contributor—and a preventable one.

As the ability to deliver oxygen diminishes, it is not surprising that smokers have an increasingly difficult time being vigorously active. Physical activity increases the oxygen demands of the muscles, including the heart, at a time when the body is being robbed of oxygen. To make matters worse, nicotine's stimulating effect burdens the circulatory system by increasing the heart rate and blood pressure.

Cancers

Cancers develop in tissues and organs you would associate with tobacco use (such as the mouth and lungs) but also in organs deep in the body that are not as obviously connected to the act of smoking. Common cancer sites include the lips, mouth, gums, esophagus, trachea (windpipe), larynx (voice box), lungs, pancreas, kidney, colon, bladder, and uterine cervix. Lung cancer is the most common cancer among cigarette smokers whereas mouth and throat cancers are more common among smokeless tobacco and pipe users. Lung cancer was a relatively uncommon disease among women until they won the dubious right to smoke; then the incidence of lung cancer tripled. Death rates for lung cancer run twenty-three times higher for male smokers and eleven times higher for female smokers compared to those persons who have never smoked.[38] Smoking accounts for 87 percent of lung cancer and 29 percent of all cancer.[39] Nor is lung cancer limited to smokers; each year about 3,000 nonsmokers who work or live with smokers die of lung cancer.[40] For more information on cancer refer to Chapter 10.

Chronic Obstructive Pulmonary Disease

COPD is a category of diseases that affect the lungs, two of the most prevalent of which are emphysema and chronic bronchitis. When new smokers take their first drag on a cigarette they usually start coughing. Why? Because the smoke irritates the airways, and the reflex is to cough the irritant back out of the body. What starts as a simple smoker's cough can become a serious lung disease. The walls of the bronchial tubes secrete a sticky mucus that helps trap foreign particles, which in turn are swept upward by hairlike cilia through the trachea (windpipe), where they are finally expelled through the mouth.

Chronic smoking eventually paralyzes, damages, and destroys the cilia, knocking out one of the body's first lines of defense. Coughing (the smoker's hack) becomes more frequent, but less effective. Additional mucus is produced, but fewer cilia are available to expel it. Long bouts of coughing will occur as the situation worsens. Smoking a cigarette may actually stop the coughing by paralyzing the cilia. This solution, however, leaves the damaging substances inside the body. Harmful bacteria normally coughed out are also trapped in the body. As the pulmonary filter breaks down, these bacteria lodge in the lungs, where they can develop into illnesses such as pneumonia.

Over time, the harmful substances in smoke will cause the bronchial tubes to thicken, lose elasticity, and weaken. Increased pressure is required to force air through this damaged system. When the walls of the air vesicles (alveoli) in the lungs are damaged and ruptured by excessive respiratory effort, the condition is called pulmonary emphysema. Emphysema patients in the latter stages of the disease gasp for air and are dependent on oxygen by mask, catheter, or respirator. Eventually they die from suffocation, pneumonia, or congestive (right) heart failure. Cigarette smokers are eighteen times more likely to die from COPD than are nonsmokers.[41]

Tobacco, Pregnancy, and Smoking's Effect on Children

Smoking while pregnant can lead to serious complications in the newborn. Nicotine, carbon monoxide, and other dangerous chemicals cross the placenta and enter the baby's body. Statistics show a direct relation between smoking during pregnancy and spontaneous abortions, stillbirths, death among newborns, and sudden infant death syndrome.[42] The babies of mothers who smoke are also often born with lower birth weights.[43] Sadly, underweight infants are more likely to die in the first month of life, to have a stunted growth pattern, to suffer respiratory illness, or to develop lifelong disabilities than are normal-weight babies. In a study involving 30,000 pregnant women, preterm babies were 20 percent more common among women who smoked a pack or more a day.[44] In other studies, babies of mothers who smoked two or more packs a day scored lower on the developmental tests administered at birth and the long-term studies in progress are showing that these children don't catch up developmentally.[45]

Nicotine can be found in breast milk. The best thing a woman can do is stop smoking when she wants to get pregnant and abstain during the pregnancy and while nursing. Although abstinence throughout is the best, stopping at any point in the pregnancy is healthier for the baby.

For those trying to get pregnant, smoking is suspected to impair fertility in both men and women. For those avoiding pregnancy, risks for heart and blood vessel disease increase for women who both smoke and use oral contraception, especially after the age of thirty-five.

Children who grow up around **secondhand smoke,** smoke they breathe because someone else in the home smokes, experience an increased number of respiratory and ear infections, are more likely to develop asthma, bronchitis, and pneumonia, and as infants have a four times greater risk of dying from SIDS.[46] The chemicals in tobacco products permeate the body so much so that traces of tobacco chemicals can be found in the hair of newborns whose mothers either smoked themselves or spent time in a smoky environment.[47] Care must also be taken when tobacco products and children inhabit the same space. Infants and toddlers who ingest tobacco suffer nicotine poisoning. Because of their smaller body size even small amounts of nicotine can be deadly.

What About Secondhand Smoke?

For a long time people assumed that only smokers were at risk for their behavior. Today clear evidence of the dangers of secondhand smoke forcefully counter the "I'm only hurting myself" argument. This has provided powerful motivation for parents, spouses, and friends to quit smoking, or at the very least, not to smoke in the presence of others.

Secondhand smoke, or *environmental tobacco smoke (ETS)* comes from two sources. Mainstream smoke is exhaled by the smoker. Sidestream smoke comes directly from a burning cigarette. Eighty-five percent of the smoke in a room is sidestream smoke. This smoke is not filtered by the filter on the cigarette or through the smoker (whose lungs act as a filter). As a result, sidestream smoke has two to three times higher concentrations of many chemicals, including nicotine, tar, and the carcinogen benzopyrene, than does mainstream smoke.

In 1992 the U.S. Environmental Protection Agency (EPA) declared ETS a carcinogen and estimated that 3,000 American nonsmokers die each year from lung cancer caused by breathing the smoke of other people's ciga-rettes.[48] In addition, environmental tobacco smoke causes an estimated 35,000 to 40,000 deaths from heart disease in people who are not currently smoking.[49]

How Do You Quit?

Constraining regulations have made life more difficult for the smoker. In order to have a cigarette, people find themselves smoking in their car, in the bathroom, in a stairwell, or outside the door where they work. Either by choice or from family pressure, smokers are increasingly finding themselves banished to the porches of their own homes. In addition to the inconvenience and increasing cost of tobacco products, many smokers feel guilty that they are continuing a habit that they know is harmful to their own health and to the health of their family and friends. Many parents also feel badly that they are poor role models for their children.

Not surprisingly, many smokers would like to quit. In 1994, 69 percent of smokers said they would like to quit completely.[50] But nicotine is difficult to give up. When people stop smoking and the level of nicotine drops in their blood, they can experience severe cravings for it, nausea, insomnia, confusion, tremors, fatigue, headache, muscle spasms, irritability, anger, and depression. A person at this stage is not an easy person to live with! The worst of these symptoms occur in the first one to two weeks. This is when understanding friends make a big difference. Although it isn't easy, quitting is certainly doable. Forty million people have succeeded in kicking the habit and many more will join this group each year.[51]

At present the most successful quitters are those who do it on their own, meaning without a treatment program, but often with the support of friends and family. Of the 60 to 80 percent who quit smoking during a cessation treatment program, 75 percent return to smoking within a year. This is a success rate of only about 5 to 6 percent. The majority of people in treatment programs may fail because the program provides a crutch (as opposed to complete personal resolve) or because the program assumes everyone is ready to quit. The new research on behavior change indicates that although people are at various stages of change, most programs are uniform in their approach—usually targeting only one stage. They assume everyone is ready to quit. As programs adjust to meet the needs of people at each stage, the success rate may improve dramatically. For example, there is evidence that moving smokers just one stage can double the chances that they will take action on their own in the near future.[52,53]

Replacement therapy is a method of quitting in which nicotine is provided through a patch or gum rather than obtained through a tobacco product. The idea behind this kind of therapy is to break the habit of smoking first and then minimize withdrawal symptoms by slowly weaning the person off nicotine. The nicotine patch placed on an individual's skin releases nicotine equal to

A Strategy for How to Quit

Just Before Quitting

- Practice going without cigarettes.
- Don't think of *never* smoking again. Think of quitting in terms of *one day at a time.*
- Tell yourself you won't smoke today and then, don't.
- Clean your clothes to rid them of the cigarette smell, which can linger for a long time.

On the Day You Quit

- Throw away all your cigarettes and matches. Hide your lighters and ashtrays.
- Visit the dentist and have your teeth cleaned to get rid of tobacco stains. Notice how nice they look and resolve to keep them that way.
- Make a list of things you'd like to buy for yourself or someone else. Estimate the cost in terms of packs of cigarettes and put the money aside to buy these presents.
- Keep very busy on the big day. Go to the movies, exercise, take long walks, go bike riding.
- Remind your family and friends that this is your quit date and ask them to help you over the rough spots of the first couple of days and weeks.
- Buy yourself a treat or do something special to celebrate.

Immediately After Quitting

- Develop a clean, fresh, nonsmoking environment around yourself, at work, and at home. Buy yourself flowers. You may be surprised how much you can enjoy their scent now.
- The first few days after you quit, spend as much free time as possible in places where smoking isn't allowed, such as libraries, museums, theaters, department stores, and churches.
- Drink large quantities of water and fruit juice (but avoid sodas that contain caffeine).
- Try to avoid alcohol, coffee, and other beverages that you associate with cigarette smoking.
- Strike up a conversation instead of a match for a cigarette.
- If you miss the sensation of having a cigarette in your hand, play with something else, such as a pencil, a paper clip, a marble.

- If you miss having something in your mouth, try toothpicks or a fake cigarette.

Avoid Temptation

- Instead of smoking after meals, get up from the table and brush your teeth or go for a walk.
- If you always smoke while driving, listen to a particularly interesting radio program or your favorite music, or take public transportation for a while, if you can.
- For the first one to three weeks, avoid situations you strongly associate with the pleasurable aspects of smoking, such as watching your favorite TV program, sitting in your favorite chair, or having a cocktail before dinner.
- Until you are confident of your ability to stay off cigarettes, limit your socializing to healthful, outdoor activities or situations where smoking is not allowed.
- If you must be in a situation where you'll be tempted to smoke, such as a cocktail or dinner party, try to associate with the nonsmokers there.
- Try to analyze cigarette ads to understand how they attempt to "sell" you on individual brands.

When You Get the Crazies

- Keep oral substitutes handy. Try carrots, pickles, sunflower seeds, apples, celery, raisins, or sugarless gum instead of a cigarette.
- Take ten deep breaths and hold the last one while lighting a match. Exhale slowly and blow out the match. Pretend it's a cigarette and crush it out in an ashtray.
- Take a shower or bath if possible.
- Learn to relax quickly and deeply. Make yourself limp, visualize a soothing, pleasing situation, and get away from it all for a moment. Concentrate on that peaceful image and nothing else.
- Light incense or a candle instead of a cigarette.
- Never allow yourself to think that "one won't hurt"—it will.

Clearing the Air, National Institutes of Health.

---

about three-quarters of a pack over the course of a day. Each stick of nicotine gum provides the chewer with the amount of nicotine of about one cigarette. Replacement therapy works for some people and is certainly an option for those who can't quit cold turkey. There are several problems associated with the patch and gum. Both can make the individual sick, the patch may irritate the skin,

and the gum may irritate the mouth. Furthermore, neither product should be used by someone who is pregnant, has ulcers, or has some forms of heart disease. If you are considering using a patch or gum, consult your physician first.

Some people can quit cold turkey. This method is most effective with someone who really enjoys cigarettes or chewing tobacco. These people have too difficult a time decreasing their intake. It is better for them to just quit all at once. Sometimes people have found it helpful to smoke excessively right before they quit or to smoke a brand they dislike in an effort to spoil the taste for smoking. Kicking the smokeless tobacco habit may be even harder. In one study only one in fourteen could stop usage for more than four hours. This may be due to the higher concentrations of tar and nicotine in these products.

Another common cessation strategy is to slowly cut down on the number of cigarettes smoked. Some people achieve this by changing to a brand they don't like. Others smoke only half of each cigarette. Smoking the same number of weaker cigarettes is another way to taper off. However, if you smoke fewer cigarettes but inhale more, you are no better off and may actually be hurting yourself more, since deep inhalations draw the harmful chemicals deeper into the body. Smoking fewer cigarettes but smoking them farther down is also more dangerous. The last third of a cigarette is far worse than the first third, because the beginning of a cigarette is drawn through and filtered by the tobacco in front of it. When you smoke the last part of a cigarette you not only lose this filtering benefit, you are also smoking more toxic tobacco since its filtering action has resulted in a more concentrated level of chemicals. When smoking a brand low in tar and nicotine, partially blocking the filter (holding your finger over some of the holes) allows more nicotine and tar to come through, which again defeats the purpose.

Additional assistance may be found in support groups, acupuncture, hypnotherapy, and behavior modification therapy. Behavior change is easier when friends, family, and coworkers support the effort. Group therapy and support groups offer additional support from people who know firsthand what the former smoker is going through.

What's So Good About Quitting?

When the body is no longer being bombarded with chemicals, it has a chance to rid itself of some of the toxins. Nicotine is actually gone from the body in two to three days. Coughing may be more frequent in the beginning, but this quickly changes as respiratory passages clear. In just a few days food will begin to taste and smell better. The lungs begin to generate new tissue and you will start to breathe easier. For a time line of improvement see Table 14.2, When Smokers Quit. In 1990 the U.S. Surgeon General's Report announced that people who quit smoking, regardless of their age, live longer than those who continue to smoke.[54] It appears that even people with chronic bronchitis and emphysema improve somewhat when they quit smoking. Ten years without tobacco restores you to the same risk level as a nonsmoker. Although it is never too late to benefit from cessation, you gain more by stopping early.

Another big benefit is the money you save. A brand name pack of cigarettes costs roughly $2.50. At a pack a

TABLE 14.2 ■ When Smokers Quit.	
Within 20 Minutes of Smoking that Last Cigarette, the Body Begins a Series of Changes that Continue for Years	
20 minutes	• Blood pressure drops to a level close to that before the last cigarette • Temperature of hands and feet increases to normal
8 hours	• Carbon monoxide level in blood drops to normal
24 hours	• Chance of heart attack decreases
2 weeks to 3 months	• Circulation improves • Lung function increases up to 30%
1 to 9 months	• Coughing, sinus congestion, fatigue, shortness of breath decrease • Cilia regain normal function in lungs, increasing ability to handle mucus, clean the lungs, reduce infection
1 year	• Excess risk of coronary heart disease is half that of a smoker's
5 years	• Stroke risk is reduced to that of a nonsmoker's 5–15 years after quitting
10 years	• Lung cancer death rate about half that of a continuing smoker's • Risk of cancer of the mouth, throat, esophagus, bladder, kidneys, and pancreas decreases
15 years	• Risk of coronary heart disease is that of a nonsmoker's

When smokers quit. Reprinted by permission of The American Cancer Society, Inc. Includes information from *U.S. Surgeon General's Report, 1988,* 1990.

day, you spend $17.50 a week, or about $900 a year. This is enough to buy two round-trip plane fares, a very nice leather jacket, an old car or insurance on a new car, or about 100 pizzas!

There is no such thing as a healthy cigarette or tobacco product. Although cigarettes low in tar and nicotine may reduce some of the health risk, and although pipes are less harmful than cigarettes, they both endanger your health. It is hard to imagine that an industry can make a profit even though each year 2 million customers quit using their product, another 400,000 customers die from use of the product, their television and radio advertising is against the law, and a warning label is stamped on every package. Yet every third adult and every fifth teenager make this possible. Will you be their next recruit? Or one of this year's 2 million people who quit? Or part of the 70 percent of the adult U.S. population that continues to say, "No thanks"?

THE USE AND ABUSE OF DRUGS

There is a poignant duality with drugs. At one extreme is legitimate use and vital health care, and at the other, human despair and violent crime. For every miracle drug that saves a life, there is an illegal one that takes a life. The power of drugs to help and to hurt affects not just the individual, but also has a rippling effect that reaches everyone in the community.

Drugs can be classified into six categories. Information on each category and the most widely used substances follows. As you read, keep in mind that, unlike prescription and over-the-counter drugs, street drugs are not regulated for content or potency. Illegal drugs are often cut (diluted or mixed) with other drugs before being sold on the street. This makes the content of the drug and its subsequent effect unpredictable. Individuals have died from added poisons, from synergistic effects of combined drugs, or from clotting of the arteries caused by added unsafe substances.

Many drugs can be injected. Whenever a drug is injected with an unclean needle there is a risk of bacterial or viral infection, septicemia (blood poisoning), hepatitis, and AIDS. Even with clean needles a person who injects frequently can suffer skin sores, scarring, and collapsed veins.

Cannabis

Drugs derived from the *Cannabis sativa* or Indian hemp plant make up the Cannabis drug category. (The plant may also be known as the marijuana plant or as American hemp, hashish, bhang, or ganja.) The most common street form of Cannabis is marijuana, but it may also be purchased as hashish or hash oil. The latter two contain higher concentrations of the psychoactive ingredient THC (delta-9-tetrahydrocannabinol) than marijuana.

Cannabis drugs have hallucinogenic properties when taken in large enough doses, but because they have a wide range of effects, not always psychedelic, many experts prefer to classify them separately under the heading Cannabis than the heading hallucinogen.

Marijuana

Street Names: Pot, Grass, Weed, Roach, Mary Jane
Marijuana is the most widely used illegal drug in the United States. Only alcohol and tobacco (both legal for adults) are more popular recreational drugs.[55] Approximately 10 million Americans use marijuana each month.[56] Increased use of marijuana is occurring among young people in the eighth through twelfth grades, and researchers from the University of Michigan Institute for Social Research think this increase is connected to a drop in the number of young people who believe illicit drugs are dangerous.[57]

Marijuana can be legally prescribed by a physician for the treatment of glaucoma (an eye disease that can cause blindness), to alleviate chemotherapy-induced nausea, and to increase appetite in some cancer patients. Marijuana has a long history as a folk medicine, and at the turn of the century in the United States many physicians used it to treat headaches, insomnia, menstrual cramps, and other ailments.[58] It was also used as an analgesic and sedative, but these practices were discontinued as its mood-altering side effects became known.

Marijuana is inexpensive, fairly simple to grow, and easy to obtain on the illicit market. The crushed leaves and flower tops of the plant can be eaten (usually in brownies or cookies or made into tea) or rolled in paper to make a smokeable joint or reefer. Smoking a joint produces stronger, quicker effects, taking roughly twenty to thirty minutes to reach a peak, followed by a sustained high for one or two hours. Marijuana produces a euphoric hallucinogenic high often followed by a period of sedation and tranquility. A sense of depersonalization can occur, with the effect of making the body seem very light, or give the user the sensation of floating above the body. This separation, especially for those accustomed to the drug, can be pleasurable, but others find it very frightening. Users also report altered perceptions of time and space and heightened sensory awareness such as keener sight or smell. The psychological effects of the drug vary, and expectation may play a role in marijuana's effect on an individual. Some first-time users do not feel the effects at all. For others, the feelings may range from deep relaxation to panicked anxiety attacks.

Short-term negative effects of marijuana include a disruption of short-term memory; interference with learning, reading comprehension, speech, and problem-solving abilities; difficulty concentrating; and periods of confusion. The drug can slow down reaction time, decrease coordination, and interfere with the ability to track a moving object—all of which make it very dangerous to drive under its influence. Marijuana users are often spotted by their red eyes, dilated pupils, and lethargic movements. They may also experience an increased heart rate, dry throat, and increased appetite.

The full ramifications of long-term marijuana use are as yet unknown. Serious studies of marijuana began thirty years ago, and the medical community warns that some negative effects may take more than thirty years to appear. (Bear in mind that some tobacco-related diseases do not surface for fifty years or more.) The potency of marijuana today is greater than that used in the 1960s, which means that the long-range effects of today's drug may be different from that of the less-potent drug of the sixties.

However, there is evidence that frequent use of marijuana can lead to serious health problems. Most marijuana smokers inhale and intentionally hold the smoke in their lungs in an effort to maximize the drug's effect; this creates a greater potential for lung tissue damage. Someone who smokes marijuana regularly may have many of the same respiratory problems that tobacco smokers have, such as a daily cough and phlegm, symptoms of chronic bronchitis, and more frequent chest colds. Continuing to smoke marijuana can lead to abnormal functioning of the lungs and airways. Scientists have found signs of lung tissue injured or destroyed by marijuana smoke.[59]

Marijuana has a dramatic effect on the brain.

THC suppresses the neurons in the information-processing system of the hippocampus, the part of the brain that is crucial for learning, memory, and the integration of sensory experiences with emotions and motivation. Researchers have discovered that learned behaviors, which depend on the hippocampus, deteriorate after chronic exposure to THC. Chronic abuse of marijuana also is associated with impaired attention and memory, while prenatal exposure to marijuana is associated with impaired verbal reasoning and memory in preschool children.[60]

A drug that negatively influences motivation, learning, and memory would seem to be an unlikely choice for college students, yet marijuana use among college students is widespread. It takes about a month to rid the body of THC after just one use, which means that if you use it more than once a month, THC will accumulate in your fatty tissues in much higher concentrations. The long-term effects of this are as yet unknown.

Psychological dependence on marijuana has been shown to occur among frequent marijuana users, and withdrawal symptoms, which include irritability, loss of appetite, sleeplessness, and nausea, have been noted when people who regularly smoke more than five marijuana cigarettes daily stop using the drug abruptly.[61] There has been much debate as to whether marijuana use leads to the use of other, more harmful drugs. Although most marijuana users do not go on to use other illegal drugs, most users of heroin, LSD, and cocaine have used marijuana.[62] This may be less a phenomenon of marijuana leading to a desire for a stronger drug and more a case of being in touch with the drug culture, which makes the next drug more accessible. Either way it acts as a conduit to more dangerous drugs.

Stimulants

Stimulants are a group of drugs that excite the central nervous system, which means that they increase heart rate, blood pressure, and body temperature. They provide extra energy, often allowing a person to continue an activity for an extended period of time with a price of deep exhaustion when the effect wears off or the body can no longer sustain it. Light to moderate use is associated with this boost of energy and feelings of pleasure and well-being. The long-term effects of heavier doses include nervousness, confusion, anxiety, loss of appetite, weight loss, malnutrition, insomnia, circulatory problems, heart complications, and strokes. Stimulants range from caffeine to amphetamines to cocaine.

Cocaine

Street Names: Coke, C, Snow, Peruvian Lady, White Girl, Happy Dust, Toot, Flake, Blow **Cocaine** is the second most popular illegal drug in the United States.[63] In 1994, almost 22 million Americans age twelve and older had tried cocaine at least once in their lifetime, about 3.7 million had used cocaine during the past year, and more than 1.3 million had used cocaine in the past month. These were significant decreases in cocaine use from its peak in 1985. Use of crack cocaine declined from 1991 to 1992, but has risen again to exceed 1991 levels. In 1994, about 4 million people had used crack cocaine at least once in their lives, and about 1.2 million people had used crack within the past year.[64]

Cocaine comes from the leaves of the coca plant found mostly in Central and South America. Just chewing the leaves can provide mild euphoria, stimulation, and increased alertness. A two-step chemical process separates the psychoactive ingredient cocaine hydrochloride, or simply cocaine, from the rest of the plant's chemicals. The drug was first isolated in 1855 and became popular as a local anesthetic in minor surgery. Although it is occasionally still used as a topical anesthetic, other drugs such as lidocaine are more widely used for anesthesia today. Cocaine has been abused for years but became a popular recreational drug in the late 1970s and 1980s. It was initially too expensive for the average drug abuser and became known as the wealthy man's drug.

Cocaine resembles flour. It is a fine, white, fluffy, odorless powder with a bitter taste. Most users snort cocaine. "Snorting" or "doing lines" means to chop the cocaine into a fine powder on a piece of glass with a razor blade, put it in a line, and then sniff it into the nose through a straw or a rolled-up dollar bill, or off a special coke spoon. The drug is absorbed through the nasal membranes, travels into the bloodstream, and hits the brain in about three minutes. The high will last between twenty minutes and several hours depending on the amount, strength, and purity of the drug. To achieve a faster, more intense rush, some abusers inject cocaine directly into their bloodstream. The effect is felt in about thirty seconds, but does not last as long as snorting. Smoking cocaine as freebase or crack results in an almost instantaneous rush. The slowest, least effective way to abuse cocaine is to swallow it. It takes ten to thirty minutes to feel the effect.

Freebase is a more powerful derivative of cocaine that is obtained by chemically separating the freebase from the street powder. In the last step of the process a fast-drying solvent like ether is added, and the mixture, usually in a water pipe, is heated with a torch and smoked. One of the dangers of freebasing is that the ether can explode in your face. The drug's effect is a powerful high that lasts for a few minutes.

Crack is a crystallized form of freebase that has rapidly gained popularity on the streets. It is sold as ready-to-smoke rocks that don't explode. Crack is 90 percent pure cocaine and about five times as potent as street cocaine. It provides an intense high that lasts longer than freebase, and is marketed in small, affordable doses. The name "crack" comes from the crackling or popping sounds it makes when it is burned. Crack appears to be less expensive than cocaine, but the illusion is similar to that of buying individual cups of coffee rather than a pound of coffee: each cup is relatively inexpensive, but you are paying more per cup. Crack users rarely stop with one purchase, so the price adds up quickly. Crack treated with PCP (see page 334) is said to be "space-based"—a combination that is both dangerous and highly unpredictable.

When smoked, crack takes only four to six seconds to hit, and the high lasts for as long as twenty minutes. The intense rush is so desirable, and the depression in between hits is so awful, that users will generally continue to smoke until they are out of the drug or out of money, or their bodies give out. A fortunate few shake their addiction in treatment programs. This is an extremely psychologically addicting drug.

Cocaine users who snort often develop a congested, inflamed, constantly running nose and eventually perforate the nasal septum (the wall between the right and left sides of the nose). High doses of cocaine can cause nervousness, dizziness, blurred vision, vomiting, tremors, seizures, high blood pressure, strokes, angina, and cardiac arrhythmias. A cocaine psychosis marked by paranoia and hallucinations may also develop. An overdose of cocaine or one of its derivatives can cause sudden death from respiratory paralysis, cardiac arrhythmias (irregular heartbeats), or severe convulsions. Len Bias, a talented University of Maryland basketball player, and Don Rogers, a professional football player, both died suddenly of cocaine-induced heart attacks in 1986. Actor John Belushi died in 1982 of an overdose when he injected a combination of cocaine and heroin called a "speedball." These deaths startled the nation and made many more people aware of the dangers of cocaine. The increasing number of babies affected by cocaine has led some states to consider legal prosecution of women who use cocaine during pregnancy. Cocaine babies are born addicted, must go through the agony of withdrawal, and often suffer long-term disabilities.

Amphetamines

Street Names: Uppers, Speed, Ups, Pep Pills **Amphetamines** are synthetic chemicals (as opposed to plant derivatives) that are strong central nervous system stimulants. Many of the amphetamine capsules look like their street names. For example, a bumblebee is a yellow and black capsule. Hearts are red, white crosses are white imprinted with an X, and black beauties are obviously black. Amphetamines can be taken as capsules, tablets, or injections or as powders inhaled through the nose. Like other stimulants, amphetamines elevate heart rate and blood pressure and in high doses can cause an irregular heartbeat. When injected, these drugs can cause a sharp rise in blood pressure, which can lead to a stroke, high fever, or heart failure. Users may feel anxious, nervous, uneasy, or restless. Long-term heavy users may develop an amphetamine psychosis characterized by hallucinations, delusions, and paranoia. These drugs are taken recreationally both for their energy-producing effect and to counteract the depressing effect of other drugs.

Methamphetamine

Street Names: Crank, Ice, Crystal Meth, Speed, Glass, Crock, Go-far, Go-fast, Batu, Cristy, Zip (These names represent a variety of drugs under the category of methamphetamine.) **Methamphetamine** is a subgroup of amphetamines that have grown rapidly in street popularity. Crank, once a street name for cocaine, is now the name of a methamphetamine commonly sold on the illegal market. It is an odorless, yellow, off-white substance that can be purchased as capsules, chunks, or crystals. It can be sniffed, inhaled, or injected, with the latter providing almost an immediate rush. The effects can last two to four hours. A day's supply is often one-eighth of an ounce, which is referred to as an "eightball." A common hallucination reported by those with crank psychosis is that of bugs crawling under the skin.

Ice or crystal meth is a crystallized form of crank that is smoked. It is very popular because it is less expensive than crack (same price per gram, but smaller doses are required), and the rush lasts as long as twenty-four hours. Unfortunately it is also more addictive than crack. It can cause lethargy, severe depression, paranoia, acute psychoses, hallucinations, and cardiopulmonary damage. One reason ice is easy to get is that it is easy to make. It is extracted from common industrial chemicals using relatively inexpensive equipment and the chemistry knowledge of a high school graduate.

Caffeine

Although **caffeine** is certainly not in the same league as crack or speed, it is considered a drug because high doses can result in dependency, tolerance, and withdrawal symptoms. Long-term heavy use of caffeine may be linked to an increased risk of cancer, heart disease, and digestive problems. Long-term abuse of caffeine may also lead to an increased risk of pancreatic cancer. Fetal growth may be retarded when caffeine is abused, but the studies at this point are inconclusive.

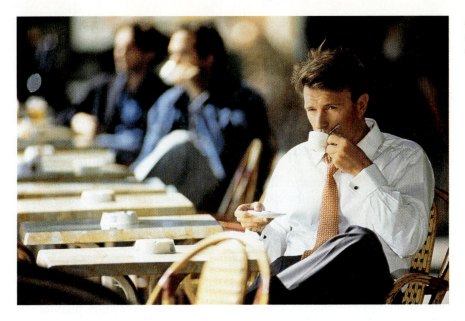

In the coffee-crazed society of late, few people acknowledge the potential hazards of caffeine.

Caffeine is attractive to many people because it increases alertness, which enhances attention and endurance during repetitive tasks, and it suppresses appetite. It also helps relieve some types of migraine headaches by constricting the blood vessels in the brain. Prescribed by a doctor, it can be used to counteract drugs that cause depression, or used to calm hyperactive children by increasing the child's ability to concentrate. Some endurance athletes have used caffeine to improve their performance, but for most people the difference it makes is too slight to be of significance. It is a diuretic, and often the urge to urinate it creates can be a nuisance.

Too much caffeine can make you nervous, jittery, anxious, or edgy. It can also upset your stomach, cause a fast and irregular heartbeat, interfere with fine motor coordination, and aggravate premenstrual symptoms. As with all stimulants, blood pressure increases; this is especially bad for people with circulatory problems, particularly hypertension. People with peptic ulcers should also avoid caffeine because of its acidic nature.

Caffeine comes from the seeds of the coffee, cocoa, and cola plants and from the leaves of the *Thea sinensis* plant from which most tea is harvested. You are probably aware that coffee, tea, caffeinated sodas, and chocolates all contain caffeine, but did you know that appetite suppressants and some over-the-counter cold and allergy medicines also contain it? It is used in cold and allergy medicines to offset the sedation effect of antihistamines. Caffeine may be taken in tablet form; two of the most common trade names are NoDoz and Vivarin. One tablet equals about two cups of coffee. During final exams or right before an assignment is due, some students pull all nighters with the use of these pills, sometimes washed down with other caffeinated products. During hot weather, iced coffee and iced tea are popular, and a lot of people inadvertently increase their caffeine intake by drinking more volume (cold drinks are served in bigger portions than hot drinks).

Although the caffeine content of all beverages is dependent on the strength with which they are made, normal daily consumption is considered to be two six-ounce cups of coffee or twenty ounces of soda. (See Table 14.3.) Heavier use can be both physically and psychologically addictive. Withdrawal symptoms of headache, fatigue, drowsiness, nausea, and a shorter attention span have been reported.

If you think you are consuming too much caffeine, here are a few quick tips that may help you cut down:

1. Dilute caffeinated coffee with decaffeinated coffee in increasing amounts.
2. Use instant coffee rather than brewed coffee, since it has about half as much caffeine.
3. Pour only half a cup of coffee or one small glass of soda at a time to make yourself aware of your consumption.
4. Drink decaffeinated iced coffees and decaffeinated or herbal iced teas when possible.
5. Limit yourself to less chocolate by trying desserts of other flavors or selecting desserts that are topped with chocolate but not made of chocolate.

TABLE 14.3 ■ Amounts of Caffeine in Various Beverages

Beverage	Caffeine (mg)
Brewed coffee	100
Instant coffee (rounded teaspoon)	55–60
Cola (12 oz)	40–50
Tea	35–40
Cocoa	5
Decaffeinated coffee	2

Hallucinogens

Hallucinogens interfere with brain chemistry by blocking or enhancing the transmission of neural signals. They do this by interfering with the neural transmitters responsible for carrying neural messages across the synapses (gaps) between nerves. The effect of a drug depends on which neural transmitters are disrupted or enhanced. A drug may block, weaken, or distort the transmission of one kind of message (for example, pain, sense of time, or coordinated movement) and enhance the transmission of another (for example, emotion, color, or movement), making it stronger than it should be. As messages are altered, a dreamlike state occurs in which reality is confused and a person may see and hear things that don't exist. In some cases people have been known to try to fly out windows and walk on water.

There are two kinds of hallucinogens—natural ones, which are found in plants, and synthetic ones, which are manufactured in a laboratory. The two most common natural hallucinogens are mescaline and psilocybin. Mescaline comes from the button-shaped crown on the peyote cactus plant and can be eaten either fresh or dried (mescal button) or brewed into peyote tea. Psilocybin is contained in a particular kind of mushroom. Users eat these so-called "magic mushrooms." LSD (lysergic acid diethylamide) and PCP (phencyclidine) are the two most popular synthetic hallucinogens. LSD is 100 times stronger than psilocybin and 4,000 times stronger than mescaline.[65]

Most hallucinogens increase heart rate and blood pressure, dilate the eyes, cause tremors, reduce appetite, and interfere with sleep. Prolonged heavy use interferes with abstract reasoning, memory, and attention span.

PCP

PCP (phencyclidine), a white powder usually referred to as "Angel Dust," is easy to make and cheap to buy. Because it was once used as a sedative by veterinarians, it also has street names like "hog" and "horse tranquilizer." (PCP is no longer used with animals.) PCP can be swallowed, snorted, injected, sprinkled on marijuana cigarettes and smoked or, taken in liquid form added to cocaine. The latter is a dangerous, often deadly combination. In very small doses PCP decreases inhibition and provides a sense of euphoria, but even a small increase in dosage can result in extremely violent and unpredictable behavior. The effects usually last between four and six hours. Other negative effects range from speech and vision impairment to convulsions, delirium, paranoia, heart and lung failure, or stroke.

Depressants

Barbiturates, Tranquilizers, Alcohol, Quaaludes

Street Name: Downers Depressants are so named because they depress the central nervous system, slowing down brain function. These drugs can have a sedating (tranquilizing), hypnotic (sleep inducing), anticonvulsant, or anesthetic effect depending on their type and dosage. Drugs in this category include alcohol, barbiturates, tranquilizers, and methaqualone (quaaludes). Alcohol is of course legal to purchase, and barbiturates and tranquilizers are available by prescription. Methaqualone, which was once a prescription drug, is no longer legally available.

Abuse of these drugs is often motivated by a desire to replace stress and anxiety with relaxation and euphoria. To achieve this people exceed the recommended dosages of prescribed drugs. Extra drugs are obtained either by visiting numerous doctors and receiving "extra" prescriptions or by purchasing them illegally. Abuse may take the form of high doses over extended periods of time or binging.

Barbiturates

Barbiturates are synthetic drugs with short, medium, or long-lasting effects. Although medicinally many of the barbiturates have been replaced by tranquilizers, some still have important medical roles. For example, phenobarbital is a long-lasting anticonvulsant used to control epileptic seizures. Secobarbital (Secodal), which lasts for two to four hours, is still used for short-term insomnia, and Thiopental, a fast-acting, short lasting barbiturate, is injected before surgery for its anesthetic qualities.

Barbiturates can cause a state of drunkenness, loss of inhibition, boisterous or violent behavior, decreased muscle control, depression, and sedation. Psychological addiction can occur in as little as three weeks, which is one reason physicians quickly switched to prescribing tranquilizers when they became available. Physical tolerance requires the person to take more drug for the same effect but it does not, in the case of barbiturates, raise the amount of drug it takes to overdose. This means that the abuser is playing with a narrower and narrower margin for error. During the mid-1980s, barbiturates were responsible for 75 percent of all drug-related deaths, mainly as a result of overdosing.[66]

Mixing barbiturates with alcohol is a lethal combination. Both are depressants and both depend on the liver to metabolize them, yet together they greatly reduce the liver's ability to function, which means the concentration levels of these drugs keeps on rising. High concentrations lead to coma and death.

Barbiturates are generally taken by capsule or pill, but they may also be injected. Some people use them with heroin to boost its effect. An addict should not try to quit these drugs without help, as this can be life threatening. Withdrawal symptoms include insomnia, convulsions, shaking, delirium, and hallucinations. Withdrawal starts about twelve to twenty-four hours after the last dose and can last as long as two weeks.

Tranquilizers

Tranquilizers are categorized as major or minor. Both types are powerful drugs. Major tranquilizers (phenothiazines) are prescribed by doctors to treat severe mental disorders, while minor tranquilizers (benzodiazepines) are used to treat anxiety, insomnia, and epilepsy. In popular usage, the term *tranquilizer* refers only to the minor tranquilizers. Trade names of some of the most commonly prescribed minor tranquilizers are Valium, Librium, Xanax, and Halcion. Even though there was a 30 percent decline in the number of prescriptions written for tranquilizers between 1975 and 1980, in the 1980s minor tranquilizers were the most frequently prescribed drugs in the United States. According to the 1990 NIDA Household Survey nearly 8.6 million Americans age twelve or older had misused tranquilizers at least once, and over one million reported misusing them in the month prior to the survey. Tranquilizers are generally used medically for very short periods of time. Physical addiction can occur with chronic use in as little as four weeks, but may take several months. Like barbiturates, tranquilizers should never be mixed with another drug without a physician's approval. Nor should alcohol be mixed with tranquilizers—the result may be a very depressing lethal dose.

Opiates and Narcotics

True opiate drugs are derived from the poppy plant, but in common usage the word *opiate* includes chemically similar synthetic drugs like methadone. A more accurate scientific term for synthetic opiates is *opioids*. Similar confusion surrounds the word *narcotic,* which is often used to refer to a spectrum of illegal drugs, but is in its strictest definition synonymous with the term *opiate*.

Opium is harvested from the pods of the poppy plant *(Papaver somniferum)* as a sticky, brownish substance. Refined it becomes heroin, morphine, and codeine. These drugs are excellent painkillers, with actions that mimic endorphins, the body's natural painkillers. Some opiates also inhibit certain muscle contractions. Morphine, for example, is used to treat severe diarrhea because it inhibits the muscle contractions behind the waves of peristalsis that move food through the digestive system. Codeine is added to some cold medicines as a cough suppressant because of its ability to inhibit the muscle contractions involved in the cough reflex. Opiates also act as a central nervous system depressant, which explains why high doses can be dangerous.

In low doses, over a short period of time, these drugs are not addictive, but high doses taken repeatedly can result in strong psychological and physical addictions. Addiction can occur in as little as two weeks of regular use. Severe nausea is common among first-time users, but as tolerance is acquired, the nausea usually subsides. Eventually the body will require more and more drug to postpone withdrawal symptoms of nausea, abdominal cramps, sweating, trembling, aching muscles, weakness, irritability, loss of appetite, and sleep interruption. Long-term users may actually reach a point where their tolerance is so great that they do not get a high from the drug—only avoidance of withdrawal symptoms. Scien-

tists are investigating whether the ingestion of opiates diminishes the number of endorphins produced by the body. If opiates are replacing endorphins, stopping or diminishing opium intake may leave the body short on painkillers. This may help explain the agony of withdrawal. Scientists are also investigating whether people with low levels of endorphins are more easily addicted to opium. The craving for opium is so strong that relapse following detoxification is common. Treatment for an opium addiction usually consists of a maintenance program on a less harmful drug such as methadone.

Opiates in the United States are generally obtained in pill form and either swallowed or ground into a powder. The powder is sniffed or mixed with water, heated, and then injected. Some abusers drink prescription cough syrups for the codeine. Opiate side effects include dizziness, nausea, sweating, uncoordinated muscle movement, and general body weakness. Heavy use can also result in loss of sexual desire. Mixing an opiate with another sedative or taking an overdose can depress the systems of the body to the point of death. Respiratory and circulatory collapse are the two most common causes of death from overdose.

Heroin

After a significant drop in popularity, heroin use is once again on the rise. Heroin can be smoked (called "chasing the dragon"), snorted, or injected. Injection is by far the most common method in the United States. Injected heroin provides a rush of pleasure followed by up to several hours of drowsy euphoria ("nodding"). Side effects include sleepiness, slow, shallow breathing, a loss of appetite, constipation, and loss of sexual desire. Malnutrition is common among addicts because they don't feel like eating. Heroin is highly addictive and the user must have some every eight to twelve hours or experience withdrawal symptoms of chills, nausea, aches, diarrhea, and muscle spasms. Withdrawal usually lasts three to five days, but some symptoms may linger for weeks.

Children born to heroin users are more likely to be premature and may get sick more often. Children may also be addicted and have to suffer withdrawal symptoms of vomiting, restlessness, and seizures, which can last for several weeks. Pregnant women who use heroin should not stop taking it on their own because of the risk of a premature birth. They should, however, see a physician as soon as they suspect they are pregnant.

Methadone

Methadone, a synthetic opium, provides relief from withdrawal symptoms, but is not euphoric. Methadone is often used in the treatment of heroin addicts. The dosage given is decreased over time. The craving for heroin, however, is so strong, even for long periods following treatment, that some professionals advocate supplying former addicts with methadone injections indefinitely. They believe that the synthetic opium is filling a need that the body can't naturally meet. Other experts see this as simply substituting one bad habit for another instead of concentrating on helping the abuser achieve a drug-free existence.

Inhalants

As the name **inhalants** indicates, the vapors of certain substances can be deeply inhaled in order to obtain a mind-altering effect. The substances used are not illegal to buy and as such are not drugs. However, when a substance like glue or aerosol paint is inhaled, it acts like a drug. People generally use inhalants to get an inexpensive high. The act of inhaling is called "huffing."

Short-term negative effects consist of nausea, nosebleeds, lack of coordination, fatigue, loss of appetite, impaired judgment, and either a quickening or depressing of heart rate and respiration. Continued use of inhalants can cause brain damage, hepatitis, kidney damage, violent behavior, disorientation, unconsciousness, asphyxiation, and death.

Designer Drugs

The chemical formula of an illegal drug is used to officially describe it. Legal restrictions are then placed on the use and sale of the substances defined by these formulas. Underground chemists alter the formulas enough to produce an analog, something that has roughly the same effects but is not "officially" restricted. These chemists are able to change the formulas faster than the U.S. Drug Enforcement Administration can write the regulations making them controlled substances.

Designer narcotics, amphetamines, and methamphetamine already exist in abundance. Synthetic heroin, China white, MPTP, EVE, PCP, PCE, and MDMA (also known as Ecstacy, Adam, or Essence) are just a few of the **designer drugs** available. The unpredictability of these drugs makes them particularly dangerous. Analogs may be hundreds of times stronger than the original drug or have unexpected side effects. China white, for example, was marketed as a safe alternative to heroin, but it turned out to be *thousands* of times more potent and has caused numerous accidental overdoses.

Over-the-Counter and Prescription Drugs

Hospital emergency rooms treat about the same number of people for misuse of legal drugs as illegal drugs. Health problems from medications can be the result of taking combinations of drugs without consulting a doctor, taking the wrong amount of a drug, or taking a drug more frequently than is recommended. Before taking two drugs together, you should check with your doctor or a pharmacist. Mixing any drug with alcohol can be dangerous. The synergistic action of two drugs can be very different and much more potent than either drug

alone. The idea that more is better does not hold with medications. Taking a higher dose than recommended can lead to side effects or overdose. Another hazard is using over-the-counter drugs or other products for purposes other than for which they were intended. For example, some people drink cough syrup, or even hairspray, for their alcohol content.

Prescription drugs need to be taken in the right dosage for a designated amount of time. Altering either of these can render the medicine ineffective or result in

Warning Signs for a Drug or Alcohol Problem

One or more of the following warning signs may indicate a drinking or drug problem. If, after reading this list, you think someone is in trouble, see the box on page 337 on how to help a friend. If you think you have a problem, talk to someone you trust about it.

- Getting drunk or high on drugs on a regular basis
- Telling lies, particularly about how much alcohol or other drugs he or she is using or what he or she has been doing
- Avoiding friends, especially friends who don't use drugs or alcohol, in order to go get drunk or high
- Giving up activities and relationships he or she used to like or used to believe were important, such as studies, sports, and family
- Planning drinking or drug use in advance, hiding alcohol, drinking or using other drugs alone
- Having a tolerance to a substance and therefore using more to get the same effect
- Complaining that activities that don't include alcohol or drugs are boring or no fun
- Frequent hangovers or other chronic conditions such as a runny, inflamed nose or chronic cough
- Pressuring others to drink or use other drugs
- Taking risks, including sexual risks
- Experiencing blackouts (forgetting what he or she did while drinking) and pretending to remember what happened or laughing it off as "no big deal"
- Change in moods and character—looking and feeling agitated, irritable, depressed, run-down, or suicidal
- Acting self-centered, not caring about others (especially if this is a dramatic change in character)
- Loss of interest in sex, food, hobbies, or friends
- Breaking the law: drinking and driving, illegally purchasing drugs and alcohol, disturbing the peace, and less respect or concern for authority
- Constantly talking about drinking or using drugs
- Asking to borrow money or having financial difficulties
- Unusually excitable behavior followed by periods of depression

complications. Imagine the effect of cutting back on an antidepressant drug in order to save money. Drugs like Prozac need to be maintained at a certain level over extended periods of time; they are not meant to be cycled. Another common abuse is the handing of prescription medications to someone else. Let's say Mary pulls a muscle and the doctor gives her some muscle relaxants. Then her friend Joe hurts his back and in trying to help him, Mary gives him some of her relaxants. But because Mary is not a doctor, she doesn't know whether this is the right treatment for Joe. He may be on other medications that will react to the prescription drug; the dosage may not be right for him; he may have a physical condition like high blood pressure that is affected by the drug; or he may be allergic to it. Joe may also have a serious back problem that is not getting proper medical attention. Prescription drugs should be dispensed only by a physician following a professional diagnosis. Responsible use can contribute to good health and quality of life.

Where Is Treatment Available?

Most drug problems require serious treatment, starting with detoxification under supervision. Withdrawal symptoms, depending on the extent of dependency and the nature of the drug, can be painful and life threatening. Immediate help and information are available by calling a hotline, visiting a hospital, going to an organizational meeting (like AA or Narcotics Anonymous), or checking into a detoxification center.

For drug treatment there are many programs, some aimed at specific addictions, and some tailored to meet specific cultural, gender, and sexual orientations. There are two basic types of programs: outpatient and residential treatment. Outpatient programs may be as informal as a drop-in center or as formal as a structured counseling and therapy program. Daily methadone injection is an example of a structured outpatient treatment. Residential programs require patients to live in a controlled environment during detoxification and counseling. This releases them from outside pressures, which frees them to deal with their problem and underlying causes. Outpatient counseling or group home living generally follow residential treatment. Many programs for drug problems also include family counseling since one person's abuse touches many lives. Family problems may also be encouraging substance abuse.

ABUSE PREVENTION: REACHING OUT

> I want to do something but I don't know what to do.
> It really isn't any of my business.
> It's not up to me.

Too often we find ourselves wanting to do something to help a substance abuser, but we are not sure what to do or when it is our place to do it. Our inaction is not intentional, but it is unfortunate. One of the things that helps people overcome addictions or bad habits is support. Friends and family members are in the best position to help because they know the individual well and are the most likely to be listened to by the person in, or on the brink of trouble. Friends and family are also the most likely to spot a problem early.

How to Talk with a Friend About a Substance Abuse Problem

If you decide to talk with your friend, here are some guidelines to help you plan how and what you could do to help:

- Pick a good time—one when you have plenty of time and your friend is sober or straight.
- Express concern, not blame. Avoid labels like "alcoholic," or "drug addict," because these can be instant turnoffs. You want the conversation to continue.
- Use a voice filled with understanding and compassion. Avoid condescension and pity.
- Start sentences with the word "I," rather than "you," because this avoids accusations and allows your friend to hear how you feel. Example: "I feel left out when you get drunk and ignore me," rather than, "You always ignore me when you are drunk."
- Give your friend specific examples of what you have seen him or her do when under the influence of an abused substance.

- Express your feelings. Tell your friend you are worried and that you want to help.
- Be prepared for denial and anger. Many abusers will say that there is nothing wrong; that they don't have a problem, you do. Don't take it personally when your friend gets angry at you.
  When confronted, many users will defend their use, blame others for the problem, or give excuses for why they drink or use other drugs.
  Behind all this your message may be getting through. Keep trying.
- Find out where help is available and offer to go with your friend. Have schedules, pamphlets, hotlines, and counseling service information available so that you can help your friend make plans.
- If your friend doesn't seek help and is under eighteen, you may need to talk to your friend's guardian or parent. If your friend is over eighteen, seek the support of other friends and family members.

BARRIER Busters

ABUSE PREVENTION

It's someone else's problem.

It's everyone's problem, but you do have to decide when your actions will make a difference. You can stop a friend from driving by taking the keys, and a stranger from putting others at risk by alerting the restaurant or bar manager or calling the police.

You may also be part of the problem. Are you helping someone continue by pretending it's OK, lending money, or providing a cover story?

It isn't my job to police other people's actions.

That depends on your position. Most of us are responsible for others, whether it is a parent-child, teacher-student, or employer-employee relationship. And if we are not in a role of authority, we still have a responsibility to help those who are. On a more personal note, a friendship and a marriage both involve being there for someone when he or she most needs it. Helping someone through a substance abuse problem or simply helping him or her get help is a job often best performed by a friend.

I might get hurt if I intervene.

Action doesn't always mean getting personally involved. Call the police, anonymously if necessary. You are not required to put yourself at risk, and in many cases you *should* contact the authorities rather than intervene. Usually the most effective personal interventions are made for family and friends, and the timing of the intervention can be made when the person is calm or not under the influence. Making plans ahead of time, such as who will be the designated driver on an evening out, can also alleviate heated arguments later.

I don't know what to do.

Ask a professional. College and university campuses are staffed with substance-abuse counselors. They can give you guidance on how to best assist a friend. Call a hotline, talk to a religious leader, or contact a doctor. Become informed and then act.

Maybe I'm wrong and there really isn't a problem.

Maybe you are right and there is a problem. Most people don't mind if you call the fire department and it turns out there isn't a fire. Sometimes taking the precaution is worth the risk of being wrong. Well-intended concern is understood by friends, whether it is accurate or not. You may also be met with a lot of denial and your friend may make you feel like you are wrong, when in fact you are not. Look to other mutual friends and professionals for input.

Whenever I bring up the subject with my boyfriend or husband, he gets mad and hits me.

Get yourself and any children out of the situation first. You may or may not be able to help him, but if you are going to try, you need to be stable first. Call a hotline for assistance. (This is also true if a man is being abused by a woman. This is statistically less common but not unknown.)

ALCOHOL

I know when I've had enough.

If you are having blackouts or hangovers, you aren't stopping soon enough. If you have ever wondered how you and the car got home, you definitely have a problem. Pay attention if friends are concerned about you or try to stop you from having another drink when you are with them. Try limiting yourself and see if you can hold to your limit or whether you rationalize your way to more drinks. Keep track of blackouts, hangovers, and risky behavior.

Drinking helps me socialize.

If you are uncomfortable at gatherings, you may need to improve your social skills. Learn communication skills (many books and courses are available), learn to dance, and attend activities that are centered around something you are comfortable with such as a recreational volleyball league, a drama or debate club, or art lessons. Avoid settings where drinking is the focus of the social gathering, such as drinking contests, drinking games, and chugging.

Alcohol helps me unwind and cope with problems.

Take a good look at the stressor and your problems. There may be other better ways to address them such as relaxation techniques, time management, and therapy. (See Chapter 11.) The problem with using alcohol as a stress and coping strategy is that when stress increases the tendency is to drink more. Drinking alcohol is not the answer to a problem.

My drinking habit is part of my ethnic heritage.

It is true that some cultures promote more drinking than others, but excessive destructive drinking is recognized as a problem worldwide. Don't use heritage as an excuse. Explore ethnic foods and celebrations rather than just the alcohol-related aspect of your heritage.

I like the taste.

When tasting fine chocolates, one savors each bite. Try drinking more slowly and enjoying the taste. Drink something nonalcoholic to quench your thirst and then sip an alcoholic drink. You may also want to try a non-alcoholic beer.

I drink to fit in. Everyone is doing it and if I don't, my friends will make fun of me or feel awkward drinking around me.

This is perhaps one of the hardest barriers to overcome. For some reason many people use excessive drinking as a way to bond together. But there are other, healthier ways to bond. Try going on a ropes course or camping trip, playing together on an intramural team, or working together on a volunteer project. At a party with alcohol you can volunteer to be the designated driver or carry around a fake drink such as nonalcoholic beer or club soda with lime. Try to interest your friends in activities that are not alcohol centered. You may be surprised at how many will be happy to join you.

TOBACCO

It's my life, and I'll live it how I want to—besides I'm only hurting myself.

Wrong. People who love you will be taking care of you when you are very sick. Unless you smoke away from everyone else, your secondhand smoke will be hurting someone else. Secondhand smoke is dangerous to all of those who share space or air with you and is especially bad for young children.

In addition, the high health care costs attributed to tobacco-related illnesses are passed on to everyone in insurance premiums. Absenteeism is also higher among smokers, so your boss may be getting a less reliable, more costly employee. If you respect your friends' right to live their own lives, you will not want to contribute to one of them dying unnecessarily. And your friends do not want anything bad to happen to you—you will cause them heartache with each puff. Children especially need healthy parents. Even if you don't have children now, a tobacco-related illness can affect you years from now when you do.

It's my decision.

Yes, it is. But make sure it *is* your decision, not a decision based on coercion from a group of friends, seductive advertising, or a habit/addiction picked up from your parents. And even if you have made the decision yourself, reevaluate periodically to make sure it is a good one.

Granddad and Aunt Mary smoked and they lived into their eighties.

Check to see what they died from. Was their quality of life in their later years as good as it could have been? Are there other smokers in the family, and are they doing as well? Do you know anyone who has suffered a to-bacco-related illness? Can you name more people who have been affected by tobacco-related illnesses than those who have smoked and escaped them?

I won't get hooked. I'll just smoke a little or chew once in a while and quit whenever I want to.

The FDA has declared nicotine an addictive drug. Many people who want to stop smoking have a great deal of difficulty doing it. Smokeless tobacco has an even greater nicotine concentration and studies suggest that it is even harder to kick this habit. It may not be so easy to stop once you start, so think twice before you do start. It's a little like getting on an express train and trying to get off at a local stop.

DRUGS

Drugs give me more confidence.

Self-confidence comes through accomplishments, developing good relationships, and learning to like yourself. Drugs can't give you confidence —only the illusion of it.

I can get more work done when I use cocaine or another stimulant.

For a while this may seem to be true, but the price is deep exhaustion later. The quality of your work also suffers.

Drugs like cocaine, crack, and crank improve sex.

Chronic use has the opposite effect, often diminishing sex drive. Fertility may also be impaired.

Drugs help pick me up when I'm feeling depressed.

The lift is temporary, and the crash usually worse than normal. The drug will not solve the problem or improve the relationship that caused the depression.

My friends all use it, and I like being one of the crowd.

Wanting to fit in is a natural human feeling. And resisting pressure from friends is very difficult. But maybe your friends need to stop using rather than you starting. Or perhaps the group you are trying to fit into isn't such a good fit if they are pushing you to use drugs. Consider joining a singing, debate, art, or athletic club in which your talent is the common criterion.

It makes me a better athlete.

It makes you an illegal athlete. Sports competitions are meant to be drug free. In addition, most drugs decrease endurance and make you more susceptible to disease and injury.

Occasional use of drugs won't hurt me.

Some drugs can kill you the first time you use them. Physical and psychological addictions can occur in relatively short periods of time. If you buy and use an illegal drug, you also risk the consequences of breaking the law.

Others think I am abusing a substance, but I know that I am in control and don't need to change.

Try quitting and see if you really are in control. Also take a good look at the people suggesting you need help. Are these people who care about you? People who have nothing to gain by sharing their concern, and who in fact risk your anger by bringing it up? Maybe their opinions are worth considering, or at least worth a heart-to-heart talk.

I plan to continue to abuse substances because they provide me the energy I need to get through the day, and the escapism I need to relax from all my stress.

Unfortunately, drugs as a solution are a short-term fix. They don't solve the underlying problems and they create problems of their own. Drug-induced energy ignores the body's natural need for rest and leads to exhaustion. Stress may be relieved during a drug high, but it returns as quickly as the drug's effect wears off, leaving you with the same problems but less time and fewer resources to cope with them. Stress management, relaxation techniques, proper nutrition, and regular exercise are much safer ways to infuse yourself with energy and reduce your stress levels.

There are a lot of things you can do to help, the first of which is to become informed. To help someone you know who is abusing alcohol, tobacco, or drugs, your first step is to find out as much as you can about the substance being abused and where your friend can get help. (For writing ease, we will refer to the person in need of help as a friend, but please read it to also mean a relative, colleague, student, life partner, or any other relationship.) To gather information, you may want to go to the library and read about the substance, or talk with a spiritual leader, social worker, health professional, counselor, hotline, or one of the support organizations. Talking with someone who has helped a friend through a similar addiction may also be helpful. All these people can help you get your friend into treatment and also support you when you are wondering if you are doing the right thing. When you feel ready, go talk to your friend either by yourself or with someone else.

There are also lots of things you can do every day to help prevent substance abuse. The problem is so pervasive that it is going to take everyone in the community working together to solve it. Prevention education programs have already made a difference, but much more is needed.

SUMMARY

Substance abuse backfires. Abusing a substance to lose weight can result in malnutrition or other life-threatening disease. Social problems aren't solved by using drugs; instead, they are complicated as debts pile up and increasing isolation occurs. Instead of helping a person escape problems, the substance becomes part of the problem and is often more difficult to overcome than the original problems. Drugs that give you energy now make you pay for it later in total exhaustion. And as you saw in Chapter 11, long-term stress relief goes well beyond the short-term relief of a tranquilizer. Drugs, including alcohol, that make you appear daring and powerful are probably also causing you to take foolish risks—risks that can lead to hurtful behavior, crime, or an overdose.

With the growing prevalence of drugs, both legal and illegal, we have to wonder if we have become a nation that solves its problems by popping a pill, having a drink, or smoking a joint. There is plenty of evidence that we are, but there is also evidence of a growing intolerance for substance dependency. More than one Olympic athlete has been stripped of a medal because of drug use, and neighbors are joining forces to drive drug dealers out of their neighborhoods and parks. More and more people are choosing to live smoke free, and programs like AA continue to grow as alcoholics take a stand against their addiction. Wellness is an outgrowth of these beliefs. Baseball great Mickey Mantle had a liver transplant in 1995—a desperate medical attempt to solve a problem caused by excessive drinking. Following the transplant, and before he died, Mickey Mantle became a wellness

advocate, using his popularity and physical condition to convince young people not to drink.

Rather than living a life that encourages health problems and then hoping a wonder drug or operation will bail you out, you can live a lifestyle that will help keep you out of the doctor's office. Then drugs can play their proper role—helping to cure *unpreventable* illnesses. When it comes to prevention, one person *can* make a difference, especially when friends talk to friends, siblings talk to siblings, and parents talk to children.

SUGGESTED READING

Alcoholic anonymous, 3rd ed. New York: Alcoholics Anonymous World Services, 1976.

Avis, H. *Drugs and life.* Dubuque, IA: Brown & Benchmark, 1990.

Blum, K. *Alcohol and the addictive brain: New hope for alcoholics from biogenetic research.* New York: Free Press, 1991.

Cocores, J. *The 800-COCAINE book of drug and alcohol recovery.* New York: Villard Books, 1990.

Dorris, M. *The broken cord.* New York: HarperCollins, 1992.

Gibbons, B. The preventable tragedy—fetal alcohol syndrome. *National Geographic* 181(2), February 1992.

Hermes, W. J. *Substance abuse (The encyclopedia of health).* New York: Chelsea House Publishers, 1993.

Nakken, C. *The addictive personality: Understanding compulsion in our lives.* Hazelton Foundation, Center City, MN. New York: Harper & Row Publishers, 1988.

Schlaadt, R. *Drugs, society and behavior.* Guildford, CT: Dushkin Publishing Company, 1992.

U.S. Department of Health and Human Services. *Healthy people 2000: National health promotion and disease prevention objectives.* DHHS Publication No. (PHS) 91-50213. Washington, D.C.: U.S. Government Printing Office, 1990.

RESOURCES

Center for Substance Abuse Prevention (CSAP)
    (301)443-0373

National Clearinghouse for Alcohol and Drug
Information (NCADI)
    (800)729-6686

Infoline
    (800)203-1234

National Council on Alcoholism and Drug Dependence
    (800)622-6255

Mothers Against Drunk Drivers (MADD)
    (800)544-3690

Behavioral Lab 14.1

What Can I Do?

At the beginning of this chapter, you determined your stage of readiness to change with regard to either substance abuse or abuse prevention. Now take out a sheet of paper and complete the corresponding section of the lab you've chosen: precontemplator, contemplator, preparer, action taker, or maintainer. The labs for substance abuse have been made general to cover alcohol, drug, or tobacco use. You may wish to complete this lab for one or more specific types of abuse. The substance abuse lab is first, followed by the one for abuse prevention.

SUBSTANCE ABUSE

Precontemplator

1. Are there any signs that your alcohol, tobacco, or drug use is having a negative impact on your life? For example,

   —Have you missed any days of work or classes because of alcohol, tobacco, or drug use?

   —Have any friends or family suggested that you have a problem? If yes, how many?

   Refer to the box on page 336 and Labs 14.2 and 14.3 for additional examples.

2. When faced with a problem, do you reach for support in the form of a "quick fix"? Do you feel like you "need" something to get you through a meeting, class, or other event?

3. Does alcoholism or any other addictive behavior run in your family? How do you feel about this?

4. Do you know if the substance you are using is psychologically or physically addictive? Are there any signs that you are physically or psychologically addicted to a substance?

5. Identify three reasons why you are using a substance.

6. Identify three side effects you don't like.

7. What are the potential health risks of using the substance? Do any of these concern you? Has use of the substance resulted in any additional medical visits?

8. Try to identify the main reasons why you are against changing or not motivated to change this habit. Refer to the Barrier Busters earlier in this chapter for ideas.

9. Can you think of any reasons why cutting down or quitting would be good for you?

10. Looking at all of your answers together, do you see any reasons to think about quitting or cutting down?

11. Is there something you would like to know more about that would help you consider whether quitting would be better for you?

Contemplator

1. What abusive habit are you thinking about changing?

2. What changes will the activity in item 1 bring about that are important to you? Why are they important?

3. Do you need help to change? If so, do you know where to get help or do you know someone who can help you find it?

4. Do you need more information about a substance or treatment program?

5. What do you need in order to consider making this change?

   Try to finish this statement:

   I would consider changing if . . .

   I had support from my friends.

   Someone would quit with me.

   There is medical evidence that I am hurting myself.

   My employer or teachers would understand if I had to miss some work or classes.

   (yours) _____

6. What might stop you from trying to change?

7. How do you think you could overcome the items in item 6? If you don't know, can you think of someone who can help you figure out a way?

Preparer

1. What do you specifically want to do? (For directions on goal setting, see Chapter 2.)

2. What type of activities will accomplish this goal?

3. Identify one or more people you could trust to help you, such as a friend, family member, clergy, counselor, or professor.

4. What is the first thing you need to do to get started toward your goal?

   Examples

   Tell someone you need help

   Call a hotline

   Throw away the substance you are abusing

5. What kinds of things might stop you from taking this first step?

6. Can you think of ways to prevent or neutralize the temptations you listed in item 5?

7. What makes you believe you can accomplish your goal(s)? *Or* What makes you believe you can accomplish this first step?

8. If your first step doesn't work, what will you do?

9. Complete the following statement:

   I am going to take my first step on _____ .
   date within 30 days

Action Taker

1. What are you currently doing that has helped you stop your substance abuse?

2. What are the positive rewards you are experiencing?

3. Are you receiving support for your effort?

   If yes, what kind?

   If no, why not? And can you change this?

4. Are you keeping track of your progress?

   If yes, how?

   > *Examples*
   >
   > Putting the money saved in a special account
   > Marking off substance-free days on a calendar
   > Keeping a journal of your feelings

   If no, would it help motivate you to keep track?

5. Do you think you will continue to stay off the substance you were abusing?

   If yes, what kinds of things are you, or those around you, doing that give you confidence to continue?

   If no, what kinds of things are you, or those around you, doing that are shaking your confidence to continue?

6. If you were to resume your abuse, what do you think would be the major reason for this relapse?

7. Is there a way to prevent this (item 6)? (barrier busting in advance)

8. How would you get yourself back on track if you did have a relapse?

9. Are you clear on what your goals are?

10. Do you believe that you can reach your goals? Why or why not?

11. If you answered no to the above question, can you think of anything or anyone who can help you work toward your goals?

Maintainer

1. For how long have you maintained your substance-free program? (If you are in a treatment program like the methadone program, you can choose to answer this in terms of being free of the original drug.)

2. What are the top two reasons that make you want to continue?

3. Have you been tempted to abuse a substance? If so, what tempted you?

4. How did you stop yourself from giving in to temptation?

5. Can you prevent such temptations? If so, how?

6. How confident are you that you can successfully do what you have listed in item 5 and stay substance free? What types of things build your confidence? Lower your confidence? How can you minimize or eliminate the latter and optimize the former?

7. Are you happy with your present behavior or is there some way in which you want to continue to improve? If you wish to improve more, can you write a goal to that effect?

8. What kind of support do you get for your efforts?

9. How have you changed? How have you changed or maintained an environment around you that promotes this healthy lifestyle?

10. Is there anything else you need to promote your continued maintenance?

11. If you listed something in the previous statement, can you think of a way to attain it or can you think of someone who can help you with it?

Note: If you do not have and never had a substance abuse problem, you are a maintainer. You may wish to work on community involvement—share with others whatever it is that is working for you.

ABUSE PREVENTION
Precontemplator

1. Why are you uninterested in learning to help others prevent substance abuse? Refer to the Abuse Prevention Barrier Busters in this chapter for ideas.

2. Have you or has anyone close to you been affected by someone who was under the influence of alcohol or drugs? How do you feel about that?

3. How do you feel toward people who are actively involved in stopping or preventing substance abuse?

   Examples

   A person who takes the car keys away from a friend who is drunk

   A person who volunteers with youth programs

   A person who won't serve alcohol to someone who is drunk

4. Who has the best chance of catching a friend's or family member's habit early? And who is the substance abuser most likely to listen to: a friend, a parent, a son or daughter, or a stranger?

5. Would you ignore it if you knew your friend, spouse, or child was using an illegal substance? (This includes underage smoking and drinking.)

6. Do your answers in items 2 to 5 outweigh your answers in item 1?

7. Professionals like the police, educators, social workers, and doctors have all been trying to deal with the problems of substance abuse and it is still prevalent. What do you think needs to be done to improve the situation?

8. Do you see any way that you can be instrumental in helping the actions you listed in item 7 to actually happen?

   Examples

   Be politically active

   Donate money

   Volunteer time

   (other) _____

Contemplator

1. Which involvement activity or activities are you thinking about trying?

2. What good will come from the activity or activities you selected in item 1?

3. Do you need help to make this change? If so, do you know someone who will help you, or who can put you in touch with other people interested in the same activity or activities?

4. Is there something you need to know more about? If yes, do you know where to get the information or do you know someone who can help you find it?

5. What do you need in order to consider getting involved?

   Try to finish this statement:

   I would consider getting involved if . . .

   A friend would do it with me.

   I could join a group already doing it.

   Someone invited me to join a project.

   I could do something that would take very little time.

   (yours) _____

6. What might stop you from becoming more involved?

7. How can you overcome the items in item 6?

Preparer

1. Community involvement takes time, so first determine how much time you have and what type of activity best fits into that time frame. For example, peer counseling requires more of a time commitment than posting information or several hours of hotline work. Some people have time each week but others may wish to commit a whole day once a month or once a year. Some things require very little extra time, like being the designated driver. How much time do you have or want to devote to abuse prevention?

2. Make a list of activities you think you would enjoy doing.

   Examples

   Prevention, for example, coaching a youth team

   Helping a friend in trouble

   Providing volunteer hours on a hotline or in a peer counseling program

3. Experiment with the activities listed in item 2.

4. Based on your answers in items 1 to 3, select one activity to focus on and decide when you will make this activity a part of your lifestyle.

5. Take the activity in item 3 and determine the first thing you need to do to get started.

6. What might cause you to put off taking the first step you listed in item 5?

7. What strategies can you use to eliminate or neutralize the temptations you listed in item 6? If you don't know, can you think of someone who can help you figure out a way?

8. If your first step doesn't work, what will you do?

9. What makes you believe you can accomplish your goals? *Or* What makes you believe you can accomplish this first step?

10. Complete the following statement:

I am going to take my first step on _____ .
date within 30 days

Action Taker

1. What are you currently doing to help someone else?

2. Do you feel as if your efforts are making a positive difference? If yes, how?

3. Have you encountered any problems? If so, can you solve them? Who can you talk to for advice?

4. Are you clear on what it is you are doing and why? If not, how can you become clearer?

5. Are you receiving support for your effort?

   If yes, what kind?

   > *Examples*
   > Financial
   > Emotional
   > Volunteers

   If no, why not? What or who can help you get support?

6. If you were to stop, what do you think would be the major reason for stopping?

7. Is there a way to prevent this (item 6)? (barrier busting in advance)

8. How would you get yourself started again if you did stop?

9. How can you change your environment or lifestyle to promote continuing this activity?

   Examples
   Set aside time
   Involve friends in the helping activity

10. Do you plan to continue? If no, examine your reasons and see if there is a way to remedy the problem. Or consider picking up a new activity that fits into your life more easily. If yes, is there anything that will make doing it easier, more comfortable, or more productive?

Maintainer

1. For how long have you maintained your involvement action?

2. What are the top two reasons that make you want to continue?

3. Have you been tempted to stop? If so, what tempted you?

4. How did you convince yourself to continue?

5. Can you prevent such temptation? How?

6. Are you happy with your present level of involvement, or do you wish to add another action? If you wish to add another action, can you write a goal to that effect?

7. What kind of support do you get for your efforts?

8. How have you changed or how have you changed the environment around you to accomplish this helping action.

9. Is there anything else you need, such as information, support, or time management, to promote your continued maintenance?

10. If you listed something in the previous statement, can you think of a way to attain it or can you think of someone who can help you with it?

LAB
14.2

Do You Have a Problem with Alcohol?

The NCADD Self-Test

Here is a self-text to help you review the role alcohol plays in your life. These questions incorporate many of the common symptoms of alcoholism. This test is intended to help you determine if you or someone you know needs to find out more about alcoholism; it is not intended to be used to establish the diagnosis of alcoholism.

Yes No

___ ___ **1.** Do you ever drink heavily when you are disappointed, under pressure, or have had a quarrel with someone?

___ ___ **2.** Have you ever been unable to remember part of the previous evening, even though your friends say you didn't pass out?

___ ___ **3.** When drinking with other people, do you try to have a few extra drinks when others won't know about it?

___ ___ **4.** Has a family member or close friend ever expressed concern or complained about your drinking?

___ ___ **5.** When you are sober, do you sometimes regret things you did or said while drinking?

___ ___ **6.** Have you sometimes failed to keep promises you made to yourself about controlling or cutting down on your drinking?

___ ___ **7.** Do you try to avoid family or close friends while you are drinking?

___ ___ **8.** Are you having more financial, work, school and/or family problems as a result of your drinking?

___ ___ **9.** Do you sometimes have the "shakes" in the morning and find that it helps to have a "little" drink, tranquilizer, or medication of some kind?

___ ___ **10.** Have any of your blood relatives ever had a problem with alcohol?

Any "yes" answer indicates you may be at greater risk for alcoholism. More than one "yes" answer may indicate the presence of an alcohol-related problem or alcoholism, and the need for consultation with an alcoholism professional. To find out more, contact the National Council on Alcoholism and Drug Dependence in your area.

Source: Excerpted by permission from National Council on Alcoholism and Drug Dependence, Inc., *What are the signs of alcoholism?* The NCADD self-test (rev. 1990). For a free copy of the complete 26-question test, call 1-800-622-6255.

Drug Awareness

Over-the-Counter and Prescription Drugs

1. List the over-the-counter and prescription drugs you are presently using or have used in the past six months.

2. Next to the items you've listed in item 1, list the benefit and possible risks of taking these drugs. The instructions with the drug, a pharmacist, and your physician can help you with this.

3. When you use an over-the-counter or prescription drug, do you follow the directions?

   Examples

   Do you continue to take the antibiotic until it is gone, even if symptoms disappear sooner?

   Do you take the prescribed amount or take more in an effort to get better faster?

   Do you consume alcohol with a medication even though the directions warn against doing so?

   Do you try to play catch-up with birth control pills if you miss one or more?

4. Have you ever used a prescription medication that did not belong to you? If yes, what prompted you to do it?

5. Do you use any prescription medicines for non-medical purposes? If yes, how often?

Illicit Drugs

1. Do you use an illegal drug? If so, how often and for how long have you been using it?

2. Do you think about quitting but feel powerless to do so?

3. Have you ever tried to cut down or control your drug use?

4. If you have tried to cut back or quit, did you experience physical withdrawal symptoms (feel poorly) or have a psychological craving for the drug?

5. Do you find you have to use more of a drug to get the same high?

6. Do you use the drug with specific people, or at a specific time or place?

7. Do you use the drug to feel confident, normal, or more energetic?

8. Do you think about the drug and where to get more, when you are not high?

9. Do you lie about where you've been, whether or not you use a drug, how much of a drug you use, or how much money you spend on drugs?

10. Do you spend money on drugs even when you can't afford to?

11. Does the drug interfere with your ability to go to school, work, or have healthy relationships?

12. Do you ever do things under the influence of the drug that you wouldn't do otherwise?

13. Do you skip other important functions in order to obtain or use the drug?

14. Do people close to you ask you about your drug use?

15. Do you use a drug even though you know it is making your condition or situation worse?

16. Are you spending more time with people who use your drug or spending less time with friends who don't use the drug or criticize your use?

17. Have you developed a mental or physical condition or disorder because of prolonged drug use?

18. Do you go to extreme lengths (for example, steal, cheat, threaten others) or put yourself in danger (go to unsafe places to purchase the drug, take high-risk loans, trade sex for drugs) in order to obtain the drug?

If you think you have a drug problem, seek out help. If you answered yes to any of the eighteen illicit drug questions, you have a problem and need help. Talk to a college counselor, a member of the clergy, a physician, or a concerned friend or family member, or call a hotline for more information and local resources.

CHAPTER 15

Living Well in Today's World

Objectives

1. Develop strategies for making long-term behavior changes.

2. Understand why relapse is common when making changes.

3. Learn how the stages of change are related to relapse.

4. Discover how your environment can influence your wellness.

5. Understand how the quality of your life requires respect for, and is influenced by, the environment.
   a. Learn how to make personal wellness decisions within the context of world wellness.
   b. Identify ways that your human-cultural environment affects your lifestyle choices.
   c. Identify ways that the natural environment affects your lifestyle choices.
   d. Learn how personal behaviors can have an impact on both your human-cultural and natural environments.

Terms

- Relapse
- World view
- Human-cultural environment
- Natural environment

Several years ago a young married man complained about having to exercise and eat a low-fat diet as part of his new weight-loss program. He complained to his wife that he was not having much fun and wondered when he could stop and go back to his old way of eating and not exercising. In his mind, his illness was excessive body weight, and the cure or treatment was diet and exercise. Once the extra weight was lost, there would be no reason to continue the treatment. Many people view aspects of wellness from the same illness/treatment perspective. Lack of physical fitness, for example, can be treated with a program of regular aerobic exercise and strength training. But once a high level of physical fitness has been achieved, many individuals stop doing the treatment.

The purpose of this chapter is to help you plan for and live a lifetime of wellness. As you may have guessed, the treatment approach is a short-term solution to problems that usually last a lifetime. Successful maintenance of a wellness lifestyle requires lifelong commitment to healthy behaviors.

In addition to successful long-term behavior change, this chapter will expose you to the idea that your personal wellness does not start and end with you, but extends to communities, cultures, cities, and the environment. Everything we do will affect other people, places, and the environment to some degree; therefore, wellness needs to include societal and environmental concerns.

MAKING BEHAVIOR CHANGE LAST A LIFETIME

Making change is rarely easy. When old behaviors are replaced with new ones, we tend to lose our sense of comfort and contentment as new and different lifestyles bring about uncertainty and anxiety. Let's face it, change is often scary. Whether starting a new job or changing the way we eat, there are obstacles and challenges to overcome. Because change is associated with both good and bad stresses, many feel that it is better and easier to leave the old behaviors just the way they are.

The Stages of Change model of behavior change that has been the focus of many labs in this text was designed to tailor behavior change to an individual's level of readiness. You will recall that the five stages of change include precontemplation, contemplation, preparation, action, and maintenance. It would be nice if we could start thinking about a new behavior, try it out for a while, and then decide to maintain the new behavior for the rest of our lives, but behavior change is rarely that simple. In the struggle for self-improvement and in the attainment of wellness, every attempt to live a healthy lifestyle may not result in a changed behavior, but every attempt is a small victory, because it brings an individual closer to becoming a maintainer. A realistic attitude toward behavior change is one that realizes that change requires time, effort, and patience. As you move closer to the main-

tainer stage, you move closer to making your behavior change last a lifetime.

RELAPSE—ACCEPT IT AND MOVE ON

The average ex-smoker attempted to quit smoking three or four times before finally succeeding. Adopting other wellness lifestyles is no different. Whether you are trying to lose weight, eat healthy, exercise, or make other lifestyle changes, research has shown that the average person will successfully move through the stages of change only to experience a setback, stop the new behavior, and **relapse** to the beginning stage. Many people who attempt to adopt a new behavior will relapse and cycle through the stages three or four times. A person can steadily move from the precontemplation stage to becoming a contemplator and an action taker who is earnestly making an effort to change. Often, however, just when things seem to be going well, a stress occurs and the new behavior is either forgotten or purposely ignored as the person slips back into the old, comfortable lifestyle, regressing into the precontemplator or contemplator stages (see Figure 15.1).

Relapsing into old behaviors can happen at any time and from any stage. Just because someone doesn't become a maintainer doesn't mean that the person has failed; it merely means that he or she has taken a temporary detour on the road to success. Detours should be accepted as part of the trip and an opportunity to recommit to doing even better next time. If you find yourself relapsing on your own wellness journey, just

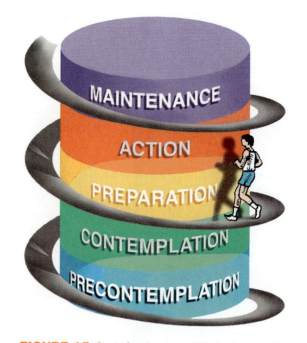

FIGURE 15.1 Relapsing into old behaviors can happen at any time. Once you have slipped backward, quickly get back into making your new behavior a permanent part of your life.

Think about a behavior change you have tried to make during this course. What are some environmental influences that have made it easier for you to change?

What environmental barriers have impeded or derailed your progress? What steps did you take to get back on the road to your personal goal?

find the main road again and get back to making your new behavior a permanent part of your life.

If you keep in mind that relapse may be part of the behavior change process, you can plan for it by preparing ways to get back on track if it happens. Most important, don't get discouraged. Most of the good aspects of our lives require large investments in time. It's all right to want to change; it's not all right to dislike yourself until you do.

Milk drinkers can relate to the effect time has on behaviors. When people who are used to drinking whole milk first try drinking skim milk to cut the fat in their diet, they all say the same thing: "Yuck, this tastes watery." From their perspective, skim milk really *is* watery. Similarly, when those who are used to skim try a glass of

whole milk, they say it's like drinking pure cream. As you can see, it's all a matter of what we are accustomed to. Just as whole-milk drinkers can gradually acquire a taste for skim by moving from whole milk to 2 percent, to 1 percent, to skim, so can we move from any undesirable behavior into a healthier one.

The passage of time gradually changes our perceptions and helps us to be comfortable with our new lifestyle. As each day passes, you will get comfortable with new behaviors, and old ways of doing things will become foreign to you. Much of your environment will also change with time. New behaviors bring about new surroundings, friends, and acquaintances.

PERSONAL WELLNESS VERSUS WORLD WELLNESS

Up to this point, we have concentrated on personal wellness with a focus on self-responsibility, self-direction, and individual improvement. But we do not live alone; we are part of something larger. We are part of the world ecosystem, a part of the United States, and a part of a society. Our environment, which includes people, places, animals, and plants, influences our behavior, and in turn our behavior has an impact on our environment. Because of this interconnectedness, it is crucial that we take a **world view**—that we make personal lifestyle decisions within the greater context of world wellness.

THE HUMAN-CULTURAL ENVIRONMENT

We human beings are social creatures—we enjoy living, playing, and working with other people. We seek out interaction, swap ideas, and ask each other's opinions. We

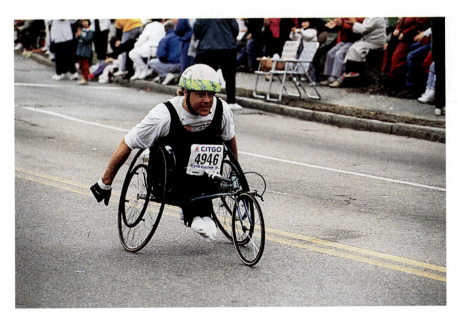

Wellness is attainable by everyone, regardless of perceived barriers. Our ability to reach and maintain personal goals depends on personal commitment and perseverance.

are immersed in a **human-cultural environment** made up of the people who surround us, plus their laws, religious beliefs, traditions, and social mores. As technology improves and the world "shrinks," it can be argued that the whole human race makes up our human-cultural environment. But when you think about behavior change, it is usually the people closest to you—the human-cultural environment of friends, family, and community—that influence you the most. If the impact (influence) is positive and supportive, the chances of maintaining a new behavior are greater.

Using this more localized focus, and recognizing the great diversity in this nation, it is easy to see how the characteristics of one human-cultural environment can be very different from another. Retirement communities offer a different environment from mixed-age neighborhoods. Ethnicity, religion, geographic location, sexual preference, and economic prosperity are a few of the many factors that help define human-cultural environments. (All that is not human, such as plants, animals, and minerals, make up the natural environment, which will be the second focus of this chapter.)

How Our Human-Cultural Environment Influences Our Wellness

The human culture in which we grow up helps shape who we are. We have learned and developed values from those around us—our parents, relatives, friends, neighbors, teachers, and spiritual leaders. How we live, what we eat, how we celebrate a marriage, how we conduct a funeral—all of these are rooted in our human culture. In fact, so ubiquitous is the nature and influence of culture that we seldom appreciate the full effect it has on us. Have you ever thought about eating something other than turkey for Thanksgiving? Vegetarians do. Do you ever question whether you can go on a date, just the two of you? The traditions in some cultures dictate that a family member must always accompany a single woman on a social outing. When you talk, are you aware that you speak with an accent and use phrases that are unique to your region and ethnic background? It is healthy to look at your culture and examine its influence on your lifestyle decisions.

Consider the different perspectives these two people would bring to a discussion on smoking:

1. Person A lives in a town supported by the tobacco industry, earns money to go to college by cutting tobacco, and has a mother and father who both smoke. Person A's friends see smoking as a rite of passage into adulthood.

2. Person B comes from a home in which both parents work in the health profession and guests who smoke are politely and firmly requested to smoke outdoors. The Walkathon for the American Cancer Society has been a family outing each year since a close friend of the family died of lung cancer. Person B's best friend quit smoking two years ago.

We have talked about awareness being the first step in the behavior change process. The following story illustrates just how important it is to step back and take an objective look at why you do what you do:

> A neighbor is visiting and watching a woman make a cake. After stirring in all the ingredients, the woman takes out and throws away one cup of the batter. The neighbor asks her why she does this. The woman's response is, "because my mother always did." Later that day the woman calls her mother and asks her the same question. The mother laughs and says, "I always did that because my baking pan was too small for the full recipe."

Family tradition was the reason for this woman's actions. What influences yours? There are several ways you can heighten your own awareness. You can write your reflections in a journal. Or you can initiate introspection through frank discussions with people whose opinions you value, especially people who are different from you. One of the best ways to make you more aware of your own culture is to experience a different one. People who travel to another country come back with a new understanding of what it is to be American. But you don't have to travel far for this experience: with so much diversity here in the United States, you can create your own cultural encounters. Here are a few ways you can meet and interact with people from other backgrounds:

- Invite a foreign student or visiting professor to have lunch or dinner with you.
- Attend folk dances and ethnic or regional food festivals.
- Visit a church or temple different from your own.
- Eat out at an ethnic restaurant or fix an ethnic food, preferably with help from someone familiar with that style of cooking.
- Take a course in comparative religion, human diversity, or world history.

When you enter college or take an adult-education class, you enter a new human-cultural environment. In many classrooms today, you will meet people from all over the country and the world; people with diverse backgrounds who express new and different ideas. These ideas raise your awareness and force you to examine your own beliefs. You may rethink some of the things you learned growing up and accepted at face value.

If you're now a college student, think about when you first entered college, and ask yourself, "Has this new environment changed my lifestyle?" If the answer is yes, try to figure out what it is in the environment that has influenced you. Then ask yourself whether the changes have been for the better.

Human-cultural environments can influence individuals in both healthy and unhealthy ways. The corporate environment offers challenge and economic advantage, but it also offers stress when job commitments are forced to take precedence over family life. Gang life offers young people a sense of belonging, but it also promotes violence. College life promotes academic learning and social opportunities, but it can also increase peer pressure to drink or use drugs. By becoming more aware of the influences of your human-cultural environment, you can draw on the positive and minimize, change, or reject the negative. Here is an example: Colleen had never had a weight problem, so she was surprised when her clothes starting feeling tight. The infamous "freshman 15" pounds had deposited themselves on *her* body. She sat down to contemplate this. At home she had played on an athletic team every season and belonged to a swim club. While she was a good athlete, she wasn't of the same caliber as the scholarship players at college, and in fact, she'd been so busy with classes and social events that she hadn't even gone for a run. Her family had insisted on sit-down family dinners and her parents always fixed nutritious, balanced meals. Campus housing had been full when Colleen applied, so she and two friends were living in an off-campus apartment. There never seemed to be enough time to shop and fix meals, so they lived on pizza, hamburgers, and ice cream. Colleen was also dating an upperclassman and at parties had been offered all the free beer she wanted.

The negative influences are obvious enough, and the need to change is clear, but how? The next day, Colleen signed up for intramural soccer and checked the free swim hours at the pool. She spoke to her boyfriend and found that he was concerned about her drinking as well as his own, and they agreed to do things together other than party. Colleen bought a meal ticket for the campus dining hall for lunches and dinners and purchased cereal and fruit for breakfast. Her roommates agreed to pitch in by buying healthier snacks.

In this example, Colleen was able to work within her environment to eliminate or modify the undermining influences and focus on the supportive ones. There are times when an environment is so destructive that individuals have to be removed, or remove themselves from it, in order to change and thrive. Alcohol and drug rehabilitation centers, for example, offer live-in programs in which a person can eliminate environmental pressures altogether, work on recovery, and then slowly reenter society.

It is easiest to make lifestyle changes when the change is aligned with the beliefs of your own human-cultural environment. Sustaining a behavior that is in conflict with your human-cultural environment, or an important element of it, can be difficult. For instance, the social acceptability of premarital sex among young adults in the United States has made it more difficult for individuals to adhere to a belief in the value of abstinence. A college student may be ridiculed for being old fashioned, while in another setting this same person might receive support, advice, and praise for the same decision. If you are choosing a wellness lifestyle that is not shared by the majority in your human-cultural environment, you will need to look for or create support. Workshops and support groups can put you in touch with other people who share your goals.

Technology's Influence on the Individual

Finally, a discussion on human-cultural influence would not be complete without mention of the technological revolution and its impact on lifestyle. From televisions and computers to faxes and call waiting, technology has changed the way we think, live, and work. We carry beepers and cell phones and talk to people all over the world via the Internet. Technology initially created more leisure time and now may actually be taking it away by making us accessible to our work twenty-four hours a day. Some forms of physical stress were decreased with the advent of modern appliances and robotics, but now new stresses, both physical and psychological, have taken their place. Computers can analyze our diets, calculate our percent body fat, and even recommend an exercise program. These are good things. But computers also make us sit for hours, both at work and at play. Has technology enabled you to live a healthier lifestyle? Or a less healthy one? Probably both. Take a good look at the technology in your life and learn to maximize the positive and minimize the negative.

Our Influence on the Wellness of Our Human-Cultural Environment

Influence works both ways. Just as the human-cultural environment has an impact on an individual, so too does the individual have an impact on the human-cultural environment. The impact is usually greatest among those people closest to us, but at times just one person can change the way a nation thinks. Can you name an individual who has changed society for the better?

The lifestyle choices you make will have an effect on the people around you; your impact can be negative or positive. As you've seen in earlier chapters, your unhealthy behaviors are a destructive force that impacts not only you but your family and friends. And when you practice wellness behaviors, you are a positive, motivating force on those around you. For example, when you exercise and eat right, others benefit from your energy and sunny disposition. If you surround yourself with healthy foods, the people for whom you cook or who join you also eat the healthy diet. If you don't smoke, those around you avoid secondhand smoke. If you practice abstinence or safer sex, you not only limit your risk of disease, but also the risk of passing it on to a loved one.

When one person makes a change, it often motivates others to do the same. You may become a test case in the eyes of those around you. People may tell you all the ways you are going to fail but watch you closely to see whether you succeed. When someone near us accomplishes something, it makes us feel as if we can do it too. You can be a catalyst for change, someone else's motivation to change. Most of us prefer to do things with the support of others. An invitation to others may encourage them to join in, providing them with an impetus to change. For example, if one person suggests going for a walk, others will almost certainly go along. If you aren't a self-starter, look for people who are and join them.

Sometimes a change one person makes will make someone else uncomfortable or embarrass them. For example, if a person quits drinking alcohol, a close friend may become embarrassed about not quitting. Instead of being supportive, this friend may even encourage the old behavior. Knowing that this can happen allows you to prepare for it in advance. Rather than letting such a person drag you down, recognize him or her as a precontemplator for whom you may be an uncomfortable but important confrontation of awareness. Encourage contemplation by being a role model for change.

Sometimes conflict arises when individuals pursuing a healthy activity disrupt others or go against traditions. Snowboarders and in-line skaters are good examples. Lots of fun and exercise is associated with both activities, but as they grew in popularity they created safety issues. Thoughtful consideration of others and a willingness to look for creative solutions can resolve such conflicts. For example, many resorts now offer special rules and spaces for snowboarders and some towns

have set up special skating areas. Other examples of conflicts that have occurred between individuals and society with positive wellness outcomes include the fight against smoke in the workplace, demands for ingredient information on food labels, and stiffer legislation concerning drinking and driving.

As we strive to improve personal wellness, it is important to be aware of, and responsible for, the impact of our actions on other people, on our culture, on our heritage, and on the rules of our society. This does not mean that we should stagnate or always follow the norm. As we learn more, we must constantly reexamine how and why we do things. Individuals that raise new issues and ideas will improve our society and our society's wellness.

Helping Others Accept Your Decision to Change

Sometimes a personal wellness lifestyle decision can upset others. When this happens, you may want to give careful consideration to how best to handle the change. It may be that educating or including those around you will ease the difficulty. For example, if you decide to abstain from sexual activity or to take part only in safer sex, explaining this decision to your partner in a calm manner may win his or her support. If you choose to add exercise to your lifestyle instead of watching TV in the evening, friends or family may be more supportive if you ask them to join you on a walk or a trip to the gym. In most cases, there is a way to create a win-win situation, in which both the individual who makes the lifestyle change and those most directly affected by his or her decision can benefit. These

---

Activity 15.2 Balancing Wellness—Me, You, and the Environment

1. Try to recall an incident in which someone placed his or her personal wellness above concern for you or someone you know. How did the situation make you feel?

3. Looking back, can you think of a way you could have achieved the same thing for yourself but not hurt someone or something else?

2. Try to recall an incident in which you placed your personal wellness above the wellness of the environment or people around you.

4. Can you think of an example of how changing a personal behavior improved the lives of those around you?

solutions can most easily be achieved when the person making a lifestyle change is open about the reasons for making the change, welcomes support from friends, relatives, and partners, and understands that others affected by the change need time to adjust.

THE NATURAL ENVIRONMENT

The previous discussion challenges you to link your wellness to other people, but for those who hold a world view (or world ecosystem view), that is not enough. They challenge you to share your wellness with the earth itself and with all that inhabits it. To achieve this, personal actions must be in harmony with the needs of the natural environment, the **natural environment** being everything nonhuman.

Our Influence on the Wellness of Our Natural Environment

It is easy to look at things from a human-centered perspective, to believe that the world exists only to fulfill human need. Many think of the earth as something to manage in a way that will produce the most usable materials for the human race. Anything that does not have a human use is automatically devalued. This belief system has unfortunately led to a depletion (and in some cases exploitation) of natural resources and disruption of animal and plant ecosystems. Encouragingly, the Trends Action Group at the 1993 National Recreation and Park Association Congress reported that "several environmental shifts have occurred during the past decade. The shifts reflect changes in how we perceive, value, and relate to the natural world. They include a move from:

- domination to stewardship
- consumption to sustainability
- 'us' to 'US'
- consequences to consciousness
- '$' greening to environmental greening
- rights to responsibilities."[1]

In modern society it is easy to live in a way that removes us from the immediacy of our natural environment. Instead of hunting or growing our food, we can go to the grocery store and then pop dinner in the microwave. And instead of the light of day dictating when we work, we can work in our electrified and temperature-regulated office or home any time we want. Test yourself: how aware are you of your natural environment? Can you name ten plants and animals that thrive in your area? Do you know when the sun rises? Sets? Where the water in the nearby river runs from and flows to?

In order to regain an awareness of the rhythms of nature and a feel for our interconnectedness with the natural world, it may be necessary to leave the comforts of home and spend time outdoors. One way to do this is to take part in an outdoor education program. These programs help strip away the layers of conventional life by allowing people to live, at least for a short time, in a new "reality." It is hoped that through activities, group discussion, and introspection the experience will allow participants to more clearly see themselves as part of an ecosystem.

Here is an example of how easily you can become aware of something when given a different reality: Joe sees the broken bottles in one parking space and quickly steers his car into another. He is annoyed by the broken glass but quickly forgets about it as he heads to work. Joe, one week later on a canoeing trip in the wilderness, catches site of an old plastic jug in the reeds along the shore of an otherwise pristine lake. Instead of quickly dismissing it, he quietly ponders the extent to which we have polluted the natural world and wonders if he is doing all that he can to prevent it. Outdoor educators hope that after such an experience an individual will be more open to, or rededicated to, taking part in things like recycling, reducing consumption, and preventing water contamination. For ideas on what you can do as a college student to care for and preserve the environment, see the box on pages 354.

How the Natural World Influences Us

The natural world is our home, and its influence surrounds us. The pattern of our lives is tied to the natural rhythms of the passing of the seasons, the rise and fall of the tides, and day's passing into night. Where we live and what natural resources we have available affect who we are and how we work and play. The natural environment of a ranch in Montana is very different from that of urban California. No matter what our setting, a wellness lifestyle can be enhanced by taking advantage of the opportunities offered by our natural world. Following are a few examples of how lifestyle can be affected by the natural environment:

The food we eat influences our health.

- Traditionally, people have eaten foods native to their geographic area. With modern refrigeration and transportation, foods from all over the world have become available to many people. This has resulted in both good and bad changes. For example, for some Native Americans a change in diet has brought a higher prevalence of obesity and diabetes. On the other hand, people who once ate a lot of red meat have learned from other cultures to modify their diets with foods lower in fat and cholesterol.

Our natural environment influences physical activity.

- Where we live and the type of weather we experience influences the activities available to us. People

You Can Make a Difference

Caring for the environment can be something as simple as recycling a soda can or as involved as organizing curbside recycling in a town. As a student you may not have a lot of time to devote to big projects, but there are still numerous meaningful things you can do that take little time. If you are interested in tackling larger projects, pool your time and energy with other motivated students and faculty members. Sharing the job makes it manageable. Consider joining or forming an environmental club. If you don't have time to be a regular member of a club or organization, consider volunteering for one of their projects. Here are a few other ways you can help the environment:

- Create less garbage by using a reusable cup or glass. Use washable silverware and dishes at home instead of plastic utensils and paper plates.
- If you commute to campus, try to carpool one or more days a week. This reduces pollution from car exhaust and will save gas money.
- Ride a bike or walk to campus whenever possible. This eliminates exhaust pollution while building in some or all of your recommended thirty minutes a day of physical activity.
- Throw beverage cans into a recycle bin instead of the trash. Many campuses locate collection boxes near soda machines. If your campus doesn't have a recycling plan, bring the idea to your student government and, if possible, volunteer to get it organized.

- Dispose of newspapers in a recycle bin. If no such bin exists, work to get one established.
- Recycling any product by passing it on to someone who can use it helps to decrease waste. Organize or propose (to the student government or other organization) the idea of a campus-wide garage sale. The sale can occur at the end of the year when students are moving out or items can be collected in the spring and sold in the fall when students move back onto campus. Students will save money by purchasing used items for their rooms and the funds raised through the sale can be used for other student-sponsored projects.
- Gather clothes that you no longer wear and recycle them to those in need.
- Help put together a map of places around town that sell used or recycled products and ask the student government for help distributing it to the student body. List on the map what kinds of things one can purchase at each location.
- If the campus bookstore is not already offering recycled notepaper and greeting cards, write a letter requesting that it do so. Encourage others to write also —preferably on recycled paper!
- Purchase recycled engine oil. Oil doesn't wear out; it simply gets dirty. Recycled oil has been cleaned and is as good as new. Look for places that sell it and pass the word.

who live in year-round warm-weather climates tend to be more physically active than those with long, cold winters. When the weather is nice, people like to be outside, go for a walk, or garden. Many people enjoy winter sports or being outdoors in a variety of weather conditions. For example, a zoo on a rainy day offers us a very different perspective. For those who don't enjoy exercising outside in inclement weather, there are a variety of home and indoor exercise and recreation facilities available.

- Our ability to be physically active is affected by heat, humidity, pollen, and air pollution. City joggers sometimes have difficulty in high-traffic areas because of carbon monoxide produced in exhaust. In some locations, people (especially those with respiratory conditions) are advised to check the air quality index before exerting themselves outdoors. Exercising early in the day before traffic builds up and temperatures rise can help reduce such problems.

The climate we live in influences the patterns of our life and sometimes our health.

- Climate influences things as diverse as construction schedules, school closings, planting and harvesting, recreational and work activities, and how we dress.

- Different kinds of weather affect people's moods. Some people love the cold, others the heat. Some tolerate rain well, others find it depressing. Air conditioning and central heat have helped modify the effects of weather; so too have opportunities to live or vacation in different climates.

- People who live in sunny climates and spend a lot of time outdoors have a higher incidence of skin cancer, while those who live in places with long, dark winters have a greater incidence of depression.[2] Making appropriate adjustments such as proper clothing, sun tan lotion, light therapy, and getting outdoors in the winter can alleviate some climate-induced problems and enhance wellness.

- Form a group of students to ask the college or university administration if you can use a plot of land for a community garden. Vegetables and flowers can be grown for personal use or donated to nursing homes and food banks. This project may lead to, or fall under, the auspices of a garden club.
- When you purchase a product and feel that the packaging around it is excessive, call the company's 800 number and let them know you are concerned. If a phone number does not appear on the product, call the toll-free directory information service at 1-800-555-1212.
- Read labels, especially on products you buy frequently. For example, a product that contains ozone-depleting chemicals like chlorofluorocarbons (CFCs) or methyl choloroform (also called 1,1,1-tricholoroethane) can often be substituted with a product that is safer for the environment. More information concerning ozone-depleters can be obtained by writing to: The Natural Resources Defense Council, 1350 New York Avenue, N.W., Washington, DC 20005 or the Environmental Defense Fund, 257 Park Ave. South, New York, NY 10010.
- On the bottom of plastic containers you will find a recycle number. Find out which numbers are being recycled in your area. Try to buy products that are packaged in containers that can be recycled in your town. Containers that are recyclable, but for which there is no recycling program, end up in landfill.
- Organize or be involved in adopting a stream or stretch of highway or portion of campus. Keep your adopted area clean by picking up debris left by others. Or simply pick up a piece of trash and deposit in a trash can on your way to class each day.
- Hiking is one of many outdoor activities that enhance personal wellness. Here are some hiking hints that give attention to maintaining environmental wellness:
  1. Stay on the trail. This minimizes plant life damage.
  2. If you are going to touch a plant, do so with an open hand, allowing the blossom or leaf to rest in your palm. Never pick flowers, leaves, or blossoms.
  3. Pack out any garbage you generate and recycle what you can.
  4. Do not feed the animals. Food meant for humans can choke or otherwise harm wildlife.
  5. Learn about fires, light one only where permitted, and be sure to bury it before you leave.
  6. Fish or boat only where permitted and throw back fish that do not meet the legal size limit.
- For additional ideas and resources read *50 simple things you can do to save the Earth* by The Earth Works Group (Berkeley, CA: Earth Works Press, 1989), and *The next step: 50 more things you can do to save the Earth* by the same publisher.

- Air pollution can make it difficult to be physically active. Natural phenomena can also affect air quality. In 1998 a number of southern U.S. areas experienced weeks of smoky air as a result of the many fires burning in South American due to El Niño.

The geography that surrounds us influences our activities.

- Many occupations such as farming, fishing, and mining are dependent on the surrounding environment and its natural resources. Others such as computer work are not tied to the land and allow people more choice in where they live.
- Different geographic settings offer different opportunities for physical activity. Water offers swimming and boating opportunities; mountains provide hiking and skiing trails; the plains are great for biking, rollerblading, and cross-country skiing. Occasionally humankind decides to create "natural" environments in the least likely places; take, for example, ice skating at a rink in California and enjoying the surf at an indoor beach in a Minneapolis shopping mall!

- Different people react to geographic conditions differently. Some people enjoy the expansiveness and freedom of the big, open spaces but feel trapped and enclosed on narrow wooded Eastern roadways. Similarly an Easterner who feels comfortable among the trees may view the open West with awe or see it as stark and empty.
- A move to, or a vacation at a high-altitude location can cause headaches or nausea until the body can adjust. Taking it slowly, staying well hydrated, and getting plenty of rest will allow for a healthy transition.

Stress and relaxation can both be products of our interaction with our natural environment.

- Noise is one of our modern stressors. Constant high levels of noise, such as city or construction noise, can be both annoying and damaging to hearing. Wearing ear plugs while mowing the lawn or working with loud appliances can help limit exposure.

- New and unfamiliar surroundings can produce stress or be enjoyable. A city dweller may enjoy a vacation in a cabin in the woods or find it isolating and fearful. A country dweller may enjoy the excitement of the city or feel serious apprehension walking down a crowded city sidewalk.

Animals and plants enrich our lives when proper precautions are taken.

- Outdoor recreation can be very satisfying but one must take into account the conditions of the physical environment. A walk in the woods, for example, can be the perfect release as long as someone knows about and takes precautions against things like poison ivy and tick bites. Dehydration, frostbite, sunburn, insect bites, and heat stroke are just a few of the problems that can avoided with proper attention and planning.

- Many people think of the natural environment only in terms of the country, suburban or undeveloped land, mountains, and forests, but cities are also home to an ecosystem of plants and animals. City wildlife thrives in parks and zoos but is also tucked into unusual places—like the falcons who nest on skyscraper ledges. Manhattan's Central Park is considered one of the best places for bird watching in the country. Plant life of all varieties can be found in city parks, as landscaping, and as gardens on balconies and rooftops. Most cities also have waterways, lakes, ponds, or ocean frontage teeming with life.

The wide variety of natural environments in the United States afford us many opportunities for enjoyment. We can ride a bike along a city or town road or up a mountain. We can hike a trail or climb the steps of a monument or tall building. We can eat fresh strawberries, peas, salmon, or trout. And we can shed our stress on a porch swing or by dancing under the stars at a rooftop party. No matter where we choose to live or recreate, the natural world touches our lives. Stop for a moment and share the next sunset as it is reflected in the thousand windows of a skyscraper, ripples quietly in a lake, or shines through your window and warms your room.

SUMMARY

You are ultimately responsible for your own behavior and in control of your lifestyle habits; however, you should recognize that your actions will be influenced by both your human-cultural and natural environments. These influences can be very positive and supportive, or they can make change difficult. Try to find ways to meld personal desires with those of people around you. This helps foster positive relationships and a healthy society. Sometimes, however, you may be faced with a destructive or hostile environment that threatens your efforts to make or sustain healthy choices. In these instances, you may have to leave the environment (such as an abusive home) or seek an intervention (such as counseling) in order to change your environment or change how you react to it. In many cases, however, a negative environment can be turned into a supportive one through communication, compromise, and positive example. Furthermore, open yourself to the possibility that you can do more to enrich, and less to harm your environment, and look for proactive ways to accomplish this. Like the ripples of a stone tossed into a pond, the positive changes you make will touch all life around you.

Lab 15.1

Where Am I?

Putting It All Together

Now that you have finished the book, it's time to reevaluate the progress you have made since you began. At the beginning of each chapter you staged yourself for each wellness area. Let's consider these your beginning stages. The table that follows shows all the wellness areas covered in this textbook. Refer back to the first part of each chapter and using the table below, mark your beginning stage for each of the wellness areas. Use the Before column for your beginning scores. In the After column mark your stages of readiness now that you have completed the class. Hopefully you will have moved toward Maintainer in one or more areas. If some areas did not show progress, you'll see where to concentrate your future efforts. Lab 15.2 will help you get started with your future activities.

Chapter	Before					After				
3. Cardiorespiratory Endurance										
Moderately Intense Activity	❏ PC	❏ C	❏ P	❏ AT	❏ M	❏ PC	❏ C	❏ P	❏ AT	❏ M
Vigorous Exercise	❏ PC	❏ C	❏ P	❏ AT	❏ M	❏ PC	❏ C	❏ P	❏ AT	❏ M
4. Flexibility	❏ PC	❏ C	❏ P	❏ AT	❏ M	❏ PC	❏ C	❏ P	❏ AT	❏ M
5. Muscle Strength and Endurance	❏ PC	❏ C	❏ P	❏ AT	❏ M	❏ PC	❏ C	❏ P	❏ AT	❏ M
6. Nutrition	❏ PC	❏ C	❏ P	❏ AT	❏ M	❏ PC	❏ C	❏ P	❏ AT	❏ M
8. Body Composition	❏ PC	❏ C	❏ P	❏ AT	❏ M	❏ PC	❏ C	❏ P	❏ AT	❏ M
9. Cardiovascular Disease	❏ PC	❏ C	❏ P	❏ AT	❏ M	❏ PC	❏ C	❏ P	❏ AT	❏ M
10. Cancer	❏ PC	❏ C	❏ P	❏ AT	❏ M	❏ PC	❏ C	❏ P	❏ AT	❏ M
11. Stress	❏ PC	❏ C	❏ P	❏ AT	❏ M	❏ PC	❏ C	❏ P	❏ AT	❏ M
12. Healthy Relationships	❏ PC	❏ C	❏ P	❏ AT	❏ M	❏ PC	❏ C	❏ P	❏ AT	❏ M
13. STDs	❏ PC	❏ C	❏ P	❏ AT	❏ M	❏ PC	❏ C	❏ P	❏ AT	❏ M
14. Substance Abuse										
Alcohol	❏ PC	❏ C	❏ P	❏ AT	❏ M	❏ PC	❏ C	❏ P	❏ AT	❏ M
Tobacco	❏ PC	❏ C	❏ P	❏ AT	❏ M	❏ PC	❏ C	❏ P	❏ AT	❏ M
Drugs	❏ PC	❏ C	❏ P	❏ AT	❏ M	❏ PC	❏ C	❏ P	❏ AT	❏ M
Abuse Prevention	❏ PC	❏ C	❏ P	❏ AT	❏ M	❏ PC	❏ C	❏ P	❏ AT	❏ M

PC = Precontemplator   AT = Action Taker
C = Contemplator   M = Maintainer
P = Preparer

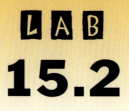

Choosing a Focus Area
for the Near Future

Look at the results of the restaging you did in Lab 15.1. If you are a maintainer in any of the areas or are at other stages of initiating change, keep up the good work. Using the space below, list each of the wellness areas in which you are *not* a maintainer.

From the above list, choose one area in which you initiated change during this course and would like to focus and work on after the class has ended, and write the area below.

Now list your goals for this area. That is, what are you working toward?

Write out your plan for achieving the goals you named above. Be sure to list supports and barriers you will encounter as you move toward your goal. (Refer back to your labs from earlier chapters as reference.)

Remember, true wellness is not just a short-term change; it requires a lifetime of good choices. Commit yourself now to a path of wellness.

Appendices

APPENDIX A

Recommended Dietary Allowances

Category	Age (yr) or Condition	Weight[a] (kg)	Weight[a] (lb)	Height[a] (cm)	Height[a] (in.)	Protein (g)	Fat-Soluble Vitamins Vitamin A (µg RE)[b]	Vitamin D (µg)[c]	Vitamin E (mg α-TE)	Vitamin K (µg)
Males	15–18	66	145	176	69	59	1000	10	10	65
	19–24	72	160	177	70	58	1000	10	10	70
	25–50	79	174	176	70	63	1000	5	10	80
	51+	77	170	173	68	63	1000	5	10	80
Females	15–18	55	120	163	64	44	800	10	8	55
	19–24	58	128	164	65	48	800	10	8	60
	25–50	63	138	163	64	50	800	5	8	65
	51+	65	143	160	63	50	800	5	8	65
Pregnant						60	800	10	10	65
Lactating	1st 6 months					65	1300	10	12	65
	2nd 6 months					62	1200	10	11	65

[a]Weights and heights of reference adults are actual medians for the US population of the designated age as reported by NHANES II. The use of these figures does not imply that the height-to-weight ratios are ideal.

[b]RE, Retinol equivalents (1 RE = 1 µg retinol or 6 µg β-carotene); α-TE, α-tocopherol equivalents (1 mg d-α tocopherol = 1 α-TE); NE, niacin equivalent (1 NE = 1 mg of niacin or 60 mg of dietary tryptophan).

[c]As cholecalciferol; 10 µg cholecalciferol = 400 IU of vitamin D.

Water-Soluble Vitamins							Minerals						
Vitamin C (mg)	Thiamin (mg)	Ribo-flavin (mg)	Niacin (mg NE)	Vitamin B_6 (mg)	Folate (µg)	Vitamin B_{12} (µg)	Calcium (mg)	Phos-phorus (mg)	Magne-sium (mg)	Iron (mg)	Zinc (mg)	Iodine (µg)	Selenium (µg)
60	1.5	1.8	20	2.0	200	2.0	1200	1200	400	12	15	150	50
60	1.5	1.7	19	2.0	200	2.0	1200	1200	350	10	15	150	70
60	1.5	1.7	19	2.0	200	2.0	800	800	350	10	15	150	70
60	1.2	1.4	15	2.0	200	2.0	800	800	350	10	15	150	70
60	1.1	1.3	15	1.5	180	2.0	1200	1200	300	15	12	150	50
60	1.1	1.3	15	1.6	180	2.0	1200	1200	280	15	12	150	55
60	1.1	1.3	15	1.6	180	2.0	800	800	280	15	12	150	55
60	1.0	1.2	13	1.6	180	2.0	800	800	280	10	12	150	55
70	1.5	1.6	17	2.2	400	2.2	1200	1200	320	30	15	175	65
95	1.6	1.8	20	2.1	280	2.6	1200	1200	355	15	19	200	75
90	1.6	1.7	20	2.1	260	2.6	1200	1200	340	15	16	200	75

Source: Food and Nutrition Board, National Academy of Sciences—National Research Council. *Recommended dietary allowances.* Washington, D.C.: U.S. Government Printing Office, 1989.

Notes: The allowances, expressed as average daily intakes over time, provide for individual variations among most normal persons as they live in the United States under usual environmental stresses. Diets should be based on a variety of common foods to provide other nutrients for which human requirements have been less well defined.

APPENDIX B1

Nutritive Value of Selected Foods

Description of Food	Serving Size	Wt (g)	Cal (kcal)	Prot (g)	Fat (g)	Sat Fat (g)	Chol (mg)	Carbo (g)	Calc (mg)	Sod (mg)
Beverages										
Beer, light	12 fl oz	355	95	1	0	0	0	5	14	11
Beer, regular	12 fl oz	360	150	1	0	0	0	13	14	18
Club soda	12 fl oz	355	0	0	0	0	0	0	18	78
Coffee, brewed	6 fl oz	180	0	0	0	0	0	0	4	2
Cola, diet	12 fl oz	355	0	0	0	0	0	0	14	32
Cola, regular	12 fl oz	369	160	0	0	0	0	41	11	18
Fruit punch drink, canned	6 fl oz	190	85	0	0	0	0	22	15	15
Gin, rum, vodka, whiskey, 80-proof	1.5 fl oz	42	95	0	0	0	0	0	0	0
Ginger ale	12 fl oz	366	125	0	0	0	0	32	11	29
Grape soda	12 fl oz	372	180	0	0	0	0	46	15	48
Lemon-lime soda	12 fl oz	372	155	0	0	0	0	39	7	33
Orange soda	12 fl oz	372	180	0	0	0	0	46	15	52
Pepper-type soda	12 fl oz	369	160	0	0	0	0	41	11	37
Pineapple-grapefruit juice drink	6 fl oz	187	90	0	0	0	0	23	13	24
Root beer	12 fl oz	370	165	0	0	0	0	42	15	48
Tea, brewed	8 fl oz	240	0	0	0	0	0	0	0	1
Wine, dessert	3.5 fl oz	103	140	0	0	0	0	8	8	9
Wine, table, red	3.5 fl oz	102	75	0	0	0	0	3	8	5
Wine, table, white	3.5 fl oz	102	80	0	0	0	0	3	9	5
Breads										
Bagels, egg	1 bagel	68	200	7	2	0.3	44	38	29	245
Bagels, plain	1 bagel	68	200	7	2	0.3	0	38	29	245
Baking powder biscuits, from mix	1 biscuit	28	95	2	3	0.8	0	14	58	262
Breadcrumbs, dry, grated	1 cup	100	390	13	5	1.5	5	73	122	736
Bread stuffing, from mix, moist	1 cup	203	420	9	26	5.3	67	40	81	1023
French bread	1 slice	35	100	3	1	0.3	0	18	39	203
Italian bread	1 slice	30	85	3	0	0	0	17	5	176
Mixed-grain bread	1 slice	25	65	2	1	0.2	0	12	27	106
Oatmeal bread	1 slice	25	65	2	1	0.2	0	12	15	124
Pita bread	1 pita	60	165	6	1	0.1	0	33	49	339
Pumpernickel bread	1 slice	32	80	3	1	0.2	0	16	23	177
Raisin bread	1 slice	25	65	2	1	0.2	0	13	25	92
Rolls, dinner, commercial	1 roll	28	85	2	2	0.5	0	14	33	155
Rolls, frankfurter & hamburger	1 roll	40	115	3	2	0.5	0	20	54	241
Rolls, hoagie, or submarine	1 roll	135	400	11	8	1.8	0	72	100	683
Rye bread, light	1 slice	25	65	2	1	0.2	0	12	20	175

Description of Food	Serving Size	Wt (g)	Cal (kcal)	Prot (g)	Fat (g)	Sat Fat (g)	Chol (mg)	Carbo (g)	Calc (mg)	Sod (mg)
Vienna bread	1 slice	25	70	2	1	0.2	0	13	28	145
Wheat bread	1 slice	25	65	2	1	0.2	0	12	32	138
Whole-wheat bread	1 slice	28	70	3	1	0.4	0	13	20	180

Cereals

Description of Food	Serving Size	Wt (g)	Cal (kcal)	Prot (g)	Fat (g)	Sat Fat (g)	Chol (mg)	Carbo (g)	Calc (mg)	Sod (mg)
All-Bran cereal	1 oz	28.35	70	4	1	0.1	0	21	23	320
Cap'n Crunch cereal	1 oz	28.35	120	1	3	1.7	0	23	5	213
Cheerios cereal	1 oz	28.35	110	4	2	0.3	0	20	48	307
Corn Flakes, Kellogg's	1 oz	28.35	110	2	0	0	0	24	1	351
Cream of wheat, cooked	1 pkt	142	100	3	0	0	0	21	20	241
Froot Loops cereal	1 oz	28.35	110	2	1	0.2	0	25	3	145
Golden Grahams cereal	1 oz	28.35	110	2	1	0.7	0	24	17	346
Grape-Nuts cereal	1 oz	28.35	100	3	0	0	0	23	11	197
Honey Nut Cheerios cereal	1 oz	28.35	105	3	1	0.1	0	23	20	257
Lucky Charms cereal	1 oz	28.35	110	3	1	0.2	0	23	32	201
Nature Valley Granola cereal	1 oz	28.35	125	3	5	3.3	0	19	18	58
Oatmeal, cooked, regular, quick, instant, w/ salt	1 cup	234	145	6	2	0.4	0	25	19	374
Oatmeal, cooked, instant, flavored, fortified	1 pkt	164	160	5	2	0.3	0	31	168	254
100% Natural cereal	1 oz	28.35	135	3	6	4.1	0	18	49	12
Product 19 cereal	1 oz	28.35	110	3	0	0	0	24	3	325
Raisin Bran, Kellogg's	1 oz	28.35	90	3	1	0.1	0	21	10	207
Raisin Bran, Post	1 oz	28.35	85	3	1	0.1	0	21	13	185
Rice Krispies cereal	1 oz	28.35	110	2	0	0	0	25	4	340
Shredded Wheat cereal	1 oz	28.35	100	3	1	0.1	0	23	11	3
Special K cereal	1 oz	28.35	110	6	0	0	0	21	8	265
Sugar Frosted Flakes, Kellogg's	1 oz	28.35	110	1	0	0	0	26	1	230
Sugar Smacks cereal	1 oz	28.35	105	2	1	0.1	0	25	3	75
Super Sugar Crisp cereal	1 oz	28.35	105	2	0	0	0	26	6	25
Total cereal	1 oz	28.35	100	3	1	0.1	0	22	48	352
Trix cereal	1 oz	28.35	110	2	0	0.2	0	25	6	181
Wheaties cereal	1 oz	28.35	100	3	0	0.1	0	23	43	354

Dairy Products

Description of Food	Serving Size	Wt (g)	Cal (kcal)	Prot (g)	Fat (g)	Sat Fat (g)	Chol (mg)	Carbo (g)	Calc (mg)	Sod (mg)
Cheddar cheese	1 oz	28.35	115	7	9	6	30	0	204	176
Chocolate milk, regular	1 cup	250	210	8	8	5.3	31	26	280	149
Cottage cheese, creamed, large curd	1 cup	225	235	28	10	6.4	34	6	135	911
Cream cheese	1 oz	28.35	100	2	10	6.2	31	1	23	84
Half and half, cream	1 Tbsp	15	20	0	2	1.1	6	1	16	6
Milk, low fat, 2%	1 cup	244	120	8	5	2.9	18	12	297	122
Milk, skim	1 cup	245	85	8	0	0.3	4	12	302	126
Milk, whole, 3.3% fat	1 cup	244	150	8	8	5.1	33	11	291	120
Pasteurized processed cheese food, American	1 oz	28.35	95	6	7	4.4	18	2	163	337
Ricotta cheese, whole milk	1 cup	246	430	28	32	20.4	124	7	509	207
Shakes, thick, chocolate	10 oz	283	335	9	8	4.8	30	60	374	314
Shakes, thick, vanilla	10 oz	283	315	11	9	5.3	33	50	413	270
Sherbet, 2% fat	1 cup	193	270	2	4	2.4	14	59	103	88
Sour cream	1 Tbsp	12	25	0	3	1.6	5	1	14	6
Swiss cheese	1 oz	28.35	105	8	8	5	26	1	272	74
Yogurt, w/ low-fat milk, fruit flavored	8 oz	227	230	10	2	1.6	10	43	345	133
Yogurt, w/ low-fat milk, plain	8 oz	227	145	12	4	2.3	14	16	415	159
Whipped topping, pressurized	1 Tbsp	3	10	0	1	0.4	2	0	3	4

Description of Food	Serving Size	Wt (g)	Cal (kcal)	Prot (g)	Fat (g)	Sat Fat (g)	Chol (mg)	Carbo (g)	Calc (mg)	Sod (mg)
Desserts, Crackers, and Snacks										
Angelfood cake, from mix	1 piece	53	125	3	0	0	0	29	44	269
Apple pie	1 piece	158	405	3	18	4.6	0	60	13	476
Blueberry muffins, from commercial mix	1 muffin	45	140	3	5	1.4	45	22	15	225
Blueberry pie	1 piece	158	380	4	17	4.3	0	55	17	423
Bran muffins, from commercial mix	1 muffin	45	140	3	4	1.3	28	24	27	385
Brownies w/ nuts, frosting, commercial	1 brownie	25	100	1	4	1.6	14	16	13	59
Carrot cake, cream cheese frosting	1 piece	96	385	4	21	4.1	74	48	44	279
Cheesecake	1 piece	92	280	5	18	9.9	170	26	52	204
Cheese crackers, plain	10 crackers	10	50	1	3	0.9	6	6	11	112
Cheese crackers, sandwich, peanut	1 sandwich	8	40	1	2	0.4	1	5	7	90
Cherry pie	1 piece	158	410	4	18	4.7	0	61	22	480
Chocolate chip cookies, commercial	4 cookies	42	180	2	9	2.9	5	28	13	140
Coffeecake, crumb, from mix	1 piece	72	230	5	7	2	47	38	44	310
Corn chips	1 oz	28.35	155	2	9	1.4	0	16	35	233
Corn muffins, from commercial mix	1 muffin	45	145	3	6	1.7	42	22	30	291
Croissants	1 croissant	57	235	5	12	3.5	13	27	20	452
Custard pie	1 piece	152	330	9	17	5.6	169	36	146	436
Danish pastry, fruit	1 pastry	65	235	4	13	3.9	56	28	17	233
Devil's food cake, chocolate frosting, from mix	1 piece	69	235	3	8	3.5	37	40	41	181
Doughnuts, cake type, plain	1 donut	50	210	3	12	2.8	20	24	22	192
English muffins, plain	1 muffin	57	140	5	1	0.3	0	27	96	378
Fig bars	4 cookies	56	210	2	4	1	27	42	40	180
French toast, home recipe	1 slice	65	155	6	7	1.6	112	17	72	257
Gingerbread cake, from mix	1 piece	63	175	2	4	1.1	1	32	57	192
Graham cracker, plain	2 crackers	14	60	1	1	0.4	0	11	6	86
Lemon meringue pie	1 piece	140	355	5	14	4.3	143	53	20	395
Oatmeal w/ raisins cookies	4 cookies	52	245	3	10	2.5	2	36	18	148
Peanut butter cookie, home recipe	4 cookies	48	245	4	14	4	22	28	21	142
Popcorn, air-popped, unsalted	1 cup	8	30	1	0	0	0	6	1	0
Popcorn, popped, vegetable oil, salted	1 cup	11	55	1	3	0.5	0	6	3	86
Pound cake, from home recipe	1 slice	30	120	2	5	1.2	32	15	20	96
Pretzels, stick	10 pretzels	3	10	0	0	0	0	2	1	48
Pumpkin pie	1 piece	152	320	6	17	6.4	109	37	78	325
Rye wafers, whole-grain	2 wafers	14	55	1	1	0.3	0	10	7	115
Saltines	4 crackers	12	50	1	1	0.5	4	9	3	165
Sandwich type cookie	4 cookies	40	195	2	8	2	0	29	12	189
Sugar cookie, from refrigerated dough	4 cookies	48	235	2	12	2.3	29	31	50	261
Toaster pastries	1 pastry	54	210	2	6	1.7	0	38	104	248
Wheat, thin crackers	4 crackers	8	35	1	1	0.5	0	5	3	69
Eggs										
Eggs, cooked, fried	1 egg	46	90	6	7	1.9	211	1	25	162
Eggs, cooked, hard-cooked	1 egg	50	75	6	5	1.6	213	1	25	62
Eggs, cooked, scrambled/omelet	1 egg	61	100	7	7	2.2	215	1	44	171
Eggs, raw, whole	1 egg	50	75	6	5	1.6	213	1	25	63
Fats, Oils, and Dressings										
Butter, salted	1 Tbsp	14	100	0	11	7.1	31	0	3	116
Corn oil	1 Tbsp	14	125	0	14	1.8	0	0	0	0
Fats, cooking/vegetable shortening	1 Tbsp	13	115	0	13	3.3	0	0	0	0

Description of Food	Serving Size	Wt (g)	Cal (kcal)	Prot (g)	Fat (g)	Sat Fat (g)	Chol (mg)	Carbo (g)	Calc (mg)	Sod (mg)
French salad dressing, regular	1 Tbsp	16	85	0	9	1.4	0	1	2	188
Italian salad dressing, regular	1 Tbsp	15	80	0	9	1.3	0	1	1	162
Margarine, imitation, 40% fat	1 Tbsp	14	50	0	5	1.1	0	0	2	134
Margarine, regular, soft, 80% fat	1 Tbsp	14	100	0	11	1.9	0	0	4	151
Mayonnaise, imitation	1 Tbsp	15	35	0	3	0.5	4	2	0	75
Mayonnaise, regular	1 Tbsp	14	100	0	11	1.7	8	0	3	80
Mayonnaise type salad dressing	1 Tbsp	15	60	0	5	0.7	4	4	2	107
Olive oil	1 Tbsp	14	125	0	14	1.9	0	0	0	0
Safflower oil	1 Tbsp	14	125	0	14	1.3	0	0	0	0
Tartar sauce	1 Tbsp	14	75	0	8	1.2	4	1	3	182
1000 island, salad dressing, regular	1 Tbsp	16	60	0	6	1	4	2	2	112
Vinegar and oil salad dressing	1 Tbsp	16	70	0	8	1.5	0	0	0	0

Fish and Shellfish

Description of Food	Serving Size	Wt (g)	Cal (kcal)	Prot (g)	Fat (g)	Sat Fat (g)	Chol (mg)	Carbo (g)	Calc (mg)	Sod (mg)
Fish sticks, frozen, reheated	1 stick	28	70	6	3	0.8	26	4	11	53
Flounder or sole, baked, butter	3 oz	85	120	16	6	3.2	68	0	13	145
Oysters, breaded, fried	1 oyster	45	90	5	5	1.4	35	5	49	70
Salmon, baked, red	3 oz	85	140	21	5	1.2	60	0	26	55
Salmon, smoked	3 oz	85	150	18	8	2.6	51	0	12	1700
Sardines, canned, oil, drained	3 oz	85	175	20	9	2.1	85	0	371	425
Scallops, breaded, frozen, reheated	6 scallops	90	195	15	10	2.5	70	10	39	298
Shrimp, canned, drained	3 oz	85	100	21	1	0.2	128	1	98	1955
Trout, broiled, w/ butter, lemon juice	3 oz	85	175	21	9	4.1	71	0	26	122
Tuna, canned, drained, oil, chunk, light	3 oz	85	165	24	7	1.4	55	0	7	303
Tuna, canned, drained, water, white	3 oz	85	135	30	1	0.3	48	0	17	468

Fruits and Fruit Juices

Description of Food	Serving Size	Wt (g)	Cal (kcal)	Prot (g)	Fat (g)	Sat Fat (g)	Chol (mg)	Carbo (g)	Calc (mg)	Sod (mg)
Apples, dried, sulfured	10 rings	64	155	1	0	0	0	42	9	56
Apple juice, canned	1 cup	248	115	0	0	0	0	29	17	7
Apples, raw, unpeeled, 3 per lb	1 apple	138	80	0	0	0.1	0	21	10	0
Applesauce, canned, sweetened	1 cup	255	195	0	0	0.1	0	51	10	8
Apricots, dried, uncooked	1 cup	130	310	5	1	0	0	80	59	13
Apricots, raw	3 apricots	106	50	1	0	0	0	12	15	1
Avocados	1 avocado	304	340	5	27	5.3	Chol	27	33	15
Bananas	1 banana	114	105	1	1	0.2	0	27	7	1
Blackberries, raw	1 cup	144	75	1	1	0.2	0	18	46	0
Blueberries, raw	1 cup	145	80	1	1	0	0	20	9	9
Cantaloupe, raw	½ melon	267	95	2	1	0.1	0	22	29	24
Cherries, sweet, raw	10 cherries	68	50	1	1	0.1	0	11	10	0
Cranberry juice cocktail w/ vitamin C	1 cup	253	145	0	0	0	0	38	8	10
Cranberry sauce, canned, sweetened	1 cup	277	420	1	0	0	0	108	11	80
Dates	10 dates	83	230	2	0	0.1	0	61	27	2
Fruit cocktail, canned, heavy syrup	1 cup	255	185	1	0	0	0	48	15	15
Fruit cocktail, canned, juice pack	1 cup	248	115	1	0	0	0	29	20	10
Grapefruit juice, canned, sweetened	1 cup	250	115	1	0	0	0	28	20	5
Grapefruit, raw, white	½ fruit	120	40	1	0	0	0	10	14	0
Grape juice, frozen, diluted, sweetened, w/ vitamin C	1 cup	250	125	0	0	0.1	0	32	10	5
Grapes, raw	10 grapes	50	35	0	0	0.1	0	9	6	1
Honeydew melon, raw	1/10 melon	129	45	1	0	0	0	12	8	13
Kiwifruit, raw	1 kiwi	76	45	1	0	0	0	11	20	4
Lemons, raw	1 lemon	58	15	1	0	0	0	5	15	1
Mangos, raw	1 mango	207	135	1	1	0.1	0	35	21	4
Nectarines, raw	1 nectarine	136	65	1	1	0.1	0	16	7	0
Orange juice, chilled	1 cup	249	110	2	1	0.1	0	25	25	2

Description of Food	Serving Size	Wt (g)	Cal (kcal)	Prot (g)	Fat (g)	Sat Fat (g)	Chol (mg)	Carbo (g)	Calc (mg)	Sod (mg)
Orange juice, frozen, concentrate, diluted	1 cup	249	110	2	0	0	0	27	22	2
Orange juice, raw	1 cup	248	110	2	0	0.1	0	26	27	2
Oranges, raw	1 orange	131	60	1	0	0	0	15	52	0
Papayas, raw	1 cup	140	65	1	0	0.1	0	17	35	9
Peaches, canned, heavy syrup	1 cup	256	190	1	0	0	0	51	8	15
Peaches, canned, juice pack	1 cup	248	110	2	0	0	0	29	15	10
Peaches, raw	1 peach	87	35	1	0	0	0	10	4	0
Pears, raw, Bartlett	1 pear	166	100	1	1	0	0	25	18	0
Pineapple, canned, heavy syrup	1 cup	255	200	1	0	0	0	52	36	3
Pineapple, raw, diced	1 cup	155	75	1	1	0	0	19	11	2
Plums, raw, 1½-in. diam	1 plum	28	15	0	0	0	0	4	1	0
Prunes, dried	5 large	49	115	1	0	0	0	31	25	2
Raisins	1 cup	145	435	5	1	0.2	0	115	71	17
Raspberries, frozen, sweetened	1 cup	250	255	2	0	0	0	65	38	3
Raspberries, raw	1 cup	123	60	1	1	0	0	14	27	0
Strawberries, frozen, sweetened	1 cup	255	245	1	0	0	0	66	28	8
Strawberries, raw	1 cup	149	45	1	1	0	0	10	21	1
Tangerines, raw	1 tangerine	84	35	1	0	0	0	9	12	1
Watermelon, raw	1 piece	482	155	3	2	0.3	0	35	39	10
Grains										
Bulgur, uncooked	1 cup	170	600	19	3	1.2	0	129	49	7
Macaroni, cooked, firm	1 cup	130	190	7	1	0.1	0	39	14	1
Noodles, chow mein, canned	1 cup	45	220	6	11	2.1	5	26	14	450
Noodles, egg, cooked	1 cup	160	200	7	2	0.5	50	37	16	3
Rice, brown, cooked	1 cup	195	230	5	1	0.3	0	50	23	0
Rice, white, cooked	1 cup	205	225	4	0	0.1	0	50	21	0
Rice, white, instant, cooked	1 cup	165	180	4	0	0.1	0	40	5	0
Spaghetti, cooked, firm	1 cup	130	190	7	1	0.1	0	39	14	1
Tortillas, corn	1 tortilla	30	65	2	1	0.1	0	13	42	1
Waffles, from mix	1 waffle	75	205	7	8	2.7	59	27	179	515
Legumes, Nuts, and Seeds										
Almonds, whole	1 oz	28.35	165	6	15	1.4	0	6	75	3
Beans, dry, canned, w/ pork + tomato sauce	1 cup	255	310	16	7	2.4	10	48	138	1181
Black beans, dry, cooked, drained	1 cup	171	225	15	1	0.1	0	41	47	1
Black-eyed peas, dry, cooked	1 cup	250	190	13	1	0.2	0	35	43	20
Brazil nuts	1 oz	28.35	185	4	19	4.6	0	4	50	1
Cashew nuts, dry-roasted, salted	1 oz	28.35	165	4	13	2.6	0	9	13	181
Cashew nuts, oil-roasted, salted	1 cup	130	750	21	63	12.4	0	37	53	814
Chickpeas, cooked, drained	1 cup	163	270	15	4	0.4	0	45	80	11
Coconut, dried, sweetened, shredded	1 cup	93	470	3	33	29.3	0	44	14	244
Filberts (hazelnuts), chopped	1 cup	115	725	15	72	5.3	0	18	216	3
Lentils, dry, cooked	1 cup	200	215	16	1	0.1	0	38	50	26
Lima beans, dry, cooked, drained	1 cup	190	260	16	1	0.2	0	49	55	4
Macadamia nuts, oil roasted, salted	1 cup	134	960	10	103	15.4	0	17	60	348
Mixed nuts w/ peanuts, dry, salted	1 oz	28.35	170	5	15	2	0	7	20	190
Peanuts, oil roasted, salted	1 cup	145	840	39	71	9.9	0	27	125	626
Peanut butter	1 Tbsp	16	95	5	8	1.4	0	3	5	75
Peas, split, dry, cooked	1 cup	200	230	16	1	0.1	0	42	22	26
Pine nuts	1 oz	28.35	160	3	17	2.7	0	5	2	20
Pinto beans, dry, cooked, drained	1 cup	180	265	15	1	0.1	0	49	86	3
Pumpkin and squash kernels	1 oz	28.35	155	7	13	2.5	0	5	12	5
Red kidney beans, dry, canned	1 cup	255	230	15	1	0.1	0	42	74	968

Description of Food	Serving Size	Wt (g)	Cal (kcal)	Prot (g)	Fat (g)	Sat Fat (g)	Chol (mg)	Carbo (g)	Calc (mg)	Sod (mg)
Sesame seeds	1 Tbsp	8	45	2	4	0.6	0	1	11	3
Walnuts, black, chopped	1 cup	125	760	30	71	4.5	0	15	73	1

Meats and Meat Products

Description of Food	Serving Size	Wt (g)	Cal (kcal)	Prot (g)	Fat (g)	Sat Fat (g)	Chol (mg)	Carbo (g)	Calc (mg)	Sod (mg)
Beef roast, eye round, lean	2.6 oz	75	135	22	5	1.9	52	0	3	46
Beef roast, rib, lean	2.2 oz	61	150	17	9	3.6	49	0	5	45
Beef steak, sirloin, broiled, lean	2.5 oz	72	150	22	6	2.6	64	0	8	48
Beef, canned, corned	3 oz	85	185	22	10	4.2	80	0	17	802
Bologna	2 slices	57	180	7	16	6.1	31	2	7	581
Brown and serve sausage, browned	1 link	13	50	2	5	1.7	9	0	1	105
Frankfurter, cooked	1 frank	45	145	5	13	4.8	23	1	5	504
Ground beef, broiled, lean	3 oz	85	230	21	16	6.2	74	0	9	65
Ground beef, broiled, regular	3 oz	85	245	20	18	6.9	76	0	9	70
Lamb chops, loin, broiled, lean	2.3 oz	64	140	19	6	2.6	60	0	12	54
Pork chop, loin, panfry, lean	2.4 oz	67	180	19	11	3.7	72	0	3	57
Pork, cured, bacon, Canadian, cooked	2 slices	46	85	11	4	1.3	27	1	5	711
Pork, cured, bacon, regular, cooked	3 slices	19	110	6	9	3.3	16	0	2	303
Pork, cured, ham, roasted, lean	2.4 oz	68	105	17	4	1.3	37	0	5	902
Pork, luncheon meat, cooked ham, regular	2 slices	57	105	10	6	1.9	32	2	4	751
Salami, cooked type	2 slices	57	145	8	11	4.6	37	1	7	607
Sandwich spread, pork, beef	1 Tbsp	15	35	1	3	0.9	6	2	2	152
Veal cutlet, med fat, braised, broiled	3 oz	85	185	23	9	4.1	86	0	9	56

Mixed Dishes

Description of Food	Serving Size	Wt (g)	Cal (kcal)	Prot (g)	Fat (g)	Sat Fat (g)	Chol (mg)	Carbo (g)	Calc (mg)	Sod (mg)
Beef and vegetable stew, home recipe	1 cup	245	220	16	11	4.4	71	15	29	292
Beef potpie, home recipe	1 piece	210	515	21	30	7.9	42	39	29	596
Cheeseburger, regular	1 sandwich	112	300	15	15	7.3	44	28	135	672
Cheeseburger, 4-oz patty	1 sandwich	194	525	30	31	15.1	104	40	236	1224
Chicken a la king, home recipe	1 cup	245	470	27	34	12.9	221	12	127	760
Chicken chow mein, canned	1 cup	250	95	7	0	0.1	8	18	45	725
Chicken and noodles, home recipe	1 cup	240	365	22	18	5.1	103	26	26	600
Chili con carne w/ beans, canned	1 cup	255	340	19	16	5.8	28	31	82	1354
Chop suey w/ beef + pork, home recipe	1 cup	250	300	26	17	4.3	68	13	60	1053
English muffin, egg, cheese, bacon	1 sandwich	138	360	18	18	8	213	31	197	832
Fish sandwich, reg, w/ cheese	1 sandwich	140	420	16	23	6.3	56	39	132	667
Hamburger, regular	1 sandwich	98	245	12	11	4.4	32	28	56	463
Macaroni and cheese, home recipe	1 cup	200	430	17	22	9.8	44	40	362	1086
Pizza, cheese	1 slice	120	290	15	9	4.1	56	39	220	699
Quiche lorraine	1 slice	176	600	13	48	23.2	285	29	211	653
Roast beef sandwich	1 sandwich	150	345	22	13	3.5	55	34	60	757
Spaghetti, tomato sauce, cheese, home recipe	1 cup	250	260	9	9	3	8	37	80	955
Spaghetti, meatballs, tomato sauce, home recipe	1 cup	248	330	19	12	3.9	89	39	124	1009

Poultry and Poultry Products

Description of Food	Serving Size	Wt (g)	Cal (kcal)	Prot (g)	Fat (g)	Sat Fat (g)	Chol (mg)	Carbo (g)	Calc (mg)	Sod (mg)
Chicken frankfurter	1 frank	45	115	6	9	2.5	45	3	43	616
Chicken, fried, batter, breast	4.9 oz	140	365	35	18	4.9	119	13	28	385
Chicken, fried, batter, drumstick	2.5 oz	72	195	16	11	3	62	6	12	194
Chicken, roasted, breast	3.0 oz	86	140	27	3	0.9	73	0	13	64
Turkey, roasted, dark meat	4 pieces	85	160	24	6	2.1	72	0	27	67
Turkey, roasted, light meat	2 pieces	85	135	25	3	0.9	59	0	16	54

Description of Food	Serving Size	Wt (g)	Cal (kcal)	Prot (g)	Fat (g)	Sat Fat (g)	Chol (mg)	Carbo (g)	Calc (mg)	Sod (mg)
Sauces and Gravies										
Barbecue sauce	1 Tbsp	16	10	0	0	0	0	2	3	130
Beef gravy, canned	1 cup	233	125	9	5	2.7	7	11	14	1305
Brown gravy from dry mix	1 cup	261	80	3	2	0.9	2	14	66	1147
Cheese sauce w/ milk, from mix	1 cup	279	305	16	17	9.3	53	23	569	1565
Chicken gravy, canned	1 cup	238	190	5	14	3.4	5	13	48	1373
Hollandaise sauce, w/ water, from mix	1 cup	259	240	5	20	11.6	52	14	124	1564
Soy sauce	1 Tbsp	18	10	2	0	0	0	2	3	1029
Soups										
Bean with bacon soup, canned	1 cup	253	170	8	6	1.5	3	23	81	951
Beef broth, bouillon, consommé, canned	1 cup	240	15	3a	1	0.3	0	0	14	782
Beef noodle soup, canned	1 cup	244	85	5	3	1.1	5	9	15	952
Bouillon, dehydrated, unprepared	1 packet	6	15	1	1	0.3	1	1	4	1019
Chicken noodle soup, dehydrated, prepared	1 packet	188	40	2	1	0.2	2	6	24	957
Chicken noodle soup, canned	1 cup	241	75	4	2	0.7	7	9	17	1106
Chicken rice soup, canned	1 cup	241	60	4	2	0.5	7	7	17	815
Clam chowder, Manhattan, canned	1 cup	244	80	4	2	0.4	2	12	34	1808
Clam chowder, New England, w/ milk	1 cup	248	165	9	7	3	22	17	186	992
Cream of chicken soup w/ milk, canned	1 cup	248	190	7	11	4.6	27	15	181	1047
Cream of mushroom soup w/ milk, canned	1 cup	248	205	6	14	5.1	20	15	179	1076
Minestrone soup, canned	1 cup	241	80	4	3	0.6	2	11	34	911
Onion soup, dehydrated, prepared	1 packet	184	20	1	0	0.1	0	4	9	635
Pea, green, soup, canned	1 cup	250	165	9	3	1.4	0	27	28	988
Tomato soup w/ milk, canned	1 cup	248	160	6	6	2.9	17	22	159	932
Tomato soup w/ water, canned	1 cup	244	85	2	2	0.4	0	17	12	871
Tomato vegetable soup, dehydrated, prepared	1 packet	189	40	1	1	0.3	0	8	6	856
Vegetable beef soup, canned	1 cup	244	80	6	2	0.9	5	10	17	956
Vegetarian soup, canned	1 cup	241	70	2	2	0.3	0	12	22	822
Sugar and Sweets										
Caramels, plain or chocolate	1 oz	28.35	115	1	3	2.2	1	22	42	64
Custard, baked	1 cup	265	305	14	15	6.8	278	29	297	209
Fudge, chocolate, plain	1 oz	28.35	115	1	3	2.1	1	21	22	54
Gelatin dessert, prepared	½ cup	120	70	2	0	0	0	17	2	55
Gum drops	1 oz	28.35	100	0	0	0	0	25	2	10
Hard candy	1 oz	28.35	110	0	0	0	0	28	0	7
Honey	1 Tbsp	21	65	0	0	0	0	17	1	1
Jams and preserves	1 Tbsp	20	55	0	0	0	0	14	4	2
Jellies	1 Tbsp	18	50	0	0	0	0	13	2	5
Jelly beans	1 oz	28.35	105	0	0	0	0	26	1	7
Marshmallows	1 oz	28.35	90	1	0	0	0	23	1	25
Milk chocolate candy, plain	1 oz	28.35	145	2	9	5.4	6	16	50	23
Milk chocolate candy, w/ almonds	1 oz	28.35	150	3	10	4.8	5	15	65	23
Milk chocolate candy, w/ peanuts	1 oz	28.35	155	4	11	4.2	5	13	49	19
Molasses, cane, blackstrap	2 Tbsp	40	85	0	0	0	0	22	274	38
Pudding, chocolate, cooked from mix	½ cup	130	150	4	4	2.4	15	25	146	167

Description of Food	Serving Size	Wt (g)	Cal (kcal)	Prot (g)	Fat (g)	Sat Fat (g)	Chol (mg)	Carbo (g)	Calc (mg)	Sod (mg)
Pudding, chocolate, instant, from mix	½ cup	130	155	4	4	2.3	14	27	130	440
Pudding, vanilla, cooked from mix	½ cup	130	145	4	4	2.3	15	25	132	178
Pudding, vanilla, instant, from mix	½ cup	130	150	4	4	2.2	15	27	129	375
Semisweet chocolate	1 cup	170	860	7	61	36.2	0	97	51	24
Sugar, brown, pressed down	1 cup	220	820	0	0	0	0	212	187	97
Sugar, white, granulated	1 Tbsp	12	45	0	0	0	0	12	0	0
Syrup, chocolate-flavored, thin	2 Tbsp	38	85	1	0	0.2	0	22	6	36
Table syrup (corn and maple)	2 Tbsp	42	122	0	0	0	0	32	1	19

Vegetables and Vegetable Products

Description of Food	Serving Size	Wt (g)	Cal (kcal)	Prot (g)	Fat (g)	Sat Fat (g)	Chol (mg)	Carbo (g)	Calc (mg)	Sod (mg)
Beets, cooked, drained, diced	1 cup	170	55	2	0	0	0	11	19	83
Broccoli, raw	1 spear	151	40	4	1	0.1	0	8	72	41
Cabbage, common, raw	1 cup	70	15	1	0	0	0	4	33	13
Cabbage, red, raw	1 cup	70	20	1	0	0	0	4	36	8
Carrots, raw, whole	1 carrot	72	30	1	0	0	0	7	19	25
Cauliflower, raw	1 cup	100	25	2	0	0	0	5	29	15
Corn, cooked from frozen, yellow	1 ear	63	60	2	0	0.1	0	14	2	3
Cucumber, w/ peel	6 slices	28	5	0	0	0	0	1	4	1
Eggplant, cooked, steamed	1 cup	96	25	1	0	0	0	6	6	3
Endive, curly, raw	1 cup	50	10	1	0	0	0	2	26	11
Lettuce, crisphead, raw, head	1 head	539	70	5	1	0.1	0	11	102	49
Lettuce, looseleaf	1 cup	56	10	1	0	0	0	2	38	5
Mushrooms, raw	1 cup	70	20	1	0	0	0	3	4	3
Onion rings, breaded, frozen, prepared	2 rings	20	80	1	5	1.7	0	8	6	75
Onions, raw, sliced	1 cup	115	40	1	0	0.1	0	8	29	2
Peas, edible pod, cooked, drained	1 cup	160	65	5	0	0.1	0	11	67	6
Peas, green, frozen, cooked, drained	1 cup	160	125	8	0	0.1	0	23	38	139
Peppers, sweet, raw, green	1 pepper	74	20	1	0	0	0	4	4	2
Peppers, sweet, raw, red	1 pepper	74	20	1	0	0	0	4	4	2
Potato chips	10 chips	20	105	1	7	1.8	0	10	5	94
Potatoes, au gratin, from mix	1 cup	245	230	6	10	6.3	12	31	203	1076
Potatoes, baked with skin	1 potato	202	220	5	0	0.1	0	51	20	16
Potatoes, boiled, peeled after	1 potato	136	120	3	0	0	0	27	7	5
Potatoes, boiled, peeled before	1 potato	135	115	2	0	0	0	27	11	7
Potatoes, french-fried, frozen, oven	10 strips	50	110	2	4	2.1	0	17	5	16
Potatoes, french-fried, frozen, fried	10 strips	50	160	2	8	2.5	0	20	10	108
Potatoes, mashed, recipe, milk & margarine	1 cup	210	225	4	9	2.2	4	35	55	620
Potatoes, mashed, from dehydrated	1 cup	210	235	4	12	7.2	29	32	103	697
Potato salad made w/ mayonnaise	1 cup	250	360	7	21	3.6	170	28	48	1323
Radishes, raw	4 radishes	18	5	0	0	0	0	1	4	4
Sauerkraut, canned	1 cup	236	45	2	0	0.1	0	10	71	1560
Snap bean, raw, cooked, drained, green	1 cup	125	45	2	0	0.1	0	10	58	4
Snap bean, frozen, cooked, drained, green	1 cup	135	35	2	0	0	0	8	61	18
Spinach, raw	1 cup	55	10	2	0	0	0	2	54	43
Squash, summer, cooked, drained	1 cup	180	35	2	1	0.1	0	8	49	2
Squash, winter, baked	1 cup	205	80	2	1	0.3	0	18	29	2
Sweetpotatoes, baked, peeled	1 potato	114	115	2	0	0	0	28	32	11
Tomato juice, canned with salt	1 cup	244	40	2	0	0	0	10	22	881
Tomato paste, canned with salt	1 cup	262	220	10	2	0.3	0	49	92	2070
Tomato puree, canned with salt	1 cup	250	105	4	0	0	0	25	38	998
Tomatoes, canned, w/ salt	1 cup	240	50	2	1	0.1	0	10	62	391
Tomato sauce, canned with salt	1 cup	245	75	3	0	0.1	0	18	34	1482

Description of Food	Serving Size	Wt (g)	Cal (kcal)	Prot (g)	Fat (g)	Sat Fat (g)	Chol (mg)	Carbo (g)	Calc (mg)	Sod (mg)
Tomatoes, raw	1 tomato	123	25	1	0	0	0	5	9	10
Vegetable juice cocktail, canned	1 cup	242	45	2	0	0	0	11	27	883
Vegetables, mixed, cooked from frozen	1 cup	182	105	5	0	0.1	0	24	46	64
Miscellaneous										
Baking powder	1 tsp	3	5	0	0	0	0	1	58	329
Catsup	1 Tbsp	15	15	0	0	0	0	4	3	156
Gelatin, dry	1 envelope	7	25	6	0	0	0	0	1	6
Mustard, prepared, yellow	1 tsp	5	5	0	0	0	0	0	4	63
Olives, canned, green	4 medium	13	15	0	2	0.2	0	0	8	312
Olives, canned, ripe	3 small	9	15	0	2	0.3	0	0	10	68
Pickles, cucumber, dill	1 pickle	65	5	0	0	0	0	1	17	928
Pickles, cucumber, fresh pack	2 slices	15	10	0	0	0	0	3	5	101
Relish, sweet	1 Tbsp	15	20	0	0	0	0	5	3	107
Salt	1 tsp	5.5	0	0	0	0	0	0	14	2132
Vinegar, cider	1 Tbsp	15	0	0	0	0	0	1	1	0
Yeast, baker's, dry, active	1 package	7	20	3	0	0	0	3	3	4

Source: Summarized from U.S. Department of Agriculture, Agricultural Research Department, 1997. USDA Nutrient Database for Standard Reference, Release 11-1. Nutrient Data Laboratory Home Page, http://www.nal.usda.gov/fnic/foodcomp.

APPENDIX B2

Nutritive Values of Selected Fast Foods

BURGER KING

ITEM *BURGERS*	Serving Size (g)	Calories	Calories From Fat	Total Fat (g)	Saturated Fat (g)	Cholesterol (mg)	Sodium (mg)	Total Carbohydrate (g)	Dietary Fiber (g)	Total Sugars (g)	Protein (g)	Vitamin A	Vitamin C	Calcium	Iron
Whopper® Sandwich	270	640	350	39	11	90	870	45	3	8	27	10	15	8	25
Whopper® With Cheese Sandwich	294	730	410	46	16	115	1350	46	3	8	33	15	15	25	25
Double Whopper® Sandwich	351	870	500	56	19	170	940	45	3	8	46	10	15	8	40
Double Whopper® With Cheese Sandwich	375	960	570	63	24	195	1420	46	3	8	52	15	15	25	40
Whopper Jr.® Sandwich	164	420	220	24	8	60	530	29	2	5	21	4	8	6	20
Whopper Jr.® With Cheese Sandwich	177	460	250	28	10	75	770	29	2	5	23	8	8	15	20
Big King Sandwich	226	660	390	43	18	135	920	29	1	4	40	8	0	25	25
Hamburger	126	330	140	15	6	55	530	28	1	4	20	2	0	4	15
Cheeseburger	138	380	170	19	9	65	770	28	1	5	23	6	0	10	15
Double Cheeseburger	210	600	320	36	17	135	1060	28	1	5	41	8	0	20	25
Double Cheeseburger With Bacon	218	640	350	39	18	145	1240	28	1	5	44	8	0	20	25
SANDWICHES/SIDE ORDERS															
BK Big Fish® Sandwich	252	720	390	43	9	80	1180	59	3	4	23	2	0	8	20
BK Broiler® Chicken Sandwich	247	530	230	26	5	105	1060	45	2	5	29	6	10	6	15
Chicken Sandwich	229	710	390	43	9	60	1400	54	2	4	26	0	0	10	20
Chicken Tenders® (8 pieces)	123	350	200	22	7	65	940	17	1	0	22	0	0	2	4
Broiled Chicken Salad†	302	190	70	8	4	75	500	9	3	5	20	100	25	15	8
Garden Salad†	215	100	45	5	3	15	110	7	3	4	6	110	50	15	6
Side Salad†	133	60	25	3	2	5	55	4	2	2	3	50	20	8	4
French Fries (Medium, Salted)	116	400	190	21	8	0	820	50	4	0	3	0	0	0	4
Onion Rings	124	310	130	14	2	0	810	41	6	6	4	0	0	10	8
Dutch Apple Pie	113	300	140	15	3	0	230	39	2	22	3	0	10	0	8

(continued)

ITEM *DRINKS*	Serving Size (g)	Calories	Calories From Fat	Total Fat (g)	Saturated Fat (g)	Choles-terol (mg)	Sodium (mg)	Total Carbohy-drate (g)	Dietary Fiber (g)	Total Sugars (g)	Protein (g)	Vitamin A	Vitamin C	Calcium	Iron
				Nutrition Facts								% Daily Value			
Vanilla Shake (Medium)	284	300	50	6	4	20	230	53	1	47	9	6	6	30	0
Chocolate Shake (Medium)	284	320	60	7	4	20	230	54	3	48	9	6	0	20	10
Chocolate Shake (Medium, Syrup Added)	341	440	60	7	4	20	430	84	2	78	10	6	6	30	6
Strawberry Shake (Medium, Syrup Added)	341	420	50	6	4	20	260	83	1	78	9	6	6	30	0
Coca Cola® Classic (Medium)	22 (fl oz)	280	0	0	0	0	@	70	0	70	0	0	0	0	0
Diet Coke® (Medium)	22 (fl oz)	1	0	0	0	0	@	<1	0	<1	0	0	0	0	0
Sprite® (Medium)	22 (fl oz)	260	0	0	0	0	@	66	0	66	0	0	0	0	0
Tropicana® Orange Juice	311	140	0	0	0	0	0	33	0	28	2	0	100	0	0
Coffee	355	5	0	0	0	0	5	1	0	0	0	0	0	0	0
Milk–2% Low Fat	244	130	45	5	3	20	120	12	0	12	8	10	4	30	0
BREAKFAST															
Croissan'wich® w/ Sausage, Egg & Cheese	163	550	380	42	14	250	1110	22	1	4	20	10	0	15	15
Croissan'wich® w/ Sausage & Cheese	106	450	320	35	12	45	940	21	1	3	13	4	0	10	10
Biscuit	93	330	160	18	4	2	950	37	1	2	6	0	0	6	10
Biscuit With Egg	150	420	220	24	6	205	1110	38	1	3	13	6	0	10	15
Biscuit With Sausage	137	530	320	36	11	35	1350	38	1	2	13	0	0	6	15
Biscuit With Bacon, Egg And Cheese	171	510	280	31	10	225	1530	39	1	3	19	8	0	15	15
French Toast Sticks	141	500	240	27	7	0	490	60	1	11	4	0	0	6	15
Hash Browns (Small)	75	240	140	15	6	0	440	25	2	0	2	0	0	0	4
A.M. Express® Grape Jam	12	30	0	0	0	0	0	7	0	6	0	0	0	0	0
A.M. Express® Strawberry Jam	12	30	0	0	0	0	5	8	0	5	0	0	0	0	0

Source: Burger King® trademarks, trade name, and Nutritional Guide are reproduced with permission from Burger King Corporation.

Note: @ Depends on the water supply.

†Without dressing.

PIZZA

Nutrient		12" Hand-Tossed Medium Pizza Serving Size 148.9 g 2 of 8 slices CHEESE PIZZA	12" Thin Crust Medium Pizza Serving Size 105.7 g ¼ of pizza CHEESE PIZZA	12" Deep Dish Medium Pizza Serving Size 180.11 g 2 of 8 slices CHEESE PIZZA	Pepperoni	Italian Sausage	Green Peppers	Onion	Extra Cheese	Anchovies
Calories	kcal	347.03	270.79	476.90	62.13	54.95	2.66	3.62	47.70	22.62
Fat–Total	g	10.68	11.76	21.56	5.63	4.34	0.05	0.03	3.78	1.05
Saturated Fat	g	5.18	5.22	8.45	2.20	1.74	—	—	2.34	0.24
Cholesterol	mg	14.55	14.54	19.11	12.99	11.41	0.00	0.00	7.27	9.16
Sodium	mg	723.32	809.34	1085.38	198.73	170.80	0.32	0.21	149.90	395.24
Carbohydrates	g	49.60	30.78	55.32	0.21	1.58	0.57	0.78	0.64	0.00
Dietary Fiber	g	2.78	1.75	3.29	0.08	0.32	0.13	0.05	0.18	0.00
Sugars	g	3.10	2.63	4.94	0.05	0.10	—	—	0.48	0.00
Protein	g	14.47	11.85	18.44	2.69	2.41	0.09	0.13	3.24	3.11
Vitamin A	IU	526.21	496.08	588.75	11.41	27.08	56.35	0.00	146.50	7.54
Vitamin C	mg	5.83	2.65	3.05	0.04	0.04	13.61	0.89	0.01	0.00
Calcium	mg	178.86	218.14	232.05	4.56	8.09	0.64	2.66	80.24	24.99
Iron	mg	3.65	0.95	3.82	0.24	0.28	0.14	0.04	0.08	0.50

Crust Type (headers: 12" Hand-Tossed Medium Pizza, 12" Thin Crust Medium Pizza, 12" Deep Dish Medium Pizza). **Add the value of each topping to the value for a cheese pizza.**

BUFFALO WINGS

Nutrient		Barbeque Wings	Hot Wings
*Serving Size	g	24.91 (1 av piece)	24.91 (1 av piece)
Calories	kcal	50.08	44.92
Fat–Total	g	2.43	2.39
Saturated Fat	g	0.65	0.65
Cholesterol	mg	25.63	25.58
Sodium	mg	175.30	354.40
Carbohydrates	g	1.58	0.50
Dietary Fiber	g	0.22	0.19
Sugars	g	1.26	0.21
Protein	g	5.50	5.46
Vitamin A	IU	42.18	135.50
Vitamin C	mg	0.07	1.13
Calcium	mg	5.66	5.44
Iron	mg	0.32	0.30

Source: © 1996 Domino's Pizza, Inc.; revised July 1997. Reprinted by permission.

Notes: Data is based on minimal portioning requirements. Nutrient values may vary slightly by location and supplier base.

*Serving size based on average wing size (edible portion only); typical order includes 10 wings.

KENTUCKY FRIED CHICKEN

CHICKEN	Original Recipe® Breast		Extra Tasty Crispy™ Breast		Tender Roast® Breast without Skin		Hot and Spicy Breast	
Serving Size								
• Grams	153		168		118		180	
• Ounces	5.4		5.9		4.2		6.5	
Amount Per Serving								
• Calories	400		470		169		530	
• Calories from Fat	220		250		39		310	
	Amount	% Daily Value*	Amount*	% Daily Value*	Amount	% Daily Value*	Amount	% Daily Value*
Total Fat	24 g	38%	28 g	42%	4.3 g	6.6%	35 g	54%
Saturated Fat	6 g	31%	7 g	35%	1.2 g	6%	8 g	42%
Cholesterol	135 mg	45%	80 mg	27%	112 mg	37%	110 mg	36%
Sodium	1116 mg	47%	930 mg	39%	797 mg	33.2%	1110 mg	46%
Total Carbohydrate	16 g	5%	25 g	8%	1 g	—	23 g	8%
Dietary Fiber	1 g	4%	1 g	4%	0 g	—	2 g	9%
Sugars	0 g	—	0 g	—	0 g	—	0 g	—
Protein	29 g	—	31 g	—	31.4 g	—	32 g	—
		% Daily Value*		% Daily Value*		% Daily Value*		% Daily Value*
Vitamin A		**		**		**		**
Vitamin C		**		**		**		**
Calcium		4%		4%		**		4%
Iron		6%		6%		**		6%

VEGETABLES	Corn on the Cob		Green Beans	
Serving Size				
• Grams	162		132	
• Ounces	5.7		4.7	
Amount Per Serving				
• Calories	150		45	
• Calories from Fat	15		15	
	Amount	% Daily Value*	Amount	% Daily Value*
Total Fat	1.5 g	3%	1.5 g	2%
Saturated Fat	0 g	0%	0.5 g	2%
Cholesterol	0 mg	0%	5 mg	2%
Sodium	20 mg	1%	730 mg	30%
Total Carbohydrate	35 g	12%	7 g	2%
Dietary Fiber	2 g	7%	3 g	12%
Sugars	8 g	—	3 g	—
Protein	5 g	—	1 g	—
		% Daily Value*		% Daily Value*
Vitamin A		2%		4%
Vitamin C		6%		4%
Calcium		**		4%
Iron		**		4%

POTATOES, BISCUITS	Mashed Potatoes with Gravy		1 Biscuit	
Serving Size				
• Grams	136		56	
• Ounces	4.8		2.0	
Amount Per Serving				
• Calories	120		180	
• Calories from Fat	50		80	
	Amount	% Daily Value*	Amount	% Daily Value*
Total Fat	6 g	9%	10 g	14%
Saturated Fat	1 g	5%	2.5 g	12%
Cholesterol	<1 mg	0%	0 mg	0%
Sodium	440 mg	18%	560 mg	23%
Total Carbohydrate	17 g	6%	20 g	7%
Dietary Fiber	2 g	8%	<1 g	0%
Sugars	0 g	—	2 g	—
Protein	1 g	—	4 g	—
		% Daily Value*		% Daily Value*
Vitamin A		**		**
Vitamin C		**		**
Calcium		**		2%
Iron		2%		6%

Source: Reprinted by permission of KFC (Kentucky Fried Chicken) Corporation.

*Percent Daily Values are based on a 2,000-calorie diet.

**Contains less than 2% of the daily value of these nutrients.

McDONALD'S

| | | | | Nutrition Facts | | | | | | | | | | | | | | % Daily Value | | | |
ITEM	Serving Size	Calories	Calories from Fat	Total Fat (g)	% Daily Value**	Saturated Fat (g)	% Daily Value**	Cholesterol (mg)	% Daily Value**	Sodium (mg)	% Daily Value**	Carbohydrates (g)	% Daily Value**	Dietary Fiber (g)	% Daily Value**	Sugars (g)	Protein (g)	Vitamin A	Vitamin C	Calcium	Iron
SANDWICHES																					
Hamburger	107 g	260	80	9	14	3.5	17	30	10	580	24	34	11	2	9	7	13	*	4	15	15
Cheeseburger	121 g	320	120	13	20	6	28	40	14	820	34	35	12	2	9	7	15	6	4	20	15
Quarter Pounder®	172 g	420	190	21	32	8	40	70	23	820	34	37	12	2	8	8	23	2	4	15	25
Quarter Pounder® with Cheese	200 g	530	270	30	46	13	63	95	32	1290	54	38	13	2	8	9	28	10	4	30	25
Big Mac®	216 g	560	280	31	48	10	51	85	28	1070	45	45	15	3	12	8	26	6	6	25	25
Arch Deluxe®	239 g	550	280	31	48	11	55	90	30	1010	42	39	13	4	16	8	28	10	10	15	25
Arch Deluxe® with Bacon	247 g	590	310	34	52	12	60	100	33	1150	48	39	13	4	16	8	32	10	10	15	25
Crispy Chicken Deluxe™	223 g	500	220	25	38	4	19	55	19	1100	46	43	14	4	14	5	26	6	8	6	15
Fish Filet Deluxe™	228 g	560	250	28	44	6	30	60	20	1060	44	54	18	4	16	5	23	6	4	8	15
Filet-o-Fish®	156 g	450	220	25	38	4.5	24	50	16	870	36	42	14	2	7	5	16	4	*	15	10
Grilled Chicken Deluxe™	223 g	440	180	20	31	3	16	60	21	1040	43	38	13	4	14	6	27	6	8	6	15
Grilled Chicken Deluxe™ (plain w/o mayo)	205 g	300	45	5	8	1	5	50	16	930	39	38	13	4	14	6	27	4	8	6	15
FRENCH FRIES																					
Small French Fries	68 g	210	90	10	15	1.5	9	0	0	135	6	26	9	2	10	0	3	*	15	*	2
Large French Fries	147 g	450	200	22	33	4	19	0	0	290	12	57	19	5	21	0	6	*	30	2	6
CHICKEN McNUGGETS®																					
Chicken McNuggets® (4 piece)	71 g	190	100	11	18	2.5	12	40	14	340	14	10	3	0	0	0	12	*	*	*	4
SALADS																					
Garden Salad	177 g	35	0	0	0	0	0	0	0	20	1	7	2	3	11	3	2	120	40	4	6
Grilled Chicken Salad Deluxe	257 g	120	10	1.5	2	0	0	45	16	240	10	7	2	3	11	3	21	120	40	4	8
BREAKFAST																					
Egg McMuffin®	136 g	290	110	12	19	4.5	23	235	78	790	33	27	9	1	6	3	17	10	2	20	15
Sausage McMuffin®	112 g	360	210	23	35	8	41	45	15	740	31	26	9	1	6	2	13	4	*	20	10
Sausage McMuffin® with Egg	162 g	440	250	28	44	10	50	255	86	890	37	27	9	1	6	3	19	10	*	25	15
English Muffin	55 g	140	20	2	3	0	0	0	0	210	9	25	8	1	6	1	4	*	*	10	8
Sausage Biscuit	127 g	470	280	31	48	9	44	35	11	1080	45	35	12	1	6	3	11	*	*	8	15
Sausage Biscuit with Egg	178 g	550	330	37	57	10	52	245	82	1160	48	35	12	1	6	3	18	6	*	15	15
Bacon, Egg & Cheese Biscuit	157 g	470	250	28	43	8	42	235	79	1250	52	36	12	1	6	3	18	10	*	15	15
Biscuit	84 g	290	130	15	23	3	16	0	0	780	33	34	11	1	6	2	5	*	*	6	10
Sausage	43 g	170	150	16	25	5	27	35	11	290	12	0	0	0	0	0	6	*	*	*	2
Scrambled Eggs (2)	102 g	160	100	11	18	3.5	17	425	141	170	7	1	0	0	0	1	13	10	*	4	6
Hash Browns	53 g	130	70	8	12	1.5	7	0	0	330	14	14	5	1	6	0	1	*	4	*	2
Hotcakes (plain)	150 g	310	60	7	10	1.5	8	15	4	610	25	53	18	2	6	11	9	*	*	10	15
Hotcakes (Margarine 2 pats & Syrup)	222 g	570	140	16	24	3	16	15	4	750	31	100	33	2	6	42	9	8	*	10	15
Breakfast Burrito	117 g	320	180	20	30	7	34	195	65	600	25	23	8	2	6	2	13	10	15	15	10
DESSERTS/SHAKES																					
Vanilla Reduced Fat Ice Cream Cone	90 g	150	40	4.5	7	3	15	20	6	75	3	23	8	0	0	17	4	6	2	10	2
Hot Fudge Sundae	179 g	340	100	12	18	9	45	30	10	170	7	52	17	1	5	47	8	10	2	25	4
Baked Apple Pie	77 g	260	120	13	20	3.5	17	0	0	200	8	34	11	<1	4	13	3	*	40	2	6
Chocolate Chip Cookie	35 g	170	90	10	15	6	28	20	7	120	5	22	7	1	4	13	2	4	*	2	6
McDonaldland® Cookies (1 pkg)	42 g	180	45	5	8	1	6	0	0	190	8	32	11	1	5	12	3	*	*	2	10
Vanilla Shake—Small	414 ml	360	80	9	14	6	30	40	13	250	10	59	20	0	0	55	11	6	2	35	2
Chocolate Shake—Small	414 ml	360	80	9	14	6	30	40	13	250	11	60	20	1	5	54	11	6	2	35	4
Strawberry Shake—Small	414 ml	360	80	9	14	6	30	40	13	180	8	60	20	0	0	55	11	6	10	35	4

Source: Reprinted with permission of McDonald's Corporation.

*Contains less than 2% of the daily value of these nutrients.

**Percent Daily Values are based on a 2,000-calorie diet.

TACO BELL

ITEM	Serving Size (oz)	Calories	Calories from Fat	Total Fat (g)	% Daily Value**	Saturated Fat (g)	% Daily Value**	Cholesterol (mg)	% Daily Value**	Sodium (mg)	% Daily Value**	Carbohydrates (g)	% Daily Value**	Dietary Fiber (g)	% Daily Value**	Sugars (g)	Protein (g)	Vitamin A	Vitamin C	Calcium	Iron
TACOS																					
Taco	2¾	180	90	10	15	4	20	25	8	330	14	12	4	3	12	1	9	10	0	8	6
Soft Taco	3½	220	90	10	15	4½	23	25	8	580	24	21	7	3	12	1	11	10	0	8	6
Taco Supreme®	4	220	120	14	22	7	35	35	12	350	15	14	5	3	12	2	10	15	6	10	6
Soft Taco Supreme®	5	260	120	14	22	7	35	35	12	590	25	23	8	3	12	3	12	15	6	10	6
Double Decker® Taco	5¾	340	130	15	23	5	25	25	8	750	31	38	13	9	36	2	14	10	0	10	10
Double Decker® Taco Supreme®	7	390	170	19	29	8	40	35	12	760	32	40	13	9	36	3	15	15	6	15	10
Grilled Steak Soft Taco	4½	230	90	10	15	2½	13	25	8	1020	43	20	7	2	8	1	15	4	0	8	8
Grilled Steak *Soft Taco Supreme®*	5¾	290	130	14	22	5	25	35	12	1040	43	24	8	3	12	4	16	8	20	10	8
Grilled Chicken Soft Taco	4½	240	110	12	18	3½	18	45	15	1110	46	21	7	3	12	2	12	15	0	8	4
BURRITOS																					
Bean Burrito	7	380	110	12	18	4	20	10	3	1100	46	55	18	13	52	3	13	45	0	15	15
Burrito Supreme®	9	440	170	19	29	8	40	35	12	1230	51	51	17	10	40	4	17	50	8	15	15
Big Beef Burrito Supreme®	10½	520	210	23	35	10	50	55	18	1520	63	54	18	11	44	4	24	60	8	15	15
7–Layer Burrito	10	530	200	23	35	7	35	25	8	1280	53	66	22	13	52	4	16	30	10	20	20
Grilled Chicken Burrito	7	410	140	15	23	4½	23	55	18	1380	58	50	17	4	16	3	17	80	2	15	8
Big Chicken Burrito Supreme®	9	510	210	24	37	7	35	95	32	1900	79	52	17	4	16	3	23	45	0	15	10
Chili Cheese Burrito	5	330	120	13	20	6	30	35	12	870	36	37	12	5	20	2	14	60	0	20	8
SPECIALTIES																					
Tostada	6¼	300	130	15	23	5	25	15	5	650	27	31	10	12	48	2	10	50	2	15	10
Mexican Pizza	7¾	570	320	35	54	10	50	45	15	1040	43	42	14	8	32	1	21	40	8	25	20
Big Beef MexiMelt®	4¾	290	140	15	23	7	35	45	15	850	35	23	8	4	16	2	16	25	6	20	6
Taco Salad with Salsa	19	850	470	52	80	15	75	60	20	1780	74	65	22	16	64	9	30	160	40	30	35
Taco Salad w/ Salsa without Shell	16½	420	200	22	34	11	55	60	20	1520	63	32	11	15	60	9	24	160	35	25	25
BORDER WRAPS™																					
Steak Fajita Wrap™	8	470	190	21	32	6	30	40	13	1190	50	50	17	3	12	3	20	30	6	15	10
Chicken Fajita Wrap™	8	470	200	22	34	6	30	60	20	1290	54	51	17	4	16	3	17	35	6	15	8
Veggie Fajita Wrap™	8	420	170	19	29	5	25	20	7	980	41	53	18	3	12	3	10	35	6	15	8
Steak Fajita Wrap™ Supreme	9	510	220	25	38	8	40	50	17	1200	50	52	17	3	12	4	21	30	10	15	10
Chicken Fajita Wrap™ Supreme	9	520	230	26	40	8	40	70	23	1300	54	53	18	4	16	4	18	40	10	15	8
Veggie Fajita Wrap™ Supreme	9	470	200	22	34	7	35	30	10	990	41	55	18	3	12	4	11	35	10	15	8
NACHOS AND SIDES																					
Nachos	3½	320	170	18	28	4	20	5	2	570	24	34	11	3	12	2	5	6	0	10	4
Big Beef Nachos Supreme	7	450	220	24	37	8	40	30	10	810	34	45	15	9	36	3	14	10	6	15	15
Nachos BellGrande®	11	770	360	39	60	11	55	35	12	1310	55	84	28	17	68	4	21	15	6	20	20
Pintos 'n Cheese	4½	190	80	9	14	4	20	15	5	650	27	18	6	10	40	1	9	50	0	15	10
Mexican Rice	4¾	190	80	9	14	3½	18	15	5	760	32	23	8	1	4	1	5	100	2	15	8
Cinnamon Twists	1	140	50	6	9	0	0	0	0	190	8	19	6	0	0	0	1	4	0	0	2

Source: Reprinted with permission of Taco Bell Corp. © 1997 Taco Bell Corp.

**Percent Daily Values are based on a 2,000-calorie diet.

WENDY'S

ITEM	Serving Size	Weight (g)	Calories	Calories from Fat	Total Fat (g)**	Saturated (g)	Cholesterol (mg)	Sodium (mg)	Total Carbohydrates (g)	Dietary Fiber (g)	Sugars (g)	Protein (g)	Vitamin A	Vitamin C	Calcium	Iron
SANDWICHES																
Plain Single	1 ea.	133	360	150	16	6	65	580	31	2	5	24	0	0	11	23
Single with Everything	1 ea.	219	420	180	20	7	70	920	37	3	9	25	6	10	13	26
Big Bacon Classic	1 ea.	282	580	270	30	12	100	1460	46	3	11	34	15	25	25	30
Jr. Hamburger	1 ea.	118	270	90	10	3.5	30	610	34	2	7	15	2	2	11	17
Jr. Cheeseburger	1 ea.	130	320	120	13	6	45	830	34	2	7	17	6	2	17	18
Jr. Bacon Cheeseburger	1 ea.	166	380	170	19	7	60	850	34	2	7	20	8	10	17	19
Jr. Cheeseburger Deluxe	1 ea.	180	360	150	17	6	50	890	36	3	8	18	10	10	18	19
Hamburger, Kids' Meal	1 ea.	111	270	90	10	3.5	30	610	33	2	7	15	2	0	11	17
Cheeseburger, Kids' Meal	1 ea.	123	320	120	13	6	45	830	33	2	7	17	6	0	17	18
Grilled Chicken Sandwich	1 ea.	189	310	70	8	1.5	65	790	35	2	8	27	4	10	10	15
Breaded Chicken Sandwich	1 ea.	208	440	160	18	3.5	60	840	44	2	6	28	4	10	10	16
Chicken Club Sandwich	1 ea.	216	470	180	20	4	70	970	44	2	6	31	4	10	11	17
Spicy Chicken Sandwich	1 ea.	213	410	130	15	2.5	65	1280	43	2	6	28	4	10	11	15
POTATOES, CHILI, and NUGGETS																
FRENCH FRIES																
Small	3.2 oz	91	270	120	13	2	0	85	35	3	0	4	0	8	1	4
Medium	4.6 oz	130	390	170	19	3	0	120	50	5	0	5	0	10	2	6
Biggie	5.6 oz	159	470	200	23	3.5	0	150	61	6	0	7	0	15	3	7
Great Biggie	6.7 oz	190	570	240	27	4	0	180	73	7	1	8	0	15	3	8
BAKED POTATO																
Plain	10 oz	284	310	0	0	0	0	25	71	7	5	7	0	60	3	21
Bacon & Cheese	1 ea.	380	530	160	18	4	20	1390	78	7	6	17	10	60	18	24
Broccoli & Cheese	1 ea.	411	470	130	14	2.5	5	470	80	9	6	9	35	120	21	25
Cheese	1 ea.	383	570	210	23	8	30	640	78	7	5	14	20	60	38	23
Chili & Cheese	1 ea.	439	630	220	24	9	40	770	83	9	7	20	20	60	33	28
Sour Cream & Chives	1 ea.	314	380	60	6	4	15	40	74	8	6	8	30	80	8	24
Sour Cream	1 pkt	28	60	50	6	3.5	10	15	1	0	1	1	4	0	3	0
Whipped Margarine	1 pkt	14	60	60	7	1.5	0	115	0	0	0	0	10	0	0	0
CHILI																
Small	8 oz	227	210	60	7	2.5	30	800	21	5	5	15	8	6	8	16
Large	12 oz	340	310	90	10	3.5	45	1190	32	7	8	23	10	10	12	24
Cheddar Cheese, shredded	2 T	17	70	50	6	3.5	15	110	1	0	0	4	4	0	12	0
Saltine Crackers	2 ea.	6	25	5	0.5	0	0	80	4	0	0	1	0	0	1	2
CHICKEN NUGGETS																
5 Piece	5	75	230	140	16	3	30	470	11	0	0	11	0	2	2	2
4 Piece Kids' Meal	4	60	190	120	13	2.5	25	380	9	0	0	9	0	2	2	2
Barbecue Sauce	1 pkt	28	45	0	0	0	0	160	10	0	7	1	0	0	1	3
Honey Mustard Sauce	1 pkt	28	130	100	12	2	10	220	6	0	5	0	0	0	1	1
Sweet & Sour Sauce	1 pkt	28	50	0	0	0	0	120	12	0	10	0	0	2	0	0

Source: Copyright © 1998 Wendy's International Inc. All rights reserved. Reprinted with permission from Wendy's International.

**Total fats are comprised of many substances other than those listed.

APPENDIX C

Common Sports Injuries

Foot Injuries

BLISTER

Definition Inflammation of the skin that results in a collection of fluid below the skin.

Symptoms Hot and red skin.

Cause Friction of the skin against something else.

Prevention Wear shoes that fit properly; wear socks. Put bandages or skin tape or rub petroleum jelly over the heel and other high-risk locations before breaking in new shoes or doing a long day of exercising.

Treatment Apply ice, rest, and put a felt or moleskin donut around the blister so that no further rubbing will occur. If the blister opens, wash with soap and water, dry, apply antibiotic ointment, and cover the area. Do not intentionally pop a blister. If it is in a very uncomfortable location and must be drained, use a sterilized needle to make a small hole in the lower side, drain, use antibiotic ointment, and cover. Do not remove the skin.

BUNION

Definition Bump that forms on the side of the big or little toe. Toe may turn inward.

Symptoms Burning, tenderness, swelling, redness, pain, and misalignment of toe.

Causes Wearing shoes that are too narrow or too short.

Prevention Wear shoes that fit well.

Treatment Reduce friction with pad or new shoes. Soak in cool water. See a physician.

METATARSALGIA

Definition Irritation of the nerves that lie between the metatarsal bones. (Metatarsals are the bones between the toes and the arch.)

Symptoms Pain under the ball of the foot.

Causes Shifting forward of the protective fat pad under the ball of the foot from excessively landing on it; overuse.

Prevention An athletic shoe with good metatarsal (forefoot) padding, good jump-landing technique, and resilient workout surfaces. Avoid overuse.

Treatment Ice, rest, and cushioned foot pads. If the pain persists, see a physician. You may need metatarsal lifts or orthotics.

PLANTAR FASCITIS

Definition Strain to the broad sheet of connective tissue that runs from the heel to the metatarsals, which supports the longitudinal arch. When weight is shifted to the ball of the foot, the tension held by this connective tissue equals twice the body's weight.

Symptoms Pain just in front of the heel where the connective tissue connects to the heel bone. May feel bruised. Pain may also radiate along the arch.

Causes A rapid increase in activity that requires pushing off the ball of the foot, particularly on a hard surface; wearing unsupportive shoes; tight calf muscles.

Prevention Work into a new program gradually. Wear shoes that support the arches. Develop calf flexibility.

Treatment Soak in cool water, buy new shoes or arch supports. If it persists, see a physician; you may need orthotics or anti-inflammatory drugs.

MORTON'S NEUROMA

Definition Localized swelling of the sensory nerve that lies between the metatarsals (bones in the ball of the foot) and innervates the toes.

Symptoms Pain radiating up between the third and fourth toes.

Causes Overuse, too much running on the ball of the foot.

Prevention Well-cushioned athletic shoes. Avoid overuse with a practical program. Use a metatarsal arch pad (a felt pad that fits under the ball of the foot).

Treatment See a physician.

Shin Injuries

SHINSPLINTS

Definition This is a general term for pain on the front or side of the lower leg. Some believe the pain comes from minute tearing of the muscle sheath from the shin bone membrane. Others believe the pain comes from damage caused by excessive vibration of the bone.

Symptoms Pain and aching in the shin area after and sometimes during exercise. May be specific areas of tenderness or swelling over the bone.

Causes Impact stress from a hard floor, poorly cushioned shoes, too much jumping, poor foot mechanics, poor posture, fallen arches, insufficient warm-up, fatigue, training too fast or too soon, poor exercise technique.

Prevention Exercise on a resilient surface with good arch-supporting shoes and proper footwork. Strengthen the foot muscles and muscles that surround the shin, especially the anterior tibialis. Stretch calves well before working out. Also keep shins warm before and during the session. Warm-up socks are helpful for this.

Treatment Ice shins for 20 to 30 minutes following exercise. You may want to freeze water in a paper cup and use it to massage your shins. Just peel down the cup as the ice melts.

If any bruising, swelling, or specific point tenderness occurs, stop exercising and rest your legs. If pain persists or worsens, consult a physician. You may need to take an anti-inflammatory drug or be fitted for orthotics.

Some individuals get relief from having their arches, shins, or both taped—consult an athletic trainer or podiatrist. Some people also get relief by running backward.

STRESS FRACTURE

Definition Very thin, undisplaced hairline break in a bone.

Symptoms Pain along the lower leg bones. If it is a stress fracture in the lower leg, it will hurt before, during, and after class and even when you get off your feet. Painful when you touch it, especially in one area.

Causes Same as shinsplints.

Prevention Wear cushioned, supportive shoes, avoid overuse and nonresilient surfaces.

Treatment See a physician. Stress fractures are difficult to diagnose because they don't show up on x-rays until calcium deposits are made during the healing process. Once diagnosed, the fractured part of the leg may be immobilized in a cast.

Knee Injuries

CHONDROMALACIA PATELLA

Definition Roughening or softening of the joint surface of the knee cap (patella).

Symptoms Pain when patella is pressed on, maybe creaking and popping noises. May hurt when climbing stairs or kneeling. Knee pain while exercising.

Causes Knee cap may be sliding out of alignment and causing irritation. Cartilage may be inflamed or degenerating. May be caused by deep knee bends or other exercises that stress the knee.

Prevention Perform a good warm-up. Avoid deep knee bends and knee hyperextension positions. Strengthen the muscles that surround and support the knee, using straight-leg exercise. Stretch legs, especially the hamstrings and calves.

Treatment Ice the knee. See a physician. Strengthen supporting muscles.

MENISCAL INJURIES

Definition Strains or tears of the cartilage that stabilizes the knee joint.

Symptoms Acute pain, popping noise, swelling, knee may "give out" or lock.

Causes Rotation or twisting of the knee joint beyond normal limitations. Foot remaining planted when the body turns so that the knee is forced to accept the rotational force. A surface with too much cushion allows the foot to sink into it and remain planted. Sticky surfaces or treaded shoes on nonslip surfaces may also cause the foot to remain planted. Injury can also be caused by working the knee joint with too much weight.

Prevention Select the appropriate shoe for the surface. Select the best possible surface. Use workout routines that don't require sudden pivots or turns, particularly on soft surfaces. Work with reasonable amounts of weight during leg exercises. Overload gradually and strengthen the supporting muscles.

Treatment Support the back of the knee and pack the knee in ice. Move the person only if the knee is supported. Keep injured person warm and call a doctor. Joint may have to be aspirated (excess fluid removed from the joint).

STRAIN

Definition Injury to a muscle or a tendon. (*Tendons* connect muscles to bone; for example, the Achilles tendon connects the calf muscle to the heel.)

Symptoms There are three degrees of injury. First-degree symptoms: local pain and tenderness usually accompanied by swelling and pain. Exercise may be continued when pain and swelling are absent and range of motion is complete. Second-degree symptoms: pain with muscle movement, muscle spasm, increased swelling, and tearing of tissue. Do not continue exercise. Third-degree symptoms: severe pain and disability, severe muscle spasms, and complete tearing of tissue. Do not continue exercise.

Causes Pushing a muscle or tendon beyond its normal range, often by a ballistic movement before the body is fully warmed up. May also occur from overuse or flinging the arms, especially when arm weights are used. Older persons are more prone to injury.

Prevention Warm up and stretch well before working out. Strengthen both agonists and antagonists.

Treatment Rest, ice, compress, and elevate (RICE) the injured muscle or tendon. If pain is acute or persists, see a physician. Do not move anyone who has a third-degree strain. Call a doctor; surgery may be necessary.

SPRAIN

Definition Injury to a ligament. (*Ligaments* attach bones to bones.)

Symptoms First-degree symptoms: twinge of discomfort, slight skin discoloration from internal bleeding, some ligament fiber damage. Exercise may be continued when pain and swelling are absent and range of motion is complete. Second-degree symptoms; pain, swelling, loss of function for several minutes, tender to the touch, loss of strength, definite tear of fibers. Do not continue exercise. Third-degree symptoms: severe pain and swelling, discoloration of skin, complete tear of the ligament, loss of function. Do not continue exercise.

Causes Any movement that pulls two connected bones apart more than a normal amount.

Prevention Warm up and stretch before working out. Exercise regularly so that ligaments are strengthened. Overload gradually and remember that ligament strength gains are usually slower than cardiorespiratory gains. When your heart says keep going, check in with the rest of your body. Strengthen muscles that surround joints so that they can minimize the stress put on the ligaments. Avoid exercises that put pressure on ligaments, and do exercises that strengthen muscles. For example, squats and lunges strengthen the legs as long as you don't bend the knee too much; deep knee bends stress the ligaments, and because the muscles are in a weak mechanical position, they can't help the ligaments.

Treatment Rest, ice, compress, and elevate (RICE) the injured part. If pain is acute or persists, consult a physician. If it is a third-degree sprain, do not move the person. Keep the person warm and call a doctor. Surgical repair may be necessary.

TENDINITIS

Definition Chronic inflammation or irritation of a tendon. Microscopic tears in the tendon tissue may be the cause of the inflammation. Some of the most commonly injured tendons are the Achilles, shoulder, and elbow.

Symptoms Area may be painful to the touch, warm, and swollen. Skin may be red.

Causes Repeated excessive stretching of a tendon, excessive running or jumping especially on hard surfaces, flinging of arms particularly when wrist weights are used.

Prevention Use careful, deliberate movements rather than flinging movements. Gradually overload. Warm up and stretch out prior to vigorous activity.

Treatment Ice and rest the tendon. If pain is acute, see a physician. May require anti-inflammatory drugs or surgery.

BURSITIS

Definition Inflammation or irritation of a bursa. Bursas are fluid-filled sacs found around the body at sites where friction might occur, such as where muscle tendons and sheaths cross over bones.

Symptoms Localized inflammation, pain, swelling, and heat.

Causes Overstretching of the Achilles tendon, direct blow to the elbow or knee, pressure on an area such as the knee, or overuse of a joint, such as the deltoid at the shoulder through unaccustomed overhead arm activity.

Prevention Avoid overuse of muscles and joints. Avoid kneeling on a hard surface. Use gradual overloads, especially when adding resistance through weights or exercise bands. Use good exercise technique.

Treatment Ice and compress the area. If pain or loss of motion persists, consult a physician.

MUSCLE CRAMP

Definition Painful muscle contraction that will not voluntarily release.

Symptoms Acute pain.

Causes Fatigue or heat induced. (Also common among pregnant women, possibly due to chemical changes.)

Prevention Warm up and stretch before vigorous exercise. Stretch a muscle following a strength workout. Stretch whenever slight muscle cramping occurs. Cool the calves in very hot weather by removing high socks and wearing lightweight tights or shorts. Hydrate with water prior to exercise and if cramps develop.

Treatment Stretch and massage the muscle. (You can also ice the opposing muscle because its contraction will cause the other muscle to stretch.)

Heat-Related Injuries

HEAT CRAMP

See Muscle Cramp.

HEAT EXHAUSTION

Definition Overheating of the body.

Symptoms Muscle spasms or cramping, cold clammy skin, chills, nausea, dizziness, and profuse sweating.

Causes Inability to dissipate heat because the environment is too hot or humid for the level of activity. Sometimes exercise rooms are not properly ventilated or the cooling systems are insufficient. Situations can also arise when the exercise room shares hot, humid air from a pool.

Prevention Exercise in a well-ventilated, controlled-temperature environment. Adjust the exercise level so that it is safe for the environment. Keep yourself well hydrated.

Treatment Drink water and cool the body by going to a cooler place or using ice. Rest.

HEAT STROKE

Definition Inability of the body to handle heat stress. This is a medical emergency. The core temperature is rising, and brain damage and death can result.

Symptoms Dry hot skin, pale or flushed skin, nausea, dizziness, faintness, weakness, or exhaustion. Skin may be hot and dry or still sweating if exercise has just stopped.

Causes Overexposure to a hot or hot and humid environment.

Prevention Keep yourself well hydrated. Do not exercise in very hot weather or when the heat and humidity combine to cause a hazardous conditon.

Treatment Immediately cool the body. Put person in a cold shower or dump cold water all over him or her. Call an ambulance immediately.

GLOSSARY

Abstinence   To refrain completely from engaging in a particular behavior.

Action Takers   People in the action stage have actually made some changes. They actually do it. However, their practices are erratic and uncommitted, and sometimes fail to become lifelong lifestyles.

Active Stretch Flexibility exercise in which a person contracts one muscle in an effort to lengthen the opposing muscle.

Adaptive Energy Reserve An individual's stockpile of energy available for adapting to situations. Each time some of it is used, according to Selye, it can't be replaced.

Addiction Compulsive and uncontrollable behavior(s) or use of substance(s), most frequently drugs.

Adenosine Triphosphate (ATP) The high-energy phosphate molecule used to make cellular energy. Muscle cells use ATP to fuel contraction.

Adiposity The number and size of fat cells, which is largely determined by genetics and the amount and type of food we consume.

Aerobic Literally "with oxygen." When applied to exercise, refers to activities in which oxygen demand can be supplied continuously by individuals during performance.

Aerobic Capacity Maximum oxygen consumption.

Aerobic System The metabolic processes of breaking down carbohydrate, fat, and protein in the presence of oxygen to produce energy (ATP).

Aerobic Target Zone The fitness target zone for aerobic activity. (*See* Fitness Target Zone.)

Aerobics Exercise that requires oxygen to produce the necessary energy (ATP) to carry out the activity.

Age Onset Obesity Increase in body fat that occurs with increased age.

Agonist Muscle that is undergoing contraction.

AIDS Disease caused by a virus (HIV) that destroys the immune system.

AIDS-Related Complex (ARC) In full-blown AIDS the person's immune system is very weak, allowing opportunistic infections to spread uninhibited. ARC is characterized by swollen lymph glands, fever, night sweats, skin rashes, diarrhea, sores, weight loss, and tiredness.

Allergens Allergy-causing substances.

Amenorrhea Cessation of regular menstrual flow.

Amino Acids Chemical compounds that contain nitrogen, carbon, hydrogen, and oxygen. Amino acids are the basic building blocks used by the body to build different types of protein.

Amphetamines Synthetic chemicals (as opposed to plant derivatives) that are strong central nervous system stimulants.

Anabolic Steroids Synthetic versions of the male sex hormone testosterone, which promotes muscle development and hypertrophy.

Anaerobic Literally "without oxygen." When applied to exercise, refers to high-intensity physical activities in which oxygen demand is greater than the amount that can be supplied during performance.

Anaerobic Glycolysis Metabolic process of breaking down carbohydrate in the absence of oxygen to produce energy (ATP).

Anaerobic System Metabolic processes that produce energy (ATP) in the absence of oxygen. (*See* Phosphagen System *and* Anaerobic Glycolysis.)

Anaphylactic Shock Life-threatening allergic response typified by a drastic drop in blood pressure.

Android Deposition of fat characteristic of males, in which fat tends to accumulate in the abdomen and upper body.

Aneurysm Weakness in the arterial wall allowing the formation of a balloonlike pouch. A ruptured aneurysm is a serious, often fatal, condition.

Angina Pectoris Chest pain.

Anorexia Nervosa Serious illness of deliberate self-starvation with profound psychiatric and physical components.

Antagonist Muscle working in opposition to the agonist. When the agonist contracts, the antagonist relaxes.

Antagonist Stretching Type of stretching in which the agonist is contracted to aid the stretch and relaxation of the antagonist. Works on the principle of reciprocal innervation.

Antioxidants Compounds that block the oxidation of substances in food or the body (examples include vitamins C and E and beta-carotene).

Arousal Form of stimulation, of stress, that affects performance. If you are excited, pumped up, and ready to go, you will perform better than if you are not particularly aroused.

Arteriosclerosis Hardening of the arteries.

Artery Major blood vessel that carries blood away from the heart.

Assisted Stretch Type of stretching in which the individual pulls or pushes a body part or has a partner pull or push the body part until stretch is achieved.

Asymptomatic Without symptoms.

Atherosclerosis Type of arteriosclerosis characterized by plaque formation or the buildup of fatty tissue in the inner layers of the wall of the arteries.

Atrophy Decrease in the size of a cell or muscle.

Autogenic Training Stress management technique. A form of self-suggestion in which an individual is able to place him- or herself in an autohypnotic state by concentrating on feelings of heaviness and warmth in the extremities.

Bacteria Microscopic organisms that can live inside the human body. Some bacteria are health promoting, whereas others act as pathogens (disease-causing agents).

Ballistic Stretch A flexibility exercise characterized by a series of bouncing or pulsing movements that alternately stretch (lengthen) and relax a muscle or muscle group.

Ballistic Stretching Technique used to develop flexibility. It is characterized by a series of bouncing or pulsing movements that alternately stretch and then relax the muscle. These movements may elicit the stretch reflex. (Opposite of static stretching.)

Barriers Circumstances, events, and obstacles that keep us from succeeding in our efforts to change behaviors.

Benign When used medically, usually refers to non-cancerous conditions.

Biofeedback Educational tool used to provide information about an individual's physiological actions.

Biopsy Cancer tissue taken using small needles or instruments and analyzed for the cancer cells. Muscle tissue sample to determine fiber makeup.

Blended Family Family formed when one or both parents bring children from a previous union.

Blood Alcohol Content (BAC) Percentage of alcohol content in the blood.

Blood Pressure Pressure the blood exerts against the walls of the arteries.

Body Building Process of developing both size and definition of muscles, mainly for competition.

Body Composition Relative amounts of lean body mass and fat in the body.

Body Mass Index (BMI) Ratio of weight to height, usually expressed in kg/meter^2.

Body Sculpting Process of developing a well-proportioned physique. Body sculpting is part of body building but may also be offered as a noncompetitive class for people who want to tone and shape their muscles.

Bulimia Eating disorder characterized by a pattern of binge eating and purging in an attempt to lose or maintain low body weight.

Caffeine Drug that stimulates the central nervous system. Most frequently found in coffee, tea, colas, and chocolate.

Calorie Common-use form of the word *kilocalorie*. A measure of the value of foods to produce heat and energy in the human body. One calorie is equal to the amount of heat required to raise the temperature of 1 gram of water 1°C.

Cancer Group of diseases characterized by uncontrolled growth and spread of abnormal cells into malignant tumors.

Candidiasis Yeast infection; type of vaginitis caused by the overgrowth of a fungus.

Capillaries The smallest blood vessels in the body. They supply blood (oxygen) to the tissues.

Carbohydrates Compounds such as sugars and starches that are made up of carbon, hydrogen, and oxygen. Serve as the primary source of energy for the body. Carbohydrates are broken down and transported in the blood as glucose; they are stored in the liver and muscles as glycogen. Dietary sources of complex carbohydrates include grains and beans; sources of simple carbohydrates include refined sugars and natural sugars.

Carbohydrate Loading Gradually reducing the amount of physical activity four days before an athletic event and consuming a diet of at least 70 percent carbohydrates.

Carcinogens Substances that contribute to the formation of cancers.

Cardiac Output Amount of blood ejected by the heart in one minute.

Cardiorespiratory Endurance The ability to perform large-muscle movements over a sustained period of time;

the ability of the circulatory and respiratory systems to deliver fuel, especially oxygen, to the muscles during continuous exercise.

Cardiorespiratory Fitness Ability of the lungs, heart, and blood vessels to deliver adequate amounts of oxygen to the cells to meet the demands of prolonged (aerobic) physical activity.

Cardiovascular Disease Disease that affects the heart and the circulatory system (blood vessels). Examples of cardiovascular diseases include coronary heart disease, peripheral vascular disease, congenital heart disease, rheumatic heart disease, atherosclerosis, stroke, high blood pressure, and congestive heart failure.

Carotid Artery Artery that runs close to the skin surface just to one side of the larynx. This artery is commonly used for counting the pulse.

Chemotherapy Use of drugs and hormones to treat various cancers.

Chlamydia Sexually transmitted disease caused by a bacterial infection that can cause significant damage to the reproductive system and may occur without symptoms.

Cholesterol Waxy substance that is technically a steroid alcohol found only in animal fats and oil.

Circuit Training Total of eight to fifteen exercises used in a circuit. The exerciser goes through the circuit with minimum rest between exercise stations.

Cocaine Addictive, illegal stimulant used in powdered form.

Cognitive Intervention Strategies Use of mental tactics to reduce psychological stress.

Complete Protein Foods that contain all nine of the essential amino acids.

Concentric Contraction Shortening of the muscle as it develops the tension to overcome an external resistance.

Connective Tissue Tissue in the body that binds, supports, and strengthens other tissues. Important in joint stability and function.

Contemplators People who are considering change. They are not only thinking about their current behavior but are also seriously considering making a change.

Cool-Down Tapering off the intensity of exercise at the end of a session instead of stopping immediately.

Coronary Heart Disease (CHD) The major form of cardiovascular disease. Involves disease of the heart or blood vessels and is the leading cause of death in the United States.

Cross Training Attainment of physical fitness through regular participation in a variety of physical activities.

Delayed Onset Muscle Soreness (DOMS) Muscle soreness that occurs up to 24 to 48 hours after the activity that caused it.

Demography Statistical study of the human population.

Depressants Commonly known as sedatives and tranquilizers, these agents slow the central nervous system.

Designer Drugs Manufactured drugs that mimic controlled substances.

Developmental Stretch The last segment of an activity session (usually considered part of the cool-down), in which flexibility exercises are used to reduce tension and elongate muscles.

Diabetes Mellitus Condition in which the blood glucose is unable to enter the cells because the pancreas either has totally stopped producing insulin or produces an amount insufficient for the body's needs.

Diastolic Pressure Pressure exerted by the blood in the arteries when the heart is filling. Diastolic pressure is represented by the denominator in the blood-pressure fraction.

Disaccharide Sugar composed of two sugar molecules. Table sugar is a disaccharide.

Distress Negative stress. Refers to unpleasant or harmful stress under which health and performance may begin to deteriorate.

Duration Length of a single exercise session.

Dynamic Exercises Exercises that move through a range of motion.

Dysfunctional Living Situation in which an individual is unable to perform activities required for daily living, such as bathing, dressing, and eating.

Eccentric Contraction Lengthening of fibers during muscle contraction.

Empty Calories Calories that provide very little if any nutritional value with the exception of providing calories found in simple sugars.

Enabling Actions Actions by others that encourage or allow abusive activities that harm oneself or others.

Endorphins Morphine-like substances released from the brain's pituitary gland during prolonged aerobic exercise. They are thought to induce feelings of euphoria and mental well-being.

Energy Balance Theory Weight-loss theory that suggests that fat is stored when more energy is consumed than is expended.

Environment The world in which we live.

Essential Fat Minimal amount of body fat needed for normal physiological functions. It constitutes about 3 percent of the total fat in men and 12 percent in women.

Eustress Positive stress. Usually health promoting.

Exercise Structured workout that usually helps make you more physically fit.

Exercise Heart Rate (EHR) The speed (contractions per minute) at which the heart beats during exercise.

Extrinsic Motivation Motivation that has its source outside the individual.

Family Violence Forms of violence that include spouse abuse, sexual abuse, marital rape, child abuse, and neglect.

Fat One of the six essential nutrients. An energy-rich compound made up of glycerol and fatty acids. A source of energy for the body, particularly during aerobic activity.

Fatty Acid Oxidation Aerobic metabolic process that produces energy through the breakdown of fatty acids.

Fiber Form of complex carbohydrate made up of plant material that cannot be digested by the human body.

Fight or Flight Physiological response of the body to stress that prepares the individual to take action by stimulating the vital defense systems.

FIT Acronym for the three variables involved in exercise overload: frequency, intensity, and time. (Sometimes called FITT, where the last T stands for type of activity.)

Fitness Target Zone Optimum intensity range for exercise. The lower limit of the zone is the threshold of training; the upper limit is the maximum amount of exercise that is beneficial for health-related fitness.

Flexibility The range of motion around a joint or group of joints.

Free Radical Substance formed during metabolism that attacks and damages proteins and lipids, in particular the cell membrane and DNA. Free radicals may lead to the development of diseases such as heart disease, cancer, and emphysema.

Free Weights Barbells and dumbbells used in resistance training.

Frequency The number of times a person exercises per week.

General Adaptation Syndrome (GAS) Series of physiological changes that occur when a stressor is encountered; the GAS is conceived of as having three phases: alarm, resistance, and exhaustion.

Glucose Simplest form of sugar. Carbohydrate is broken down into glucose before being absorbed into the bloodstream and taken to the cells for the production of energy.

Gonorrhea Sexually transmitted bacterial disease that can lead to serious complications if left untreated, including sterility and scarring of the heart valves.

Gynoid Fat deposition characteristic of women, in whom fat tends to accumulate on the hips and thighs.

Hallucinogens Group of illegal drugs that create a euphoric or dreamlike state. Examples include mescaline, mushrooms, LSD, and PCP.

Headache Common discomfort often caused by distress, tension, and anxiety; may be the result of injury or brain disease.

Health Balance of the physical, mental, emotional, social, and spiritual components of personality, resulting in optimal well-being and a higher quality of life.

Health-Related Components of Physical Fitness Cardiorespiratory endurance, body composition, flexibility, muscular endurance, and muscular strength.

Heart Rate Number of times a person's heart beats in one minute.

Heart Rate Reserve Difference between the maximum heart rate and the resting heart rate.

Hepatitis B Viral disease that can be transmitted sexually.

Herpes Sexually transmitted disease caused by a viral infection (herpes simplex virus types I and II). The disease is characterized by the appearance of sores on the mouth, genitals, rectum, or other parts of the body. There is no known cure, but treatments exist to help control symptoms.

High Density Lipoproteins (HDL) Complex of lipids (fat) and proteins that picks up cholesterol in the blood and carries it to the liver. Exercise increases the amount of HDL in the blood.

HIV Virus that causes acquired immunodeficiency syndrome (AIDS).

Hives Skin discoloration or rashes that are a result of an allergic reaction.

Homeostasis State of balance or constancy; the body is continually attempting to maintain homeostasis.

Human Papilloma Virus (HPV) Causative agent of genital warts.

Human-Cultural Environment People who surround and influence a person through their actions, laws, beliefs, traditions, and social mores.

Hydrostatic Weighing Method of estimating body fat. Also referred to as underwater weighing.

Hyperplasia Increase in the number of cells.

Hypertension Chronically elevated blood pressure.

Hypertrophy Increase in the size of cells and muscles.

Hypoglycemia Low blood sugar (glucose).

Hypostress Inadequate stimulation.

Imagery Cognitive stress management technique involving the use of visualization to imagine yourself in, and successfully handling, stressful situations. Also used for relaxation.

Immunotherapy Powerful cancer treatment that stimulates the body's own immune system to attack cancer cells.

Incomplete Proteins Foods that do not contain all the essential amino acids.

Individuality Principle that no two people react exactly the same way to exercise.

Infatuation Strong initial physical attraction.

Inhalants Substances that can cause druglike effects when inhaled.

Insoluble Fiber Part of foods that cannot be digested.

Intensity Level of exertion during exercise.

Interval Training Anaerobic method of conditioning that alternates short, high-intensity exercise bouts with short rest periods.

Intimate Relationships High degree of closeness that can exist in the form of friendship, relationship, or association.

Intrinsic Motivation Motivation that arises from within a person; self-motivation.

Inverse Myotatic Reflex Protective mechanism that stops a muscle contraction before the tension is great enough to rip all or part of the tendon from the bone.

Inverted "U" Hypothesis Describes the relationship between arousal and performance.

Irradiation Exposure of foods like grains, flour, fruits, and vegetables to low doses of ionized radiation or other forms of electromagnetic radiation in order to prolong their shelf life.

Ischemia Lack of blood flow (oxygen).

Isokinetic Contraction Muscle contraction during which the speed of the contraction is held constant and the resistance varied to match the force exerted.

Isokinetic Exercises Muscular strength and endurance exercises performed using special equipment that exerts a resistance equal to the force placed on it and that controls the speed of a movement.

Isometric Contraction Muscle contraction during which the muscle fibers contract but the length of the muscle does not change.

Isometric Exercises Muscular strength and endurance exercises during which muscles exert force against an immovable object.

Isotonic Contraction Muscle contraction during which muscle tension is held constant throughout a full range of motion.

Isotonic Exercises Muscular strength and endurance exercises in which the tension of the muscle remains the same throughout the range of motion.

Karvonen Formula Method of calculating the intensity target range for aerobic work using a percentage of the heart rate reserve.

Kyphosis Permanent rounding of the upper spine.

Lactic Acid By-product of high-intensity anaerobic exercise. Accumulation of lactic acid is associated with muscle fatigue and "burn."

Lean Body Weight Body weight without body fat.

Learned Tolerance Characteristic in which a person learns to tolerate the fact that he or she will not always get what he or she wants.

Leukemia Cancers that originate from and spread through the blood-forming systems of the body.

Ligament Fibrous tissue that connects bones to bones.

Loneliness Personal situation in which there is little or no close emotional or social support from others.

Lordosis Condition in which there is excessive curvature in the lower back.

Low Density Lipoproteins (LDL) Complex of lipids and proteins that carries cholesterol and deposits it along the walls of the arteries. High concentrations of LDL are associated with an increased risk of heart disease.

Low-Impact Aerobics Type of aerobics in which the participant keeps one foot on the floor at all times. It is often characterized by moderately paced, full range of motion movements with a lot of upper body work.

Lymphomas Tumors originating from lymphatic tissue.

Maintainers People who have made a new behavior part of their permanent lifestyle.

Malignant Cancer capable of spreading.

Malignant Melanoma Malignant tumor of the skin that originates from pigmented cells, usually a mole.

Mammogram X-ray examination of the breast to detect cancer.

Marijuana Psychoactive drug from the hemp plant, *cannabis sativa*. Also referred to as pot, grass, and mary-jane.

Maximum Heart Rate (MHR) Maximum number of times a person's heart can beat in one minute. Estimate by subtracting your age from 220.

Maximum Heart Rate Formula Method of estimating the intensity range for an aerobic workout using a percentage (70 to 85 percent) of the maximum heart rate.

Meditation Stress-management technique used to gain control over one's attention, clearing the mind and blocking out the stressors responsible for increased tension.

Mega Dose Large doses of vitamins, usually in the form of supplements.

Metabolism All necessary energy and material transformations that occur within living cells to sustain life.

Metastasis Process by which cancerous cells spread from their original location to another location in the body.

Methamphetamine Subgroup of amphetamines that has grown rapidly in street popularity.

Migraine Headaches Headaches characterized by throbbing pain that can last for hours or days, sometimes accompanied by nausea and vomiting. Migraines are thought to be the result of dilation of blood vessels in the head.

Monogamous Relationship Sex with only one partner.

Monosaccharides Simplest carbohydrates (sugars) formed by five- or six-carbon skeletons. The three most common monosaccharides are glucose, fructose, and galactose.

Motivational Syndrome Syndrome characterized by a loss of motivation, dullness, apathy, and no interest in the future.

Motor Unit Combination of a motor neuron and the muscle fibers that it innervates.

Muscle Fibers Muscle cells.

Muscle Wasting Conversion of muscle protein into energy; this conversion removes protein from muscles and weakens them.

Muscular Endurance Ability of a muscle to exert a submaximal force repeatedly over a period of time and/or maintain a submaximal force for an extended period of time. The term usually implies a specific muscle group, such as chest, thighs, or abdominals.

Muscular Power Combination of strength and speed expressed as work (force × distance) divided by time.

Muscular Strength Maximum force that a muscle or muscle group can exert in a single contraction.

Myocardial Infarction Heart attack; death of heart muscle tissue.

Narcotics *See* Opiates.

Natural Environment Everything nonhuman that surrounds and influences a person.

Nonessential Fat Any body fat that is more than what we need for normal physiological function.

Noninfectious Diseases that cannot be passed to another individual through casual contact.

Nutrients Substances found in food that provide energy, regulate metabolism, and help with growth and repair of body tissues.

Obesity Accumulation of excess fat. Usually defined as 20 percent above the ideal weight or above 30 percent fat for women and above 25 percent fat for men.

Oncogene Cancer-causing gene.

Opiates/Narcotics Controlled substances that are excellent painkillers with actions that mimic endorphins, the body's natural painkillers. Some opiates also inhibit certain muscle contractions.

Osteoporosis Progressive decrease in the mineral content of bone, resulting in brittle bones.

Overfat An excessive percentage of body weight that is fat weight.

Overload Key training concept that states that the demands placed on the cardiovascular or muscular system must be systematically and progressively increased over a period of time to cause physiologic adaptation (that is, development or improvement).

Overuse Injuries that result from violating the principle of overload by overdoing.

Overweight Excessive weight for one's height without regard for body composition.

Oxygen Consumption Rate at which oxygen is used to produce energy. Measured in liters per minute or milliliters per kilogram body weight per minute.

Passive Stretch Flexibility exercise in which the stretch (lengthening) of the muscle(s) is created by an outside force such as a partner or gravity. Also known as an assisted stretch.

Pelvic Inflammatory Disease (PID) Chronic condition of infection in the uterus, fallopian tubes, and upper reproductive areas; the leading cause of infertility in women.

Percent Body Fat Term used in body composition assessment. It represents the total amount of fat in the body based on the person's weight. It includes both essential and storage fat.

Perception Way a person interprets and mentally frames things; a person's frame of reference.

Phosphagen System Anaerobic system that rapidly produces energy through the breakdown and resynthesis of high-energy phosphagens (not carbohydrate). This system can supply only a few seconds of energy.

Physical Activity Any bodily movement produced by skeletal muscles that results in energy expenditure.

Physical Dependency Having a physical addiction to a substance such as alcohol or tobacco.

Physical Fitness Capacity to adapt and respond favorably to physical effort. Individuals are considered physically fit when they can meet the ordinary as well as the unusual demands of daily life safely and effectively without being overly fatigued and still have energy left for leisure and recreational activities.

PNF Stretching Method of stretching that uses Proprioceptive Neuromuscular Facilitation (PNF); a combination of isometric contractions and active and passive stretches.

Precontemplators Individuals who are not yet thinking about making any changes.

Preparers Individuals who are actively preparing and making plans to change behavior.

Principle of Individuality Exercise principle that states that any two people can react differently to the same exercise.

Principle of Overload Exercise principle that states that a physiological system or organ of the body repeatedly subjected to greater than normal stress will adapt to the stress. A proper amount of overload results in positive adaptations.

Principle of Overuse Exercise principle that states that too much stress over a period of time can result in fatigue and injury.

Principle of Progression Exercise principle that states that the gradual increase (or overload) of the intensity, frequency, or duration of exercise will improve physical fitness.

Principle of Reversibility Exercise principle stating that a physiological system or organ that is not repeatedly subjected to normal amounts of stress will adapt by deconditioning. (Also known as use/disuse principle.)

Principle of Specificity Exercise principle that states that physiological adaptations are specific to the systems that are overloaded with exercise.

Progression Series of small changes that lead to a major change.

Progressive Relaxation Stress-management technique. It involves progressive contraction and relaxation of muscle groups throughout the body.

Proteins Complex organic compounds containing nitrogen and formed by combinations of amino acids. Proteins are the main substances used in the body to build and repair tissues such as muscles, blood, internal organs, skin, hair, nails, and bones. They are also part of hormones, antibodies, and enzymes.

Psychoactive Drug One that can alter feelings, moods, and/or perceptions.

Psychological Dependence An intense mental (psychological) craving or compulsive desire for something.

Psychological Headaches Headaches caused by mental and emotional strain.

Pubic Lice Parasites (insects) that breed in the pubic hair.

Pulse The wave of pressure felt in the arteries when the heart beats.

Resting Heart Rate The number of heart contractions needed per minute to supply oxygen to the resting body.

Quality of Life Form of living that allows a person to feel good about him- or herself and do most of the things a person wants to do despite any limitations the person may have.

Radiation Therapy Use of radiation either to destroy cancer cells or to destroy their reproductive mechanism so they cannot replicate.

Range of Motion (ROM) The amount of mobility a joint or group of joints has; degree of movement.

Ratings of Perceived Exertion (RPE) Method of estimating the intensity of an exercise session. A scale of numbers with brief qualifiers, developed by Borg, is employed.

Reciprocal Innervation Contraction of one muscle while the nervous system signals its paired muscle to relax and lengthen. For example, as your biceps flexes, your triceps accommodates by relaxing and lengthening. The result is smooth, coordinated movement.

Recommended Dietary Allowances (RDAs) Daily recommended intakes of nutrients for normal, healthy people in the United States.

Reframing Ability to reduce stress by seeing the positive side to a situation.

Relapse Reverting to old behaviors that a person has worked through previously.

Repetitions Number of times an exercise is performed (for example, ten repetitions on the bench press).

Resistance Training Training that includes both strength and endurance training.

Resting Heart Rate (RHR) Number of times a person's heart beats in one minute when the person is at complete rest.

Resting Metabolic Rate The energy required to maintain vital functions when the body is at rest.

RICE (Rest, Ice, Compression, Elevation) Immediate first aid for injuries like sprains, strains, and contusions.

Safety Net A network of close personal friends who can provide emotional and physical support.

Sarcomas Cancers arising from bone, cartilage, or muscle.

Saturated Fat Fatty acids with carbon atoms fully saturated with hydrogens; therefore only single bonds link the carbon atoms on the chain. High intake of saturated fats increases the risk for coronary heart disease.

Scoliosis, Structural Condition in which the spine takes on a C or S curve because of anatomical defects such as incorrect bone formation, a short limb, and so on.

Secondary Headaches Headaches that are a side effect of some other underlying condition.

Secondhand Smoke Other people's tobacco smoke.

Selfishness A human characteristic in which an individual is concerned only about his or her wants, needs, and desires.

Selflessness A characteristic in which a person puts the needs and desires of others first.

Self-Responsibility An individual's taking increased responsibility to prevent or manage certain health conditions.

Set-Point Theory Weight control theory that presumes that the body has an established weight and strongly attempts to maintain that weight.

Sets Number of repetitions (for example, three sets of twelve repetitions).

Sexually Transmitted Diseases (STDs) Diseases spread through sexual contact, such as AIDS, chlamydia, gonorrhea, and herpes.

Shinsplints A general term for pain on the front or side of the shin. A common overuse injury.

Skill-Related Components of Physical Fitness Agility, balance, coordination reaction time, power, speed, and sometimes kinesthetic awareness.

Skinfold Technique Method of estimating a person's percentage of body fat. Subcutaneous fat is measured using a skinfold caliper.

Smokeless Tobacco Tobacco used in the form of chew or snuff. It is generally held in the mouth instead of smoked. It is thought to be more addictive than smoking tobacco.

Soluble Fiber Gels and pectins found in the foods we eat. They dissolve in water and add bulk to the contents of the stomach, giving a feeling of fullness.

Specificity Refers to placing a specific demand on the body that results in a specific adaptation.

Spot Reducing Theory that claims that exercising a specific body part (for example, abdominal or midsection of the body) will result in significant fat reduction in that area. Contrary to popular opinion, spot reducing is not effective.

Static Exercise Exercise that is performed without movement.

Static Stretch Flexibility exercise in which a muscle or muscle group is held in a lengthened position for approximately 10 to 60 seconds.

STD Risk Assessment A physical examination and laboratory tests to detect sexually transmitted diseases, including those that are asymptomatic.

Stimulants Drugs that speed up the central nervous system.

Strain Overstretching or tearing of a muscle or tendon, resulting in swelling, discoloration, and pain.

Strength *See* Muscular Strength.

Strength Training Conditioning program that requires resistance to help increase muscular strength, power, or body size.

Stress Nonspecific response of the body to any demands made on it.

Stress Response Physical reaction to a stimulus (stressor).

Stressor Any physical, psychological, or environmental event or condition that initiates the stress response.

Stretch Reflex Automatic muscular contraction that occurs when a muscle is suddenly stretched.

Stretching Slowly lengthening a muscle to increase flexibility.

Strict Vegetarian Individual who refrains from eating any animal product, including milk, meat, poultry, and egg products.

Stroke Condition caused by a lack of oxygen to the brain cells.

Stroke Volume Amount of blood ejected by the heart in one beat (contraction).

Subcutaneous Located immediately below the skin.

Substance Abuse Use of a substance even though the substance is harmful to the user or to the people around the user.

Supports Special attention, improved self-esteem, improved health, better grades, more social approval, or improved quality of life resulting from our efforts to change our behaviors.

Syphilis Sexually transmitted disease caused by a bacterial infection. During the last stage of the disease, some people will suffer from paralysis, crippling, blindness, heart disease, brain damage, insanity, and even death.

Systolic Pressure The pressure exerted by the blood in the arteries when the heart is contracting. Systolic pressure is represented by the numerator in the blood pressure fraction.

Target Heart Rate Range (THR) *See* Target Heart Rate Zone.

Target Heart Rate Zone Optimum intensity range for aerobic exercise using the exercise heart rate as the indicator of intensity. Training within the range improves cardiorespiratory endurance.

Tendinitis Inflammation of a tendon. A common overuse injury.

Tendons Fibrous tissue that connects muscle to bone.

Tension Headaches Headaches that result from muscle tension.

Threshold of Aerobic Training Fifty percent of VO$_2$max, the minimum amount and intensity of aerobic exercise required to improve aerobic fitness.

Threshold of Training The minimum amount and intensity of exercise required to produce an increase in physical fitness.

Thrombosis Blood clot that forms in the arteries.

Time Length of a single exercise session.

Traditional Family A relationship involving a working father, a homemaker wife, and children.

Training Heart Rate Range (THR) *See* Target Heart Rate Zone.

Trichomoniasis STD caused by the parasite *Trichomonas vaginalis,* a protozoan that thrives in warm, moist places.

Tumor Single mutated cell that continues to divide, eventually forming clusters of abnormal cells.

Type I and Type II Diabetes Type I diabetes is also known as insulin-dependent diabetes and is the result of destruction of the insulin-producing cells of the pancreas. Type II diabetes results from a decrease in insulin sensitivity and production.

Underwater Weighing *See* Hydrostatic Weighing.

Use/Disuse Principle *See* Principle of Reversibility.

Vegetarian Individual whose diet consists of plant products, including grains, fruits, vegetables, nuts, seeds, and legumes. Some vegetarians also consume dairy products and eggs.

Vein Vessel that carries blood toward the heart.

Venous Pump Action of the muscles that helps to massage blood up the veins against gravity.

Very Low Calorie Diet (VLCD) Diet that limits daily total caloric intake to between 400 and 800 calories.

Viruses Submicroscopic organisms made up of complex proteins that can grow and multiply inside living cells and cause infectious diseases.

Vitamins Organic compounds that help release energy from food and act as metabolic regulators. Vitamins A, D, E, and K are fat soluble. The rest are water soluble.

VO$_2$max Largest amount of oxygen the body can consume in one minute. Measured in liters per minute or milliliters per kilogram body weight per minute.

Warm-up Period of time used to prepare the body for vigorous activity. Stretching movements and easy-range-of-movement exercises that raise the core temperature of the body are performed. A gradual increase in activity level that allows the heart and lungs to make a smooth transition into more vigorous activity/exercise.

Weight Cycling Phenomenon of successfully losing weight only to gain it back within a few months, followed by renewed dieting, weight gain and loss, and so on. Also known as yo-yo dieting.

Weight Lifting Exercise in which the objective is to lift as much weight as possible each time.

Weight Training Conditioning program that requires the use of weights to help increase muscular strength, endurance, power, or body size.

Wellness Constant and deliberate effort to stay healthy and to achieve the highest potential for well-being. Implies the adoption of healthy lifestyle factors that will decrease the risk for disease and enhance quality of life.

Workout The physical activity/exercise that follows the warm-up and precedes the cool-down. (Some definitions include the warm-up and cool-down as part of the workout.)

World View View that encompasses and considers all that is living and nonliving. Not human-centered.

ENDNOTES

Chapter 1

1. Anderson, R. N., K. Kochanek, and L. Murphy. The report of the final mortality statistics 1995. *Monthly Vital Statistics Report,* Vol. 45, No. 11, Suppl. 2, Report of Final Mortality Statistics, Publication (PHS) 97-1120, 1995.
2. Erikson, P. Unpublished analysis of vital statistics and National Health Interview Survey data, 1990.
3. U.S. Department of Health and Human Services, *Physical activity and health: A report of the Surgeon General.* Centers for Disease Control and Prevention, National Center for Chronic Disease Prevention and Health Promotion. Atlanta: The President's Council on Physical Fitness and Sports, 1996.
4. Murphy, T. A., and D. Murphy. *The wellness for life workbook,* 4th ed. San Diego: Fitness Publications, 1987.
5. Pate, R. R., et al. Physical activity and public health: A recommendation from the Centers for Disease Control and Prevention and the American College of Sports Medicine. *Journal of the American Medical Association* 273(5):402–407, 1995.
6. Blair, S. N., H. W. Kohl III, R. S. Paffenbarger, Jr., D. G. Clark, K. H. Cooper, and L. W. Gibbons. Physical fitness and all-cause mortality: A prospective study of healthy men and women. *Journal of the American Medical Association* 262(17):2395–2401, 1989.
7. Ibid.
8. Ibid.
9. American Cancer Society. *Cancer facts and figures.* Atlanta, 1995.
10. Ibid.
11. Williams, R. B., Jr. Hostility, anger, and heart disease. *Drug Therapy* August 1986, p. 43.
12. Justice, B. *Who gets sick: Thinking and health.* Houston: Peak Press, 1987.
13. Siegel, B. S. *Love, medicine, and miracles.* New York: Harper & Row, 1986, p. 181.
14. Justice, *op. cit.*
15. Murphy and Murphy, *op. cit.*
16. Prochaska, J. O., and C. diClemente. Toward a comprehensive behavior change. In *Treating Addictive Behaviors,* W. Miller and N. Healther, eds. New York: Plenum, 1986.
17. Rossi, S. R., S. S. Jonnalagadda, and P. M. Kris-Etherton. Dietary interventions. In N. Jairath, ed. *Coronary heart disease and risk factor management: A nursing perspective.* Philadelphia: W. B. Saunders, 1998.

Chapter 2

1. U.S. Department of Health and Human Services. *Physical activity and health: A report of the Surgeon General.* Centers for Disease Control and Prevention, National Center for Chronic Disease Prevention and Health Promotion. Atlanta: The President's Council on Physical Fitness and Sports, 1996.
2. Ibid.
3. Stephens, T. Secular trends in adult physical activity. *Research Quarterly for Exercise and Sport* 58:94–105, 187.
4. Corbin, C. B., and R. Lindsey. *Concepts of physical fitness with laboratories.* Dubuque, IA: William C. Brown, 1970.
5. Caspersen, C. J., K. E. Powell, and G. M. Christiansen. Physical activity, exercise, and physical fitness. Definitions and distinctions for health-related research. *Public Health Reports* 100:126–131, 1986.
6. American Alliance of Health, Physical Education, Recreation, and Dance. *Health related physical fitness: Test manual,* 1980.

7. American College of Sports Medicine. The recommended quantity and quality of exercise for developing and maintaining cardiorespiratory and muscular fitness in healthy adults. *Medicine and Science in Sports* 22(2):265–274, 1990.

8. U.S. Department of Health and Human Services. *Healthy people 2000: National health promotion and disease prevention objectives.* DHHS Publication No. (PHS) 91-50213. Washington, D.C.: U.S. Government Printing Office, 1990.

9. Pate, R. R., et al. Physical activity and public health, a recommendation from the Centers for Disease Control and Prevention and the American College of Sports Medicine. *Journal of the American Medical Association* 273(5):402–407, 1995.

10. International Society of Sport Psychology. *Physical activity and psychological benefits: Position statement* 20:179, 1992.

11. Martinsen, E. W., and T. Stephens. Exercise and mental health in clinical and free-living populations. In R. K. Dishman, ed. *Advances in exercise and adherence.* Champaign, IL: Human Kinetics, 1994, pp. 67–69.

12. Bova, B. *The beauty of light.* New York: Wiley, 1998, pp. 88, 89.

13. Shellock, F. G., and W. E. Prentice. Warming up and stretching for improved physical performance and prevention of sports-related injuries. *Sports Medicine* 2:267–278, 1985.

14. Paffenbarger Jr., R. S., R. T. Hyde, A. L. Wing, and C. C. Hsieh. Physical activity, all-cause mortality, and longevity of college alumni. *New England Journal of Medicine* 314:605–613, 1986.

Chapter 3

1. Dishman, R. K., ed. *Advances in exercise and adherence.* Champaign, IL: Human Kinetics, 1994, pp. 374–375.

2. Wilmore, J. H., and D. L. Costill. *Training for sport and activity: The physiological basis of the conditioning process.* Champaign, IL: Human Kinetics, 1993, p. 162.

3. Portions of this section are taken from J. G. Bishop, *Fitness Through Aerobics,* 3rd ed. Scottsdale, AZ: Gorsuch Scarisbrick Publishers, 1995, pp. 18–22.

Chapter 4

1. Shephard, R. J. Exercise prescription for the healthy aged: Testing and programs. *Clinical Journal of Sport Medicine* 1(2):88–99, 1991.

2. Stamford, B. A stretching primer. *The Physician and Sportsmedicine* 22(9):85–86, 1994.

3. Munns, K. Effects of exercise on the range of joint motion in elderly subjects. In E. Smith and R. Serfass, eds. *Exercise and aging.* Hillside, NJ: Enslow Publishers, 1981.

4. Alter, M. J. *Science of stretching.* Champaign, IL: Human Kinetics, 1988.

5. Ross, J. G., and G. G. Gilbert. The national children and youth fitness study: A summary of findings. *Journal of Physical Education, Recreation, and Dance* 56:45–50, 1985.

6. Ross, J. G., and R. R. Pate. The national children and youth fitness study II: A summary of findings. *Journal of Physical Education, Recreation, and Dance* 58:51–56, 1987.

7. Docherty, D., and R. D. Bell. The relationship between flexibility and linearity measures in boys and girls 6–15 years of age. *Journal of Human Movement Studies* 11:279–288, 1985.

8. Payne, V. G., and L. D. Isaacs. *Human motor development: A lifespan approach.* Mountain View, CA: Mayfield, 1995.

9. Germain, N. W., and S. N. Blair. Variability of shoulder flexion with age, activity and sex. *American Corrective Therapy Journal* 37:156–160, 1983.

10. Low back pain. *Mayo Clinic Health Letter* 7:4, 1989.

11. Burkett, L. N. Investigation into hamstring strains: The case of the hybrid muscle. *Journal of Sports Medicine* 3(5):228–231.

12. Shellock, F. G., and W. E. Prentice. Warming-up and stretching for improved physical performance and prevention of sports-related injuries. *Sports Medicine* 2:267–278, 1985.

Chapter 5

1. American College of Sports Medicine. The recommended quantity and quality of exercise for developing and maintaining cardiorespiratory and muscular fitness in healthy adults. *Medicine and Science in Sports* 22(2):265–274, 1990.

2. Wilmore, J. H., and D. L. Costill. *Training for sport and activity,* 3rd ed. Champaign, IL: Human Kinetics, 1988, p. 10.

3. Strength training. *Mayo Clinic Health Letter* 8:2–3, 1990.

4. Tortora, G. J., and N. P. Anagnostakos. *Principles of anatomy and physiology.* New York: Harper & Row, 1984.

5. Ibid.

6. Wilmore and Costill, *op. cit.,* p. 10.

7. Costill, D. L., J. Daniels, W. Evans, W. Fink, G. Krahenbuhl, and B. Saltin. Skeletal muscle enzymes and fiber composition in male and female track athletes. *Journal of Applied Physiology* 40:149–154, 1976.

8. Costill, D. L., W. J. Fink, and M. L. Pollock. Muscle fiber composition and enzyme activities of elite distance runners. *Medicine and Science in Sports* 8:96–100, 1976.

9. Wilmore and Costill, *op. cit.,* p. 35.

10. Gollnick, P. D., R. B. Armstrong, C. W. Saubert IV, K. Piehl, and B. Saltin. Enzyme activity and fiber

composition in skeletal muscle of untrained and trained men. *Journal of Applied Physiology* 33:312–319, 1972.

11. Gettman, L. R., and M. L. Pollock. Circuit weight training: A critical review of its physiological benefits. *The Physician and Sportsmedicine* 9:44–60, 1981.

12. Anspaugh, D. J., M. H. Hamrick, and F. D. Rosato. *Wellness: Concepts and applications*, 2nd ed. St. Louis: Mosby, 1994, p. 103.

13. Laubach, L. L. Comparative muscular strength of men and women: A review of the literature. *Aviation, Space and Environmental Medicine* 47:534–542, 1976.

14. Fleck, S. J., and W. J. Kraemer. *Designing resistance training programs*, 2nd ed. Champaign, IL: Human Kinetics, 1997.

15. Cureton, K. J., M. A. Collins, D. W. Hill, and F. M. McElhannon. Muscle hypertrophy in men and women. *Medicine and Science in Sports and Exercise* 20:338–344, 1988.

16. Fleck and Kraemer, *op. cit.*

17. Brooks, G. A., and T. D. Fahey. *Exercise physiology: Human bioenergetics and its application.* New York: Wiley, 1984.

18. Fleck and Kraemer, *op. cit.*

19. Ibid.

20. Baechle, T. R., and B. R. Groves. *Weight training steps to success.* Champaign, IL: Leisure Press, 1992.

21. Fleck and Kraemer, *op. cit.*

22. Ibid.

23. American College of Sports Medicine, *op. cit.*

24. Ibid.

25. Ibid.

Chapter 6

1. U.S. Department of Health and Human Services. *Healthy people 2000: National health promotion and disease prevention objectives.* DHHS Publication No. (PHS) 91-50213. Washington, D.C.: U.S. Government Printing Office, 1990, pp. 16–20.

2. Kuczmarski, R. J., K. M. Flegal, S. M. Campbell, and C. L. Johnson. Increasing prevalence of overweight among U.S. adults. The national health and nutrition examination surveys, 1960–1991. *Journal of the American Medical Association* 272:205–211, 1994.

3. Tucker, L. A., and M. J. Kano. Dietary fat and body fat: A multivariate study of 205 adult females. *American Journal of Clinical Nutrition* 56:616–622, 1992.

4. Consumer's Union. Are you eating right? *Consumer Reports* 57(10):645–648, 1992.

5. Thompson, L. Potential health benefits of whole grains and their components. *Contemporary Nutrition* 17(6):1, 1992.

6. Wardlaw, G. Eating vegetarian. *Healthline* 10(July):2–4, 1991.

7. McArdle, W. D., F. I. Katch, and V. L. Katch. *Exercise physiology: Energy nutrition, and human performance,* 3rd ed. Philadelphia: Lea & Febiger, 1991.

8. Heaney, R. P., et al. Menopausal changes in calcium balance performance. *American Journal of Clinical Nutrition* 36:986, 1982.

9. Williams, S. R. *Nutrition and diet therapy,* 7th ed. St. Louis: Mosby, 1994.

10. Mayer, J. How fast food figures. *Tufts University Diet and Nutrition Letter* 8(1):7, 1990.

11. Neiman, D. C., D. E. Butterworth, and C. N. Neiman. *Nutrition.* Dubuque, IA: William C. Brown, 1990.

12. American Heart Association and adapted with permission of Tufts Health and Nutrition Letter from *No more label fables, Tufts University Diet and Nutrition Letter* 10, February 1993, phone 1-800-274-7581.

13. Sherman, W. M. Muscle glycogen supercompensation during the week before athletic competition. *Sports Science Exchange, Sports Nutrition* 2(16):June 1989, Gatorade Sports Science Institute.

Chapter 7

1. McArdle, W. D., F. I. Katch, and V. L. Katch. *Exercise physiology: Energy nutrition, and human performance,* 3rd ed. Philadelphia, PA: Lea & Febiger, 1991.

2. Margaria, R., et al. Energy cost of running. *Journal of Applied Physiology* 18:367, 1963.

3. Kuczmarski, R. J., K. M. Flegal, S. M. Campbell, and C. L. Johnson. Increasing prevalence of overweight among U.S. adults. The health and nutrition examination surveys, 1960–1991. *Journal of the American Medical Association* 272:205–211, 1994.

4. Ibid.

5. Folsom, A. R., S. A. Kaye, T. A. Sellers, et al. Body fat distribution and 5-year risk of death in older women. *Journal of the American Medical Association* 269:483–487, 1993.

6. National Center for Health Statistics. *Health, United States, 1987.* DHHS Publication No. (PHS) 88-1232. Public Health Service. Washington, D. C.: U.S. Government Printing Office, March 1988.

7. Ross, J. G., R. R. Pate, T. G. Lohman, and G. M. Christenson. Changes in the body composition of children. *Journal of Physical Education, Recreation, and Dance* November/December: 98–102, 1987.

8. Manson, J. E., G. A. Colditz, M. J. Stampfer, et al. A prospective study of obesity and risk of coronary heart disease in women. *New England Journal of Medicine* 322:882–889, 1990.

9. Garrison, R. J., and W. P. Caselli. Weight and thirty-year mortality of men in the Framingham Study. *Annals of Internal Medicine* 103:1006–1009, 1985.

10. Haffner, S. M., M. P. Stern, H. P. Hazuda, J. Pugh, and J. K. Patterson. Do upper-body and centralized

adiposity measure different aspects of regional body-fat distribution? Relationship to non-insulin-dependent diabetes mellitus, lipids and lipoproteins. *Diabetes* 36:43–51, 1987.

11. Pi-Synyer, F. X. Medical hazards of obesity. *Annals of Internal Medicine* 119(7, Part 2):655–660, 1993.

12. Gortmaker, S. L., A. Must, J. M. Perrin, A. M. Sobol, and W. H. Dietz. Social and economic consequences of overweight in adolescence and young adulthood. *New England Journal of Medicine* 329:1008–1012, 1993.

13. Cooper, K. H. *The aerobics program for total well-being: Exercise, diet, emotional balance.* New York: M. Evans, 1982.

Chapter 8

1. Harris, L. *Inside America.* New York: Louis Harris, Random House, 1985.

2. Bovsun, M. The diet dilemma. *Medical World News,* May 1992.

3. National Center for Health Statistics. *Health, United States, 1993.* Hyattsville, MD: Public Health Service, 1994.

4. Kramer, F. M., R. W. Jeffery, J. L. Forster, and M. K. Snell. Long term follow-up of behavioral treatment for obesity: Patterns of weight regain among men and women. *International Journal of Obesity* 13:123–136, 1989.

5. Kuczmarski, R. J., K. M. Flegal, S. M. Campbell, and C. L. Johnson. Increasing prevalence of overweight among U.S. adults. The health and nutrition examination surveys, 1960–1991. *Journal of the American Medical Association* 272:205–211, 1994.

6. Ravussin, E., and C. Bogardus. A brief overview of human energy metabolism and its relationship to essential obesity. *American Journal of Clinical Nutrition* 55:242S–245S, 1992.

7. Serdula, M. K., D. Ivery, R. J. Coates, D. S. Freedman, D. F. Williamson, and T. Byers. Do obese children become obese adults? A review of the literature. *Preview of Medicine* 22:167–177, 1993.

8. Ibid.

9. Martin, E. M. Prevalence of eating disorders such as anorexia and bulimia nervosa among the college population. *College Student Affairs Journal* 12:77–80, 1993.

10. Shisslak, C. M. Body weight and bulimia as discriminators of psychological characteristics among anorexic, bulimic, and obese women. *Journal of Abnormal Psychology* 99(4):380–384, 1990.

11. Adapted from Diagnostic criteria for eating disorders. *American Psychiatric Association: Diagnostic and statistical manual,* 4th ed. Washington, D.C.: American Psychiatric Association, 1994.

12. Davis, J. M., S. P. Bailey, F. J. Galiano, et al. Increased free fatty acid and glucose availability and

fatigue during prolonged exercise in man. *Medicine and Science in Sports and Exercise* 24(5): S71, 1992.

13. Adapted from Ornish, D. *Eat more, weigh less: Dr. Dean Ornish's life choice program for losing weight safely while eating abundantly.* New York: Harper-Collins, 1993.

14. Gray, G. A. Pathophysiology of obesity. *American Journal of Clinical Nutrition* 55:488S–494S, 1992.

15. Foster, G. D., T. A. Wadden, I. D. Feurer, et al. Controlled trial of the metabolic effects of a very low calorie diet: Short and long term effects. *American Journal of Clinical Nutrition* 51:167–172, 1990.

16. Kirshner, M. A., G. Schneider, H. N. Ertel, and J. Gorman. An eight year experience with a very low calorie formula diet for control of major obesity. *International Journal of Obesity* 12:69–80, 1988.

17. Lissner, L., P. G. Odell, R. M. D'Agostino, J. Stokes, M. E. Kregar, B. E. Belanger, and K. D. Brownell. Variability of body weight and health outcomes in the Framingham population. *New England Journal of Medicine* 324:1839–1844, 1991.

18. Brownell, K. D. The good and bad of dieting: Applying knowledge from work on weight cycling. Paper presented at the Society of Behavioral Medicine/NAASO Colloquium, Washington, D.C., March 1991.

19. Zuti, W. A., and L. A. Golding. Comparing diet and exercise as weight reduction tools. *The Physician and Sportsmedicine* 4:49–53, 1976.

20. Kramer et al., *op. cit.*

Chapter 9

1. Enos, W. F., R. H. Holmes, and J. Beyer. Coronary disease among United States soldiers killed in action in Korea. *Journal of the American Medical Association* 152:1090–1093, 1953.

2. National Center for Health Statistics. Annual summary of births, marriages, divorces, and deaths: United States, 1993. *Monthly Vital Statistics Report,* Vol. 42, No. 13. Hyattsville, MD: Public Health Service, 1994.

3. Goldman, L., and E. F. Cook. The decline in ischemic heart disease mortality rates. *Annals of Internal Medicine* 101:825–836, 1984.

4. Centers for Disease Control and Prevention. Prevalence of sedentary lifestyle. *Morbidity and Mortality Weekly Report* 42:576–679, 1993.

5. National Heart, Lung, and Blood Institute. *The fifth report of the Joint National Committee on Detection, Evaluation, and Treatment of High Blood Pressure.* National Institutes of Health Publication No. 93-1088. Hyattsville, MD: Public Health Service, 1993.

6. Garraway, W. M., and J. P. Whisnant. The changing pattern of hypertension and the declining incidence of stroke. *Journal of the American Medical Association* 258:214–217, 1987.

7. American Heart Association. *Heart and stroke facts.* Dallas, TX, 1994.

8. National Center for Health Statistics, *op. cit.*

9. Ross, R. The pathogenesis of atherosclerosis: An update. *New England Journal of Medicine* 314:488–500, 1986.

10. Expert Panel on Detection, Evaluation, and Treatment of High Blood Cholesterol in Adults. Summary of the second report of the National Cholesterol Education Program (NCEP) Expert Panel on Detection, Evaluation, and Treatment of High Blood Cholesterol in Adults (Adult Treatment Panel 11). *Journal of the American Medical Association* 269:3015–3023, 1993.

11. Lipid Research Clinics Program. The Lipid Research Clinics coronary primary prevention trial results, II. The relationship of reduction in incidence of coronary heart disease to cholesterol lowering. *Journal of the American Medical Association* 251–365, 1984.

12. Fuster, V., L. Badimon, J. J. Badimon, and I. H. Chesebro. The pathogenesis of coronary artery disease and the acute coronary syndromes. *New England Journal of Medicine* 326:242–249, 1992.

13. PDAY Research Group. Relationship of atherosclerosis in young men to serum lipoprotein cholesterol concentrations and smoking. *Journal of the American Medical Association* 264:3018–3024, 1990.

14. Perkins, K. A. Family history of coronary heart disease: Is it an independent risk factor? *American Journal of Epidemiology* 124:182–194, 1986.

15. Hager, T. High-risk "heart" families: A genealogical look. *Journal of the American Medical Association* 250:1663–1664, 1983.

16. Jacobsen, B. K., and D. S. Thelle. Risk factors for coronary heart disease and level of education. *American Journal of Epidemiology* 127:923–932, 1988.

17. National Center for Health Statistics. *Health, United States, 1994.* Hyattsville, MD: Public Health Service, 1995.

18. Tucker, L. A., and S. G. Aldana. Family history of heart disease and hypercholesterolemia. *Health Values* 14(2):38, 1990.

19. National High Blood Pressure Education Program. *The fifth report of the Joint National Committee on Detection, Evaluation, and Treatment of High Blood Pressure.* National Heart, Lung, and Blood Institute, National Institutes of Health Publication No. 93-1088. Bethesda, MD: National Institutes of Health, 1993.

20. Kuczmarski, R. J., K. M. Flegal, S. M. Campbell, and C. L. Johnson. Increasing prevalence of overweight among U.S. adults. The national health and nutrition examination surveys, 1960–1991. *Journal of the American Medical Association* 272:205–211, 1994.

21. Centers for Disease Control and Prevention, *op. cit.*

22. Doll, R., and R. Reto. The causes of cancer: Quantitative estimates of avoidable risks of cancer in the United States today. *Journal of the National Cancer Institute* 66:1191–1308, 1981.

23. Centers for Disease Control and Prevention. Cigarette smoking among adults—United States, 1990. *Morbidity and Mortality Weekly Report* 41(20), 1992.

24. Glantz, S. Passive smoking and health disease: Epidemiology, physiology, and biochemistry. *Circulation* 1:1–12, 1991.

25. Scherwitz, L. E., L. E. Graham, and D. M. Ornish. Self involvement and the risk factors for coronary heart disease. *Advances* 2:6–18, 1985.

26. Kaplan, G. A., J. T. Salonen, R. D. Cohen, et al. Social connections and mortality from all causes and from cardiovascular disease: Prospective evidence from Eastern Finland. *American Journal of Epidemiology* 128:370–380, 1988.

27. Expert Panel on Detection, Evaluation, and Treatment of High Blood Cholesterol in Adults, *op. cit.*

28. Eichner, E. R. Exercise and heart disease: Epidemiology of the "exercise hypothesis." *American Journal of Medicine* 75:1008–1023, 1986.

29. National Heart, Lung, and Blood Institute, *op. cit.*

30. Ibid.

31. American Cancer Society. *Cancer facts and figures.* Atlanta, 1994.

32. Treatment of Mild Hypertension Research Group. The treatment of mild hypertension study: A randomized, placebo-controlled trial of a nutritional-hygienic regimen along with various drug monotherapies. *Archives of Internal Medicine* 151:1412–1423, 1991.

33. Ornish, D. *Dr. Dean Ornish's program for reversing heart disease.* New York: Ballantine Books, 1992.

Chapter 10

1. Amler, R. W., and H. B. Dull, eds. Closing the gap: The burden of unnecessary illness. *American Journal of Preventative Medicine* 3(Supplement 5), 1987.

2. National Center of Health Statistics. *Health United States, 1994 and prevention profile.* DHHS Publication No.(PHS)90-1232. Hyattsville, MD: U.S. Department of Health and Human Services, 1995.

3. Nieman, D. C. *Fitness and sports medicine: A health-related approach.* Palo Alto, CA: Bull Publishing, 1995.

4. American Cancer Society. *Cancer facts and figures.* Atlanta, 1995.

5. Boring, C. C., T. S. Squires, and T. Tong. Cancer statistics, 1993. *California Cancer Journal for Clinicians* 43:7–26, 1993.

6. Eliopoulos, C., J. Klein, K. M. Phan, and B. Knie. Hair concentrations of nicotine and cotinine in

women and their newborn infants. *Journal of the American Medical Association* 271:621–623,1994.

7. National Center of Health Statistics, *op. cit.*

8. Reichman, M. E. Alcohol and breast cancer. *Alcohol Health & Research World* 18:182–183, 1994.

9. Hunter, D. J., and W. C.Willett. Diet, body size, and breast cancer. *Epidemiology Review* 15:110–132, 1993.

10. NCI replaces guidelines with statement of evidence. *Journal of the National Cancer Institute* 86:14, 1994.

11. Greenwald, P., and E. Sondik. Diet and chemoprevention in NCI's research strategy to achieve national cancer control objectives. *Annual Review of Public Health* 7:267–291, 1986.

12. American Cancer Society. Cancer prevention study, II. The American Cancer Society prospective study. *Statistical Bulletin of the Metropolitan Insurance Company* 73:21–29, 1992.

13. Doll, R., and R. Reto. The causes of cancer: Quantitative estimates of avoidable risks of cancer in the United States today. *Journal of the National Cancer Institute* 66:1191–1308, 1981.

14. Roebuck, B.D., J. McCaffrey, and K. J. Baumgartner. Protective effects of voluntary exercise during the postinitiation phase of pancreatic carcinogenesis in the rat. *Cancer Research* 50:6811–6816, 1990.

15. MacNeil, B., and L. Hoffman-Goetz. Chronic exercise enhances in vivo and in vitro cytotoxic mechanisms of natural immunity in mice. *Journal of Applied Physiology* 74:388–395, 1993.

16. Blair, S. N., H. W. Kohl III, R. S. Paffenbarger, Jr., D. G. Clark, K. H. Cooper, and L. W. Gibbons. Physical fitness and all-cause mortality: A prospective study of healthy men and women. *Journal of the American Medical Association* 262(17):2395–2401, 1989.

17. Lee, I. M. Physical activity, fitness and cancer. In C. Bouchard and R. J. Shephard eds. *Exercise, fitness, and health: A consensus of current knowledge.* Champaign, IL: Human Kinetics, 1994.

18. Bernstein, L., B. E. Henderson, R. Hanisch, J. Sullivan-Halley, and R. K. Ross. Physical exercise and reduced risk of breast cancer in young women. *Journal of the National Cancer Institute* 86:1403–1408, 1994.

19. Shephard, R. J. Physical activity and cancer. *International Journal of Sports Medicine* 11:413–420, 1990.

20. Sternfeld, B. Cancer and the protective effect of physical activity: The epidemiological evidence. *Medicine and Science in Sports and Exercise* 24:1195–1209, 1992.

21. Shephard, R. J. Exercise in the prevention and treatment of cancer. An update. *Sports Medicine* 15:258–280, 1993.

22. Lee, *op. cit.*

23. Davis, D. L., D. Hoel, J. Fox, and A. Lopez. International trends in cancer mortality in France, West

Germany, Italy, Japan, England and Wales, and the USA. *Lancet* 336:474–481, 1990.

24. U.S. Department of Health and Human Services. *Health United States, 1994.* Public Health Service, Centers for Disease Control and Prevention, National Center for Health Statistics. DHHS Publication No. (PHS)95-1232. Hyattsville, MD, May 1995.

25. Farrell, P. A., A. L. Caston, D. Rodd, and J. Engdahl. Effect of training on insulin secretion from single pancreatic beta cells. *Medicine and Science in Sports and Exercise* 24:426–433, 1992.

26. Yamanouchi, K., H. Nakajima, T. Shinozaki, et al. Effects of daily physical activity on insulin action in the elderly. *Journal of Applied Physiology* 73:2241–2245, 1992.

Chapter 11

1. Time out. *U.S. News & World Report*, December 11, 1995, p. 90.

2. Mason, J. W. A historical view of the stress field. *Journal of Human Stress* 1:6–27, 1975.

3. Lazarus, R. S., and S. Folkman. *Stress, appraisal and coping.* New York: Springer, 1984.

4. Ibid.

5. Tkrubin, R. The biochemistry of touch. *U.S. News & World Report*, November 10, 1997, p. 62.

6. Ellis, J. A. Community interventions for helping isolated and underserved elders. *Journal of Gerontological Social Work* 26(3–4):145–157, 1996.

7. DeBerard, S. M., and R. A. Kleinknecht. Loneliness, duration of loneliness, and reported stress symptomatology. *Psychological Reports* 76:1363–1369, June 1995, part 2.

8. Hu, U. R., and N. Goldman. Mortality differentials by marital status: An international comparison. *Demography* 27(2):333–350, 1990.

9. Gjerdingen, D. A., D. G. Froberg, and P. Fontaine. The effects of social support on women's health during pregnancy, labor and delivery, and the postpartum period. *Family Medicine* 23(5):370–375, July 1991.

10. Snowdon, D. A., S. J. Kemper, J. A. Mortimer, L. H. Greiner, D. R. Wekstein, and W. R. Markesbery. Linguistic ability in early life and cognitive function and Alzheimer's disease in late life. Findings from the nun study. *Journal of the American Medical Association* 275(7):528–532, February 21, 1996.

11. Selye, H. *The stress of life*, 2nd ed. New York: McGraw-Hill, 1976, p. 74.

12. Magill, R. A. *Motor learning: Concepts and applications*, 4th ed. Dubuque, IA: Brown & Benchmark, 1993, pp. 129–130.

13. Rice, P. L. *Stress and health*, 2nd ed. Pacific Grove, CA: Brooks/Cole, 1992, pp. 27–28.

14. Ibid., p. 5.

15. Cannon, W. B. *The wisdom of the body.* New York: Norton, 1932.

16. Selye, H. *Stress without distress.* Philadelphia & New York: J. B. Lippincott, 1974.

17. Ibid., pp. 26–27.

18. Aldwin, C. M. *Stress, coping and development: An integrative perspective.* New York: Guilford Press, 1994.

19. Seyle, 1974, *op. cit.,* p. 17.

20. Insel, P. M., and W. T. Roth. *Core concepts in health,* 7th ed. Mountain View, CA: Mayfield, 1994, pp. 34–35.

21. Mason, *op. cit.*

22. Lazarus, R., and R. Launier. Stress-related transactions between person and environment. In L. A. Pervin and M. Lewis, eds. *Perspectives in interactional psychology.* New York: Plenum, 1978, pp. 287–327.

23. Lazarus and Launier, *op. cit.*

24. Coyne, J. C., and K. Holroyd. Stress, coping, and illness: A transactional perspective. In T. Millon, C. Green, and R. Meagher. *Handbook of clinical health psychology.* New York: Plenum, 1982, pp. 103–127.

25. Fischman, J. Type A on trial. *Psychology Today* 21(2):42–64, 1987.

26. Friedman, M., and R. Roseman. *Type A behavior and your heart.* New York: Alfred A. Knopf, 1984.

27. Kobasa, S. Stressful life events, personality, and health: An inquiry into hardiness. *Journal of Personality and Social Psychology* 37:1–11, 1979.

28. Rice, *op. cit.*

29. Kanner, A. D., J. C. Coyne, C. Schaefer, and R. S. Lazarus. Comparisons of two modes of stress measurement: Daily hassles and uplifts versus major life events. *Journal of Behavioural Medicine* 4:1–39, 1981.

30. Rice, P. L. *Stress and health,* 2nd ed. Pacific Grove, CA: Brooks/Cole Publishing, 1992, p. 36.

31. *Merriam-Webster's collegiate dictionary,* 10th ed. Springfield, MA: Merriam-Webster, 1993, p. 78.

Chapter 12

1. Brown, P. *The death of intimacy: Barriers to intimate relationships.* New York: Haworth Press, 1995.

2. Lynch, J. J. *The broken heart: The medical consequences of loneliness.* New York: Basic Books, 1977.

3. Sagan, L. A. *The health of nations.* New York: Basic Books, 1987.

4. Heisel, J. S., S. E. Locke, L. J. Kraus, and R. M. Williams. Natural killer cell activity and MMPI scores of a cohort of college students. *American Journal of Psychiatry* 143:1382–1386, 1986.

5. Curran, J. P. Dating anxiety. *Medical Aspects of Human Sexuality* 37:160–175, 1982.

6. National Center for Health Statistics. *Annual summary of births, deaths, marriages, and divorces—1991.* Washington, D.C.: Department of Health and Human Services, 1992.

7. Davis, M. Living arrangements and survival of middle-aged men. American Public Health Association Meeting, October 1990.

8. Ibid.

9. Rosengren, A., H. Wedel, and L. Wilhelmsen. Marital status and mortality in middle-aged Swedish men. *American Journal of Epidemiology* 129:54–64, 1989.

10. Sarason, B. R., I. G. Sarason, and G. R. Pierce. *Social support: An interactional view.* New York: Wiley, 1990.

11. Folkenberg, J. Fighting to save your marriage. *Alcohol, Drug Abuse, and Mental Health Administration Headlines,* January 1992.

12. U.S. Bureau of the Census. *Marital and living arrangements: March 1990.* Current Population Reports, Series P-2. Washington, D.C.: U.S. Government Printing Office, 1991.

13. Ibid.

14. Olson, D., and J. DeFrain. *Marriage and family.* Mountain View, CA: Mayfield, 1994.

15. Men's transition to parenthood: Longitudinal studies of early family experience. Hillsdale, NJ: Erlbaum Associates, 1987.

16. National Center for Health Statistics, *op. cit.*

17. Saluter, A. F. *Singleness in America. Studies in marriage and the family.* Current Population Reports, Series P-23, No. 162. Washington, D.C.: U.S. Department of Commerce, Bureau of the Census, 1990.

18. Hu, U. R., and N. Goldman. Mortality differentials by marital status: An international comparison. *Demography* 27(2):333–350, 1990.

19. Kaslow, F. The thirty-something women: Companionship, children, and career choices. Presented at the American Psychological Association Meeting, Boston, 1990.

20. U.S. Bureau of the Census, *op. cit.*

21. Lynch, *op. cit.*

22. Walker D., and R. E. Beauchene. The relationship of loneliness, social isolation and physical health to dietary adequacy of independent living elderly. *Journal of the American Dietetic Association* 91:300–306, 1991.

Chapter 13

1. Centers for Disease Control. *Division of STD/HIV Prevention annual report, 1989.* Atlanta, GA: U.S. Department of Health and Human Services, 1990.

2. Holmes, K. K., P-A. Mardh, P. F. Sparling, P. J. Wiesner, W. Cates, Jr., S. M. Lemon, and W. E. Stamm, eds. *Sexually transmitted diseases,* 2nd ed. New York: McGraw-Hill, 1990.

3. U.S. Department of Health and Human Services. *Medicine for the public: Sexually transmitted diseases.* Public Health Service, National Institutes of Health Publication No. 93-3057, April 1993, p. 5.

4. U.S. Department of Health and Human Services. *HIV infection and AIDS: Are you at risk?* Public Health Service. Available on the World Wide Web at www.cdcnac.org.

5. U.S. Department of Health and Human Services, *op. cit.*, p. 7.

6. Ibid.

7. Insel, P. M., and W. T. Roth. *Core concepts in health,* 7th ed. Mountain View, CA: Mayfield, 1994, p. 479.

8. Leppart, P. C., and F. M. Howard. *Primary care for women.* Philadelphia: Lippincott-Ravin, 1997.

9. Ibid.

10. Newkirk, G. R. Pelvic inflammatory disease. A contemporary approach. *American Family Physician* 4(53):1127–1135.

11. Leppart and Howard, *op. cit.*

12. Ibid.

13. Ibid.

14. Newkirk, *op. cit.*

15. Leppart and Howard, *op. cit.*

16. U.S. Department of Health and Human Services, *op. cit.*, p. 13.

17. Division of STD Prevention. *Sexually transmitted disease surveillance, 1995.* U.S. Department of Health and Human Services. Atlanta: Centers for Disease Control and Prevention, September 1996.

18. Ibid.

19. Ibid.

20. Centers for Disease Control. Chlamydia trachomatis infection. *Mortality and Morbidity Weekly Report* 33:805–807, 1985.

21. Ibid.

22. Ibid.

23. U.S. Department of Health and Human Services, *op. cit.*, p. 9.

24. Ibid.

25. Ibid., p. 7

26. Ibid., p. 4.

27. Insel and Roth, *op. cit.*

28. U.S. Department of Health and Human Services, *op. cit.*, p. 9.

29. U.S. Department of Health and Human Services, *op. cit.*, p. 11.

30. Mertz, G. J., et al. Risk factors for the sexual transmission of genital herpes. *Annals of Internal Medicine* 116: 197–202, February 1992.

31. U.S. Department of Health and Human Services, *op. cit.*, p. 15.

32. Ibid.

33. Leppart and Howard, *op. cit.*

34. Ibid.

Chapter 14

1. Gibbons, B. Alcohol the legal drug. *National Geographic* 181(2): 2–35, February 1992.

2. Larson, D. E., ed. *The Mayo Clinic family health book.* New York: William Morrow and Company, 1990.

3. Ibid., p. 419.

4. Kendler, K. S., A. C. Heath, M. C. Neale, R. C. Kessler, and L. J. Eaves. A population-based twin study of alcoholism in women. *Journal of the American Medical Association* 268:1877–1882, 1992.

5. National Institute on Alcohol Abuse and Alcoholism. Alcohol and minorities. *Alcohol Alert* No. 25, July 1994.

6. National Institute on Alcohol Abuse and Alcoholism. *Eighth special report to U.S. Congress on alcohol and health,* September 1993.

7. Ibid.

8. Connecticut Clearinghouse. *Prevention works!* Plainville, CT, 1993.

9. Ibid.

10. Bausell, C. R., et al. *The links among drugs, alcohol and campus crime.* Towson, MD: Towson State University Center for Study and Prevention of Campus Crime, 1990.

11. U.S. Department of Health and Human Services, Office of the Inspector General. *Youth and alcohol: Dangerous and deadly consequences.* Washington, D.C.: April 1992.

12. Presley, C., and P. Meilman. *Alcohol and drugs on American college campuses.* Carbondale, IL: Student Health Wellness Center, Southern Illinois University, July 1992.

13. Frezza, M., C. DiPadora, G. Pozzato, M. Terpin, E. Barano, and C. S. Lieher. High blood alcohol levels in women: The role of decreased alcohol dehydrogenase activity and first-pass metabolism. *New England Journal of Medicine* 32:95–99, April 11, 1990.

14. National Institute on Alcohol Abuse and Alcoholism, *op. cit.*

15. Thomasson, H. R., and T-K. Li. How alcohol and aldehyde dehydrogenase genes modify alcohol drinking, alcohol flushing, and the risk for alcoholism. *Alcohol Health & Research World* 17(2):167–172, 1993.

16. National Institute on Alcohol Abuse and Alcoholism. Alcohol and minorities. *Alcohol Alert,* No. 23, PH 347, January 1994.

17. Meier-Tackmann, D., R. A. Leonhardt, D. P. Agarwal, and H. W. Goedde. Effect of acute ethanol drinking on alcohol metabolism in subjects with different ADH and ALDH genotypes. *Alcohol* 7(5):413–418, 1990.

18. National Institute on Alcohol Abuse and Alcoholism. *Sixth special report to U.S. Congress on alcohol and health,* January 1987.

19. Filmore, K. M., E. Hartka, B. M. Johnstone, E. V. Leino, M. Motoyoshi, and M. T. Temple. A meta-analysis of life course variation in drinking: The

collaborative alcohol-related longitudinal project. *British Journal of Addiction* 86(10):1221–1268, 1991.

20. Substance Abuse and Mental Health Services Administration. *Preventing perinatal abuse of alcohol, tobacco, and other drugs.* U.S. Department of Health and Human Services Technical Report No. 9, 1993, p. 1.

21. Substance Abuse and Mental Health Services Administration. *National household survey on drug abuse: Main findings 1992.* U.S. Department of Health and Human Services, January 1995, p. 152.

22. U.S. Department of Health and Human Services. *The health benefits of smoking cessation: A report of the Surgeon General.* Public Health Service. Washington, D.C., 1990.

23. Centers for Disease Control and Prevention. Cigarette smoking among adults—United States, 1994. *Morbidity and Mortality Weekly Report* 45(27):588–590, 1996.

24. American Cancer Society. *Cancer facts and figures—1997.* Atlanta, 1998.

25. Johnston, L., J. Bachman, and P. O'Malley. *Cigarette smoking among American teens rises again in 1995.* Ann Arbor, MI: University of Michigan News and Information Services, December 11, 1995.

26. U.S. Department of Health and Human Services, *Health benefits of smoking cessation, op. cit.*

27. Centers for Disease Control and Prevention. Tobacco use and usual source of cigarettes among high school students—United States, 1995. *Morbidity and Mortality Weekly Report* 45(20):413–418, 1996.

28. Centers for Disease Control and Prevention. Use of smokeless tobacco among adults—United States, 1991. *Morbidity and Mortality Weekly Report* 42:263–266, 1993. Erratum: 42:382, 1993.

29. Insel, P. M., and W. T. Roth. *Core concepts of health.* Mountain View, CA: Mayfield Publishing, 1994.

30. Gingiss, P. L., and N. H. Gottlieb. A comparison of smokeless tobacco and smoking practices of university varsity and intramural baseball players. *Addictive Behaviors* 16:335–340, 1991.

31. U.S. Department of Health and Human Services, Public Health Service. *Preventing tobacco use among young people: A report of the Surgeon General.* Centers for Disease Control and Prevention Atlanta, 1994.

32. American Cancer Society. *Questions about smoking, tobacco, and health . . . and the answers.* Atlanta, 1982.

33. Ibid.

34. American Cancer Society, *Cancer facts, op. cit.*

35. American Heart Association. Cigarette smoking and cardiovascular diseases, *Heart & stroke A–Z guide,* 1996.

36. American Heart Association. *Heart and stroke facts: 1996 statistical supplement.* Dallas, TX, 1996.

37. American Cancer Society, *Questions, op. cit.*

38. American Cancer Society, *Cancer facts, op. cit.*

39. Ibid.

40. Ibid.

41. Insel and Roth, *op. cit.*

42. American Cancer Society, *Questions, op. cit.*

43. Cook, P. S., R. Petersen, and D. T. Moore. *Alcohol, tobacco, and other drugs may harm the unborn.* U.S. Department of Health and Human Services, DHHS Publication No. (ADM) 90-1711. Washington, D.C.: U.S. Government Printing Office, 1990.

44. Ibid.

45. Ibid.

46. U.S. Department of Health and Human Services. *Healthy people 2000: National health promotion and disease prevention objectives.* DHHS Publication No. (PHS) 91-50213. Washington, D.C.: U.S. Government Printing Office, 1990.

47. Eliopoulos, C., J. Klein, K. M. Phan, and B. Knie. Hair concentrations of nicotine and cotinine in women and their newborn infants. *Journal of the American Medical Association* 271:621–623, 1994.

48. American Cancer Society, *Cancer facts, op. cit.*

49. Ibid.

50. U.S. Department of Health and Human Services, *Cigarette smoking among adults, op. cit.*

51. Larson, *op. cit.*

52. Prochaska, J. O., and C. C. DiClemente. Stages of change in the modification of problem behaviors. In M. Hersen, R. M. Eisler, and P. M. Miller, eds. *Progress in behavior modification.* Sycamore, IL: Sycamore Publishing Company, 1992.

53. DiClemente, C. C., J. O. Prochaska, S. K. Fairhurst, W. F. Velicer, M. M. Velasquez, and J. S. Rossi. The process of smoking cessation: An analysis of precontemplation, contemplation, and preparation stages of change. *Journal of Consulting Clinical Psychology* 59:259–304, 1991.

54. U.S. Department of Health and Human Services, *Health benefits, op. cit.*

55. Sweeting, R. *A values approach to health behavior.* Champaign, IL: Human Kinetics, 1990.

56. U.S. Department of Health and Human Services, *Health benefits, op. cit.*

57. Mathias, R. Student's use of marijuana, other illicit drugs, and cigarettes continued to rise in 1995. *NIDA Notes,* January/February 1996. Available on the WWW at www.nida.gov.

58. Hermes, W. J. *Substance abuse (the encyclopedia of health).* New York: Chelsea House Publishers, 1993.

59. Facts about marijuana and marijuana abuse. *NIDA Notes,* March/April 1996. Available on the WWW at www.nida.gov.

60. Ibid.

61. Hermes, *op. cit.*

62. Zimmer, L., and J. P. Morgan. *Marijuana myths, marijuana facts: A review of the scientific evidence.* New York: Open Society Institute, 1997.

63. Schlaadt, R., and P. Shannon. *Drugs,* 3rd ed. Englewood Cliffs, NJ: Prentice-Hall, 1990.

64. U.S. Department of Health and Human Services. *The 1994 national household survey on drug abuse,* 1997.

65. Schulman, S. *A guide to drugs: Use, abuse, and effects.* London: Davis-Poynter, 1991.

66. Hermes, *op. cit.*

Chapter 15

1. DeGraaf, D. G., and D. J. Jordan. Our environment in crisis—We can change the future. *Journal of Health, Physical Education, Recreation, and Dance,* October 1994.

2. Millin, J., E. Mellerup, T. Bolwig, T. Scheike, and H. Dam. *Journal of Affective Disorders* 37(2–3):151–155, April 12, 1996.

INDEX